HANDBOOK OF PSYCHIATRY · 1
GENERAL
PSYCHOPATHOLOGY

HANDBOOK OF PSYCHIATRY

General Editor: Professor M. Shepherd

Edited by: Professor N. Garmezy, Dr L. A. Hersov, Professor M. H. Lader, Professor P. R. McHugh, Professor G. F. M. Russell, Professor J. K. Wing, Professor O. L. Zangwill

Assisted by the Editorial Board and International Advisory Board of *Psychological Medicine*

Volume 1: General psychopathology
Edited by M. Shepherd and O. L. Zangwill

Volume 2: Mental disorders and somatic illness
Edited by M. H. Lader

Volume 3: Psychoses of uncertain aetiology
Edited by J. K. Wing and L. Wing

Volume 4: The neuroses and personality disorders
Edited by G. F. M. Russell and L. A. Hersov

Volume 5: The scientific foundations of psychiatry
Edited by M. Shepherd

Handbook of
PSYCHIATRY
Volume 1

GENERAL
PSYCHO-
PATHOLOGY

Edited by
M. Shepherd, *Professor of Epidemiological Psychiatry, Institute of Psychiatry, London*
and
O. L. Zangwill, FRS, *Professor of Experimental Psychology University of Cambridge*

CAMBRIDGE UNIVERSITY PRESS
Cambridge
London New York New Rochelle
Melbourne Sidney

Published by the Press Syndicate of the University of Cambridge
The Pitt Building, Trumpington Street, Cambridge CB2 1RP
32 East 57th Street, New York, NY 10022, USA
296 Beaconsfield Parade, Middle Park, Melbourne 3206, Australia

First published 1983

Printed in the United States of America

Library of Congress catalogue card number: 81-21575

British Library cataloguing in publication data
Handbook of psychiatry
Vol. 1; General psychopathology.

1. Psychiatry
I. Shephard, M.   II. Zangwill, O. L.
616.89   RC454
ISBN 0 521 23649 5 hard covers
ISBN 0 521 28137 7 paperback

Contents

Contents

Contributors

W. F. Bynum, MD, PhD,
Head, Unit of History of Medicine,
Department of Anatomy and Embryology,
University College, London
and
Assistant Director (Research),
Wellcome Institute for the History of Medicine,
183 Euston Road, London, NW1 2BP

R. H. Cawley, BSc, MB, PhD, FRCP, FRCPsych,
Joint Professor of Psychological Medicine,
King's College Hospital Medical School and Institute of
Psychiatry
Institute of Psychiatry
De Crespigny Park, Denmark Hill, London SE5 8AF

J. E. Cooper, FRCP, FRCPsych, DPM,
Professor of Psychiatry,
University of Nottingham,
Professorial Unit, Mapperley Hospital,
Porchester Road, Nottingham, NG3 6AA

Esther Fischer-Homberger
Professor of the History of Medicine
University of Berne
Medizinhistorisches Institut
CH-3012, Berne, Bühlstrasse 26, Switzerland

T. C. N. Gibbens, MD, FRCP, FRCPsych, DPM,
Emeritus Professor of Forensic Psychiatry,
London University
31 College Road, London SE21 7BG

J. Hoenig, MD, FRCP, FRCPsych, FRCP(C),
Professor of Psychiatry,
Memorial University,
St John's, Newfoundland, Canada, A1B 3V6

R. E. Kendell, MD, FRCP, FRCPsych,
Professor of Psychiatry,
University Department of Psychiatry,
(Royal Edinburgh Hospital),
Morningside Park, Edinburgh, EH10 5HF

Edgar Miller, BSc, MPhil, PhD, FBPsS
Top Grade Clinical Psychologist,
Addenbrooke's Hospital
Cambridge, CB2 2QQ

H. B. M. Murphy, MD, PhD, DPH,
Professor,
Department of Psychiatry,
McGill University,
1033 Pine Avenue West, Montreal, PQ, Canada H3A 1A1

Felix Post, MD, FRCP, FRCPsych,
Emeritus Physician,
The Bethlem Royal Hospital and the Maudsley Hospital,
Denmark Hill, London, SE5 8AZ

T. W. Robbins, MA, PhD (Cantab),
University Lecturer in Experimental Psychology,
Psychological Laboratory,
Downing Street, Cambridge CB2, 3ER

Christian Scharfetter, DR MED,
Professor of Psychiatry,
University of Zurich,
Psychiatric Clinic, Research Department,
8029 Zurich, Lenggstrasse 31, Switzerland

Michael Shepherd, DM, FRCP, FRCPsych, DPM,
Professor of Epidemiological Psychiatry,
University of London, Institute of Psychiatry,
Institute of Psychiatry,
De Crespigny Park, Denmark Hill, London SE5 8AF

Jean Starobinski, Docteur de lettres et Docteur en médecine,
Professor of the History of Ideas,
Faculté des Lettres,
University of Geneva,
12 rue de Candolle, CH-1205, Geneva, Switzerland

F. Kräupl Taylor, MD, FRCPsych, DPM,
Emeritus Physician,
The Bethlem Royal Hospital and the Maudsley Hospital,
22 Redington Road, London, NW3 7RG

Owsei Temkin, MD, LLD (hon.), ScD (hon.),
William H. Welch Professor Emeritus of the History of
Medicine,
419 Alabama Road, Towson, MD, 21204, USA

Maria A. Wyke, MA, PhD,
Senior Lecturer in Psychology,
Institute of Psychiatry,
De Crespigny Park, Denmark Hill, London, SE5 8AF

O. L. Zangwill, MA, FRS,
Professor of Experimental Psychology, University of Cambridge
and
Head of the Cambridge Psychological Laboratory (until 30
September 1981)
King's College,
Cambridge CB2 1ST

Foreword

The idea of this handbook originated from a survey of the available British books on psychiatry in the late 1960s (1). It became apparent then that the post-war development of the subject as a major, independent branch of medicine had been accompanied by a spate of textbooks and specialized monographs from the rapidly increasing number of academic and clinical departments. The time seemed ripe 'to compile the comprehensive authoritative multi-authored handbook which has yet to appear in this country' (2).

In the event almost another decade was to pass before the enterprise was to be realized. During this time the climate of opinion has come to favour the appearance of a representative statement of what has been termed the 'Maudsley' approach to psychological medicine. Modern British psychiatry, as Lord Taylor has pointed out, is 'largely the product of the Maudsley Hospital' (3). It embodies not so much a national school of opinion as a continuation of the broad, central tradition of psychiatric theory and practice which originated on the European mainland, was transported through the psychobiology of Adolf Meyer to North America and returned to Europe via the United Kingdom, where its pre-eminent representative has been Sir Aubrey Lewis (4). At its core is an adherence to the principles of scientific enquiry in clinical and basic research, with due acknowledgement of the role played by social and psychological investigation as well as by the natural sciences.

The prospects for the production of a handbook were further improved by the creation in 1969 of *Psychological Medicine,* a journal devoted to research in the field of psychiatry and the allied sciences, which brought together an editorial board which has played an important part in this undertaking. The participation of the journal's international advisory board also helped to ensure a wide base for the work which, from its inception, has received sympathetic encouragement from Cambridge University Press.

Why call a handbook what is clearly so much more than a manual or guide which can be held in the hand? If the term is a misnomer it is one which has been blessed by tradition and usage. In the German-speaking countries, where so many of the roots of modern psychiatry are embedded, a *Handbuch* is much weightier than a *Lehrbuch* and the massive volumes associated with the names of Aschaffenburg and Bumke exemplify the fruits of German scholarship at its most diligent. The format has, of course, been applied to other medical disciplines in other languages, largely to meet a need which has been clearly expressed in the preface to the *Handbook of Clinical Neurology,* now comprising some forty volumes: 'only a Handbook designed on the principle of exhaustive, critical, balanced and comprehensive reviews written by acknowledged experts, is in the position of reflecting the state of neurology in the second half of the twentieth century' (5).

While the *Handbook of Psychiatry* has a similar objective, it is less expansive in content and more ambitious in form. An encyclopaedic compilation of all the theories and speculations which impinge on contemporary psychiatry would call for more than forty volumes, but would become outdated very soon. Here we have preferred to concentrate on the fabric of psychological medicine and the loom of observations and concepts on which it has been woven. Accordingly, volumes 2–4 contain the clinical substratum of the subject, flanked by one volume devoted to general psychopathology and another to the various scientific modes of enquiry on which the discipline is founded.

A full list of contents, with titles of chapters and names of authors, is provided in each volume. An outline of the material contained in all five volumes is as follows:

Vol.1 General Psychopathology
Editors: M. Shepherd and O. L. Zangwill
Part I
The historical background
Part II
The clinical phenomena of mental disorders
Part III
Taxonomy, diagnosis, and treatment

Vol.2 Mental Disorders and Somatic Illness
Editor: M. H. Lader
Part I
General medical disorders
Part II
Neurological disorders
Part III
Drug-induced disorders
Part IV
Severe subnormality

Vol.3 Psychoses of Uncertain Aetiology
Editors: J. K. Wing and L. Wing
Part I
Schizophrenia and paranoid psychoses
Part II
Affective psychoses
Part III
Psychoses of early childhood

Vol.4 The Neuroses and Personality Disorders
Editors: G. F. M. Russell and L. Hersov
Part I
Concepts, assessments, and treatments
Part II
Disorders specific to childhood
Part III
Neurotic states, sexual disorders, and drug-dependence
Part IV
Personality disorders

Vol.5 The Scientific Foundations of Psychiatry
Editor: M. Shepherd
Part I
Philosophy and psychiatry
Part II
Epidemiology and genetics in relation to psychiatry
Part III
Social science, psychology, and ethology in relation to psychiatry
Part IV
The neurosciences in relation to psychiatry

All the volumes are self-contained and edited separately, but they are intended to reinforce one another. Every effort has been made to avoid overlap and duplication of material, and the inclusion of cross-references, some in the text and others at the back of each volume, should facilitate the process of integration. The whole is designed to be more than the sum of its parts.

Michael Shepherd
Institute of Psychiatry
1981

References

(1) Shepherd, M. (1969) British books on psychiatry, I & II. *British Book News,* Feb/Mar., pp. 85–8 and 167–70

(2) Shepherd, M. (1980) Psychiatry: personal book list. *Lancet,* i, 937

(3) Taylor, Lord (1962) The public, parliament and mental health, In *Aspects of Psychiatric Research,* ed. Richter, D., Tanner, J. M., Taylor, Lord & Zangwill, O. L., p. 13. London: Oxford University Press

(4) Shepherd, M. (1977) *The Career and Contributions of Sir Aubrey Lewis.* Bethlem Royal & Maudsley Hospitals

(5) Vinken, P. J. & Bruyn, G. W. (1969) Preface to *Handbook of Clinical Neurology,* vol. I, p. v. Amsterdam: North Holland

Introduction: The sciences and general psychopathology

MICHAEL SHEPHERD

The subject-matter of this volume develops the map charted by Karl Jaspers in his *General Psychopathology*, which remains the clearest and most convincing outline of the whole field (Jaspers, 1963). Jaspers nowhere provides a clear-cut definition of psychopathology, and points out that its 'essence . . . as a study can only emerge from a composite framework'. Inveighing against the futility of 'endlessness', the attempt to establish absolute knowledge through the application of any one scientific discipline, he urges the psychiatrist to 'acquire some of the view-points and methods that belong to the world of the Humanities and Social Studies . . . since the methods of almost all the Arts and Sciences converge on psychopathology'. With this ambiguous phrase Jaspers indicates the complex nature of a discipline which, in his view, extended the notion of scientific enquiry as it is usually understood.

Jaspers refers to science in relation to psychopathology repeatedly but disconnectedly throughout the several sections of his text. While claiming scientific status for psychopathology he also asserts that 'Science is wrongly identified with Natural Science . . . natural science is indeed the groundwork of psychopathology and an essential element in it but the humanities are equally so and, with this, psychopathology does not become in any way less scientific but scientific in another way'. According to Jaspers there are no fewer than four modes of scientific thought which are relevant to psychopathology:

descriptive phenomenology, causal explanation, genetic understanding (the psychology of meaningful connections), and the construction of complex unities.

The phenomenological approach to psychopathology, involving as it does the careful analysis of the phenomena of mental disorders, constitutes a basic contribution to clinical knowledge. The careful and systematic delineation of abnormal forms of experience and behaviour provides the descriptive groundwork of the subject but even though such material can be given quantitative expression its heavily subjective nature has led some observers to distinguish it from scientific enquiry proper. According to Zubin, for example, 'Science deals with public events while phenomenology deals with the still private events' (Zubin, 1972). To Jaspers, on the other hand, phenomenology remained not only a form of scientific enquiry but one which, by its very nature, separated itself from the study of all infra-human organisms, lacking as they do capacity for comparable self-expression. 'In psychopathology', he maintains, 'the human being has himself become the object of scientific study and thus observations on animals do not contribute anything essential . . .' Further, he speaks pointedly of 'physical findings that have or may have some relation to psychic events but they do not portray them nor reveal them in any sense which we can understand'.

From this point it is a short step to his distinction between 'explanatory' and 'understandable' processes in the sphere of psychopathology, a dichotomy borrowed from Dilthey and Weber who applied it originally to philosophy and the social sciences. For Jaspers the establishment of 'explanatory' connections in psychopathology belongs to the sphere of natural science, leading to the formulation of rules and eventually to mathematical laws. Here he comes close to a generally held opinion, summarized by Oakeshott, for whom 'The explicit character of scientific experience is a world of absolutely stable and communicable experience: the explicit purpose in science is to conceive the world under the category of quantity' (Oakeshott, 1978). In psychopathology, by contrast, Jaspers asserts that particular causal connections and some general laws are attainable but that the discovery of more specific, immutable laws 'would presuppose a complete quantification of the events observed and since these are psychic events which by their very nature have to remain qualitative, such quantification would as a matter of principle remain impossible without losing the actual object of the enquiry'.

In Jaspers' schema natural science is equated with biology. 'It is an absolute necessity', he says, 'for the psychopathologist to *see life* the way biologists do'. Inasmuch as this statement implies the subordination of the physical sciences his meaning is clear enough: 'The concrete phenomenon is part of a living whole and it never permits the isolation of a simple fact, a simple cause which operates like a cannoning billiard-ball; it can be conceived only as a *complex event* taking place among a host of conditioning factors'. This distinction between inanimate mechanisms and a living biological causality, however, runs counter to the outlook of many practising biologists. To Mainz, for example, biology 'has developed special methods and special subdivision, but these are nevertheless not different in principle from those of other natural sciences' (Mainz, 1955). And for Monod: 'Science rests upon a strictly *objective* approach to the analysis and interpretation of the universe, including Man himself and human societies. Science ignores, and must ignore, value judgements' (Monod, 1971). Jaspers, on the other hand, rejects the need to suspend value judgements except when attempting causal explanations and regards this view of science as insufficient: 'Psychopathological phenomena may also be reinterpreted as *biological events* against a general ground of biological theory, e.g. genetics, where human existence and mental illness can be studied from this point of view. Only when the biological aspects have been clearly distinguished can we proceed to discuss what essentially belongs to man. Whenever the object studied is Man and not man as a species of animal, we find that psychopathology comes to be not only a kind of biology but also one of the Humanities'.

It is on this proposition that Jaspers bases his argument for the need of a science of 'understanding', as opposed to 'explanation', in which meaningful psychic connections can be established because 'psychic events "emerge" out of each other in a way which we understand'. This form of 'genetic' or 'psychological' understanding underpins the empathic, interpersonal components of Jaspers' schema: 'The scientific attitude suspends all value-judgement in order to arrive at knowledge. But though this is possible when attempting causal explanation it is not possible with empathic understanding, at least not exactly in the same sense. We can, however, make an analogous claim to impartiality when we have shown an understanding that is fair, many-sided, open and critically conscious of its limitations. Love and hate bring values which are indeed the pacemakers of understanding but their suspension brings us a clarity of understanding that amounts to knowledge'. The application of psychological understanding, however, extends only to the field of 'empirical experiment and free existential achievement'. Beyond this knowledge is derived only from 'metaphysical' understanding which is attainable by philosophy rather than by any form of scientific enquiry.

According to Jaspers, 'Metaphysical understanding (as distinct from psychological understanding) reaches after a meaning into which all the other limited meanings can be taken up and absorbed. Metaphysical understanding interprets the empirical facts and the free achievement as the language of unconditioned Being. This interpretation is not a mere device of reason, something futile, but the illumination of fundamental experiences with the help of symbol and idea. As we look at the inanimate world, the cosmos, the landscape, we experience something we call "soul" or "psyche" '. And what is 'psyche'? '1) Psyche means *consciousness*, but just as much and, from certain points of view it can even, in particular, mean "the unconscious". 2) Psyche is not to be regarded as an object with given qualities but as "being in one's own world", the integrating of an inner and outer world. 3) Psyche is a becoming, an unfolding and a differentiating, it is nothing final nor is it ever fully accomplished'. The concept of psyche, therefore, is the gateway to an existentialist universe: 'There is no valid theory of the psyche, only a philosophy of human existence'.

Here is the language of Kierkegaard and Nietzsche, a transcendentalism which Jaspers was later to develop at length in his philosophical writings but which is also central to his outline of psychopathology: 'The sciences through knowledge provide a springboard for thought which transcends. It is only where scientific knowledge is at its fullest that we first have the experience of *really not knowing* and in this not knowing we transcend the situation with the help of specific, philosophic methods. But the sciences also tend to *obscure Being itself* by the knowable facts and keep us tied to preliminaries without end. They tend to make absolutes of our limited insights and convert them into a supposed knowledge of Being itself'. Again: 'Human beings . . . constantly transcend their own empirical human self which is the only self that scientific research can

recognise and grasp'. Within this context Jaspers also develops his notion of 'wholes' in relation to science, the 'whole' being 'the proper theme for philosophy whereas science is only concerned with particular aspects of the whole'. He argues that '. . . science, if it is to be productive, will vacillate constantly between the elements and the whole' and goes on to conclude: 'Some exact experiment in biological research may often make us feel that we have grasped life in its original wholeness and that we have at last penetrated it through and through and yet in the end we find it is still only a widening of the mechanistic insight . . . In the end we have comprehended only elements and the problems of the whole appears again in new form'. As for the scientific method with its reliance on hypothesis-formation: 'Where our theories may seem to have some kinship with the natural sciences it is in the forming of tentative hypotheses, which we make for limited research ends only and which have no application to the psyche as a whole'.

In sum, then, Jaspers enlarges the field of general psychopathology to extend from the natural sciences, and in particular biological science, via descriptive phenomenology to existentialist philosophy. The psychopathologist employs the scientific method and the scientific attitude even when dealing with phenomena like subjective experience or meaningful connection, but his own position is ultimately non-reductionist and transcendental. In the preface to the seventh edition of his book, written in 1959, Jaspers acknowledged that after 65 years his methodological principles had remained largely unchanged but that there was room for modification in the light of recent research. The hypsography and the contours of his map have both been modified by the evolution of new areas of scientific enquiry, many of which have emerged since the completion of the final revision of his text. Some of these have developed as a result of new techniques of investigation, and the intensive study of the central nervous system and its functions has led to the recognition that many traditional areas of psychopathology involve a variety of disciplines not traditionally associated with psychopathological enquiry. The investigation of memory, to take one example, now involves the microbiologist, the physiologist, the anatomist, and the pharmacologist as well as the clinician (Brazier, 1979). In consequence, psychopathology has been subject to a series of shifting 'paradigms' which, as Kuhn has so convincingly argued, indicate the turmoil of a science on the move (Kuhn, 1970). The boundaries between the older scientific disciplines have been re-drawn to generate the emergence of new, compound sciences whose nature is tellingly indicated by a multiplicity of prefixes – 'neuropsychopharmacology', 'neuropsychoendocrinology', 'psychobiology', 'socio-biology'.

The bearing of these scientific methods and disciplines on general psychopathology has already been profound. Detailed consideration is given to them in volume 5 of this Handbook. In this volume a brief general account of their impact on the clinical and basic sciences is more appropriate.

Clinical sciences

Chapters 3, 4, 5, and 6 present the principal phenomena associated with mental disorders. Jaspers' outline of the clinical conditions calling for psychopathological investigation corresponds to most of the widely accepted classifications. He grouped the conditions into three broad categories:

Group I. Known somatic illness with psychic disturbances

    Cerebral illnesses

    Systemic diseases with symptomatic psychoses

    Poisons

Group II. Major psychoses

    Genuine epilepsy

    Schizophrenia

    Manic-depressive illness

Group III. Personality disorders

    Isolated abnormal reactions that do not arise on the basis of illnesses belonging to Groups I and II

    Neuroses and neurotic syndromes

    Abnormal personalities and their developments

It may be noted that this scheme is hierarchical, that precise diagnosis is feasible only in Group I, and that classification in Group II is least satisfactory. The somatic basis of the diagnoses in Group I brings these conditions most intimately into the orbit of conventional scientific enquiry, where advances in the spheres of physical investigation and treatment have proved to be most fruitful. At the same time, however, these advances have underlined the need to re-categorize the major 'functional psychoses' in Group II. In the case of epilepsy, for example, while Jaspers originally stated that the diagnosis is psychological, 'made on the basis of convulsive attack linked with a psychological diagnosis', the introduction of electroencephalography has pro-vided a physical substrate for the disorder in the form of cerebral dysrhythmia (Commission on Terminology, 1969). Similarly, the work of Gjessing demonstrated the importance of metabolic disorders in the genesis of periodic catatonia, thereby rekindling interest in the physiobiology of the schizophrenias (Gjessing, 1976).

New knowledge has stimulated an increasing awareness of the need to establish the principles of psychiatric diagnosis and classification which in general follow conventional lines (see chaps. 7, 8, and 9). An exception, however, has been provided by the claims of psycho-analysis which, because of their radical nature, calls for separate mention (Menninger, 1963). The complicated system derived from psycho-analytical theory and practice does not lend itself to a detailed summary (see vol. 5, Kräupl Taylor). Essentially, however, it is a reductionist schema which, to Freud, was 'a dynamic conception which reduces mental life to an interplay of reciprocally urging and checking forces'. These forces are conceived in terms of a schema of 'libidinal' energy which ultimately determines the basic attributes of the individual and is dependent on a variety of postulated 'mechanisms', such as sublimation, repression, and fixation. One of the suggested contributions to general psychopathology has been the hypothesis that some of these 'mechanisms' are causally related to particular phenomena of mental disease, e.g. the links between hostility and depression. Another major implication of psycho-dynamic theorizing for general psychopathology has been the proposed nexus between early childhood experience and mental disorder in later life, e.g. maternal attachment and adult homosexuality.

Jaspers was one of the first to point out the fundamentally unscientific nature of 'psychodynamic' theory, to which he allocated the limited role of establishing meaningful connections by way of genetic understanding. This view has been vigorously contested by Hartmann who, while accepting the value of the phenomenological method, asserted that psycho-analysis 'has come to see the most essential processes of the human mind from the causal point of view' (Hartmann, 1964). The goal of psychoanalysis according to Hartmann, is not the understanding of the mental, but rather the explanation of its causal relationships, for psycho-analysis is '. . . a science which proceeds inductively and is rooted in biology . . . a natural science not only in its manner of conceptualization . . . but also in the scientific goals it sets itself – namely the knowledge of laws and regularities', '. . . an inductive science of the connections between complex mental structure'. Closer examination, however, has shown that these constructs are metaphors rather than models and are not susceptible to operational definitions so that they cannot be subjected to scientific enquiry. The protean theoretical system has none the less led to a vast amount of experimental work, only a small proportion of which has supported the operationally derived hypotheses (Fisher & Greenberg, 1977), even when the work can overcome the twin methodological problems of poor interobserver agreement and the confusion between 'interpretation' and observation. A great deal of ingenuity has been expended in an effort to render these studies scientific, and the psycho-dynamic model has probably been of most value as a stimulus to provoking such work rather than as an accurate picture of human behaviour.

Perhaps the impact of 'psychodynamic' theorizing would have been greater if its therapeutic claims had been substantiated (Cawley, 1970). In the event, the efficacy of psychotherapy has been rendered questionable by the application of techniques of evaluation to new forms of treatment which have themselves exercised a major impact on psychiatry and psychopathology as a clinical science (see vol. 1, chap. 10, by Cawley). For Jaspers, physical treatment occupied a tiny section of his discussion and was confined to a brief mention of anticonvulsants, opiates, diet, and the shock-therapies. He was unable to take account of recent advances in the pharmacological therapy of the functional psychoses which were introduced in the early 1950s (Shepherd *et al.*, 1968) and whose implications for psychopathology have been twofold. On the one hand, by modifying the outcome of many forms of these disorders medication has provided another axis of classification in an area where prognosis is a central issue: the postulate, for example, of a 'drug-responsive' or 'non-responsive' depression (Freyhan, 1978) has been to introduce a novel dichotomy far removed from the traditional, clinically-based endogenous–exogenous or neurotic–psychotic type of categorization. Secondly, and still more important, the apparent response of the functional psychoses to substances acting on the central nervous system has raised the possibility of identifying a physico-chemical basis for these disorders via the mode of drug-action. The older idea of psychosis resulting from a 'metabolic disorder' or a 'biochemical lesion' has been superseded by the modern concept of disorders of neuro-transmitters (Legg, 1978) in which the functional psychoses take their place alongside neurological and other medical conditions. The 'dopamine hypothesis' of schizophrenia (Carlsson, 1977) and the 'catecholamine hypothesis' of the affective disorders (Maas, 1975) exemplify this mode of thinking (see below).

The other large area of clinical science which receives inadequate consideration in Jaspers' schema is epidemiology, the study of the nature and distribution of disease in populations, whose methods and techniques have been applied increasingly to non-infectious as well as infectious conditions (see vol. 5, chap. 2). Jaspers' account of the need to establish the demographic and social associations of disease and his searching discussion of the methods of correlation are close to the core of the epidemiological method. What is lacking, however, is an explicit awareness of the role which can be played by epidemiology in establishing causal connections, as in the cases of pellagra (Shepherd, 1978) or twin-research in schizophrenia (Rosenthal & Kety, 1968), as well as in extending the scope of descriptive enquiry. The central part played by epidemiology in the development of the controlled clinical trial is also missing, understandably, from a text which pays so little regard to treatment.

Yet though Jaspers nowhere uses the term, an epidemiological perspective is apparent in his chapter on heredity (devoted largely to population genetics), on eidology, on the social and historical status of the individual and on diagnosis and classification. Indeed, he explicitly extends the boundaries of general psychopathology to cover the population at large: '. . . our science starts in the field of the "normal" and with the study of personality. Once psychiatry began to designate personalities as "sick" it became simply a practical matter where to draw the line in regard to all the individual variations'. And he goes on to say that 'the personality disorders (the psychopathies and neuroses) and the psychoses are veritable sources of human possibilities, not only deviations from a healthy norm'. Within this framework the socio-cultural contributions to psychopathology fall naturally into place, as illustrated in this volume by chapters 2 and 5 (see also vol. 5, chap. 4).

Basic sciences

Alongside the advances in the clinical study of psychopathology which have been made in recent years must be placed the contributions from the so-called basic sciences, each elaborating on its concepts and techniques to demarcate an area of relevance. In general, the representatives of these disciplines proceed not so much by tackling clinical phenomena directly as by constructing 'models'. Jaspers, while referring to the significance of 'analogy' in the study of biological processes, does not discuss the value of scientific models which are susceptible to experimental manipulation. As Alinstein (1965) has pointed out, such models possess four attributes: (1) a set of assumptions about the subject under investigation; (2) the derivation of properties of hypotheses derived from these assumptions which can be tested; (3) the view that the model employed is an approximation to the 'true' model which excludes other theories; and (4) the analogical nature of the model employed. Having constructed the model the scientist has to establish its reliability and validity by appropriate examination and then to test its applicability, being prepared to discard or modify it when the limits of its relevance have been determined.

The broad objective of experimental science in using its models is to investigate the mechanisms of disease by the controlled manipulation of relevant variables and then to test these directly on the human subject. The mechanisms in question may be neurobiological or behavioural, according to the methods and standpoint adopted. The use of infra-human species plays a large part in such work and the question of the degree to which the animal model can be regarded as a homologue for the study of human psychopathology has constantly to be considered.

1. *The neurobiological sciences*

The recent explosion of research in the neurosciences has impinged on psychopathology in a number of ways. First in order of significance is the impact of psychopharmacology following the introduction of a variety of new drugs in the 1950s. The scientific significance of these compounds has extended beyond their use in clinical practice to involve their mode of action and, by implication, the biological mechanisms assumed to underlie the conditions for which they are used therapeutically. The case of schizophrenia may be taken to illustrate the issues: 'Insofar as schizophrenia is not a purely linguistic disorder, but involves abnormalities in more elementary perceptual, attentional, and cognitive processes, such paradigms can be used to investigate the anatomical, physiological and neurochemical

mechanisms underlying the disease' (Matthysse, 1977). Translating this view into testable hypotheses, Matthysse and Haber (1975) lay down four minimum and essential requirements for a model of schizophrenia: (1) that aberrant animal behaviour should be restored to normal, at least in part, by drugs which are therapeutically effective in schizophrenia; (2) that substances which are chemically similar to antipsychotic drugs but are therapeutically ineffective in schizophrenic psychoses should fail to normalize aberrant behaviour in the model-animal; (3) that drug-tolerance, which does not develop to antipsychotic drugs, should not develop in the animals; (4) that the effect of drugs on abnormal animal behaviour should not be counteracted by anticholinergic agents. The underlying assumption in such reasoning is that schizophrenia results from a defect of neuro-transmission, as exemplified by the 'dopamine hypothesis' (Carlsson, 1977).

Clearly, however, the gap between a basically neurochemical disorder and the complex symptoms associated with schizophrenia is difficult to close conceptually without the postulation of mediating mechanisms, such as elementary psychological processes which may be studied in terms of either experimental biology or the phenomena of the disease itself. Thus from the biological standpoint it has been suggested that relevant dopamine-related behaviour includes stereotypy and motor disinhibition (Matthysse, 1978), corresponding to perseveration of thought and distractibility respectively; the clinical features of the psychosis have, in turn, been related to the psychology of attention and its disturbances (Matthysse *et al.*, 1979), especially since the identification of 'focal attention' neurons in the parietal lobe (Lynch *et al.*, 1977). Whatever their detailed nature such psychological mechanisms could thus be associated with anatomico-physiological systems utilizing neuro-transmitters or even constitute predisposing factors to overt disease in a manner akin to the inherited 'risk factors' in some physical diseases.

A model of this type, which has been applied to other forms of functional psychoses and to the neurotic disorders, refurbishes the old notion of mental disorder as dependent on cerebral dysfunction. The concept of the 'lesion' however, has become more complex, reflecting a multi-factorial framework which incorporates neurochemical, endocrinological, genetic, psychological, and even environmental factors. A major emphasis here is on the elucidation of physical mechanisms which have been extended to traditionally psychological domains. In the field of memory, for example, animal experiments have been carried out to examine the hypothesis that nucleic acids or protein molecules synthesized in the learning process may constitute a chemical basis for memory (Squire, 1976). Anisomycin and cyclohexicide, both of which suppress cerebral protein synthesis, have been used for this purpose in the study of discrimination-tasks and habituation; the results have then been compared with the retrograde amnesia which follows the administration of ECT to human subjects to construct a model for short-term memory in terms of synaptic conductance.

2. *The behavioural sciences*

For the advocates of a behavioural approach to psychopathology the subject has been defined, significantly, as 'the scientific study of disordered behaviour' (Maher, 1970). Without minimizing the importance of biological disorders, these workers concentrate on the overt behavioural disturbances which characterize many forms of psychopathology, and attempt to reproduce them in the laboratory with animal or human subjects by experimental means. Perhaps the most fundamental examples of the behavioural approach have come from the field of genetics. While the study of population genetics has successfully demonstrated through pedigree analyses and twin studies the hereditary basis for much human variation, including several forms of mental disorder, geneticists have also turned their attention to behavioural syndromes. Recognizing that such syndromes are multifactorial in aetiology, they have attempted to identify controlling factors by taking advantage of the fact that some genetic polymorphisms can be used as linkage markers; the use of these in conjunction with the familial distribution of a syndrome renders it possible to construct a genetic taxonomy within the syndromal spectrum. Several different psychopathological areas have already been explored along these lines. Animal models for epilepsy, for example, have been developed through the study of mice which carry a gene for susceptibility to audiogenic seizures (Ginsburg *et al.*, 1969). Again, the genetic selection of aggressive animals has received an impetus from the suggested association of the extra Y-chromosome with aggression in human males, while breeding experiments and the cross-fostering of mice indicate that certain Y-chromosomes are associated with a propensity for aggressive behaviour in combination with certain autosomal genes, possibly by regulating the testosterone-level of puberty (Ginsburg, 1971).

So far, though, perhaps the most promising application of behavioural genetics relating to mental disease has been in the area of drug-response to a drug as a phenotypic property, the resultant of a genotype modified by a change in the internal milieu induced by drugs (Broadhurst, 1978). The marked individual variation in response to drugs and in the exhibition of their adverse effects has drawn attention to differences in pharmacokinetics, susceptibility of cell-receptors and the physiopathology of psychiatric syndromes. The well-established tendency for alcoholism to occur in families, for example, has been matched by the breeding of mouse strains which vary in their ability to metabolize ethanol, to exhibit preference for alcohol, and to exhibit widely differing behavioural responses to low doses of alcohol (Ginsburg *et al.*, 1975). Again, the biochemical effects of morphine on inbred strains of mice have shown that analgesia and locomotor activity can be genetically differentiated, suggesting that striatal dopaminergic systems are involved in the latter, and cholinergic neurones in the former, syndrome (Racagni *et al,.* 1977). In the field of mental disorder attention has been drawn to the inactivation of isoniazid and related drugs by the liver by an acetylating enzyme because of the use of monoamine oxidase inhibitors in the treatment of depression. 'Slow' acetylation, a trait determined by a simple gene and attributable to less enzymic activity, has been reported to be associated with greater therapeutic effectiveness of phenelzine in the treatment of neurotic depression among patients carrying the genetic predisposition to acetylate slowly (Johnstone, 1975). Another example is minimal brain dysfunction, a condition which is known to respond unpredictably but strikingly to stimulants like amphetamine and methylphenidate. Attempts to reproduce the syndrome have been made by breeding hyperactive beagle hybrids whose response to large doses of amphetamine have been used as analogues to the human condition (Ginsburg *et al.*, 1976).

Other significant behavioural approaches to clinical conditions have been via the conflict paradigms of 'experimental' neurosis (Gantt, 1944) and the various uses made of the conditioned reflex in relation to schizophrenia (Lynn, 1963) and phobias (Marks, 1969). In addition, attempts at behaviour modification by means of psychological techniques derived from learning theory have introduced new notions about the genesis and outcome of such disorders as the phobias and the obsessional states (Beech & Vaughan, 1978).

By way of a more detailed example **depression** stands out with particular clarity. Though the response to ECT and to certain psychotropic drugs have pointed to a biological substrate in some forms of depression, the phenomena of the disorder also lend themselves to behavioural analysis by meeting 'the assumption that the variables controlling normal behaviour also control deviant behaviour' (Maher, 1970). This outlook represents the application of principles developed from the laboratory study of normal behaviour in terms of learning, motivation, and perception as developed in the laboratory. For depression the model becomes most telling when the behavioural analogues can be most closely approximated to the conditions under study, as is the case with two currently productive concepts, namely 'learned helplessness' and 'separation'.

(a) *'Learned helplessness' and depression.* The experimental observations here are based on the defective escape-avoidance behaviour of infra-human organisms after receiving inescapable traumata; e.g. electric shocks. Those animals which make no attempt to escape from the traumatic situation, passively accept the noxae, and learn the effectiveness of response with difficulty are said to exhibit 'learned helplessness' (Miller *et al.*, 1977). They also exhibit other deficits in adaptive behaviour, e.g. food-seeking, appetite, and aggression, and depletion of norepinephrine has also been established. A comparable state induced in human subjects exposed to inescapable high noise or electric shocks exhibits several parallel features characterizing morbid depression – inertia, passivity, retardation, slowness, and negative attitudes. The suggested links between depression and a diminution of norepinephrine at receptor-sites in the brain have also been adduced as a further feature of similarity. On the other hand, the associations of intense anxiety and of peptic ulceration with 'learned helplessness' in the laboratory animal do not find a counterpart in depression, and the treatment measures which prove effective in clinical practice cannot be fitted readily to the model.

(b) *'Separation' and depression.* Most of the work on separation has centred on the so-called anaclitic or dependency depression which can occur in some very young children as a consequence of prolonged separation from the mother (Spitz, 1946). Clinicians have described a sequence of 'protest' leading to 'despair' and eventually to a state of 'detachment', characteristically responding to maternal reunion. Since this constitutes a model in pre-verbal subjects it can be established in purely behavioural terms with a causal factor, a natural history, and a response to 'treatment'. Such a situation suggests the possibility of creating laboratory models with subhuman primates and this objective has been pursued by animal ethologists (Hinde & Davies, 1972). The complexities and limitations of employing monkey analogues of depression have been carefully summarized by Suomi and Harlow (1977) who conclude that despite certain defects the model can be defended.

Conclusion

As a ground-plan of the current status of general psychopathology the foregoing outline may serve to introduce the content of this volume. Several of the themes point to gaps in knowledge which are developed further in a clinical context in volumes 2, 3 and 4, while the various scientific disciplines which contribute to the subject are considered in greater detail in volume 5. It remains to be emphasized that the area between the formal methods of science and those areas of psychopathology which Jaspers regarded as the province of philosophical enquiry has become an area of study in its own right (Bolton, 1979). Against the various reductionist theories of physicalism and behaviourism may be ranged such concepts as non-reductive materialism (Margolis, 1978), transcendentalism, phenomenology, and emergent biology (Thorpe, 1974), all in their various ways attempting to account for those aspects of human activity which have still to be incorporated satisfactorily in any holistic schema of psychopathology. At present these issues remain unresolved and necessarily a matter of personal bias. Meanwhile the contributions of scientific research continue both to consolidate the foundations of psychopathology and to open new fields of enquiry.

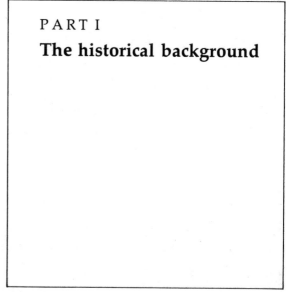

PART I

The historical background

1
Psychiatry in its historical context

W. F. BYNUM

Historiographical introduction

Psychiatry is a medical speciality with a long cultural, social, and intellectual history. Psychiatry's importance in contemporary life is undisputed, but its claims to scientific legitimacy are presently being challenged – and defended – in writings sometimes polemical in character and historical in conception (Szasz, 1973; Scheff, 1966; Scull, 1977; Clare, 1976). The historical dimensions to these contemporary debates illustrate the fact that history is not some fixed body of knowledge about the past but a vital, flexible dialogue between the present and the past.

There is nothing new in the use of history to leaven contemporary psychiatric concerns, for the appearance of a formal historiography of psychiatry in the nineteenth century coincided with the rise of the modern psychiatric profession. This historical literature was produced by individuals instrumental in these professional developments, and it played a strategic role in the medical, philanthropic, humanitarian, and political activities of these early psychiatric historians (e.g. Friedreich, 1830; Friedreich, 1836; Leidesdorf, 1865; Tuke, 1882: see Mora, 1966; Mora, 1970).

Until relatively recently, the history of psychiatry continued to be written primarily by practising psychiatrists and reflected to a large extent the professional preoccupations of its authors. Thus, the culmination of Daniel Hack Tuke's historical writings was the well-ordered Victorian asylum, whereas a generation of post-Freudian psychiatrists viewed the history of their discipline as a series of blind alleys and flashes of insight eventually leading to the creation of dynamic psychiatry (Tuke, 1882; Zilboorg, 1935; Zilboorg, 1941; Leibbrand & Wettley, 1961; Alexander & Selsnick, 1966). Other general surveys embody more eclectic approaches, although their authors are clearly sympathetic to the triumphs of modern psychotherapy (Schneck, 1960; Bromberg, 1954). Psychiatry's historical relationship to medicine is cogently shown by Ackerknecht (1968), in a short monograph which contains more information than many general histories several times as long. This work may now be supplemented by Mora's (1975) account which is particularly rich bibliographically, and by Ellenberger's historical introduction to the field (Ellenberger, 1974). The multi-authored volume edited by Howells (1975) provides brief histories of the evolution of psychiatry in specific nationalistic contexts, and supplements the many monographs devoted to the history of psychiatry in particular countries. For England, the work of Hunter and Macalpine (especially Hunter & Macalpine, 1963; Macalpine & Hunter, 1969) is important; other examples include Deutsch (1949) for America; Sémelaigne (1930) and Baruk (1967) for France; Henderson (1963) for Scotland; and Leigh (1961) and Skultans (1979) for Britain.

Increasingly, however, the history of psychiatry has not been the exclusive domain of the psychiatrist, as social, intellectual, and legal historians, sociologists, criminologists, anthropologists, philosophers, and historians of medicine, among others, have examined many cultural and historical aspects of mental disorders. (For a small sample of this literature not referred to elsewhere in this chapter, see Favazza & Oman, 1977; Brody & Engelhardt, 1980; Eliade, 1964; Kiev, 1964.) This literature has raised many issues about the historical delineations of mental disorders; the nosological status of psychiatric diagnoses (Kräupl Taylor, 1979); the political and social uses to which these diagnoses are put (Bloch & Reddaway, 1977); and the wider ramifications of psychiatry's medical, cultural, and ethical past (Kiell, 1965; Laehr, 1900; Engelhardt & Spicker, 1976).

Many of these issues can be dealt with only tangentially, if at all, in the present chapter, which seeks merely to describe some of the historical themes in Western psychiatry. It is hoped that some of its obvious limitations will be partially compensated for by the bibliographical guides to fuller accounts. The omission of Near Eastern and Oriental cultures is dictated by considerations of space and by the extent to which Greek medicine seems a natural origin for many of the attitudes which permeate our own grapplings with the problems of mental disorders. (For the Near East, see Rosen, 1968; for the East, see Reynolds, 1976; Howells, 1975.)

Greek psychiatry in Greece and Rome

Like so much of our science, medicine, and philosophy, Western psychiatry stems primarily from the Greeks, who elaborated a conceptual framework and vocabulary which permeated psychiatry until the nineteenth century, and whose clinical attitudes are still of relevance today. Significantly, these developed as an integral part of Greek medicine, and it is more accurate to say that the Greeks established a rational medicine which could accommodate forms of disease that would later be called 'mental' than that Greek doctors were concerned with psychiatry as we know it.

It is sometimes forgotten that a millennium separates Homer (eighth century B.C.) from Galen (A.D. 129–*c*.200), and that the small fraction of surviving literary, philosophical, and medical texts embodies a rich variety of approaches to madness. A most decisive contrast is that between Homer and the authors of the Hippocratic corpus, a series of medical treatises composed from the fifth to the first centuries B.C. Little is known with certainty about Hippocrates himself, but his dates (*c*.460–377 B.C.) make him the contemporary of Socrates and slightly older than Plato and Aristotle. The thought forms of the earlier period, from Homer to about the sixth century B.C., are conveniently referred to as 'archaic', and share much with those of other predominantly oral societies. In terms of Dodds' nice distinction, Homer described a shame-culture; Plato lived in a guilt-culture (Dodds, 1951). This transition from the archaic to the classical involved, in the words of other scholars, the discovery of the mind, the genesis of the concept of individuality, and the birth of philosophy (Rohde, 1925; Jaeger, 1939–45). For Homer, the *psyche* was more like a double self, or alter ego, and Homeric man was not the introspective, internalized being enjoined by Socrates to know himself. Indeed, there is no word in Homer for 'person' or 'oneself', and he ascribed human behaviour and mental activity, both 'normal' and 'abnormal', to the operation of external forces (Simon, 1978). In archaic Greek culture, the underlying assumption was that men are literally driven mad, just as they are driven to acts of valour, heroism, or cowardice. During this early period, as Lain Entralgo has pointed out, the spoken word, in the form of the charm, incantation, or even poetry, played an important role in the prevention and treatment of disease and madness (Lain Entralgo, 1970). Although we may legitimately speak of such activity as a kind of psychotherapy, it has little formal connexion with the medical world of the classical Hippocratic doctor.

The Hippocratics considered diseases as natural occurrences, amenable to rational, material explanations, and to cure through the ministrations of doctors, generally acting in concert with the body's own innate tendencies ('the healing power of nature') (Neuburger, 1943). Their principal aetiological framework was the famous doctrine of the humours, whereby diseases were described as caused by excesses or deficiencies of physiologically active body fluids, such as blood, yellow bile, black bile (melancholia), and phlegm. The details of the humoral doctrine are too well known to need explication, for it remained a cornerstone of Western medicine until the eighteenth century, and our everyday speech still retains its reverberations. The doctrine's staying power depended on both its elegant simplicity and its convenient elasticity, for it was easily adaptable to observations made at the sickbed, where sweating, diarrhoea, jaundice, vomiting, and other common features of disease involve bodily fluids.

There is no surviving Hippocratic treatise on psychiatric disorders, nor is there evidence that one was ever written, for the humoral doctrine explained disturbances of affect, behaviour, and consciousness within the same precise interpretive system as other diseases such as fevers, phthisis, and dropsy. The Hippocratics were aware of the importance of this innovation, as the author of the treatise *On the Sacred Disease* made clear. The 'sacred disease' was epilepsy, a condition which has frequently been associated historically with madness. The opening lines of this work are as familiar as they are significant:

> I am about to discuss the disease called "sacred". It is not, in my opinion, any more divine or more sacred than other diseases, but has a natural cause, and its supposed divine origin is due to men's inexperience, and to their wonder at its peculiar character. . . . My own view is that those who first attributed a sacred character to this malady were like the magicians, purifiers, charlatans and quacks of our

own day, – men who claim great piety and superior knowledge. Being at a loss, and having no treatment which would help, they concealed and sheltered themselves behind superstition, and called this illness sacred, in order that their utter ignorance might not be manifest. (Hippocrates, 1923–31, II, pp. 139–41)

This strongly aggressive treatise, defending a pervading naturalism, also claims the brain as the organ of thought, feeling, and perception, and by extension, of disorders of these functions.

> Men ought to know that from the brain, and from the brain only, arise our pleasures, joys, laughter and jests, as well as our sorrows, pains, griefs and tears. Through it, in particular, we think, see, hear, and distinguish the ugly from the beautiful, the bad from the good, the pleasant from the unpleasant, in some cases using custom as a test, in others perceiving them from their utility. It is the same thing which makes us mad or delirious, inspires us with dread and fear, whether by night or by day, brings sleeplessness, inopportune mistakes, aimless anxieties, absentmindedness, and acts that are contrary to habit. These things that we suffer all come from the brain, when it is not healthy, but becomes abnormally hot, cold, moist, or dry, or suffers any other unnatural affection to which it was not accustomed. Madness comes from its moistness. (Hippocrates, 1923–31, II, p. 175)

This striking example of what William James was later to call 'medical materialism' embodies the general professional claim of medical jurisdiction over diseases of the brain (including madness), and the specific counter to an alternative Greek interpretation (held by Aristotle, among others) that the heart is the seat of intellectual and emotional life (Harris, 1973). Galen was to side firmly with the Hippocratics and Plato on the issue, but Shakespeare could still ask rhetorically:

> Tell me, where is fancy bred,
> Or in the heart, or in the head?
> (*Merchant of Venice*, III, ii)

Despite the effective triumph of the Hippocratic view, the heart still had deep symbolic meaning for Shakespeare's younger contemporary, William Harvey (Pagel, 1967).

The easy naturalism of much Greek medical writing may be one reason why psychiatric disorders were not commonly singled out for special comment.

Rather, scattered through this corpus we find descriptions of several conditions which later writers identified as psychiatric. These include mania, melancholia, phrenitis, and hysteria. The latter disease was frequently attributed to a wandering uterus even by authors whose basic commitment was to humoral aetiologies, though suppression of the menses was also invoked as a causative factor (Veith, 1965). The Hippocratic abiding interest in veterinary medicine might have provided them with a reasonable analogical basis for the wandering uterus theory, since prolapsed uteri are common among goats, sheep, and other farm animals, and the Hippocratics occasionally made use of animal observations in explaining human diseases. In any case, the Greeks identified a complex of symptoms associated with hysteria – palpitations, migratory pain, breathing difficulties, the *globus hystericus* – and they implicated its sexual nature through their recommended treatments, including marriage and sexual intercourse. Hysteria is often found in societies and situations where women are devalued and denied sexuality, while still being subjected to a great deal of sexual innuendo and stimulation; classical Athens was no exception (Simon, 1978; Dover, 1978).

The other conditions mentioned above – mania, melancholia, and phrenitis – were freely harmonized within the humoral framework, and we have relatively full descriptions of them from later medical authors, especially Celsus (*c.* A.D. 40), Aretaeus of Cappadocia (*c.* A.D. 150) and, *en passant*, Galen (Drabkin, 1955). As Ackerknecht has pointed out, it is incorrect to attempt to translate these conditions into modern diagnostic categories, for the Greeks frequently used mania simply to describe any agitated form of insanity, and melancholia for any quiet one (Ackerknecht, 1968). The author of *On the Sacred Disease* suggested that 'those who are mad through phlegm are quiet, and neither shout nor make a disturbance; those maddened through bile are noisy, evil-doers and restless, always doing something inopportune'. Galen held that mania was a chronic disease of the brain and hot humour (yellow bile) or the vital spirits in the heart (Jackson, 1969; Galen, 1928, p. 211). This latter interpretation was closer to an alternative to the humoral scheme which Galen used to explain physiological, and less often, pathophysiological, phenomena. It involved three kinds of spirit or *pneuma* (natural, vital, and animal), each associated with a major organ (liver, heart, and brain); Galen left a particularly full exposition of this phys-

iological system in his work *De Usu Partium* (Galen, 1968; Temkin, 1977). Whether the ultimate cause was an excess of a hot humour or of vital spirit, the general therapeutic principle adopted by Galen in common with the Hippocratics and other Greek doctors – the restoration of an equilibrium through the use of opposites – dictated a cooling regimen, for mania was a 'hot' disease. This principle of treatment by opposition, long the basis of orthodox Western medicine, is an *allopathic* one, in contrast to the *homeopathic* theories of Samuel Hahnemann (1755–1843) and his followers.

Melancholia has attracted a particularly rich historical literature (Klibansky *et al.*, 1964; Lewis, 1967; Flashar, 1966; Starobinski, 1960). Galen's views were not entirely consistent, but they illustrate several features of the Greek conceptions of the condition. Galen considered it to be a chronic, non-febrile disorder, ultimately derived from black bile. Kudlien and, more recently, Simon have suggested that for some earlier Greek authors such as the Hippocratics and Aristotle, black bile was rarely, if ever, identified with any particular physical substance (Kudlien, 1967; Simon, 1978). Rather, it played a somewhat hypothetical, and richly symbolic role for these writers who incorporated, perhaps unconsciously, magical and religious elements into their work. By the time of Galen, though, this fourth humour had been rendered substantial, Galen holding that black bile results from either the cooling and thickening of the blood, or the overheating of yellow bile. The consequent disorder, melancholia, could take a variety of chronic, non-febrile forms. Cooled, thickened blood yielded a primary brain disorder, whereas the bilious form affected the upper abdominal organs (hypochondrium) primarily, the brain being only secondarily disturbed. The latter condition merged into what was called hypochondriasis, in which flatulence, bloating, and other abdominal symptoms combined with additional aspects of melancholia – fearfulness, misanthropy, and (often) delusions – to produce the clinical syndrome so frequently described in the medical, as well as popular, literature from Antiquity to the Renaissance. Galen believed that the sedentary, intellectual life was frequently associated with melancholia, a theme later elaborated in much detail by Robert Burton. Like the Hippocratics, Galen held that melancholia and epilepsy were closely related disorders, the former sometimes turning into the latter. We should also recall that the humoral framework provided Galen and its other exponents with a guide to everyday behaviour and personality, for each person 'naturally' had a dominant humour, helping to shape his temperament. In melancholics black bile prevailed, though with careful diet, life-style, and other preventative measures, the melancholic might hope to avoid the full-blown clinical consequences of his temperament. Sanguine, phlegmatic, or choleric persons could also hope to preserve their own health through appropriate hygienic measures related to the individual peculiarities of their own temperament.

Galen's therapeutic recommendations for cases of melancholia included blood-letting if the entire blood was affected, purgatives, exercise, fattening foods, sexual intercourse, music, dramatic poetry, and drugs to counter the black bile. His therapeutics have a good deal in common with those of Soranus (A.D. 100), a Greek physician whose views on acute and chronic disease survive in a Latin author Caelius Aurelianus (*c.* A.D. 500) (Aurelianus, 1950). However, Soranus used a completely different theoretical framework, based on the solid rather than the fluid parts of the body. Soranus followed Asclepiades in attributing disease to the praeternatural striction of the body's pores; in his opinion melancholy was caused not by black bile but by an emotion which he called 'black rage'. That the theoretical differences between Galen and Soranus were greater than the practical, therapeutic ones is a commonplace in the history of medicine.

Galen's other principal diagnostic category was phrenitis, an acute, febrile condition which involved agitation and delirium. Historians have found what they believe to be meningitis, malaria, and typhoid among Galen's case histories of phrenitis, though retrospective diagnosis can be a treacherous activity which may blind us to the genuinely historical context of our material. Galen's own descriptions of the condition cannot be fitted into a modern nosological slot and attempts to do so fall victim to the fact that distinctions between organic and psychological diseases are not part of the Greek medical world. For Galen, prodromal symptoms of phrenitis include insomnia, nightmares, forgetfulness, and inappropriate behaviour. The acute attack could involve clouding of consciousness, picking at the bedclothes (carphology), and agitation. Unlike its opposite disease – lethargy – phrenitis was a hot, dry condition, attributed by Galen to either an excess of yellow bile or (according to his alternative system) a deficiency of animal spirit. Dodds has called this tendency,

common among the Greeks and their successors, to 'explain' a single phenomenon with a variety of sometimes incompatible interpretative systems, *overdeterminism* (Dodds, 1951).

These descriptions of disease are scattered through many of Galen's writings, which occupy twenty volumes in the standard edition. Though his clinical histories frequently contain shrewd insights into human behaviour – as when he diagnosed a lady's insomnia not as a case of melancholia but of 'love sickness' by feeling her pulse quicken when the name of her secret lover was mentioned – his medical world amply illustrates the truth of Lain Entralgo's remark that 'Medicine has always been, and has always had to be, in one way or another, "Psychosomatic"; this has not always been the case of pathology' (Lain Entralgo, 1955). Galen's pathology technically made psychotherapy irrelevant, indeed, impossible, though as a shrewd clinician, undoubtedly he often employed what we would call psychotherapy, and occasionally emphasized that psychic conditions such as stress and anxiety can cause disease (Galen, 1956). His treatise, *On the Passions and Errors of the Soul* (1963), is sometimes cited as evidence that Galen possessed a concept of mental disease, but as Garcia Ballester has shown, this work falls within the tradition of Stoic philosophy rather than medicine (Ballester, 1974; Starobinski, 1960). Exponents of Stoic philosophy urged the use of words (*lógos*) to avoid error and excess passion. But this was a moral, not a medical, injunction, and this aspect in later history of the Stoic tradition belongs rather to Christian writers of devotionals and moral tracts than to doctors.

Greek and Roman literature also yield some evidence about popular attitudes to madness, and in Roman times the mad were sometimes imprisoned and whipped. Yet in certain contexts, madness took on positive connotations, as in Plato's description of 'divine madness' (enthusiasm), or the corybantic activities of religious groups. The transition from a culture of archaic shame to one of classical guilt did not put paid to the Greek fascination with the irrational; indeed, as Nietzsche pointed out, the opposing strands of Apollonian and Dionysiac elements in Greek life were united in Attic tragedy (Simon, 1978, pp. 44–5; North, 1966). Of particular medical relevance were the Aesculapian temples, which flourished even as the Hippocratic corpus was being written. The priests of these healing temples employed symbolic dream interpretations and incantations in their activities. Aesculapian shrines can only in a loose sense be considered as the ancestors of hospitals, and even the Romans, who developed the military hospital, or *valetudinarium*, did not make any special institutional provision for the mad. We know but little of the way the mad were actually treated in Greek and Roman society, though imaginative literature and legal writings suggest a variety of social attitudes and practices ranging from the brutal to the humane and sympathetic. The insane were generally the responsibility of their families (Rosen, 1968).

The Christian era
Greek medical writings continued to be preserved, translated, and commented upon for some time after Galen's death around A.D. 200; indeed, our fullest ancient account of mental disorders is the fifth century A.D. work of Caelius Aurelianus. Nevertheless, the rise of Christianity as the dominant European religion and the crumbling of the vast empire of Rome, produced profound changes in social, intellectual, and religious values (Kroll, 1973). Although historians of psychiatry have often dismissed this as a period of virtual darkness – Zilboorg's chapter is entitled 'The great decline' – the mingling of Judo-Christian and Graeco-Roman elements produced some intricate formulations of the soul, its functions and disorders (Zilboorg, 1941). Lain Entralgo has insisted that the Old Testament tendency to equate disease with sin was reversed by the message of the New Testament and that the early Church Fathers created the intellectual possibility of a genuine psychosomatic medicine through their progressive 'Hellenization of the primitive Christian idea of a disease' (Lain Entralgo, 1955). Other historians, such as Doob, have emphasized the extent to which medieval attitudes towards madness – and disease in general – embodied specific theological and moral dimensions, even when the resulting process was described in humoral terms. Ultimately, disease was a legacy of Original Sin and could be inflicted for purposes of punishment, purgation, or testing (Doob, 1974).

Despite certain unique aspects of the Christian world view, there are basic continuities between the classical and Christian eras, as is evident in the literature relating to epilepsy, or in the psychological theories of a number of Christians between St Augustine (354–430) and St Thomas Aquinas (1225–74). Positive antipathy towards pagan classical writers was unusual, and both theologians and physi-

cians (sometimes they were one and the same) generally discussed mental functions in terms of humours and spirits (*pneuma*). One other particularly influential tradition, with Greek antecedents but formally elaborated by Nemesius, Augustine, and other Church Fathers, located the psychological functions of sensation, reason, and memory in the anterior, middle, and posterior ventricles or cells of the brain, respectively (Clarke & Dewhurst, 1972). Galen's suggestion that the animal spirits are elaborated in the *rete mirabile* continued to be repeated until early modern times, even after Vesalius (1514–64) demonstrated that the human brain contains no such vascular structure. Even though these spirits were conceived as being exceedingly subtle and rarified, their very existence and assigned functions and seats of action remind us of the extent to which Christian thinkers could accommodate a thoroughgoing psychophysiology. Aquinas, deeply indebted to Aristotle, accepted that matter and form, structure and function, body and mind, are to be considered as unities, not opposites (Mora, 1978).

Aquinas had the works of a number of classical authors available to him. Much earlier, most classical works had disappeared from European culture, though still being preserved, studied, and extended in Byzantium and Islam. Probably the first hospitals devoted to the care of the insane were established in the Islamic world as early as A.D. 800 in Damascus, and by the thirteenth century several were in existence. The Arabs added little to Greek formulations and classifications of mental disorders; even less did their European contemporaries. However, one particular condition, *acedia* or sloth, was differentiated from melancholia, despite the fact that many of its symptoms (boredom, anxiety, obsessions) were common to both diagnoses (Wenzel, 1967). *Acedia* was also one of the Seven Deadly Sins, in itself a comment on the integration of theology and medicine during the European Middle Ages (Bloomfield, 1967; Altschule, 1977). By the Renaissance the word had been shorn of many of its theological connotations, and Petrarch used it to describe a secular condition of listlessness and enervation (Wenzel, 1961).

By the twelfth century the recovery and study of classical texts was underway, largely in southern Europe; a few key medical works, such as the Hippocratic *Aphorisms* and Avicenna's *Canon*, acquired special status (Reynolds & Wilson, 1974). At the same time, occult beliefs, such as astrology or the attribution of curative or preventative powers to charms and amulets, were common, and the phases of the moon were thought to be especially significant in cases of lunacy. Among the learned, the occult was generally an integral accretion to, rather than a displacement of, humoralism or other naturalistic explanations of health and disease: either as another kind of over-determinism, or formulated within a framework of remote and proximate causes (Thorndike, 1923–58).

As always, we know more about what was said than what was done, and for most of the mentally disturbed or subnormal, the physician or medically literate scholar was a remote irrelevancy. Laws and legal records may bring us closer to what Acker-knecht has called 'behavioural' medicine, as Walker, Clarke, and others have shown (Walker, 1968; Clarke, 1975; Pickett, 1952). Clarke has used Celtic, Anglo-Saxon, as well as later medieval material for his stud-ies, which document the existence of special legal provisions for the insane from an early date. For instance, the tenth-century Welsh 'Laws of Hywel Dda' exclude the relatives of an idiot from seeking active revenge in cases of homicide, and insanity precluded one from becoming a judge. Insanity was a ground for divorce in much of early medieval Europe, though it is not always clear how the diag-nosis was made. What would today be considered brutal social and legal discrimination or physical treatment sometimes emerges in a clear, unselfcon-scious form in these early documents, as in a tenth-century leechbook which states categorically: 'In case a man be lunatic (*monath-seóc*), take the skin of a mere-swine, or porpoise, work it into a whip. Swinge the man therewith, soon he will be well. Amen.' (Clarke, 1975, p. 45). On the other hand, sacred wells, shrines, and saints' relics also were important at the popular level, and while some of these acquired spe-cial significance for the epileptic, mentally subnor-mal, or mad, more often holy places and objects were deemed to have powers, the operation of which would not discriminate between our own categories of physical and mental disorder.

The insane were also cared for in monasteries and other religious institutions, and as an offshoot of the emergence of hospitals in Europe, specialized hospitals for the insane appeared, most systemati-cally in Spain, where Islamic influence was strong (Burdett, 1893). An asylum for the insane was founded in 1365–7 in Granada, and during the next century others were opened in Valencia, Saragossa, Seville, Barcelona, and Toledo (Chamberlain, 1966; Domin-guez, 1967). In London, St Mary of Bethlem (popu-larly known as Bedlam) is known to have housed psychiatric patients as early as 1403, and psychiatric wards or departments existed in hospitals in many major European cities, including Paris, Montpellier, Munich, Zürich, and Basle (O'Donoghue, 1914; Rosen, 1968). The colony at Gheel, Belgium (still in existence), where the insane lived with the local inhabitants, can be traced back at least to the thir-teenth century (Roosens, 1979).

From the twelfth century, the formal medical literature becomes richer, either in the form of com-mentaries on Greek or Arabic authors, or in general encyclopaedic compilations. Typical was the *Com-pendium Medicinē* (*c.*1230) of Gilbertus Anglicus where, under diseases of the head, he described a variety of disorders including mania, melancholia, lethargy, epilepsy, and demoniac possession. While locating mania and melancholia in the anterior and middle cells respectively, he also discussed them in terms of humours, temperaments, psychological fac-tors, and demons. His therapeutic recommendations were also an eclectic mixture of drugs, diet, exercise, and psychological and environmental manipula-tions. As Clarke has noted, Gilbertus seemed aware that he was dealing with a range of disorders embracing illness, social disturbance, and theologi-cal deviation (Clarke, 1975).

The early modern period
1. *Renaissance psychiatry*

It is no longer possible to accept Zilboorg's portrait of a barbaric and superstitious medieval psychiatry giving way to the 'first psychiatric revo-lution' in the sixteenth century. Zilboorg underesti-mated the extent to which naturalistic explanations of mental disorders persisted throughout the Middle Ages and failed to appreciate that the lot of the insane was no better in 1600 than it had been 500 years before (Zilboorg, 1941). Nevertheless, the scientific and medical achievements during the period from Co-pernicus (1473–1543) and Vesalius (1514–64) to Gali-leo (1564–1642) and Harvey (1578–1657) justify the description 'Scientific Revolution', and the psychi-atric writings of the times display a richness and variety which set them apart from earlier work. It is not possible to grasp the formal psychiatric thought apart from its medical and social context. In this sense, new developments in the printing and distribution of books, or changes in medical education and the medical profession are more than simply background issues. We should not overlook the extent to which religion still permeated much that was thought and written. The Reformation left many people with difficult personal decisions and lingering anxieties. Theological debates touch many basic areas of human existence, including individualism, free will, responsibility, sin, and suffering. On the other hand, the continued recovery and study of classical texts was accompanied by a certain recovery of nerve and critical independence (Neugebauer, 1979).

There is no way easily to summarize without distortion the many complicated and often contradictory psychiatric themes of the period. Renaissance innovations in anatomy were more striking than those in either physiology or pathology, and the widespread veneration of Galen guaranteed the persistence of a basic vocabulary of humours, temperaments, and vital spirits (Temkin, 1973). In Paris, for instance, Jean Fernel (1497–1558) remained faithful to a fundamentally Galenic pathophysiology even while expounding a comprehensive medical synthesis. He accepted the division of mental faculties into reason, imagination, and memory, and described phrenitis, delirium, melancholia, mania, and lycanthropy in humoral terms (Sherrington, 1946). Another energetic traditionalist, Felix Platter (1536–1614), Dean of the Medical Faculty at the University of Basle, left extensive accounts of psychiatric disorders in his general medical treatises, especially *Praxis Medica* (1602) and *Observationes* (1614). He left a pioneering classification of psychiatric illness, his main divisions being mental weakness, mental consternation, deep sleep or coma, and mental alienation. He fully discussed hysteria and sexual disorders, described cretinism, and advocated a variety of psychological, pharmacological, and physical therapies (Diethelm & Heffernan, 1965). Platter worked within the humoral framework, but his own powers of observation were formidable and the many editions and translations of his books together with a considerable range of theses of psychiatric relevance presented at Basle and elsewhere attest to his European influence (Diethelm, 1971).

During the same period, the Aristotelian corpus was central to the intellectual life of many Italian and northern universities, and Renaissance psychology often bears marks of Aristotelian hylomorphism. The mortalism of Italian philosophers like Pomponazzi (1462–1525) falls within this spectrum, as does the suggestion of Girolamo Mercuriale (1530–1604) that melancholia is a disturbance of the imagination and can be located in the heart (Randall, 1961).

Humanism infused much medical writing and men like Johannes Weyer (below, p. 21), Juan Luis Vives (1492–1540) and Juan Huarte (1529–88) were active in reform movements of their day. Vives was concerned with the education and social status of women, in welfare, and in the role of instinct and the passions in health and disease. He protested against physical abuse of the mentally disturbed. Although born in Spain, Vives spent his adult life largely in England and Flanders and was intimate with Erasmus, Thomas More, Linacre, and other humanists of northern Europe (Clements, 1967). Huarte's *Examination of Men's Wits* (1575) expounded its author's psychological and educational theories and included a long section on physiognomy, a subject of continuing interest during the period (e.g. Savonarola, 1478; Gratarolus, 1554; J. B. della Porta, 1586) (Mora, 1977). Physiognomy – the doctrine of correspondence between physical form and moral and psychological characteristics – appealed to an age which found analogy everywhere: between the 'signatures' of plants and their medicinal properties; between an environment and its flora and fauna; and above all, between the microcosm and macrocosm (Debus, 1978).

Renaissance neo-Platonism, mysticism, hermeticism, and occultism nourished many of these latter themes, even if their reverberations can be found almost everywhere. Modern scholarship has sympathetically explored this 'softer' side of Renaissance thought, both as an integral aspect of the period and as a genuine source of the 'positive' achievements of the Scientific Revolution. The neo-Platonist Marsilio Ficino (1433–99) related melancholia to the influence of Saturn (as well as to the action of black bile), and men like Paracelsus (*c.* 1493–1541) and Jerome Cardan (1501–76) sought to create a new medicine for a new age (Klibansky *et al.*, 1964; Walker, 1958).

Like many other intellectual rebels who have eschewed the knowledge of books in favour of the direct, unmediated study of Nature, Paracelsus was an inveterate scribbler whose collected writings run to more than twenty volumes. A visit to the village of Einsiedeln, his Swiss birthplace, can still help us appreciate the roots of his thought. Always an individualist, he rejected humoral theory and substituted instead three principles – salt, sulphur, mercury – as the regulative substances of health and disease. *On the Diseases which deprive Man of Reason* (1526) was his most systematic treatise of psychiatric relevance, but pregnant passages occur in many of his works, including a cogent description of mass psychic contagion in a treatise on St Vitus's dance. He there insisted that this dancing mania was a natural phenomenon, caused by physical or psychological disturbances. Elsewhere, however, he suggested that the devil was behind St Vitus's dance. Paracelsus recognized five primary psychiatric diseases: mania, epilepsy, 'true insanity', St Vitus's dance, and *suffocatio intellectus* (the old hysteria). He associated cretinism with goitre, and distinguished between mental deficiency and insanity. His approach to patients was holistic, and Coulter has recently stressed the extent to which empirical, therapeutic experience informed his more theoretical pronouncements (Coulter, 1973–7). A master of the memorable epigram ('The physician is only the servant of nature, not her master', 'Every physician must be rich in knowledge, and not only of that which is written in books; his patients should be his books, they will never mislead him'), Paracelsus has been adopted as a forerunner of dynamic psychiatry, particularly by Jungians (Pagel, 1958; Paracelsus, 1941; Leibbrand & Wettley, 1961; Ellenberger, 1970).

Jerome Cardan was another magus-figure in the Paracelsian mould. His *Autobiography*, a work of impressive psychological subtlety, describes Cardan's own emotional development, his relationships with his father and his son, and the neurotic symptoms which coloured family life for these three generations of Cardans. He also experimented with hallucinogenic drugs, cautioned against witchcraft persecutions, and advised his readers how to maintain mental health. Like Cardan, François Rabelais (*c.* 1483–1553) and Michel de Montaigne (1533–92) are other authors whose lives, letters, and reflective writings illustrate the Renaissance discovery of selfhood. Many of their doubts and anxieties, as well as their astute psychological perceptions, induce sympathetic resonances in the modern reader (Batisse, 1962; Chesney, 1977; Screech, 1979).

This small sample of psychiatric authors demonstrates the variety of Hippocratic, Aristotelian, Galenic, and neo-Platonic strands in Renaissance medicine, although clearly there were many novel features as well. The art and imaginative literature of the period frequently depict fools, melancholics, and madmen: Sebastian Brant, Bosch, Dürer, Erasmus, Cervantes, and Shakespeare, to name just a few, have left us their own creative insights into the nature of abnormal mental states. Foucault has stressed the

public visibility of madness during the period, but much more needs to be known before his own stark vision can be properly evaluated. Foucault's suggestion that the leper was replaced by the madman as an object of collective aggression is superficially attractive but historically untenable, and not only because more than a century separated the European disappearance of leprosy from the psychiatric literature and iconography of the high Renaissance (Foucault, 1971).

What is certain is that the attitudes reflected in both the literature and the increased institutional involvement show an ambiguous mixture of brutality, suspicion, fear, and sympathy. The number of psychiatric hospitals and psychiatric wards in general hospitals grew; chains and close confinement were common, and many stereotyped characteristics of the mad – insensitivity to cold and pain, praeternatural strength, dominance of animal over human attributes – found repeated expression in medical and non-medical writing. The word 'bedlam' acquired many of its wider connotations during the sixteenth century and the official privilege of discharged Bethlem patients to identify themselves for purposes of begging encouraged ordinary vagabonds to exploit the perquisite (O'Donoghue, 1914; Rosen, 1968). Tom O'Bedlam became a well-known figure, even if Foucault's vision of gangs of roving madmen is undoubtedly exaggerated and the ship of fools was a literary and artistic device probably without historical reality (Midelfort, 1980).

2. *The European witch-craze*

Historians have not failed to appreciate the irony in the fact that the 'first psychiatric revolution' coincided temporally and geographically with the wave of mass hysteria, brutality, and social dislocation known as the European witch-craze. Occult and magical beliefs had been common in the Middle Ages, and lycanthropy was a favourite medieval diagnosis (Villeneuve, 1956; Jackson, 1972). However, the social consequences of occult beliefs between about 1460 and 1680 were utterly different from those of earlier times. Despite the biblical injunction that 'Thou shalt not suffer a witch to live' (Exodus xxii 18), medieval doctrine firmly declared belief in witchcraft to be heretical (Russell, 1972; Kieckhefer, 1976). This had changed by the late fifteenth century, and a Papal Bull of 1484 deplored the spread of witchcraft itself and authorized the vigorous extermination of its practitioners. Two years later, the *Malleus Maleficarum* of the two Dominican monks Krämer and Sprenger brought an aggressive note of urgency to the scene. It became a handbook for witch-finders, passing through more than twenty editions and translations during the following two centuries (Hansen, 1900).

Despite gaps in our knowledge, the contours of the craze are well established. The widespread accusations of witchcraft began in mountainous regions such as the Alps and Pyrenees, and probably at some level was related to much earlier Albigensian and Cathar heresies, against which the Dominican order had been particularly active. Ultimately, however, virtually no area of Europe escaped, and the total number of accusations, trials, and executions, though episodic from region to region, increased steadily throughout the sixteenth and early decades of the seventeenth century. It has been estimated that more than 50 000 people were tried for witchcraft during the period.

Historical explanations of the craze have involved a variety of causal factors and interpretive frameworks. Some recent historiography has employed the insights of anthropology and the broader perspectives of contemporary social history in an effort to get behind more traditional accounts which stressed the intellectual theological contexts (Thomas, 1973; Macfarlane, 1970; Monter, 1972). Local studies undermine sweeping interpretations such as the tensions of Protestant–Catholic interactions, and even the general historical literature on the economic turmoils of the sixteenth century and the *crise de la conscience européenne* of the seventeenth sometimes appears remote when the particular and idiosyncratic features of local witch-hunting outbreaks are examined (Rabb, 1975). It is for this reason that geographically constrained studies such as Macfarlane's on Essex, Midelfort's on south-west Germany, and Boyer and Nissenbaum's on Salem, Massachusetts, are so valuable (Macfarlane, 1970; Midelfort, 1972; Boyer & Nissenbaum, 1974; Monter, 1976).

There are many points at which the language of disease seems appropriate for describing the events of the witchcraft era. Nineteenth-century psychiatrists and rationalist historians suggested that most of those accused of being witches were mentally disturbed, their confessions of participation in sabbaths, possession of familiars, intercourse with the devil, and other aspects of occult activity resulting from hallucinations, delusions, and other symptoms of mental derangement (Schoeneman, 1977). It is true that many of the victims of accusations lived marginal existences, encumbered with a variety of mental, physical, and social vulnerabilities. Some of the victims actively courted their status, and epilepsy and hysteria were two conditions which might have encouraged charges of witchcraft or possession. But the simple scapegoat theories of the nineteenth century are not completely persuasive; no more than the recent versions of them which Szasz and others have advanced. They are too rigidly polemical, overlook too many local exceptions, and excessively simplify the historical nuances and contingencies of the accusations.

Alternatively, the charge of psychopathology has been levelled primarily at the witch-hunters rather than the victims. The printed works of men such as Krämer, Sprenger, and Matthew Hopkins reveal much about their authors, who frequently manifest high degrees of masochism, paranoia, misogamy, and sexual frustration. Men like these helped create a stereotype of the witch, a process which, as Cohn's researches have shown, had many structural similarities with earlier stereotypes which had developed for the Jews or the Knights Templar. Once in existence, these stereotypes influenced perceptions and behaviour, even though their objects possessed none of the characteristics attributed to them. Cohn speculates that much of the aggression directed against witches resulted from displaced – and largely unconscious – resentment at the asceticism and devaluation of sexuality inherent in Christian doctrine (Cohn, 1976; Cohn, 1970). These psychosexual conflicts were exacerbated by the positive secular achievements of this age of exploration, invention, and material progress.

The rhetoric and drama of the denunciations and formal accusations themselves also generated social unrest and group paranoia. Witch-finders often catalysed outbreaks of mass hysteria, as wholesale trials in the Pyrenees (1609–10), Essex (1645), and Salem (1692) testify. The episode at Salem, Massachusetts, had small beginnings but large consequences and is a cautionary tale with disturbing twentieth-century analogues in McCarthyism and persecution of minority groups (Rosen, 1968).

Though the witchcraft phenomenon is much more than simply an episode in the history of psychiatry, some physicians were among those who remained sceptical about the wisdom or legitimacy of the witchcraft accusations. Trevor-Roper has identified common sense, Paduan science, and Platonic metaphysics as three major sources of the scepticism, the most significant medical expression of which was contained in *De Praestigiis Daemonum* (1563) of Johannes Weyer (1515–88) (Trevor-Roper, 1967). Weyer, an Erasmian Platonist, was a town medical officer of Arnhem before becoming personal physician to Duke William of Jülich-Cleve-Berg. In his book, he cautioned against the ease with which illness could be mistaken for witchcraft. The devil, he insisted, does exist and can influence human behaviour. However, since his power is ultimately limited by God, he choses melancholics and others prone to disturbances of the imagination on whom to work. Witches simply imagine many of the things which they confess: the results of hallucinatory drugs or fantasies. Likewise, many of the deeds of which they are accused – causing sudden death, impotence, crop failure, or other misfortunes – are natural occurrences. Witches are thus to be pitied and treated rather than feared and punished (Zilboorg, 1941; Cobben, 1976).

Although it would be anachronistic to make of Weyer a modern rationalist, his book was a considerable achievement, coming as it did in the wake of renewed witch-hunting. Many of his arguments had been used before – by his teacher Agrippa, among others – and were to appear later in the works of other sceptics of witch-hunting such as Reginald Scot (1538?–99). During the period, though, Weyer's views were more often refuted than espoused and it was only later generations which fully appreciated the quality of his thought, based as it was on shrewd insights into human nature, sound clinical judgement, and wide medical experience.

Significant regional variations in the patterns of witchcraft accusations make generalization hazardous. For instance, *maleficium* was the usual charge laid against witches in England, whereas heresy was of greater consequence in many Continental trials. Economic factors are constitutive to Boyer and Nissenbaum's persuasive account of Salem, while Midelfort has insisted that the panic reactions which led to wholesale trials and executions in south-west Germany served no identifiable social functions. Further, witch beliefs sometimes persisted as part of popular culture long after trials and executions ceased, and even the latter did not die out in parts of Eastern Europe until the early nineteenth century (Burke, 1978). By 1700, though, in most of Europe and America, these beliefs had lost currency among educated élites, and the medical, legal, and theological machinery which adjudicated over witchcraft trials

was dismantled. Thus, while both individual and mass psychopathology may frequently be invoked in historical accounts, psychiatric factors represent only part of the complicated texture of the epoch, which was a tragic episode in the ongoing Western dialectic between disease and sin, the natural and the supernatural.

3. *The seventeenth century*

The exponential growth of medical and scientific activities characteristic of modern Western culture is already evident in seventeenth-century Europe through the foundation, from mid-century, of a number of scientific societies (e.g. the Royal Society of London and the *Académie des Sciences* in Paris), and the regular publication of scientific journals (e.g. *Philosophical Transactions* and *Journal des Savants*). Much has been written about the religious and theological background to this systematic exploration of the natural world, and shows a continuing historical preoccupation with themes which, in a slightly different context, Max Weber long ago developed in *The Protestant Ethic and the Spirit of Capitalism* (1904–5) (Weber, 1930). Among Protestant groups, the Puritans elaborated a philosophy which most overtly justified the study of nature (and the accumulation of wealth) (Merton, 1970). Puritan values can be found in the writings of Francis Bacon (1561–1626), who was widely accepted in England as a spokesman for the New Science (Webster, 1975). Bacon held that man's mastery of nature could be achieved by careful and unprejudiced observations which through the principles of induction could help man formulate more general laws. Among medical men, Thomas Sydenham (1624–89) acknowledged his deep debt to Bacon (Wolfe, 1966). One manifestation of the premium placed on Baconian observationism was the frequency with which doctors published detailed case histories, including those of patients suffering from psychiatric disorders.

As always, psychiatric theories of the period can be related to broader formulations of health and disease. The century was one of exuberant innovation in both medicine and science, and while the Hippocratic writings continued to exert influence, the power of Galenism declined (Debus, 1974). The Baconian programme encouraged the rejection of the Galenic concept of the 'faculty' as a sterile, meaningless abstraction (although Molière's satires show it a fit subject for caricature), and Harvey's discovery of the circulation put paid to the strict adherence to

Galen's doctrines of natural and vital spirits. On the other hand, *animal* spirits (sometimes identified in part with the cerebral spinal fluid) were functionally invoked in many seventeenth- and eighteenth-century theories of brain and nervous action (Clarke & O'Malley, 1968). Galenism retreated before a number of alternative medical philosophies, some drawing inspiration from the chemical doctrines advanced by men such as Paracelsus and Van Helmont (1577–1644); other medical philosophies were inspired by the mechanical traditions of Galileo and Descartes (1596–1650) (King, 1978).

Descartes, whose opinions were particularly important for subsequent explanations of mind, divided the world into two incommensurable categories: body and mind (Descartes, 1967, 1972). Among terrestrial beings, only human beings possessed minds, the behaviour of animals being completely explicable in terms of matter and motion. He thus conceived animals as simply complicated machines, devoid of feeling, will, or consciousness. Descartes equated *mind* with the theological soul; mind endowed men and women with consciousness, rationality, moral responsibility, and immortality. Although, as an immaterial principle, mind could not be precisely located in space, Descartes felt that its operations were most intimately connected with the pineal gland (a unitary, mid-line structure). The *sensorium commune* was the general term given to the brain site where sensation was supposed to terminate and movement to originate. While Descartes favoured the pineal gland, other areas of the brain, including the *medulla oblongata* (Malpighi, Willis), the *corpora striata* (Vieussens) and the *corpus callosum* (Lancisi) were advanced by other seventeenth-century doctors as the seat of the human soul (Clarke & Dewhurst, 1972).

The psychiatric implications of Descartes' physiological psychology were considerable, for it is difficult to see how his dualistic philosophy was logically compatible with primary mental disease. Certainly psychiatrists with a concern for the theological implications of the concept of mind tended to assume that insanity was always connected with physical disease of the brain (Bynum, 1972). The potential explanatory power of Cartesian mechanistic physiology encouraged such an assumption, although the direct neuropathological evidence was missing in most cases of insanity, and Cartesian dualism never satisfactorily came to grips with the issue of how the mind and brain actually interacted (Vartanian, 1953).

In fact, Descartes was also concerned with the passions and came close to suggesting that the passions were instrumental in connecting the mind to the body (Levi, 1964; Riese, 1965). The passions were implicated in cases of madness by many doctors throughout the seventeenth and eighteenth centuries (Neu, 1977).

We must not modernize Descartes into a cryptic materialist whose dualism served as a decoy against political or religious persecution. Nevertheless, materialists like Thomas Hobbes (1588–1679), drawing inspiration from the mechanistic writings of both Descartes and Galileo, tackled the formidable implications of a materialistic psychology (Peters, 1962). Much of the work of Cambridge Platonists such as Henry More (1614–87) and Ralph Cudworth (1617–88) was directed against what they saw as the rising tide of mortalism and materialism (Passmore, 1951). On the Continent, Pierre Gassendi (1592–1655) and Nicolas Malebranche (1638–1715) extended the philosophical and psychological ramifications of Cartesianism.

Thomas Willis (1621–75) was probably the most distinguished neuroscientist working within the Cartesian tradition. He brought a new rigour to neuroanatomy and neurophysiology (circle of Willis, use of the term 'reflex'), and clinical neurology (epilepsy, progressive paralysis, myasthenia gravis) (Hierons, 1967). His clinical descriptions include cases of psychiatric interest, such as mental deficiency and what may well have been schizophrenic and manic-depressive psychoses. Willis attempted to localize a number of mental functions to particular areas of the brain; his theories of many central, and most peripheral, neurological activities depended on animal spirits (Meyer & Hierons, 1965; Bynum, 1973). These spirits were a kind of half-way house between body and mind but capable of being affected by either. He believed that patients suffering from mania should be forcibly restrained, but recommended a variety of other somatic and psychological measures, including drugs, travel, and baths, for other psychiatric disturbances (Isler, 1968; Jackson, 1978).

During the period, a number of monographs were written on individual psychiatric diseases, beginning (in England) with Timothy Bright's *Treatise on Melancholy* (1586). In fact, a number of historians have described what is sometimes called an epidemic of melancholia during Elizabethan and Jacobean England (Babb, 1951, 1959; Lyons, 1971). Certainly, if literary evidence may be taken, melancholia was a fashionable condition, even before Robert Burton's *Anatomy of Melancholy* (1621, see 1955) etched it into the English reading public's consciousness (Evans, 1972). Melancholy continued to be discussed primarily in humoral terms, though Bright, Laurentius, and Burton all offered a variety of other psychological, theological, and astrological explanations of its aetiology. In literary works, the melancholic was frequently called the *malcontent*. Jacques in *As You Like It* is a particularly well-developed example, but both comedy and tragedy during this golden period of English drama are replete with this stock character. Hamlet's madness (if madness it was) fits no stereotyped mould and has been a source of fascination for literary critics and psychiatrists alike (Wilson, 1935; Jones, 1949; Bradley, 1955; Lidz, 1976).

Hypochondriasis was conceived as closely related to melancholia on the one hand, and to hysteria, on the other. As the name suggests, hypochondriasis was often described primarily in terms of abdominal complaints such as epigastric pain, bloating, and loss of appetite, together with more general symptoms still associated with the term. Under names such as the vapours, or the spleen, the condition was a favourite diagnosis in the following century, by which time, as Fischer-Homberger has shown, it was thought of as a nervous rather than humoral disorder (Fischer-Homberger, 1970). 'Nostalgia' or *Heimweh*, a condition to which the Swiss seem particularly prone, was another form of hypochondriacal sadness described first in 1678 and 1685 by two Swiss doctors, J. Hofer and J. J. Harder respectively (Rosen, 1975).

Hypochondriasis was considered to be a predominantly (or exclusively) male disorder, and sometimes identified as the male equivalent of hysteria. The little monograph on hysteria (1603) by Edward Jordan (he called it 'suffocation of the mother') was written in direct response to a witchcraft trial of 1602 at which he had given evidence. Jordan believed that hysteria is principally a disease of the uterus, the symptoms of which can be explained by reference to the humours or to the notion of sympathy. Other seventeenth-century authors (e.g. Lepois, 1618; Highmore, 1640; Willis, 1676: see Boss, 1979) denied this traditional uterine aetiology, either because they held that the disease could appear in both men and women, or because they recognized that the wandering uterus theory of earlier writers was anatomically impossible. Willis stressed its neurological derivation. Thomas Sydenham left a partic-

ularly full discussion of hysteria, and it is usually from him that modern formulations of the disease are seen to arise (Dewhurst, 1966). Sydenham's achievement lay in the precision with which he distinguished hysteria from other disorders; in his emphasis on the interplay of psychological and physiological factors; and in the care with which he observed his hysterical patients. He described a full range of behavioural and pathophysiological symptoms, from emotional lability and inappropriate affect to migratory pains, hyperventilation, muscle weakness, and diarrhoea. The passing of large quantities of clear urine was, according to Sydenham, almost pathognomonic of hysteria or its male equivalent, hypochondriasis. This belief was consistent with his opinion that diseases could be described by doctors in the same way as botanists describe species of plants, and he devoted the same care to delineating other diseases (smallpox, measles, gout) as to hysteria. His therapeutic recommendations were eclectic and for the most part, straightforward: he valued fresh air and horseback riding, milk diets and iron preparations. Boss has recently suggested that Sydenham went beyond Willis and others who had discarded the old uterine theories of hysteria in favour of a disease located in the brain: Sydenham recognized the condition as one of the whole person (Boss, 1979).

This heightened medical concern with neuroses may well reflect the rise in middle-class demand for medical care. At the same time, the social upheavals of the century, together with the modernization of the State machinery for dealing with disruptive behaviour, led to the tightening of public control on the insane. Legal psychiatry was explored in Paolo Zacchia's (1584–1659) *Questiones Medico-Legales* (1621–35) (Ackerknecht, 1950). Zacchia, personal physician to the Pope, was involved in many high-level legal proceedings. He championed the idea of the medical expert when crime was complicated by insanity or mental incompetence. He divided mental disease into three categories – *fatuity, insanity*, and *phrenitis* – and laid down criteria for judging the extent of legal and social responsibility for people afflicted with each disorder (Cranefield & Federn, 1970; Mora, 1975). Zacchia's influence was naturally greater in countries where Roman Catholicism was strong, but his work is generally reckoned to be the foundation of modern legal medicine and psychiatry. In England, Sir Matthew Hale delivered judgements about the criminal responsibility of the insane which continued to be cited till the nineteenth century

(Walker, 1968). Suicide was a topic of considerable interest to doctors, theologians, and lawyers; it was increasingly viewed as evidence of insanity rather than as a sin or crime (MacDonald, 1977; Rosen, 1971).

Legal psychiatric issues were complicated by the absence of separate provision for the criminally insane. From the middle of the century, however, the number of general custodial institutions increased, particularly on the Continent. The *Hôpital Général* in Paris dates from 1656, and other *Hôpitaux Généraux, Zuchthäusern,* and workhouses were built with some regularity during the closing decades of the century. These institutions housed an undifferentiated mixture of humanity: the insane, orphans, beggars, petty thieves, prostitutes, unmarried mothers, the chronically ill. Foucault has called this concern by the State for the containment of its deviants, 'the Great Confinement' and has related it to the acceptance of the Puritan work ethic by Government officials who now possessed the power to control social dependants by these new repressive means (Foucault, 1971). Foucault's case rests primarily on the French evidence, which is more impressive than that for England, whose public houses of confinement were on a much smaller scale and were often employed for individuals awaiting other dispositions rather than as places of long-term confinement (Ignatieff, 1978). Indoor relief (support within a place of confinement or correction) was encouraged through various amendments of the Poor Laws until their complete revision in 1834, but it is clear that the original Acts of 1597 and 1601 were envisaged by Parliament as a stopgap to be used only when private charity was inadequate (Checkland & Checkland, 1974). Most of the insane continued to be the primary responsibility of their families, and recent work on folk medicine and religious healers substantiates the distance between élite and popular approaches to illness, including psychiatric disorders (Thomas, 1973; Burke, 1978). An insight into the nuances of ordinary medical practice is possible through the extensive case records of Richard Napier (1559–1634), currently being systematically explored by MacDonald (MacDonald, 1981).

On the other hand, formal psychiatric institutions assumed increased significance. There are occasional seventeenth-century references to private madhouses; part of the action of Thomas Middleton's *The Changeling* (1624) takes place in one (Reed, 1952). In 1676 a much enlarged Bethlem Hospital was opened 'for the relief and cure of persons distracted'. Despite its specialized function, none of its

seventeenth-century physicians published anything of consequence in psychiatry, although Edward Tyson (1650/51–1706; physician from 1684) was a distinguished comparative anatomist.

The eighteenth century
We still tend to view eighteenth-century psychiatry through lenses polished by nineteenth-century psychiatric reformers. These later individuals were anxious to set their own activities into sharp focus and consequently sometimes exaggerated the novelty of their theories and treatments. They emphasized the brutality and callousness of eighteenth-century attitudes towards the insane as a way of magnifying their own humanity. The reality was undoubtedly more complex. Eighteenth-century doctors did sometimes insist that madness results from the loss of reason, that attribute which sets a man apart from the brutes. Physical restraint could thus be justified on the same grounds as those appropriate when chaining an animal. In practice, however, more subtle theoretical formulations or more prosaic exigencies lay behind Enlightenment attitudes towards the mad. The century, after all, fostered many new schemes and institutions aimed at bettering the lot of man on earth; it saw the rise of companionate marriages and closer ties between parents and their children; and it nourished a wide range of secular values and attitudes. The decline of the Calvinistic emphasis on original sin enabled apostles of an optimistic environmentalism to speculate on mankind's potential perfectibility. These and many other aspects of Enlightenment culture must be assimilated before a fuller understanding of the century's psychiatry is achieved (Gay, 1967–9; Stone, 1977; Passmore, 1970).

Much of the formal psychiatric vocabulary of the earlier 1700s was mechanical, for Newton's achievements provided a model which many physiologists and physicians sought to emulate. Nicholas Robinson (*A New System of the Spleen,* 1729) argued that nerve fibres control behaviour, a pathological laxity in them being the primary cause of melancholia. On the Continent, Friedrich Hoffmann (1660–1742) developed a systematic solidist pathology based on the fibres and pores, while Herman Boerhaave (1668–1738) used the Newtonian banner for much of his own work. Both men discussed certain aspects of mental disorders within their more general medical writings (Jobe, 1976; King, 1978; Schofield, 1970; Bynum, 1980; Rousseau, 1980).

A richer, subtler, and ultimately more innovative tradition derived from the philosophical writings of Thomas Hobbes (1588–1679) and John Locke (1632–1704). Both men stressed the secular character of insanity and incorporated it into their broader observations on human psychology. Hobbes divided insanity into two varieties, melancholy (caused by dejection and 'causeless fears') and rage or fury (caused by pride and excessive passion or anger). Hobbes deemed that a rampant imagination or fancy was instrumental in both kinds of insanity, theories which he integrated into a faculty psychology (De Porte, 1974). Locke contemplated the relative importance of the reason and the imagination in cases of insanity, finally opting for the priority of the latter in a passage frequently quoted during the eighteenth century: '[Madmen] do not appear to me to have lost the faculty of reasoning, but having joined together some ideas very wrongly, they mistake them for truths; and they err as men do that argue right from wrong principles. For by the violence of their imaginations, having taken their fancies for realities, they make right deductions from them' (Locke, 1890, I, 209; Tuveson, 1960). Significantly, it was primarily to explain lunacy that Locke introduced the principle of the association of ideas (a psychological mechanism already described by Hobbes and others) (Warren, 1921). Locke divorced the role of the passions from his proposed aetiology of insanity, a move whereby he sought to extricate madness from the province of the clergyman or moralist. Many subsequent psychiatric writers continued to see the passions as central to the problem of madness; and the associative principle was used by numerous authors, including John Gay (1699–1745), David Hartley (1705–57), Joseph Priestley (1733–1804), Erasmus Darwin (1731–1802), and the Abbé de Condillac (1714–80), as the principal, or even sole, mechanism of the normal and abnormal mind. The importance of associationism in the psychiatric literature of the period has been established by Hoeldtke (1967). In the early nineteenth century, it almost disappeared from psychiatry, but James Mill (1773–1836), John Stuart Mill (1806–73), Herbert Spencer (1820–1903), and Alexander Bain (1818–1903) used the association of ideas in their psychological writings (Young, 1973).

In early Georgian Britain, madness was a potent cultural emblem, used by men like Jonathan Swift, Alexander Pope, Tobias Smollett, and Laurence Sterne in a variety of ways. Swift's famous 'Modest Proposal' could have been written by a Lockean mad-

man correctly reasoning from false premises, and Swift's personality was a particularly dark one. He saw madness lurking everywhere in Dissenters, atheists and social schemers (De Porte, 1974; Byrd, 1974). Dr Johnson's own fear of madness symbolizes the terror which many of his contemporaries found in the darker reaches of the mind, and three of the well-known poets of the century – William Collins, William Cowper, and Christopher Smart – had incapacitating bouts of mental disorder (Ober, 1979). Hogarth's depiction of the *Rake's Progress* was remorseless in its evocative precision; his *Gin Lane* captures the essence of alcohol abuse, especially during the decades before the Gin Acts of the 1740s and 50s discouraged excessive consumption of spirits through taxation (George, 1966). Sterne's attitudes to madness were more gentle, bound up with his conviction that this world ought to make any sensitive person a little desperate and melancholy at times. On the Continent, Diderot used an imaginative work like *D'Alembert's Dream* as a vehicle for exploring his own materialistic philosophy through his perceptive understanding of the twilight world of sleep and dreams (Diderot, 1966).

By mid-century, there is evidence of a fairly extensive network of private madhouses aimed at providing psychiatric care on a formal basis. Arrangements varied, from the accommodation of one or two patients in the proprietor's own house, to more extensive and (by the end of the century) purpose-built establishments capable of housing one hundred or more patients (Parry-Jones, 1972; Phillips, 1973; Morris, 1958). Clergymen and doctors became particularly active in the private sector, but the absence of any regulatory laws before 1774 meant that anyone could receive lunatics in such a house (Jones, 1972). Some proprietors aimed at the middle and upper classes while others specialized in the mad poor who through the century were still mostly confined in poorhouses, bridewells, or workhouses, even if the extent of long-term confinement appears to have been less in England than in many places on the Continent (Ignatieff, 1978).

St Peter's Hospital, Bristol, founded in the seventeenth century for paupers, became essentially a psychiatric institution during the Enlightenment, and asylums and psychiatric wards in voluntary hospitals (e.g. Norwich, 1724; Manchester, 1766; Newcastle, 1767; York, 1777; Liverpool, 1790) attest to abundant activity in the public sector. Most famous of these was St Luke's Hospital (1750) in London, established primarily through the exertions of William Battie (1703–76), a successful physician (President of the Royal College of Physicians), proprietor of a private madhouse and a governor of Bethlem Hospital. Inevitably, St Luke's became a kind of rival to Bethlem. Conditions for patients were probably better at the newer hospital, where Battie pioneered clinical psychiatric teaching. His *Treatise on Madness* (1758, see 1962) relied on his own psychiatric experience, though the theoretical views expressed in it were not strikingly profound. His simple division of madness into 'original' (functional) and 'consequential' (organic) was easier to use than some of the more complicated psychiatric nosologies of the next generation (e.g. Thomas Arnold, 1782–6; William Cullen, 1784). He believed that 'deluded imagination' was the essential feature of madness and insisted on the importance of management over medicine in such cases. The physician to Bethlem, John Monro (1715–91), was provoked into response over Battie's monograph which had hinted at too much reliance at Bethlem on routine medical measures such as bleeding and purging. Monro placed the lesion of madness more in the judgement or reason than the imagination. The Battie–Monro exchange has more symbolic than intrinsic significance, as indicative of a growing professional concern with psychiatric disorders and as the first literature on these disorders to come from a Bethlem physician. John Monro was the second of four successive Monros (son succeeding father) to hold that post at Bethlem (Battie, 1962).

Serious mental disorders thus attracted considerable medical, philanthropic, and literary attention during the first two-thirds of the century. At the same time, what were later called the 'neuroses' were apparently widespread among certain social groups and were the object of minute analysis by both doctors and laymen. Under a variety of terms – hypochondriasis, the vapours, the spleen, melancholy, low spirits, etc., – these conditions seemed particularly prevalent in England, where climate, temperament and life-style were deemed capable of producing what George Cheyne (1733) called the 'English malady' (Fischer-Homberger, 1972; Rousseau, 1976). Those of sedentary habits and 'refined sensibilities' were most susceptible to this cluster of disorders, the treatment for which often involved visits to the spas at Bath, Harrogate, or one of the Continental watering places such as Baden-Baden. Aetiological frameworks were frequently eclectic, sometimes incorporating logically incompatible explanatory schemes. The humoral

vocabulary survived, but the growth of mechanical physiological models encouraged both literal and metaphorical uses of the concept of 'spirits'. In addition, both the passions and the imagination were frequently invoked in the causation of hypochondriacal afflictions and as the century progressed (particularly after Haller's 1752 work on the distinction between irritability and sensitivity (Haller, 1936)) the nervous system rather than the fluids (humours) or blood vessels was more often posited as the seat of what could then be called 'nervous disorders' (Lawrence, 1979; Macalpine & Hunter, 1969). When William Cullen (1710–90) in 1783 introduced the term 'neurosis', he meant it to refer, in a precise physiological sense, to a group of diseases in which the nervous system was disordered in the absence of fever (Lopez Piñero, 1963; Lopez Piñero & Morales Meseguer, 1970). The word neurosis continued to be used in general medicine as a description of functional diseases of the nervous system until J. M. Charcot (1825–93) popularized the notion of the ideational aetiology of neurotic conditions (Ellenberger, 1970). It is really only from this middle third of the eighteenth century that patients were said to be suffering from 'nervous' conditions in the modern sense. By the 1770s Cullen's pupil, John Brown (1735–88), had elaborated a system of medicine (particularly influential in Italy and the German-speaking lands) in which virtually all diseases were described in terms of excess or deficiency of 'irritability', a property of all living organisms which Brown believed was intimately connected with nervous activity (Risse, 1970). The nineteenth-century concept of 'neurasthenia' stems from this intellectual tradition (Sicherman, 1977).

This Enlightenment preoccupation with the nervous system allowed for a subtler interplay between psychological and physiological factors in the aetiology of madness and the hypochondriacal disorders, although the emotions were still frequently associated with the visceral nerves (and indeed hypochondriasis still carried a rather literal meaning with some nineteenth-century authors) (Fischer-Homberger, 1970). Ackerknecht (1968) has suggested that Georg Ernst Stahl's (1660–1734) theories of animism increased the attractiveness of psychogenic theories of insanity during the latter part of the Enlightenment, but Stahl's direct psychiatric influence is not easy to document in Britain.

What is certain, however, is that King George III's illness – accepted at the time as a 'mania' – was of paramount significance in drawing widespread public and medical attention to psychiatric disorders; and the fact that the 'mad king' recovered from his incapacitating attack of 1788 encouraged an aura of optimism in the spate of psychiatric writings of the following decades (Macalpine & Hunter, 1969). It is a fine historical irony that among the products of this heightened medical concern with the plight of the insane were the rotary machines, douches, and restraining chairs which later psychiatrists were to look upon as symptomatic of all that was wrong with Enlightenment psychiatry (Hunter & Macalpine, 1963). In practice, however, these instruments and therapies are simply parts of a rich and subtle cultural texture which cannot be dismissed as a sterile detour from mainline psychiatric progress (Porter, 1980; Mora, 1979).

The nineteenth century

1. *1800–1850*

Common to British, American, and French society of the period was the 'discovery of the asylum' (Rothman, 1971). Although general custodial institutions had been built with some frequency during the previous hundred years and more, these new asylums were to be both specialized and therapeutic, housing only the insane and designed to create a physical and moral environment capable of curing, and not simply containing them. The psychiatric reformers of the early nineteenth century were convinced that the altered institutional arrangements and the new therapeutic forms – particularly moral therapy – could reclaim a large proportion of the insane for socially productive and happy lives (Scull, 1979; Grob, 1973; Grob, 1962).

Despite the novelty of much of this psychiatric theory and practice, there are also striking continuities. The career of Philippe Pinel is a case in point. Born in 1745, he was a middle-aged physician before the circumstances of the French Revolution brought him the chair of hygiene in the reformed medical school (1794), a year after he had been placed in charge of the *Bicêtre* (Ackerknecht, 1967). One of the general custodial institutions (the *Hôpital Général*) of the *ancien régime*, the *Bicêtre*, like its equivalent for females, the *Salpêtrière*, was altered during the Revolution to cater exclusively to the needs of the insane. Pinel brought to the *Bicêtre* (and to the *Salpêtrière*, where he became head in 1795) many of the characteristics which shaped his earlier medical career. Despite his lasting fame as a psychiatrist, internal

medicine was always his primary professional preoccupation and his *Nosographie* (1798, 6th ed., 1818), and *La Médecine clinique* (1804) were produced during the same years as his *Traité médico-philosophique sur l'aliénation mentale, ou la manie* (1801, 2nd ed., 1809). Pinel's psychiatric and medical writings reflected a number of his Enlightenment traits: intense admiration for Hippocrates and an emphasis on clinical observations numerically expressed, combined with a diffidence about overt speculation (Lewis, 1967). The stress which he laid on psychogenic factors in the causation of insanity rested on cogent Enlightenment foundations – because observations failed to detect any underlying structural abnormalities in the brains of dead lunatics: 'Derangement of the understanding is generally considered as an effect of an organic lesion of the brain, consequently as incurable; a supposition that is, in a great number of instances, contrary to anatomical fact' (Pinel, 1962, p. 3).

Philosophically, Pinel was an *idéologue*, influenced by John Locke and the British empirical tradition, especially as interpreted by Condillac. Pinel's preference for a 'moral regimen' also has Enlightenment reverberations, for the word 'moral' meant more to Pinel than simply 'psychological'. As Grange has pointed out, Pinel's *traitement moral* was most directly related to the affective, as opposed to the intellectual, portions of mental life. Seventeenth- and eighteenth-century philosophers such as Descartes, and doctors such as Alexander Crichton, had produced a rich literature, from which Pinel could draw, implicating the passions in human motivation and action, and in the causation of insanity (Grange, 1961; Grange, 1963). Finally, Pinel's striking off the chains was no revolutionary gesture; rather, it was a series of cautious, deliberate, and prudent acts completely consistent with his ideals as a man of reason (Doerner, 1981).

Nevertheless, the cumulative impact of his careful work at the *Bicêtre* and *Salpêtrière* was considerable, and the contemporary recognition of the *Traité*'s worth was substantiated by translations into English, Spanish, and German. In his book Pinel described the path by which he came to his ideas on the moral causation and moral treatment of insanity. They were rooted in his own experiences in the asylums, experiences which convinced him of the need for a different kind of asylum milieu, new techniques in constructing, maintaining, and 'policing' these institutions, and greater demands on staff and patients alike. Above all, moral methods required asylum staff to take seriously each patient's individuality.

Perhaps surprisingly in a general physician who had published a standard work on disease classification, Pinel was content to retain the relatively simple Greek division of insanity into melancholia, mania (with or without delirium), idiocy, and dementia. Despite this traditional nosology, Pinel's discussions of these disease types contained elements of the optimistic and broadened definitions of insanity widely adopted by early nineteenth-century doctors. Werlinder has called them the twin doctrines of *partial* and *affective* insanity (Werlinder, 1978). Both concepts are central to the *Traité. Manie sans délire*, later to be called *manie raisonnante* or *folie raisonnante*, was a partial insanity in that the understanding remained unaffected. These patients were, Pinel insisted, under the 'domination of instinctive and abstract fury', and his case histories remind us that he invoked the passions or emotions as the primary source of this condition. When the English physician James Cowles Prichard (1786–1848) consolidated in 1835 earlier formulations of affective disorders by the phrase 'moral insanity', he acknowledged Pinel's work, while insisting on the originality of his own somewhat sharper delineations (Prichard, 1835).

Pinel's psychiatry was optimistic in that while he considered organic brain disease incurable, functional disorders were demonstrably responsive to moral methods in cases of melancholy and in mania without delirium. While Pinel was not impressed with the elevation, by late eighteenth-century Anglo-American physicians such as Rush, Cullen, and Darwin, of traditional vices such as drunkenness and masturbation to disease status, his own work did much to broaden the concept of insanity to include affective as well as intellectual disorders. Thomas Sutton's description of delirium tremens heightened medical interest in both acute and chronic forms of alcohol abuse (Bynum, 1968; Levine, 1978). Masturbatory insanity also attracted a considerable literature during this period (Hare, 1962; Neuman, 1975; Gilbert, 1975).

Pinel was fluent in English and kept abreast of British medical literature. Consequently he was aware at first hand that, by 1801, moral therapy already enjoyed some vogue in the British Isles. His principal British authorities, however, were Francis Willis, Alexander Crichton, and John Ferriar; he placed the York Retreat in Scotland and professed to find philanthropy but no originality in an article on the Retreat which he incorrectly attributed to its first physician, Thomas Fowler. Pinel's comments on the British scene are understandable, for the Quaker institution, though opened in 1796, did not achieve wide prominence until 1813, when Samuel Tuke published his *Description of the Retreat*. That book, with its favourable reviews in national periodicals, placed the Tukes in the public view; the testimony which Samuel and his grandfather William Tuke presented to the 1815 Parliamentary Select Committee on the Better Regulation of Madhouses in England further sharpened the family's public visibility as leaders of an energetic group of reformers – largely laymen – concerned with the condition of the insane in Britain. The evidence collected by the Committee in 1815 and 1816 – when its brief was extended to include Soctland – laid the framework within which the insane and their problems were discussed for almost half a century. Though the York Retreat came to stand for much which the reformers sought, its beginnings were local, rather parochial, and almost accidental, for its origin resulted from the mysterious death of a Quaker patient in the York Asylum, a subscription hospital for the insane which, as subsequent events proved, had been grossly mismanaged by two successive physicians, Alexander Hunter and Charles Best. The twenty-year-old feud between the physicians at the Asylum and the Tukes, Godfrey Higgins, and others identified with the Retreat, formed part of the backdrop to the 1815 Committee investigations (Scull, 1979).

The printed volumes of testimony still make compelling reading. Three themes emerged: the reformers' belief in the superiority of moral over medical therapy in the treatment of the insane; the extent to which moral therapy was identified with the humanitarian values of the reformers who were mostly laymen rather than doctors; and the general acceptance that the insane were best treated in institutions of which the York Retreat and one or two private madhouses provided the best examplars (Bynum, 1974; Scull, 1981).

Moral therapy had been a major motif in Tuke's *Description*, and, like Pinel before him, he justified it on the twin grounds of humanity and efficacy. The Retreat was organized around the ideal of middle-class family life; sashes replaced iron bars and, when restraint was necessary, strait-jackets replaced chains. Whenever possible, patients and staff dined together, and by accepting the analogy between insanity and childhood, the Tukes sought to create an environment where the lunatic could be re-educated, through the dynamics of approbation for good behaviour, into the responsible, sober, and industrious habits of the mature Quaker. Self-control was the proclaimed goal of the Retreat's moral regimen. Samuel Tuke believed that the question whether insanity was a physical or mental condition was beside the point: medical therapy did not work, and the physicians to the Retreat were employed primarily to look after the patients' bodily ills. Most of the daily therapeutic responsibility rested with the resident steward and his wife, George and Katherine Jepson. It was recognized at the time, and has been reiterated since, that comparisons between the well-endowed, exclusively Quaker Retreat and badly crowded public institutions like Bethlem were not entirely apposite. Even the reformers shied away from recommending that pauper lunatics be treated precisely as their more genteel counterparts at the Retreat. Nevertheless, Tuke's *Description* provided both a language and an ideal for early nineteenth-century philanthropists (Tuke, 1964).

Their language was still that of disease, treatment, and cure. Insanity was a disease, not a sin, and the lunatic had the same claim to treatment as the patient with a fever or broken leg. But neither the Retreat nor the evidence collected by the Parliamentary Select Committee established a case for the medical control of insanity. Some of the worst scandals reported to the Committee involved establishments like the York Asylum and Bethlem which were run by physicians, and the testimony presented by the doctors themselves would not have increased anyone's confidence in the effectiveness of standard medical remedies such as blood-letting and purgatives. But the obvious alternative to a medical vocabulary was a theological one, and even religiously motivated laymen did not want a return to the Inquisition. By assuming that the brain is the instrument through which the immaterial mind or soul operates, medical and lay writers of the period discussed insanity in the putatively neutral language of structural or functional disorders of the brain. Moral therapy thereby could be advocated for its humanity and its demonstrably better results (Scull, 1975; Walk, 1954).

Furthermore, the York Retreat was an institution which, despite its special features, did not fundamentally challenge the ideal of treating the insane in hospitals. Samuel Tuke was not dismissive of doctors to the extent that his grandfather William continued to be, and most lay reformers had neither the

time nor the inclination to devote themselves wholly to the study and care of the insane. On the other hand, medical men had economic as well as humanitarian and scientific reasons for involving themselves in the plight of the mad. After 1815 in particular, there was a dramatic increase in the output of books, pamphlets, and articles on insanity, virtually all of it from the pens of doctors. In addition, medical men lobbied against lay inspection of institutions for the insane and pushed for greater medical powers in the bills introduced into the House of Commons in 1816, 1817, and 1819, in the wake of public concern over the revelations of the 1815–16 Parliamentary Committee. As early as 1808, the Wynn Act had permitted counties to divert public money into specialized asylums for the mad poor, but the response had been sporadic, and none of the legislation of the 1810s got past the House of Lords. A decade later, the Metropolitan Commissioners in Lunacy, established by the 1828 Act, replaced the old committee operating under the 1774 Act; five of the Metropolitan Commission's fifteen members were medical and were paid for their services. This 1828 Act increased the powers of inspection and the Annual Reports of the Commissioners provided more comprehensive statistics of insanity (Mellett, 1981). Medical involvement with the care of the insane continued to grow steadily over the years and the formation, in 1841, of the Association of Medical Officers of Asylums and Hospitals for the Insane provided a forum for the discussion of educational, practical, and professional matters relating to mid-century Victorian psychiatry. Small at first, the Association met each year at a different asylum; its peripatetic format was modelled on the British Association for the Advancement of Science and, more relevantly, on the Provincial Medical and Surgical Association (now the B.M.A.). After a precarious first decade, the Association began to grow, starting its own publication, the *Asylum Journal*, in 1853. The Association and its journal became the Royal Medico-Psychological Association and the *Journal of Mental Science* (Walk, 1959; Walk, 1961; Walk, 1978).

These manifestations of professional activity were evident by mid-century, and it was unsurprising that when the 1845 Act at last compelled each county to erect, at public expense, an asylum for the pauper insane, these institutions were to be provided with a Resident Medical Officer whose duties included the keeping of a medical case book for each patient. As late as 1844, no fewer than 9339 out of

20 893 institutionalized pauper lunatics in England were contained in workhouses, so that some, though not all, of the subsequent growth in late Victorian asylums resulted from the simple transfer of patients from general to specialized institutions. By the mid-1840s, much of British psychiatry could be identified with the public asylums, for the private 'trade in lunacy' was beginning to decline, both relatively and absolutely, and there was no appreciable or systematic development of specialized psychiatric practice outside the institutional setting (Scull, 1979; Parry-Jones, 1972). By the 1840s, physicians such as Marshall Hall and John Russell Reynolds were establishing reputations in 'nervous disorders', including hysteria and epilepsy, but there seems to have been relatively little formal interchange between this type of physician and those with asylum affiliations.

The outstanding British psychiatrist of the early Victorian period was undoubtedly John Conolly (1794–1866), noted for his introduction of complete non-restraint at the large public asylum at Hanwell, in Middlesex (Conolly, 1964; Conolly, 1968; Conolly, 1973). Conolly had been preceded in this by Robert Gardiner Hill (1811–78), who from 1835 had abolished mechanical restraint at the Lincoln Asylum (Walk, 1970). Though medically qualified himself, Gardiner Hill put a low premium on the relevance of medical knowledge in the treatment of the insane. Consequently, his writings met with little approbation from the medical profession at large and he spent a rather isolated and fruitless old age monotonously advancing his priority claims for the introduction of the non-restraint system. Conolly on the other hand achieved professional and public eminence, and his *Inquiry concerning the Indications of Insanity* (1830, see under 1964) and *Treatment of the Insane without Mechanical Restraints* (1856, see under 1973) document the extent to which the ideal of moral therapy was integrated into an institutional context most easily achieved by the asylum under the control of the physician:

> . . . in all cases of mental disorder, the regular life led by patients in asylums is to a great extent remedial; the diet and exercise contributing to physical improvement, and the absence of all ordinary causes of violent emotions keeping the brain in a tranquil condition, favourable to the recovery of healthy mental action. For these reasons, a residence in a well-ordered asylum deserves to be ranked, in relation to a majority of cases of insanity, among the most efficacious parts of direct treatment.

Properly constructed and professionally run, the asylum was to live up to its name as a place where disordered minds could be restored.

Conolly was not a particularly sophisticated theorist, though his case histories document his sensitivity to the interplay of psychological and social factors in the backgrounds of his patients. Like a number of other psychiatrists of the period (including his predecessor at Hanwell, Sir William Ellis, and W. A. F. Browne), Conolly was heavily indebted to the phrenological doctrines of Franz Joseph Gall (1758–1828) and J. C. Spurzheim (1776–1832). Gall and Spurzheim sought to develop an empirically-grounded psychology based on three related propositions: (1) that the brain is the organ of the mind; (2) that the brain is an aggregate of several parts, each subserving a distinct mental faculty; (3) that the size of the cerebral organ is, *caeteris paribus*, an index of power or energy of function. Gall believed that the specific organs of the mental faculties were located in the cerebral and cerebellar cortices, and that skull shape accurately reflected the underlying cortical contours, thereby justifying minute facial and skull measurements as a means of quantifying psychological propensities. Phrenology provided Conolly and other alienists with a framework in which to consider the healthy and disordered human personality; furthermore, the doctrine was easily consistent with the notion of partial insanity and helped provide a rationale for the effectiveness of moral therapy. Though phrenologists believed that basic psychological traits were innate, their concept of human nature was flexible enough to underpin the vigorous employment of education and occupational and other forms of milieu therapy among the insane. The nexus between phrenological theory and psychiatric practice was of course not an inflexible one, and the same therapeutic programmes could be backed by other conceptual schemes. Indeed, by the end of his career Conolly was distinctly less enthusiastic about phrenology than he had been when he wrote his first books. Nevertheless, the impact of phrenology during the 1820s and 30s was considerable, in France and America as well as Britain (Cooter, 1976; Shapin, 1975; Cantor, 1975; Young, 1970; Temkin, 1947).

The ties between British and American psychiatry were fairly close, and the absence of copyright laws made it easy to publish British authors such as Samuel Tuke and Prichard in America. The Hartford Retreat, founded in 1824, was one of several psychiatric institutions explicitly modelled on the York Retreat, and Jacksonian Americans discovered the asylum at about the same time and for many of the same reasons as the early Victorians in Britain. But American psychiatry was not simply a case of adapting imported ideas to a local setting, for Benjamin Rush had published his consequential *Medical Inquiries and Observations upon the Diseases of the Mind* in 1812. Rush (1745–1813) has been described as a backward-looking physician and forward-looking psychiatrist; certainly his medical writings, with their emphasis on a single cause of all disease and a favoured remedy of massive, repeated blood-lettings, were not long esteemed by nineteenth-century physicians. Through his practical activities on behalf of the insane at the Pennsylvania Hospital, as well as his formal psychiatric publications, though, Rush has acquired a lasting reputation. He campaigned for the separation of patients by sex and the better classification of them by diagnosis and severity of their disease; he advocated an increased number of attendants and more adequate heating of the hospital's psychiatric wards; and, like Pinel, he elaborated notions of both partial and affective insanity. His own variety of 'moral therapy' employed physical restraint and fear as therapeutic agents, and despite his insistence that psychological factors can cause insanity, his enthusiasm for blood-letting also extended to his psychiatric practice (Dain, 1964; Goodman, 1934; Noel & Carlson, 1973).

As in Britain, the early asylum era in America was attended by the emergence of a group of specialists in mental disorders. Among the most distinguished were Samuel B. Woodward (1787–1850) at the Worcester State Hospital; and Pliny Earle (1809–92) of the Bloomingdale Asylum in New York (Grob, 1962; Grob, 1966). These American physicians effected a relatively easy integration of medical and moral therapies, and recorded their basic therapeutic optimism in numerous papers and books as well as in their annual asylum reports during the years before mid-century (Waldinger, 1979). They were among the thirteen originators of the Association of Medical Superintendents of American Institutions for the Insane, established in 1844 (Deutsch, 1949; Schneck, 1975). One of the group, Amariah Brigham (1798–1849), had established the journal the *American Journal of Insanity* (now the *American Journal of Psychiatry*) in the same year, and it became quickly identified with the AMSAII (Carlson, 1956–7). Yet another 'founding father', Isaac Ray (1807–81) had already acquired a reputation as an expert in medico-legal matters (Quen, 1974; Fullinwider, 1975). Prichard's notion of moral insanity was crucial in this area, and

the insanity plea received wide public airing in both Britain and America during the 1840s. The 1843 trial of Daniel McNaughton for the murder of Sir Robert Peel's Private Secretary (the victim was actually mistaken for Peel himself) was effectively stopped on the grounds of McNaughton's insanity. Appeals went to the House of Lords, where the issues were clarified by what became known as the McNaughton Rules (West & Walk, 1977). Although these Rules have until recently been the primary formal guidelines in America and Britain for the determination of criminal insanity, they have been subjected to much psychiatric and legal criticism since they were laid down. An intellectual rather than a moral or affective definition of insanity dominated the formulation of the Rules, for the absence of a knowledge of right and wrong was the principal ground on which the insanity plea could be based. The insanity defence involved medical testimony, and physicians figure prominently in a number of famous nineteenth-century trials, though conflict between the medical and legal professions was not uncommon (Walker, 1968; Smith, 1979, 1981). In Britain, Forbes Benignus Winslow (1810–74) probably did more than anyone else to familiarize the public with the concept of criminal insanity, though Winslow himself was a rather self-important doctor whose work on behalf of the psychiatric profession carried a large element of self-advertisement. Winslow founded the *Journal of Psychological Medicine* in 1848. McNaughton himself was transferred from Bethlem to Broadmoor in 1864, shortly after the latter was opened as a specialized asylum for the criminally insane (Alldridge, 1974; Walton, 1979).

By 1850, then, the presence of professional societies and journals, and a body of legislation concerning the insane, testify to the establishment of a definite asylum psychiatry in both Britain and America. Still basically optimistic, these psychiatrists pinned much therapeutic hope on the specific architectural and domestic features of their asylums and much of the literature was given over to the construction of these institutions (Hurd, 1916–17; Jetter, 1971; Thompson & Goldin, 1975). Similar concerns can be discovered among psychiatrists in France, where in 1838 each Department was required to build a public asylum for the pauper insane (Baruk, 1967). There was fairly general agreement that asylums should not be too large – (200 was frequently mentioned as a good size); that adequate provision should be made for the segregation of noisy patients from quiet ones, and acute from chronic ones; that patients should be shielded from the home environments in which they had fallen ill; and that moral measures such as occupational therapy, re-education, and incentives for self-discipline should conspicuously feature in asylum life. It is perhaps unsurprising that Lord Shaftesbury (1810–85), the philanthropist who devoted so much of his life to the problems of the insane, could comment in 1850 that the reforms of half a century had achieved what common sense should have dictated in the first place.

At the same time, considerable clarification of psychiatric thought had been achieved by men like Jean-Etienne Dominique Esquirol (1772–1840), Pinel's pupil but a major figure in his own right. Esquirol has been called the 'first complete psychiatrist' (Mora, 1972). Like so many of his colleagues, he was particularly interested in the details of asylum design and he travelled extensively in France, Belgium, and Italy, observing psychiatric institutions and using his knowledge to campaign, from the second decade of the century, for the improvement of psychiatric facilities and the standardization of admission procedures. The 1838 Code incorporated many of Esquirol's recommendations. In addition, he began formal psychiatric lectures in 1817 at Charenton, the large Paris asylum which he headed for many years and whose rebuilding in the 1830s he oversaw. Esquirol continued to work within the intellectual framework laid down by Pinel, though his major work, *Des Maladies mentales* (1838) has fair claim to the outstanding synthesis of the period. While insisting on the ultimate organic nature of psychiatric disorders, Esquirol provided impressive individual and statistical documentation of their social and psychological roots. He coined the term 'monomania' to describe a kind of partial insanity which eventually came to be principally identified with affective disorders, especially those involving paranoia. He also left accurate descriptions of puerperal psychoses and epilepsy. He and his pupils dominated French psychiatry during the middle decades of the century, maintaining its close ties with the best of French hospital medicine and its emphasis on close clinical observation, routine autopsy, and an open but rather sceptical attitude towards traditional therapeutic measures. Esquirol's pupils included E. J. Georget (1795–1828), who wrote on legal psychiatry and cerebral localization; Jean-Pierre Falret (1794–1870), author of a classic description of circular insanity; Louis Florentin Calmeil (1798–1895), who described dementia paralytica as a separate disease; Jules Baillarger (1809–90),

first to note the pupillary changes in general paresis; and J. J. Moreau de Tours (1804–84), one of the early 'degenerationists'. The latter two founded the *Annales Médico-Psychologiques* in 1843. General paresis had already been described as a separate clinical entity in 1822, by Antoine Laurent Bayle (1799–1858). Although the causative organism of syphilis was not known, the particular psychological and neurological features of general paresis, combined with its distinctive organic changes as revealed by autopsy, gave great encouragement to physicians who believed that psychiatric diseases could be effectively described using the same techniques as those employed so successfully by French doctors including Laennec and Pierre Louis in diseases such as tuberculosis, typhus, and typhoid. The early volumes of the *Annales* reflect this clinico-pathological orientation very well, for the best French psychiatrists during those decades were rather better integrated into mainstream medicine than their British or American counterparts. Although this integration gave it an organic orientation, Esquirol and many of his pupils continued to refine many of the moral and psychological therapies associated with Pinel and earlier reformers (Baruk, 1967; Ackerknecht, 1967; Ackerknecht, 1968).

In the German-speaking countries, however, there developed a much sharper demarcation between the organic and psychological traditions, although the work of J. C. Reil (1759–1813) (see Lewis, 1959) is not easily made the exclusive province of either. Reil's psychiatric text books developed a holistic approach, and the journal which he co-founded in 1805 – *Magazin für die psychische Heilkunde* – acted as an early vehicle for German psychiatric activity. The psychological tradition, associated with the work of physicians such as J. C. A. Heinroth (1773–1843) and Karl Ideler (1795–1860), was closely identified with German Romanticism, with its speculative abstractions, and glorification of the individual and his emotions. Heinroth, a pious Catholic, viewed mental disorder within a religious context, as the ultimate result of sin. Both priests and psychiatrists such as Kerner and Eschenmeyer were actively concerned with possession and exorcism (Marx, 1965; Harms, 1959). Other 'psychicists' as they were called, were less doctrinal and viewed their practices within a more secular ethical context. Although their language abounded with neologisms and is not immediately intelligible to those reared in more empirical Anglo-American attitudes, romantic German medicine and psychiatry still have their modern sympathetic advocates, and Ellenberger's work documents its importance for the development of psycho-analysis (Ellenberger, 1970; Leibbrand & Wettley, 1961).

Other German psychiatrists regretted the obvious speculative tendencies of the psychicists and sought to cultivate a firmer organic orientation in the subject. Maximilian Jacobi (1775–1858) was probably the most important of these somatists. Not surprisingly, his work showed considerable French influence, particularly in his concern with physical diagnosis (Kraepelin, 1962). Ultimately, though, no group had a monopoly on speculation, and concern with unidentified toxic chemicals or electrical activity can be just as abstract as discussions of souls or polarities. Towards the middle of the century, men like the Viennese physician, Ernst von Feuchtersleben (1806–49), attempted to synthesize the psychic and somatic strands into a personality-based psychiatry. The title of his major work, *Lehrbuch der ärztlichen Seelenkunde,* is significant, for he attempted an ambitious synthesis of neurophysiology, psychology, psychopathology, and psychotherapeutics, always within a psychosomatic context. Feuchtersleben still held to a rather pure doctrine of the temperaments and made use of the notion of *coenaesthesis* (common feeling) so favoured by Pinel's friend P. J. G. Cabanis. 'Psychopathy' to Feuchtersleben meant a disease of the whole personality, and he first employed the concept of psychosis in roughly its current usage. Curiously, Kraepelin never mentioned him in his *One Hundred Years of Psychiatry,* and though the 1847 English translation of Feuchtersleben's *Medical Psychology* was prefaced by warm words of praise, Feuchtersleben seems to have had no lasting influence either at home or abroad, perhaps because he died prematurely in 1849 (Lesky, 1976). At any rate, another German work which first appeared in 1845, Wilhelm Griesinger's *Pathologie und Therapie der psychischen Krankheiten,* more nearly came to represent for European psychiatrists the definitive arrival of a mature German psychiatry on the international scene.

2. *1850–1900*

The contextual relationship between the medicine and psychiatry of particular times and places is nowhere more historically apparent than in the emergence in Germany, during the second half of the nineteenth century, of what Karl Jaspers called university psychiatry, for this kind of psychiatry developed as part of those twin German pillars of medical education, practice and research, the polyclinic and

the research institute. As Jaspers remarked, the major university psychiatrists, unlike their colleagues in the asylums, did not share their patients' lives day and night. Their concern was not solely always immediately pragmatic or therapeutic, for psychiatry in the university setting had as its more basic goal the scientific understanding of psychiatric disorders through detailed observation, dissection, measurement, and experimentation (Jaspers, 1963). Exemplars of this academic tradition such as Wilhelm Griesinger, Theodor Meynert, and Karl Wernicke sought to create a rigorous psychiatry wedded to neurology and neuropathology and rooted in the scientific materialism which from Feuerbach onwards, pervaded so much of post-Romantic German thought (Gregory, 1977).

Griesinger (1817–68) spent only five years in full-time psychiatric practice and teaching, two years at the beginning (with Zeller at Winnenthal), and three years at the end, of his career, when he occupied the newly-created chair in psychiatry and neurology at the University of Berlin. However, he continued to lecture on psychiatric disorders, and occasionally to admit mentally disturbed patients to his medical services at Tübingen and Zürich where he was successively professor of medicine from 1854 to 1864. His 1854 textbook is most easily recalled for its ringing slogans ('Psychological diseases are diseases of the brain' and 'Insanity itself, an anomalous condition of the faculties of knowledge and will, is only a symptom') and for its firm critique of romantic psychiatry. In fact, Griesinger's work demonstrates the extent to which a thorough organic commitment was still compatible with astute analyses of psychological processes and symptoms. He derived much of his psychology from J. F. Herbart (1776–1841), the German psychologist and educationalist, who had held that psychology was empirical, even mechanical, but could never be properly experimental (Littman, 1979; Boring, 1950). Griesinger's ideas of the ego and its functions were sophisticated and he was sensitive to the workings of the unconscious and the symbolic nature of dreams. Heavily indebted in his clinical orientation to the French school of Pinel and Esquirol, he criticized the latter's concept of monomania, along with Prichard's of moral insanity, since in Griesinger's opinion the unified ego could not contain single fixed ideas or partial insanity. He identified British psychiatry primarily with Conolly's non-restraint system which he eventually championed on the German scene. Above all, though still principally as clinician rather than experimentalist, he played key roles in the reform of German medicine and the establishment of psychiatry in an academic setting. At the time of his premature death, he was actively campaigning for the integration of psychiatry and neurology, and for the establishment of urban neuropsychiatric clinics, a campaign conducted partially in the pages of the *Archiv für Psychiatrie*, which he had established in 1868 (Marx, 1972; Mette, 1976). His successor in Berlin, Karl Westphal (1833–90), assumed the editorship of the *Archiv* and continued in Griesinger's tradition, publishing a number of monographs on diseases of the brain and spinal cord, and a classic study of agoraphobia (Wolf, 1976).

Theodor Meynert (1833–92) was the product of the famous medical school in Vienna and spent his entire career there, first as an assistant to the pathologist Rokitansky, and then from 1870 in the chair of psychiatry. Although he succeeded in formally combining neurology into his service only in 1887, his organic commitment was even more dogmatic than Griesinger's. Essentially a neuropathologist, he subtitled his textbook (1884) *A clinical treatise on the diseases of the forebrain* as a protest against the mentalistic connotations of the word 'psychiatry'. In practice, Meynert's attempt at a synthetic organic framework was less than satisfactory, and he introduced various rather vague entities – such as the primary and secondary ego – in order to describe the behavioural and thought disorders of his patients. His psychiatric nosology, based on the idea of local hyperaemia, did not even have the merit of originality. Nevertheless, he made many fundamental discoveries in neurophysiology. It was his laboratory more than his clinic which established his reputation and attracted a steady stream of students who included August Forel, Karl Wernicke, and Freud (Lesky, 1976; Levin, 1978; Marx, 1971; Marx, 1970).

Wernicke (1848–1905), who trained with both Heinrich Neumann (1814–84) and Meynert, probably represents the apogee of nineteenth-century German neuropsychiatry. His lifelong interest in aphasia (he gave the first full description of sensory aphasia) was part of a more general concern with cerebral localization. He helped establish the concept of cerebral dominance and carefully delineated the symptoms following vascular insult from several cerebral arteries, including the posterior inferior cerebellar artery. The original case of 'Wernicke's encephalopathy' followed sulphuric acid ingestion, though the condi-

tion is more commonly found in chronic alcoholics. His three-volume *Lehrbuch der Gehirnkrankheiten* (1881–3) – published, incidentally, while he was still in private practice – was encyclopaedic in scope, and his *Grundriss der Psychiatrie* (2nd ed., 1906) has been described by Jaspers as intellectually one of the most significant works ever published in psychiatry (Jaspers, 1963; Marx, 1970; Kleist, 1959; Eggert, 1977; Geschwind, 1974).

Characteristically, brain psychiatrists possessed considerable confidence in the ability of their science to provide material explanations of the pathophysiological mechanisms of psychiatric disorders; they were less sanguine about the curative capacities of their medicine. This attitude derived in part from the nature of their patient populations, for nineteenth-century psychiatric asylums and clinics contained a high percentage of patients with irreversible organic disease, including many tertiary syphilitics (Hunter & Macalpine, 1974). One manifestation of this therapeutic pessimism is reflected in the role assigned to heredity in the genesis of the spectrum of disorders coming under their ken. 'Nature–nurture' controversies are still with us, but nineteenth-century debates were beset with difficulties of a different magnitude, for 'heredity' was then an elastic concept which could 'explain' as much or as little as the individual author desired. At one level, though, the nature–nurture formulation is a modern gloss, for until late in the nineteenth century most doctors, biologists, and social thinkers accepted as unproblematic the belief that characteristics acquired by the parents could, under certain circumstances, be passed on to the offspring. Since this was assumed to apply equally to physical and moral, and desirable as well as undesirable, traits, the science of heredity seemed to many in an increasingly secular society to provide the key to a naturalistic ethic. Psychiatrists routinely came into contact with those on the margins of social acceptability, and psychiatric comment on these issues was common (Rosenberg, 1974).

The early advocates of asylum reform and moral therapy were not overtly hostile to the notion that certain aspects of behaviour and mental disorder were mediated by heredity, but they placed confidence in the efficacy of early treatment and environmental manipulation. In the 1830s, Esquirol listed 'heredity' as an important remote physical cause of insanity, particularly common among the rich, though seen in all classes. By mid-century, however, silting-up in the asylums had taken much of the edge off the earlier optimism, and closer attention to family backgrounds seemed to have documented the extent to which asylum inmates had relatives also suffering from some form of psychiatric or social taint. These observations were systematically cast into a degenerationist mould by two French psychiatrists, J. Moreau de Tours (Esquirol's pupil) and Benedict Augustin Morel (1809–73). Morel, successively physician to large asylums in Mareville and Saint-Yon, made degeneration into a powerful explanatory principle with wide medical, psychiatric, anthropological, and social applications (Friedlander, 1973). Caused by either physical or moral factors, or more usually a combination of the two, hereditary degeneration was cumulative from generation to generation, characteristically ending in the ultimate extinction of the afflicted family through sterile imbecility or idiocy. A 'typical' generational history would pass through excessive nervousness or neurasthenia through drug or alcohol dependence with associated prostitution and criminality to overt insanity and, finally, idiocy. The cycle could be broken in its early stages, but since the effects were progressively inherited, the outcome was not hopeful once a family had started on the road to dissolution. Alcoholism served as a particularly powerful paradigm for a degenerative disease, since it combined the physical and the moral, was prevalent among pauper lunatics and their families, and was deemed by a series of authorities from the Bible and Hippocrates down to Erasmus Darwin to lead to deterioration in subsequent generations. Valentin Magnan (1835–1916), in particular, placed Morel's theories into the explicit context of evolutionary biology with its message of improve or perish; Magnan's ideas in turn were given artistic expression in the novels of Emile Zola, particularly *L'Assommoir* where Magnan himself appears thinly disguised as the doctor at the Asylum of Sainte-Anne (Sérieux, 1921).

These French attitudes took root in German, Italian, and, with some qualifications, Anglo-American soil. Griesinger openly acknowledged his debt to Morel, and Meynert, Wernicke, Gudden, and other brain psychiatrists placed hereditarian categories among the prominent 'causes' of insanity. Heinrich Schuele (1840–1916), director of the asylum in Illenau, and Richard von Krafft-Ebing (1840–1902), Meynert's successor in Vienna, exemplify in psychiatry the fullest extent of degenerationist thought in the German-speaking lands. Though Krafft-Ebing was best known for his *Psychopathia sexualis* (1886),

both his textbook (1879; 1903, 7th ed.) and his monograph of forensic psychiatry were outstanding. He classified a whole group of disorders as *psychische Entartungen*, constitutional degenerations of those 'whose central nervous system has always been in a state of labile equilibrium'. Others, including Paul Möbius (1853–1907) and Max Nordau (1849–1923) popularized the wider connotations of degenerationist thought, particularly in the presumed connexions between the extremes of genius and insanity. Through his series of essays on Goethe, Rousseau, and, above all, Nietzsche, Möbius developed what he called 'pathography', an early version of psychohistory (Lange-Eichbaum, 1931).

In Italy, the psychiatrist and criminologist, Cesare Lombroso (1836–1909), was Morel's most ardent disciple. Lombroso saw criminals and most psychiatric patients as degenerates, evolutionary throwbacks identifiable by a variety of physical stigmata which he believed he had codified through comparative measurements. Many of these physical evidences of degenerative taints could also be found in non-European races, in apes, and, to a certain extent, in children. Haeckel's famous phrase 'Ontogeny recapitulates phylogeny' seemed to many during the closing decades of the century to be a grand synthetic truth which linked the medical, biological, and social sciences. Gould has recently traced the impact of the idea in a variety of thinkers, including Lombroso and Freud (Gould, 1977).

Anglo-American psychiatry did not escape hereditarian modes of analysis. George M. Beard (1839–83) popularized the concept of 'neurasthenia' as a condition of nervous weakness which many saw as an early stage of progressive hereditary degeneration (Macmillan, 1976). Neurasthenia and various so-called 'traumatic neuroses' were frequently described as products of advanced 'civilization', with its enhanced pressures and pace of life (Fischer-Homberger, 1975). There was widespread fear that the incidence of insanity was on the rise, a notion reinforced by the fact that asylums, however fast they were built, immediately filled up (Tyor & Zainaldin, 1979; Rosenkrantz & Vinovskis, 1978). The 1881 trial of Charles Guiteau, the assassin of President Garfield, gave the issues of heredity, criminality, and insanity (particularly moral insanity) wide public airing. Though the nature of his crime almost guaranteed Guiteau's execution, several young psychiatrists, including J. G. Kiernan and Edward Spitzka (fresh from three years' study in Leipzig and Vienna) based defence testimonies on their conviction that the assassin was an atavistic degenerate (Rosenberg, 1968). Richard Dugdale's subsequent investigation of *The Tukes: a Study in Crime, Pauperism, Disease, and Heredity* (1887), with H. H. Goddard's work on the Kallikak family (1912) documented the cost to society of 'degenerate' families, though Dugdale's neo-Lamarckianism led him to propose environmental reforms aimed at preventing vicious habits becoming ingrained and hereditary. By the turn of the century, of course, more active eugenic measures were being advocated (Haller, 1963; Fox, 1978).

The evolutionary philosophy of Herbert Spencer (1820–1903) was at least as influential in America as in Britain (Hofstadter, 1955; Bannister, 1979). His vision of the inevitability of cosmic progress was often called upon to justify *laissez-faire* in economics, politics, and medicine, though by the end of Spencer's life August Weismann's (1834–1914) doctrines of the continuity of the germ plasm were becoming scientific orthodoxy. Weismann's theories, together with the rediscovery of Mendel's work in 1900, permitted a modern science of genetics; and while putting paid to classic formulations of degeneration theory, and leading to a re-evaluation of the whole question of heredity in mental disorder, in the short run the decline of Lamarckianism seemed merely to increase the cogency of eugenic arguments (Allen, 1976; Searle, 1976). Earlier, John Hughlings Jackson (1834–1911) had used Spencer's evolutionary biology as the basis for describing neurological function and dysfunction in the hierarchical vocabulary of evolution and dissolution (Lassek, 1970). Remembered principally for his work on epilepsy (a disease commonly found in nineteenth-century asylums), Jackson was a neurologist of great originality who achieved an international reputation despite the obscurity of some of his writing. Like Meynert, Wernicke, and other German neuropsychiatrists, Jackson held that the reflex arc is the basic functional unit at all levels of the nervous system; he consequently drew on the earlier physiological discoveries of Marshall Hall (1790–1857), Johannes Müller (1801–58), and Thomas Laycock (1812–76), integrating whenever possible reflex physiology with the newer work on cerebral localization of G. T. Fritsch (1838–1927) and E. Hitzig (1838–1907) in Germany and David Ferrier (1843–1928) in England (Young, 1970; Hearnshaw, 1964). Jackson attempted to resolve the mind–body quandary through his doctrine of concomitance, whereby he sought to recognize the autonomy of mental events

(and hence of psychology) without violating his own firm commitment to a material substratum for all biological phenomena, including consciousness (Engelhardt, Jr, 1975). His comments on jokes and puns, on dreams, and on the stream of consciousness were shrewd. Various psychiatrists, including Freud, have made use of this fertile clinician's work (Stengel, 1963).

Henry Maudsley (1835–1918) also used the reflex concept in his own explorations of mental disorder in its relation to evolutionary biology, psychology, and criminal responsibility (Lewis, 1967). Like several other outstanding British psychiatrists of the period, e.g. J. C. Bucknill (1817–97), Daniel Hack Tuke (1827–95), James Crichton-Browne (1840–1939), Maudsley found the professional opportunities of asylum practice limited by routine administration. These men sought instead to carve out careers in private practice, lecturing, writing, and governmental service, although Crichton-Browne's years (1866–75) as medical superintendent at the West Riding Asylum at Wakefield were marked by the establishment of a research laboratory there and the publication, under his editorship, of the *West Riding Lunatic Asylum Medical Reports* (1871–6). The journal *Brain*, cofounded in 1878 by Crichton-Browne, Hughlings Jackson and David Ferrier, further linked the psychiatric and neurological sciences in late Victorian Britain. Maudsley's own ideals were best perpetuated through his endowment (1907) which permitted the establishment of the Maudsley Hospital and the Maudsley Hospital Medical School, later to be renamed the Institute of Psychiatry, in London, where graduate psychiatric training and research were pursued in conjunction with a large psychiatric hospital. F. W. Mott's (1853–1926) researches on neurosyphilis, neuropathology, and endocrinology quickly secured an international reputation for the Maudsley Hospital, whose laboratories Mott directed (Meyer, 1973). Both Maudsley and Mott were explicitly inspired by the institutional achievements of Emil Kraepelin.

Kraepelin (1856–1926) brought descriptive clinical psychiatry and psychiatric nosology to new heights, especially in the fifth (1890) and successive editions of his *Textbook*. Building on Karl Kahlbaum's (1828–99) conception of the disease entity, (to be distinguished from the patient's psychopathological state) he approached his patients as collections of symptoms (Kahlbaum, 1973). His case histories minimized idiosyncratic and particular features and concentrated on what he believed to be the core symptoms of each disorder. Kraepelin's classification is in its essential elements still in use. In particular, he pulled together earlier descriptions by Kahlbaum (catatonia), Morel (*démence précoce*), and Hecker (hebephrenia) into a single category which he called dementia praecox and which he demarcated from the manic-depressive psychoses (the old 'circular insanity'). His interest in the 'natural history' of mental disorders frequently involved him in the entire life-histories of his patients. This longitudinal perspective entailed prognosis, with its inherent danger of reformulating the original diagnosis in the light of subsequent events. Nevertheless, he recognized the deficiencies of his descriptive classification, insisting that the current knowledge of neuroanatomy, physiology, biochemistry, and pathology was inadequate to justify these disciplines as nosological or aetiological foundations for psychiatry. This he saw only as a practical difficulty, and as befitted a student of the great experimental psychologist Wilhelm Wundt (1832–1920), Kraepelin pioneered the use of psychological testing in psychiatric patients and he attempted quantitative correlations of body habitus with mental disorders (Hearst, 1979). He actively encouraged integrative psychiatric research, and his Munich clinic with its attached Research Institute – founded under his impetus – was an international attraction and the inspiration for similar establishments elsewhere, including the Institute of Psychiatry in London. Kraepelin's Institute contained clinical, neuropathological, serological, and genealogical divisions. Among his colleagues were Alois Alzheimer (1864–1915) and Franz Nissl (1860–1919) (Havens, 1973).

Kraepelin was critical of the degenerationists, though heredity still played its part in his general conceptual framework. He and Freud viewed each other with some suspicion; in fact, Kraepelin had only nominal interest in any kind of therapy, psycho-analytical or otherwise (Decker, 1977). He was less than sanguine about the therapeutic outcome of most major psychiatric disorders, especially dementia praecox, the literal meaning of which was pregnant for him. With his usual insight, Jaspers placed Kraepelin with the descriptive rather than analytical thinkers, but he also recognized that Kraepelin and Wernicke between them irrevocably changed the face of psychiatry (Jaspers, 1963). Like Sydenham and Laennec, Kraepelin demonstrated that descriptive clinical diagnosis can be an activity worthy of the first class mind.

Dynamic and early twentieth-century psychiatry

The historical origins of dynamic psychiatry are so well known as not to need detailing here. Ellenberger's work documents various intellectual, social and cultural continuities between Franz Anton Mesmer's (1734–1815) use of 'animal magnetism' as a therapeutic agent and the development of psychoanalysis just over a century later (Ellenberger, 1970). Animal magnetism was known by a variety of names before the psychological processes associated with it were called hypnotism by the Manchester surgeon James Braid (1795–1860). Interest in dynamic aspects of the human psyche was often associated with the more general nineteenth-century fascination with the supernatural and occult (clairvoyance, mediums, etc.), but physicians like A. A. Liebault (1823–1904) and H. M. Bernheim (1840–1919) in Nancy more carefully explored the therapeutic potentials of hypnotism. J. M. Charcot (1825–93) gave hypnotism the authority of his own international reputation in connexion with his studies of hysteria (Havens, 1973; Owen, 1971; Glaser, 1978). His clinic at the *Salpêtrière* attracted large professional audiences to whom Charcot demonstrated the diagnostic value of hypnotism and suggestion and expounded his notions of the ideational aetiology of hysteria and related neuroses. The months which Sigmund Freud (1856–1939) spent in Paris in 1885 were crucial to his own development.

Freud received early training in neuroanatomy, neurophysiology and neuropsychiatry in Vienna. He never lost his conviction that all mental processes are rooted in the nervous system, psychopathology in theory being describable in material terms. In practice, of course, he elaborated his therapeutic techniques and psycho-analytical theories without explicit reference to his remarkable metapsychological essay, 'Project for a scientific psychology', written in 1895 but not published in Freud's lifetime (Freud, 1954; Pribram & Gill, 1976). The essay was composed during what was effectively Freud's self-analysis, for which the otorhinolaryngologist Wilhelm Fliess (1858–1928) acted as friend and confidant (Jones, 1956–7; Schur, 1972). During this period Freud went beyond his early joint work with Josef Breuer (1842–1925) on the sexual aetiology, and the treatment by hypnosis and suggestion, of hysteria, to extend his theories of childhood sexuality and the childhood origin of neuroses, and his techniques of psycho-analysis such as free association and dream interpretation (Hirschmüller, 1978; Levin, 1978). Many of his major writings (e.g. *The Interpretation of Dreams, Psychopathology of Everyday Life, Three Essays on the Theory of Sexuality*) date from the first decade of the twentieth century, and by 1907 the first formal psycho-analytical society had been formed in Vienna. From the very beginning, the psycho-analytical movement contained seeds of dissent and many of the original members of the Viennese Psycho-analytical Society (e.g. Alfred Adler (1870–1937), Otto Rank (1884–1939), and Carl Jung (1875–1961)) eventually broke with Freud and developed their own ideas. Freud himself continued to elaborate his own theories of individual psychology (e.g. Oedipus complex, developmental phases of maturation, death instinct, ego, superego, and id) and to extend his insights into social, historical, cultural, and anthropological spheres (e.g. psychohistorical studies on creative geniuses such as Leonardo da Vinci and Dostoevsky, the origins of incest taboos, patriarchy, and monotheism). Although Freud cherished the image of himself as a natural scientist he did much to ensure that the impact of his ideas extended far beyond medicine and psychiatry (Rieff, 1979; Fisher & Greenberg, 1978). He sometimes generalized too readily on the basis of limited or personal data (e.g. the Oedipus complex), and his therapeutic successes were achieved with a relatively narrow range of neurotic disorders; but there can be no doubt that he was one of the creators of the modern world view.

Psycho-analysis was particularly influential in the United States, where a number of pioneer analysts emigrated – Adler, Helene Deutsch (1884–1982), Paul Schilder (1886–1940) – and where Freud's one trip to the New World (1909) left a lasting impression. James J. Putnam (1846–1918), Adolf Meyer (1866–1950), and Harry Stack Sullivan (1892–1942) were among those who adapted psycho-analysis to the American scene and helped establish dynamic psychiatry within an academic context (Gifford, 1978; Hale, 1971a, b; Burnham, 1967; Mullahy, 1970; Rieber & Salzinger, 1977; Townsend, 1978). Its uptake in Germany was limited by the strength of the indigenous university psychiatry and by resistance to what was seen as its Jewish origins (Decker, 1977). In Switzerland, Jung's influence was considerable, and although he broke with Freud from about 1912, Jung attempted to apply the perspective of psycho-analy-

sis to the understanding of psychotic disorders during his years on the staff of Burghölzli, the Zürich psychiatric hospital (McGuire, 1974). Jung's chief at Burghölzli, Eugen Bleuler (1857–1939), also used psycho-analytic theories in his classical descriptions of schizophrenia (which term he coined) (E. Bleuler, 1950; M. Bleuler, 1979). August Forel (1848–1931) was another Swiss psychiatrist of the period who made major contributions to the treatment of sexual disorders and alcoholism (Wettley, 1953; Walser, 1968). Early British psycho-analysis coalesced around Ernest Jones (1879–1958), Freud's biographer. Later, Melanie Klein (1882–1960) and Anna Freud (b.1895) enhanced the scene, the latter coming to England with her father in 1938 (Jones, 1959).

In France, Pierre Janet (1859–1947) elaborated his own theories of personality development and mental disorders which dominated French dynamic psychiatry for many years. Like Freud (but independent of him), Janet explored many facets of the unconscious and left sensitive clinical descriptions of psychiatric conditions (hysteria, anorexia, amnesia, obsessional neuroses) and of their treatment with hypnosis, suggestion, and other psycho-dynamic techniques (Ellenberger, 1970; Prévost, 1973).

There can be no doubt that psycho-analysis has immeasurably increased public awareness of modern psychiatry. However, the various systems of dynamic psychiatry have been created at a cost, for the ties between medicine and psychiatry have thereby been loosened. None the less, many facets of the rapid growth of psychiatric services and research during the present century have developed cheek by jowl with medical science and clinical medicine. Microbiology, biochemistry, genetics, physiology, pharmacology, epidemiology, endocrinology, neurology, radiology, and surgery are just some of the medical disciplines with direct relevance to the understanding and treatment of mental disorders (Clare, 1976; Hirsch & Shepherd, 1974; Wing, 1978; Ayd & Blackwell, 1970). The sophisticated application of knowledge derived from these disciplines to psychiatry dates largely from the present century. At the same time, the issues which practising psychiatrists daily confront guarantee that psychiatry must be, and must continue to be, a broadly based social enterprise with much to learn from its own past (Shepherd, 1977; Hill, 1969; Lewis, 1979).

2
The evolution of some basic clinical concepts

2.1
Psychosis
CHRISTIAN SCHARFETTER

The term psychosis was originally used by alienists in the first half of the nineteenth century. Feuchtersleben (1845), for example, refers to it as a common term for a variety of mental and personality disorders (p. 260). At that time the term was not restricted to particular patterns of symptomatology nor to aetiological theories. Some authors regarded all types of psychotic experience and behaviour as the expression of different stages of a single mental disorder (*Einheitspsychose*) seen as a disease process (Neumann, 1822; Griesinger, 1861). Griesinger postulated an underlying cerebral dysfunction (excitation or retardation) as the common somatic basis for the *Einheitspsychose*. The postulate of a somatic disturbance arising from brain disease as the prerequisite for applying the term psychosis to a behaviour disturbance led to much neuropathological theorizing (Meynert, 1884; Wernicke, 1881–83; Kleist, 1908). Kurt Schneider (1967), the best-known modern exponent of this view, argued that only when a somatic disease can be identified or, as with the so-called endogenous psychoses, at least reasonably postulated should it be permissible to utilize the category of Psychosis. According to Schneider, even the most severe psycho-reactive and psycho-dynamically understandable behaviour disorders fail to qualify as 'psychoses' or even diseases.

The exclusively somatic approach to psychosis was opposed by workers with an interest in the psyche, e.g. Heinroth (1818–25), who assumed madness to be a disorder of the soul, a notion corresponding to the modern concept of personality. Möbius (1886) distinguished between endogenous and exogenous and psychogenic disorders. Whereas Kraepelin (1887) and Bleuler (1911) presented the classical descriptions of endogenous psychoses, Bonhoeffer (1910) was responsible for the representative study of exogenous (symptomatic) psychoses. E. Bleuler (1911) took a pragmatic view of psychosis, focusing on the degree of malfunctioning in an individual who had not been formerly so severely impaired. He was well aware of the need for social criteria in categorizing patients as psychotic. For Jaspers (1910, 1913, 1959), the criterion for psychosis is the psychiatrist's incapacity to understand meaningful connections relating an individual's experience and behaviour to the context of his life. Freud (1924) advanced a metapsychological concept of psychosis as the reflection of a conflict between the ego and the outside world. Birnbaum (1923) proposed a structural analysis of psychoses, differentiating pathogenic from pathoplastic factors. Psychogenic or reactive psychoses are seen by some workers as conditions in which various forms of psychotic symptom patterns emerge in response to overt or intimate and covert (unconscious) life-events (see paranoia (p. 46) and Faergemann, 1963). The old idea of psychic contagion has been re-examined (Scharfetter, 1970) to support the role of psychosocial factors in the induction of psychosis.

At the present time, therefore, 'psychosis' is a loosely defined term distinguishing severe mental illness from neuroses, personality disorder and mental retardation. Psychotic patients, in general, suffer from a serious loss of ability to cope with the task of life through impairment of intellectual and cognitive functioning, or of consciousness (acute and chronic brain syndromes), or of severe mood changes (affective disorder of depressive or manic type), or of schizophrenic states with an impairment of sense of reality, delusions (paranoid states), hallucinations, or psychomotor, obsessional, or phobic symptoms. Combinations of these symptom-patterns can occur.

2.2
Neurosis
ESTHER FISCHER-HOMBERGER

The modern term 'neurosis' designates a group of psychiatric disturbances commonly regarded as psychogenic and usually manifesting themselves in the form of particular groups of psychical and physical symptoms. This notion of 'neurosis', like any of our conceptual tools, has several historical roots, for neither the idea of psychogenesis nor its various symptoms were always associated with it.

The word 'neurosis', derived from the Greek 'neuron' (=nerve) and the suffix '-osis' was coined by William Cullen (1710–90) in his *Synopsis Nosologiae* of 1769 and *First Lines of the Practice of Physick* (1777). For Cullen 'neuroses' constituted a class of diseases attributable to disordered motions or sensations of the nervous system which, in the century of emergent neurophysiology, embraced a very wide range of disturbances. *Sensu strictu* the 'neuroses' included comas, the adynamias (including hypochondriasis), the spasms (including hysteria) and the vesanias (madness). After Cullen the term 'neurosis' was seldom used and then usually to designate disturbances which were considered to be nervous in origin, but for which no physical substrate could be demonstrated. Thus it included considerably more than it does today: Philippe Pinel (1745–1826), translator of Cullen, subsumed all forms of madness – including dementia, idiocy and rage, comas, many forms of sensory and motor disturbances, and disturbances of vital functions, e.g. deafness, blindness, tetanus, paralysis, whooping-cough and ileus

– under the *'névroses'* (*Nosographie philosophique,* first published in 1798). Only towards the end of the nineteenth century did 'neurosis' gradually come to acquire the more restricted meaning which the twentieth century attributes to it. The organic causes of many former 'neuroses' having been ascertained, 'neurosis' has become associated more closely with 'hysteria', 'neurasthenia', 'nervousness', and especially 'traumatic neurosis'. Through Sigmund Freud's (1856–1939) psycho-analysis 'neurosis' then became the frequently used and misused diagnosis of to-day.

Thus the word 'neurosis' has become the receptacle of a traditional syndrome embracing a characteristic cluster of psychological and bodily phenomena, namely moodiness, fixed ideas, unpleasant and disturbing feelings and behaviour, manifold disturbances of digestion and circulation, flatulence, eructations, uneven pulse, palpitations, etc. For many centuries this syndrome had gone by its ancient name of 'melancholy' (derived from black bile); in the eighteenth century it had been called 'hypochondriasis' and was derived mainly from the upper abdominal organs (see p. 47). In the later eighteenth and in the nineteenth century, however, physicians preferred to derive it from disturbances of the nervous system (after the discovery of the spinal reflex often as a type of abnormal reflex action) and called it by a variety of names, of which Cullen's 'neurosis' was but one among others like 'spinal irritation' (probably coined by John Burns, 1775–1850, in 1809), 'cerebral irritation' (Wilhelm Griesinger, 1817–68), *'névrospasmie'* (Jean-Louis Brachet, 1789–1858). From 1880 onwards all these conditions, as well as the older hysteria and hypochondriasis, merged into George Miller Beard's (1839–83) 'neurasthenia' ('Neurasthenia, or nervous exhaustion' in the Boston Medical and Surgical Journal of 1869; *A Practical Treatise on Nervous Exhaustion* (*Neurasthenia*) of 1880, and *American Nervousness* of 1881, reprinted in 1972). Beard supposed his 'neurasthenia' to be caused by some neurochemical alterations of the nervous system which would be demonstrable in time. Others stressed the hereditary, constitutional, or degenerative basis of 'nervous' disturbances.

When, towards the turn of the century, the term 'neurosis' became associated with the psychosomatic syndrome of the melancholia–hypochondriasis tradition there was characteristically another change of opinion about its cause, which was then supposed to be psychological. The idea that the physician has to treat maladies which do not originate in the body but

in the psyche is as old as medicine itself, but only since the development of modern determinism and materialism has it been given a theoretical expression which separates psychological causes of disease from somatic causes. With the 'animism' of Georg Ernst Stahl (1660–1734) the dissolution of the old psychosomatic entity was complete and the idea of 'psychogenic' diseases was definitely introduced into medicine. Thus in the course of the eighteenth and, especially, of the nineteenth century the antithesis between somatogenesis and psychogenesis became increasingly stressed, and while within this frame of thought psychiatrists at first tended predominantly to accept the somatic roots of the 'neuroses', towards the turn of the nineteenth century they began to agree about the psychogenesis of 'neurosis'. This development had its point of departure in the *Salpêtrière* in Paris, where it was slowly associated with the work of the neuropathologist Jean Martin Charcot (1825–93) and the philosophically trained Pierre Janet (1859–1947), and in the 'Nancy School' with Hippolyte-Marie Bernheim, an internist (1840–1919). It assumed spectacular forms in the German-speaking countries which had perhaps been most fascinated by the somato-psychic dichotomy, and Sigmund Freud (1856–1939) gave it a revolutionary aura. The failure of neuropathology and neurophysiology to identify the causes of the neuroses may have helped to bring about this change. Furthermore, there was a growing tendency to dispute the monopolistic claims of the neurologists to attribute the highest functions and command of the whole organism to the nervous system, and, lastly, there were certain social and economic factors. These factors led to a fierce dispute about 'traumatic neurosis' which at the time had become an acute problem because of its involvement with insurance. This dispute centred on the question of whether traumatic neurosis had any physical basis and thus entitled the patient to indemnity or not; it was resolved by an agreement that though the neuroses might lack a physical basis they were not necessarily simulated, since they might be psychogenic diseases. The rise of hysteria to the status of a paradigmatic neurosis is of course closely related to this replacement of somatogenesis by psychogenesis. With its traditional roots in the unsatisfied woman and the womb (hystera=womb), in the female imagination and female sexuality, hysteria has long and intimate connections with the concept of psychogenesis. It was therefore consistent that Freud, when he took hysteria as the model of neurosis and psychologized the doctrine concerning neuroses in general, replaced the physical accident occasioning traumatic neurosis by the sexual trauma and sexuality at large.

The subsequent tendency of psycho-analysis to dominate the understanding of neuroses has led to neglect of the psychosomatic, physiological and psychosocial concepts of neurosis. Within the body of psycho-analytical theory psychosomatics were more or less reduced to conversion symptoms; only later, after the two world wars, did more complex psychosomatic concepts emerge from psycho-analysis. A neurophysiological concept of neurosis has survived in the socialist countries in form of the Pavlovian doctrine, according to which neuroses are caused by the collision of mutually exclusive conditioned reflexes (Ivan Petrowitsch Pawlow, 1849–1936). This notion re-entered Western psychiatry in the 1950s, linked up with a more behaviouristic approach going back to John Broadus Watson (1878–1958) and Burrhus Frederic Skinner (born 1904) (see Hans Jurgen Eysenck: *The Causes and Cures of Neurosis. An Introduction to Modern Behaviour Therapy based on Learning Theory and the Principles of Conditioning*. London; Routledge & Kegan Paul, 1965). The sociological interpretation of the phenomena of 'neurosis', first explicitly taken up in connection with the debate over traumatic neurosis at the end of the nineteenth century, has also been systematically developed only recently.

If the term 'neurosis' seems to have lost some of its original medical character in the last two decades, this may be partly due to behaviouristic influences on medicine, partly to the development of social psychiatry and anti-psychiatry, and more generally to the influence of diverse claims by non-medical professionals to competence in various aspects of theory and practice in psychiatry. There now seems to be a tendency on the part of physicians to prefer the adjective 'neurotic' to the noun 'neurosis' and to ascribe to themselves integrative rather than controlling functions in the handling of these disorders. (For further discussion see also vol. 4.)

2.3
Mania and depression
JEAN STAROBINSKI

The Greek word *mania* (from *mainesthai*) describes a state of madness, enthusiasm, or passion. This word, which denotes a form of behaviour, is applied alike to the fury of warlike heroes and to divine inspiration (as in the theory of the four types of *maniai* presented by Plato in *Phaedrus*); but it applies equally to the excitement caused by drunkenness. According to Plato (1) it shares a linguistic heritage with *mantis* (a prophet) and *manteia* (an act of prophecy). Figures used to illustrate *mania* include *Sibyls* and *Bacchantes*, the former inspired by Apollo, the latter possessed by Dionysus. The word has thus a wide acceptance in the cultural field of Greek thought. The *Maniai* have even been personified as the Goddesses of Insanity, who are akin to Lyssa, the Goddess of Rage, and to the Eumenides (2).

Hippocratic medicine makes frequent mention of states of agitation, but does not give them the status of a separate morbid entity. Aetiological involvement varies: cerebral attack, excess of yellow or black bile. The idea of a spontaneous cure by evacuation (dysentery) was generally accepted up to the nineteenth century, within a framework of more systematic concepts.

The 'classical' clinical picture of mania, an amalgam of several symptoms, was established in late antiquity (Aretaeus of Cappadocia, 3; Soranos, as translated by Caelius Aurelianus, 4). Ancient medicine was careful to distinguish between agitation accompanied by fever (phrenitis) and agitation not accompanied by fever (mania).

The clinical definition of mania remained practically unchanged up to the end of the nineteenth century; it covered all states of agitation and delirium, except those arising from somatic conditions caused by infection. The spectrum covered, which was very wide for Pinel (5), became narrower with the removal of the agitated forms of general paralysis, identified in the nineteenth century, and later with the creation of separate nosological categories for hebephrenia, and finally for the 'group of schizophrenias' (Bleuler) (6). As can be seen from the works of John Haslam (1764–1844) (7), Beddoes (1760–1808) (8), Guislain (1797–1860) (9), Griesinger (1817–69) (10), and J.-P. Falret (1794–1870) (11), medical opinion came to isolate a type of psychosis covering principally the affective or *thymic* state. Mania and melancholia, until then described respectively as '*délire universel*' and '*délire partiel*', came together to form the bipolar entity of manic-depressive psychosis, a subgroup of which was the regularly alternating and prognostically unfavourable 'circular insanity' described by Falret. Kahlbaum (12) later introduced the concept of 'cyclothymia'.

Historically the concept of melancholia differs from that of mania in that it relates not to a form of behaviour but to an aetiological hypothesis: black bile (*melaine chole*) is responsible for various mental disorders characterized by 'sadness and fear' (Hippocrates). Having its principal seat in the spleen, and endowed with qualities of dryness and coldness, melancholia ranks alongside blood, phlegm, and bile as one of the four humours whose balanced mixture constitutes the temperament (crasis) of the normal man. The pseudo-Aristotelian *Problemata* (13) includes a text (presumed to have been written by Theophrastus) which states that all superior men are melancholic; this was to exert a considerable influence on Western thought, particularly at the time of the Renaissance (Ficino, 14). Some early authors attribute to black bile the property of easily becoming incandescent and of rapidly cooling again; this idea of heat change explains alternating agitation and stupor, and may be regarded as an intuitive forerunner of manic-depressive bipolarity. Later, towards the end of the era of Ancient Medicine, the idea of the *melancholic man* emerged: this was a variant of the normal man but with a predisposition to pathological excesses. Galen (15) drew a distinction between three types of melancholia: one in which the entire

blood supply becomes melancholic, one in which the melancholic blood affects only the brain, and one in which black bile emits exhalations from the stomach and the hypochondrium. This accounts for the concepts of spleen, hypochondria, and 'vapours', all of which are satellites of melancholia in the history of medical thought. It explains, too, why treatment was for a long time limited to evacuant remedies, and to humidifying and warming preparations (since the dryness and coldness of black bile had to be treated by their opposites); as the doctrine of solidism came to be applied to the causes of mental illness, remedies came into use which were either *relaxing* (where the contraction of the fibres was incriminated) or *tonic* (where their lack of tension was thought to be to blame).

Considered as a possible cause of manic excitement (when it is 'inflamed') or of stupor (when it 'freezes'), and regarded also as the source of hallucinations, *black bile* continued, for as long as medicine was dominated by the humours, to preside over an aetiological empire that embraced all the manifestations of mental pathology. This medical concept made it possible for the adversaries of the legal and religious persecution of witches to exculpate those accused of such crimes by presenting them as the victims of delusions and hallucinations.

Robert Burton's *Anatomy of Melancholy* (1621) (16) affords a good illustration of this trend. But humoral aetiology, tied as it was to the very definition of melancholia, was to be questioned in all areas from the seventeenth century onwards and was to share in the decline of Galenic medicine (17). The nosographic classifications of the eighteenth century – Sauvages (18), Linnaeus (19), Cullen (20), E. Darwin (21), Pinel (22) – which were based in general on symptomatology, made of melancholia a form of 'délire partiel', considered by some clinicians to be a subgroup of mania. A terminological debate followed in which it was suggested that the word melancholia should be replaced by such terms as '*mono-manic sadness*' or lypemania (Esquirol, 23), which prevailed for a few decades in France. The word *depression* made its appearance during the nineteenth century and received recognition within the Kraepelinian system, with its category of manic-depressive illness. It was Kraepelin (24), too, who clearly delineated the concept of *mixed states* (*Misch-zustände*).

In Pinel's view (25) melancholia was due to an abnormal nervous excitation of epigastric origin. In

Germany the debate continued throughout the nineteenth century between those who favoured a psychological aetiology (Heinroth, 26) and the partisans of a somatic aetiology (an extreme example being found in Meynert's (27) vascular theory). Towards the end of the nineteenth century the familial incidence of depressive illnesses gave way to the concept of endogenous depression, which owes all its meaning to the contrast with exogenous depression (of toxic or infectious origin) and with the more complex concept of reactive depression. Without denying the role of somatic factors, Freud in his *Mourning and Melancholia* (1917) (28) introduced the causal concept of a form of narcissistic libidinous cathexis, detached from the object and turned round upon the subject's own self, which is subject to aggression and punishment by moral conscience. The existential school of *Daseinsanalyse* (Binswanger, 29), relies on phenomenology to describe the experience of time in manic and depressive states.

Electro-convulsive treatment (1938) was the sole new therapeutic method used until imipramine and its derivatives were introduced in the 1950s, together with monoamine oxidase inhibitors. Lithium carbonate made its appearance a little over ten years ago and continues to be actively studied. (For further discussion in detail see also vol. 3, Part II.)

2.4
Schizophrenia
CHRISTIAN SCHARFETTER

The term 'dementia praecox' was employed by Kraepelin in 1899 to subsume catatonia, hebephrenia and dementia paranoides under one category of the functional ('endogenous') psychoses. In 1903 he also included dementia simplex which had been previously described by Pick (1891) and Diem (1903). As a concept 'dementia praecox' had several precursors. Pinel (1801) used the word 'démence' for a group of psychoses, and Morel (1852, 1860) spoke of *'démence précoce'* when he reported psychotic illness commencing at the age of 14. Snell (1865) emphasized primary paranoid psychoses (monomania, *primäre Verrücktheit*) as one fundamental type of mental disorder, alongside melancholia and mania. Kahlbaum (1874) devoted a monograph to the subject of catatonia, and his pupil Hecker (1871) discussed the phenomena of hebephrenia. Fink (1881) described mixtures of a catatonic and hebephrenic symptomatology, stressing the relationship between these two types of psychoses, which had previously been regarded as representing separate disease entities.

Eugen Bleuler (1911) introduced the term 'schizophrenias' to replace Kraepelin's (1899: see 1909) 'dementia praecox'. The word 'schizophrenia', 'splitting of the mind', stresses the dissociation of psychic functions (associations), which to Bleuler was the feature common to a group of heterogeneous psychoses. Phenomenologically the outstanding *symptoms* are a disintegration of personality with disturbances of thinking, perception and sense of reality and an incongruous affect. These symptoms usually occur in clear consciousness and without signs of organic brain disorder (see vol. 3 chap. 1). Bleuler (1911) also attempted to construct a subdivision of primary and secondary symptoms. The primary symptoms (disorders of thinking and affect) were seen as an expression of the basic schizophrenic disturbance (*Grundstörung*). The secondary or accessory symptoms were conceived as psycho-dynamically understandable. Bleuler was one of the first clinical psychiatrists to pay serious attention to Freud's theories. Kurt Schneider (1950) weighted the symptoms intuitively according to their diagnostic importance, distinguishing between first and second rank symptoms (see vol. 3 chap. 1). Numerous other attempts have since been made to categorize and sub-classify the polymorphic features of schizophrenic illness (WHO, 1973, 1977), including Scharfetter's construct of five basic dimensions of ego-vitality, ego-activity, ego-consistency, ego-demarcation and ego-identity (1976). (For further discussion in detail see also vol. 3, Part I.)

2.5
Paranoia

CHRISTIAN SCHARFETTER

The word paranoia, derived from the Greek *para* (=beside) *noos* (=mind), indicates a mode of thinking and conceptualizing the world in an idiosyncratic, private, alien fashion. It became widely adopted as a general term for madness and in this sense was used during the eighteenth and nineteenth centuries to designate many forms of mental disorder characterized by queer, uncommon, or crazy styles of thought, perception, or behaviour. Heinroth (1818) regarded paranoia as a disorder of the intellect (*Verrücktheit*). Kahlbaum used the term to describe delusional psychoses. For Griesinger (1861) paranoia (*Verrücktheit*) was secondary to an underlying affective disturbance, while Snell (1865) postulated a monomania, i.e. a delusional psychosis with hallucinations without other gross mental disturbance, as a primary form of mental disorder.

Kraepelin (1896) used the term only for incurable chronic systematized delusional systems without severe personality disorder. Taking up the theoretical constructs advanced by Magnan and Jaspers of disease process versus personality development, Kraepelin later allocated (1913, see under 1896) paranoia to the latter category, thereby separating it from dementia paranoides; paraphrenia, on the other hand, was given an intermediate position between paranoia and paranoid schizophrenia. However, this distinction was challenged by several authorities, and Kolle (1931) was able to demonstrate that patients suffering from supposedly pure paranoia frequently

developed paranoid schizophrenia; further the incidence of schizophrenics among the blood relatives of
his paranoiacs was the same as that estimated for the
relatives of schizophrenic probands. This evidence
was taken to argue for the nosological status of paranoia as a special form of schizophrenia, developing
in individuals with a relatively well-preserved ego-
structure.

The patient's personality is central to the clinical concept of paranoia, whether the delusional psychosis be centred on love, jealousy, religion, invention, litigation, or persecution. The content of the
delusions is in most cases understandable and can be
traced back to an important event, overt or intimate,
in the life-history of the patient. This key-event
(*Schlüsselerlebnis*) was regarded by Kretschmer (1918)
as provoking sensitive delusions of reference in
unusually sensitive personalities. In this way paranoia has been interpreted as a special paranoid
development of personality (Kretschmer, 1918, see
1950; Gaupp, 1920). Freud (1911, see 1968) in his
analysis of Schreber, assumed that an internal conflict over homosexuality was central to the development of male paranoia.

The evolution of the notion of paranoia thus
brings together the history of ideas on delusion,
'endogenous' psychosis and psycho-dynamic theory
(Kehrer, 1928, Berner, 1965, Lewis, 1970). (For further
discussion see also vol. 3, chap. 5.)

2.6
Hypochondriasis
ESTHER FISCHER-HOMBERGER

The term 'hypochondriasis' is derived from the
Greek *hypo* (=under) and *chondros* (=cartilage),
hypochondrion signifying the region under and behind
the costal cartilages with liver, spleen, and stomach;
originally it also included the heart, which is separated from these organs by only the diaphragm. Thus
hypochondriasis was originally a disease deriving
from the central region of the body and of human
existence. Today, by contrast, it designates merely
the state of nosophobia, the fear of being ill without
foundation in reality. The two meanings, different as
they appear, are connected by the historical development of the concept.

'Hypochondriasis' is a descendant of the classical 'hypochondriac melancholy' of Galen (*c.* A.D.
130–*c.* 200). Galen distinguished three forms of melancholia, that is, of pathological states caused by an
excess of black bile in the human organism (Greek
melas = black; Greek *chole* = bile): first, a universal
form, with bile diffusing throughout the body; secondly, a form with biliary concentration in the head;
and, thirdly, the hypochondriacal form, with its seat
in the stomach. This 'hypochondriac melancholy'
manifested itself in the form of flatulence, 'winds',
abdominal pain, sour eructations and psychological
symptoms. It was logical that melancholic disturbances should manifest themselves as psychological,
as well as physical, phenomena, because the classical
concept of melancholia was in fact an all-embracing
psychosomatic concept. 'Black bile' was not merely a

material humour, with its seat and fountain in the liver, spleen, and stomach, but also a dark and gloomy humour originating in the centre of the body which was at the time also seen as a centre of psychic forces. The liver was a seat of psychic forces in the Babylonic and Platonic tradition (cf. Plato's *Timaeus*); the Greek *phrenes* meant both 'diaphragm' and 'mind', and the heart was the Egyptian, Aristotelian, and one of the Platonic seats of the soul.

In the course of the replacement of humoral pathology by pathological anatomy the attention of physicians was drawn to organs more than to humours. In addition, neither the black bile nor the corresponding duct leading from the spleen to the stomach could be demonstrated by means of dissection. The dark humour therefore declined in importance whereas the organs of the upper abdomen became more significant, and 'melancholy' became 'hypochondriasis'. Because of its intimate connection with the splenic organ it was also called 'the spleen'. The term 'vapours', (French *vapeurs*, German *Windsucht*,) was derived from one of its most prominent symptoms. Historically, the 'winds' of eighteenth century hypochondriasis can be viewed as the dematerialized, evaporated form of the original melancholic humour.

Hypochondriasis remained an essentially psychosomatic disease throughout the eighteenth century. Psychological factors were seen as causal for this affliction, partly in the form of pathogenic fixed ideas and imaginations, partly in form of the strain that civilization (e.g. traffic, tea, wealth, and coffee) then imposed on human beings. The upper abdomen seems still to have been the favoured recipient for such influences as well as an important source of psychophysical malaise, since the time of Thomas Willis (1621–75), along with the nervous system. Thus classical hypochondriasis consisted in a cluster of digestive, cardiovascular, and mental disturbances, flatulence, sickness, indigestion, palpitations, irregularities of the pulse, moodiness, fixed ideas, and classical 'ennui'. After Thomas Sydenham's (1624–89) letter to Dr. William Cole 'concerning. . . . hysterick diseases', (1681–2) hypochondriasis merged with hysteria. Thus headaches, cramps, imaginations (often with a sexual colouring), and a pronounced multiplicity and changeability of symptoms all went into the concept of eighteenth-century hypochondria, actually a hysterohypochondriasis (cf. Robert Whytt: *Observations on the Nature, Causes, and Cure of those Disorders which*

have been commonly called Nervous Hypochondriac, or Hysteric . . . Edinburgh, 1765.) In the eighteenth century this malady was very fashionable and widespread, indeed almost universal, as Johann Ulrich Bilguer (1720–96) put it (*Nachrichten an das Publikum in Absicht der Hypochondrie* . . . Kopenhagen, 1767). This was due partly to the multiplicity and variability of its symptoms, which rendered it a widely applicable diagnosis for doctors and patients, partly to its status. Since hypochondriasis was held to be the consequence of civilization, it was also considered a sign of civilization and was valued highly in the Enlightenment. Thus the English often proudly called it 'the English Malady' (George Cheyne: *The English Malady; or, a Treatise of Nervous Diseases of all kinds, as Spleen, Vapours, Lowness of Spirits, Hypochondriacal and Hysterical Distempers, etc.* London, 1733).

In the course of the later eighteenth century, however, hypochondriasis began to go out of fashion and to disintegrate into the term 'hypochondriasis' on the one hand and the hypochondriacal syndrome, as one might call it, on the other. The term became more and more associated with the symptom 'nosophobia' (*vide* the nosologists of the 18th century), whereas the syndrome, still recognized as a real and common disease, was now generally traced back to nervous disorders. For, as had been the case with black bile, exact methods had not furnished proof of any organic substrate for hypochondriasis in the upper abdomen. Physicians in the nineteenth century thus preferred to call the former hypochondriasis by a variety of new names, alluding to its nervous origin (see p. 41). In the 1880s George Miller Beard's (1839–83) notion of 'neurasthenia' assumed dominance. Neurasthenia strikingly resembled the old hypochondriasis, but it was seen to be caused by a weakness of the nerves due to organic though invisible causes; it was not an 'English' malady, but an 'American nervousness', for the Americans had by now laid claim to being the most civilized people of the world. The appearance of 'neurasthenia' was a turning point in the history of hypochondriasis. Before 1880 hypochondriasis still existed as a sort of disease in its own right, mostly defined as a more or less nervous complaint mediated by disturbances of the digestive functions. After that date it became 'nosophobia', a mere symptom of neurasthenia and a psychiatric *Zustandsbild* at large. Robert Wollenberg (1904) therefore distinguished between a pre-neurasthenic and a post-neurasthenic period in the history of hypochondriasis. It is interesting to note that hypochondriacal fears at first tended to concentrate on the gastro-intestinal tract. The background of this development is complex, being related to the ascendancy of the nervous system to a commanding position within the human organism during the eighteenth and nineteenth centuries, to an inflation of the over-used and misused diagnosis of 'hypochondriasis' during the eighteenth century, and to the general devaluation of the concept of 'imagination'. Up to the middle of the eighteenth century imagination was still regarded as exercising a profound influence on corporality – to the point of causing monsters and diseases. The concept then lost its power; 'imagination' was used in the pejorative sense of the word and hypochondriasis became a *'maladie imaginaire'*. The splenic organ, formerly the seat of black bile and pathogenic ideas, became the 'spleen', deprived of a real basis. In the nineteenth century only hysterical women were seen as still harbouring genuine pathogenic imaginations, and they were not too highly estimated for this capacity.

In the twentieth century hypochondriasis has generally been equated with nosophobia, a neurotic fear of being ill, not based on reality. It may be questioned, however, whether the dichotomy 'with' and 'without' a material basis will do as a frame of thought for hypochondriacal clinical pictures. Perhaps one would do better to reconstruct the original hypochondriacal experience, evaluate hypochondriasis in the light of the actual revision of psychosomatic thought and view it primarily as a mode of being, as Ladee has proposed (1966). This train of thought has been pursued throughout this century by those French authors who have associated hypochondriasis with the 'coenaesthopathia', those who have tried to establish connections between the psycho-physiological basis of bodily perceptions (and the concept of a 'body scheme') and those who from the 1950s have tried to work out the peculiar hypochondriacal *'Leibbezogenheit'* in its philosophical, psychological and semantic aspects. (For further discussion see also vol. 4.)

2.7
Sexology
J. HOENIG

Introduction

The single most important event in the history of the study of sexual life, in particular of the abnormal variants of it, is probably the appearance of Krafft-Ebing's *Psychopathia Sexualis* in 1886. In this comprehensive arraignment of the sexual disorders, presented in brilliant clinical descriptions of cases largely seen by himself during his medico-legal practice he offered a summary of contemporary knowledge of these disorders. Their classification and the approach to their study which he introduced was fundamentally the same as that used for psychiatric disorders in general. He thus drew the study of sexual disorders entirely into the discipline of psychiatry.

Krafft-Ebing (1840–1902) in his *Psychopathia Sexualis* mentions as his predecessors only J. J. Moreau de Tours (1844–1908) and B. Tarnowsky (1886) who was Professor at the Medical Academy in Petersburg in Russia. However, the historical reality is more complex. He drew on the work and ideas of many others and the earlier literature on sexual disorders both inside and – largely – outside medicine was much wider. Wettley and Leibbrand (1959) have traced to those earlier writings the historical roots of many current theories, and have been able to shed much light on the development of ideas held at present and in the past.

The history will take us through four fairly distinct phases. The first precedes the publication of

Krafft-Ebing's *Psychopathia Sexualis;* the second straddles the turn of the century and, although it brings a variety of approaches, is generally dominated by the idea of degeneracy; the third phase begins with Bloch's emancipation from the essentially biological approach and prepares the ground for the post-Freudian schools; the fourth phase brings a rich harvest of scientific advances contributed largely by workers outside psychiatry. It ushers in the present, with its empirical clinical and other research work.

Earlier work

The term 'Psychopathia Sexualis' was introduced in 1844 by H. Kaan (1844), a Ruthenian physician who dedicated his book, which was written in Latin, to the Czar's physician of the time. The book, however, deals mainly with masturbation, its allegedly pathological causes and deleterious consequences. The view of masturbation as a serious danger and pathogenic factor had dominated medical thought as well as general opinion since the publication by Tissot in 1766 of a book called *L'Onanisme, ou Dissertation Physique sur les Maladies Produites par la Masturbation.* The vast influence of this popular science book on almost two centuries of European thought has been reviewed by Hare (1962). The idea is originally an English one and had been put forward in three books: one ascribed to Dr Bekkers appeared in the early eighteenth century under the title of *Onania,* one by D. M. Robinson called *A New Method of Treating Consumption,* and one by Lewis called *A Practical Essay upon the Tabes Dorsalis,* the last two published in London in 1727 and 1748 respectively. It fell largely to another Englishman at the beginning of the twentieth century, Havelock Ellis, to dispel the devastating influence of these books.

As Wettley and Leibbrand (1959) have shown, much of what was absorbed into the *Psychopathia Sexualis* of Krafft-Ebing and into the subsequent writings of the other great pioneers of modern sexology was the work of earlier writers such as Johann Häussler in 1826, an assistant of J. B. Friedreich in Würzburg, of the French writers, F. J. Gall (1758–1828), who in his *Phrenology* had also dealt with the cerebral localization of the sexual instinct, and his eminent pupil, Auguste Comte (1798–1857), who in his monistic philosophy built on Gall's work, and by his emphasis on the importance of affects and passions had anticipated much of Freud's views (Wet-

tley, 1959a). Among other earlier workers, C. H. Ulrichs (1825–95), a lawyer who published under the name of Numa Numantius, should be mentioned. Himself a homosexual, he fought against the persecution of homosexuals. He devoted himself to the study of homosexuality which he called Uranismus. (The term 'homosexuality' was introduced later in 1869 by a physician writing under the pseudonym M. Kertbeny). Ulrichs writes about an address he gave to a congress of German lawyers, 'Right to my last day will I be proud of having to my undying fame found the courage on August 29th, 1867 to face that millennial, thousand-headed furious hydra, which verily for far too long a time had been spitting poison and slime at myself and my natural comrades, had driven many a man to suicide, and poisoned their life's happiness. Yes, I am proud to have found the strength to thrust a first lance into the belly of that hydra of public humiliation.' (Ulrichs, 1898).

Dégénérescence

But the greatest influence undoubtedly came from the French writers Morel (1809–73) and Magnan (1835–1912) and their theory of *'dégénérescence'* which dominated medical thinking of the time. Morel had given this idea, which had long preceded him, a new meaning. His ideas were religious in nature. He conceived the degenerative types as deviations from Adam, the first man created in the image of God. Humanity after the fall became exposed to factors in the environment outside paradise which caused man to change – to change also into illness, physical and mental. The adverse influences were those of civilization which were seen as evil; a view which in other guises is still with us, and – it appears – keeps on being dished up again and again to each new generation, every time as a brand-new revelation. Magnan, who was strongly influenced by Charles Darwin, modified this view by secularizing it. According to Magnan, healthy humanity is set on a course of progressive evolution, but individuals can be affected in such a way that their ascending evolution is arrested and they then embark on a degenerative course. The degeneration is passed on by heredity, becoming more severe with each generation, until it leads to sterility, and hence to the end of the line. Degeneration which was conceived as a constitutional abnormality was seen as the underlying cause of many illnesses, physical as well as mental.

Magnan's degeneration theory was taken up by Krafft-Ebing and applied by him to the sexual disorders. The concept of degeneration as held by Krafft-Ebing is much more nebulous than and quite different from the scientific concept of heredity, and the two were not always kept separate by him. The final crystallization of modern genetic concepts of heredity as opposed to the idea of degeneracy was provided very much later by Bumke in 1924 (Wettley, 1959b).

It was held that degeneration could be brought on by a variety of traumata (most of them the outcome of civilization) such as, to name but a few, alcohol, phthisis, epilepsy – and masturbation.

The classical period from Krafft-Ebing to Bloch

The publication of *Psychopathia Sexualis* ushered in a golden era of the study of the sexual disorders (Hoenig, 1977a). Now established as a primary medical interest, and assigned a particular methodology, namely that of psychiatry, the study of these disorders became an increasing concern of medicine. It attracted brilliant workers and so successful were their efforts that soon their findings were to have an impact not only on the whole of medicine but also on the entire culture of the time (Hoenig, 1977b). The aftermath of this impact seems still to be growing, alas, not always with the most salutary results.

At the turn of the century the workers in the field seemed to fall into two opposing groups, one tending to ascribe the aetiology of most sexual perversions to inborn, the other to environmental, factors. There was of course a third group which was seeking a compromise between the two. Amongst the most important representatives of the environmentalists are Tarnowsky, Binet, and von Schrenck-Notzing. Amongst those of the first group there is Moll, Ellis, Hirschfeld, and Eulenburg. Freud's position in this dichotomy is not quite as clear – he changed his views very often – but would seem closer to the group who stress the importance of inborn or constitutional factors (Hoenig 1976).

Such polarizations are of course over-simplifications. The decisive question is not whether perversions as such are inherited or not, but *what* precisely is inherited. Furthermore the term perversions subsumes several diverse conditions with possibly different aetiologies. Thus many would concede that Binet's (1857–1911) view of association as a cause for the origin of fetishism has great claims to validity, but would deny that such faulty learning is likely also to underlie homosexuality. Perhaps a better way of

evaluating the historical position of each worker is to assess his relationship to the theory of *dégénérescence*. In fact the history of sexology in the later part of the nineteenth century and the early part of the twentieth can be seen as the history of attempts at emancipation from the French idea of degeneracy.

Albert Moll (1862–1939) saw as the starting point for the origin of sexual perversions a change in the sexual drive because of cultural influences, which leads to a weakening of the natural stimuli and their replacement by artificial and insecure stimuli like clothes, etc. However, the additional and indispensable factor is always degeneration which makes the person vulnerable to these changes. At the same time Moll accepts the possibility that for instance homosexuality can sometimes arise without degeneracy, such as when men are cut off from women (as in prisons), or under certain cultural conditions like those in Hellenic Greece.

Similarly, Albert Eulenburg (1840–1917) considers perversions as illnesses due to a primary neuropathic or psychopathic constitution. There is usually hereditary loading and the afflicted show the signs of degeneracy, but unfavourable circumstances are usually necessary to bring about the actual manifestation of the perversions.

Henry Havelock Ellis (1858–1939) also emphasizes the preponderance of inborn factors, but narrows the concept of degeneracy by admitting it only if definite signs can be demonstrated. He separates constitutional abnormalities from degeneracy. He stresses that homosexuality, although due to an inborn predisposition, can nevertheless occur in otherwise healthy and normal people. Ellis moves considerably away from the ideas of degeneracy by his concept of 'erotic symbolism' whereby each perverse act is thought to be a symbol for the ordinary love object although not entirely explained by this.

Magnus Hirschfeld (1868–1935) revives the old theory of the bisexual *Anlage* to explain the perversion of homosexuality. The idea of bisexuality is as old as humanity itself. In modern science Darwin had already pointed to the bisexual anatomical disposition of vertebrates. The application of this idea to explain the origin of homosexuality has been made in America in 1888 by Frank Lydston (1857–1923) and J. G. Kiernan (1852–1923). Hirschfeld's view of the 'Intersexes' rests on the same embryonic bisexual morphological basis. He believes that everyone inherits both male and female potentialities and the particular mixture in which they are activated by hypothetical substances called by him *'andrein'* and *'gynäcin'* will determine the particular syndrome of hetero-, homo- and bisexuality. He finds that homosexuality is often accompanied by a general instability in the nervous system and sees here a manifestation of degeneracy. He conceives homosexuality to be a substitute for degeneracy. Magnus Hirschfeld used advances in endocrinology to underline his theory. He was greatly impressed, as were Freud and many others, by the experiments of Eugene Steinach (1861–1944) in Vienna, who had succeeded in transplanting testicles or ovaries into young animals whose own reproductive glands had been removed first. He showed that such animals developed cross-sexual, physical and behavioural characteristics. Steinach unfortunately drew conclusions from his results which were far ahead of the facts and are now clearly seen to have been erroneous. But at the time Hirschfeld accepted them and saw in them a strong support for his own views.

Sigmund Freud (1856–1939) has become the best-known worker of that period and his influence on our time is greater than that of any of the others. This is perhaps mainly due to the compactness of his comprehensive theory of the origin and nature of sexual disorders and his success in relating these to the normal development of the sexual instinct. His acolytes however have modified and – as he would feel – often distorted or mutilated his original views so that it often becomes difficult to assess accurately his historical position. As regards degeneracy, he, like Ellis, wants to see the concept much restricted and accepted only if definite signs are present. At the same time, like Ellis, he does not entirely dismiss it. (Hoenig, 1976). Freud takes as the starting point for his views on the origin of perversions the theory of 'partial sexual instincts'. These partial instincts, conceived as basically biological entities, undergo changes during early life before the genital instincts gain dominance over the others as the individual reaches maturity. If this development is impaired because one or another partial instinct is too strong and cannot be subordinated to the genital instinct or the latter is relatively too weak to attain hegemony over the others, 'fixation' of the libido occurs at an earlier level and a perversion can result. Freud with his theory of libido development goes beyond the confines of psychopathia sexualis and its disorders; he uses it to propose an explanation of the entire range of psychiatric disorders. If the fixated instinct meets with repression, but the repression succeeds only

partly, a neurosis (called by him 'a negative perversion') will result. Similar mechanisms explain the origin of certain psychoses and, in the area of psychosomatic medicine, even physical illnesses.

Thus the study of the sexual disorders had turned a full circle. Having started out with Krafft-Ebing applying psychiatric methodology to the study of sexual disorders, psycho-analysis claims that sexual disorders underly the entire range of psychiatric disorders and to some extent that of medical illnesses as well. A great deal of this has been dropped by Freud's successors and, indeed much to his regret, had never been accepted even by contemporary admirers of his work. Its validity is as contentious now as it has ever been. But it had another effect which is greatly influencing the position of patients afflicted with sexual disorders in society. By providing a developmental theory of the cause of sexual perversions he succeeded better than anyone else in narrowing or eliminating the gap between these disorders and the variations of normal sexuality. This, however, as we shall see later, has in turn created new theoretical and practical difficulties.

We can see that most of the workers from Krafft-Ebing to Freud, while making important contributions to the study of psychopathia sexualis never managed to break through the confines of the essentially biological approach laid down by Krafft-Ebing. This breakthrough was achieved for the first time by Iwan Bloch (1872–1922). Bloch wrote 'Up to now, clinical purely medical concepts have dominated the study of sexual abnormalities . . .' and he continues, 'So as to fully appreciate the entire significance of the love life for the individual and for society, as well as for the entire cultural development of humanity, its study has to be arraigned with the study of man as such, in which and towards which all disciplines combine; general biology, anthropology, ethnology, philosophy, psychology, medicine and literary and cultural history in its entirety'. This provided sexology with a new framework and methodology, and Bloch pleaded for the acceptance of a new name for the new discipline, namely that of *'Sexualwissenschaft'* or sexology, which was to replace *'Psychopathia Sexualis'*.

The post-Freudians and the existentialists

The new era ushered in new problems foremost among them a need to develop the application of the methods provided mainly by the humanitites and by cultural anthropology to this as yet uncharted field. In the United States, where psycho-analysis had been more firmly entrenched than anywhere else, we find what has come to be called the post-Freudian schools, whereas in Europe, the modern philosophy and psychology of Edmund Husserl (1859–1938) and his followers came to play an increasing role in psychiatric thinking. The post-Freudians had taken over from Freud his psychology, but not his biological sexual theories. Freud (1943) complained wistfully after the first world war '. . . not all parts of the teachings [of psycho-analysis] have met the same fate. The purely psychological findings of psychoanalysis . . . enjoy a growing acceptance . . . Those parts of the teachings, however, which border on biology, and which are presented here . . . continue to evoke undiminished objections . . .'. Freud having as it were sexualized the whole of psychiatry, we find that the post-Freudians do not pay a great deal of attention to the study of the sexual disorders as such. Outstanding exceptions are Karen Horney (1885–1952), Wilhelm Reich (1897–1957), Erich Fromm (1900–1980), and I. Bieber (1962) who consider all sexual abnormalities to be the result of various disturbances in personal relationships, mostly with the parents, or as the result of the socio-economic structure of society.

Not so the Europeans. Here we find contesting schools speculating on the nature of these disorders. There are mainly three 'schools' contesting the field. They consider themselves philosophically emancipated from psycho-analysis, but use many of its ideas, and do not clearly define the way they differ from psycho-analysis. There is the 'anthropological theory of the perversions' held by E. V. von Gebsattel (1932), by E. Strauss (1930), by H. Kunz (1942) and by O. Schwarz (1935) among others. The second group led by Medard Boss (1966) relates itself to the school of 'existential analysis' which sees itself as an application of the philosophy of Martin Heidegger (1889–1977), and lastly there is L. Binswanger (1949/50) whose 'phenomenological school' is derived from the psychology of Husserl, in particular its ontological aspects.

What they have in common is that they see in the Freudian theory a fragmentation of the sexual experience, which loses sight of the totality of the very human experience of love. There is a search for the *meaning* of the erotic experience, for its *essence*. Whereas anthropological psychiatry sees in the perversions a destruction of this love, Boss emphasizes that within the perversion there is still contained an attempt to love, a limited or truncated attempt to be

sure, but a positive element nevertheless. This seems to Boss an important factor in seeking a starting point in the therapeutic approach. The central concern of all these schools is the concept of normality. Where does sexual abnormality start and when is medical intervention ethically justified? The shift from a mainly biological approach makes a criterion like procreation, as it was still used by Freud, too narrow. No doubt the noise of battle between militant permissiveness and its equally militant backlash penetrate to even the most remote ivory tower of the theoreticians of sexology, and make the question of normality one of great importance and actuality. We find that this normality is often defined simply in terms of contemporary mores which in the light of theology are given the character of timelessness. The controversies have a certain fierceness and seem full of life but have somehow failed to bring new scientific knowledge. Sexology with its promising start seemed to have led to nothing but a noisy silence.

Empirical sexology

This vacuum was suddenly filled not by psychiatry but from outside its ranks. Scientific investigations were set in motion by members of other disciplines. Alfred C. Kinsey (1894–1956), a zoologist, created instruments to conduct the first large-scale epidemiological studies. N. Tinbergen (1951) and K. Lorenz (1953), both ethologists, brought to light the extraordinary forms of mating behaviour in various species. W. H. Masters and V. E. Johnson (1966), a gynaecologist and a psychologist, conducted experimental clinical studies on sexual behaviour; molecular biologists provided new knowledge of the chromosomes. Bronislaw Malinowski (1884–1942), Margaret Mead (1901–78) and Ruth F. Benedict (1887–1948), all anthropologists, studied sexual behaviour in primitive societies. Alex Comfort (1972) and H. Benjamin (1966), both geriaticians, contributed, one in the field of sex education, and the other by detailed follow-up studies, after surgical intervention, of the syndrome of transsexualism. The discovery of the masculinizing locus on the Y chromosome was made by Jirásek (1967). Money (Money *et al.*, 1955) and Ehrhard (Erhard *et al.*, 1968), both psychologists, conducted their startling studies on the development or maldevelopment of gender identity in hermaphrodites, and the effect of steroids during pregnancy on certain aspects of gender behaviour in the offspring. These are merely illustrative examples of much other important work, published around the middle of our century.

Psychiatry seemed to have needed this push from outside to return to its proper task of empirical research, and indeed much promising research of that kind is in progress, using a variety of approaches and methods, be they biological, medical, sociological, psychological or other, working freely together thanks to the framework given us by Iwan Bloch.

2.8
Epilepsy
OWSEI TEMKIN

Originally, the Greek word *epilèpsiē* meant a seizure; later, it also replaced the popular name 'sacred disease' for epilepsy as a nosological entity. Defying all magic implications, Hippocratic physicians presented epilepsy (idiopathic with grand mal seizures) as a natural disease with hereditary predisposition, and with its seat in the brain. (For details here and throughout the article, see Temkin, 1971.) With improving anatomical knowledge, Galen distinguished two main forms. In 'idiopathic' epilepsy the brain was primarily diseased, a viscous humour blocking the ventricles; in 'sympathetic' epilepsy the brain was secondarily affected from the stomach, or from some other part from which a qualitative change or some substance ascended that poisoned or irritated the brain.

Though epilepsy, under the vague name of the falling sickness, was sometimes confused with other disorders, its clinical forms and pathological physiology became better known from the Renaissance on. After post-mortem examinations had failed to reveal a blocking humour, the idea of an irritation of the brain was favoured for idiopathic epilepsy, especially after more mechanistic explanations, such as an explosion of chemical particles, had gone out of fashion in the eighteenth century. However, before Fritsch and Hitzig, in 1870, proved the excitability of the cerebral cortex, it seemed unavoidable to attribute convulsions and loss of consciousness to different parts of the brain.

On the clinical side, such terms as grand mal, petit mal, absence, epileptic vertigo, partial epilepsy, and status epilepticus were well established by the middle of the nineteenth century. Tumours and other lesions of the brain, as well as diseases like syphilis, were known to cause 'sympathetic' or 'symptomatic' epilepsy. But since in idiopathic epilepsy, the 'true' epilepsy, anatomical lesions usually were absent, this was concluded to be a functional disease on the basis of molecular changes, a disease with a genetic factor but otherwise unknown cause.

Taking his departure from epileptiform seizures, where gross lesions on the surface of the brain were associated with partial convulsions, Hughlings Jackson (1835–1911) elaborated a general theory of epilepsy: damaged nerve tissue becomes unstable, liable to discharge explosively. The convulsion spreads with the spread of the discharge. The location of the lesion, the strength of the discharge, the path and extent of its spread, and the parts of the brain involved determine the clinical features of the fits. The definition made the distinction of genuine epilepsy and of other forms a matter of mere practical convenience. Scientifically speaking, epilepsy was 'the name for occasional, sudden, excessive, rapid, and local discharges of gray matter' (Jackson, 1973).

Modern concepts have largely followed Jackson but have replaced grey matter by neurons, and discharge has come to mean electrical depolarization. Though epilepsy has not regained the status of a 'disease', human electroencephalography (Berger, 1929) has made the term a common denominator for current attacks of cerebral dysrhythmias. (For further discussion see also vol. 2, chap 13.)

2.9
'Psychosomatic'
W. F. BYNUM

The term *psychosomatic* – from the Greek *psychè* (soul) and *soma* (body) – was coined first in German by J. C. A. Heinroth (1773–1843) (Heinroth, 1818) and popularized by K. W. M. Jacobi (1775–1858) (Jacobi, 1822); 'psychosomatic' was gradually adopted into English, largely through the French *psychosomatiatrie* (Mayne, 1860; Kaplan, 1980). It originally meant simply 'belonging both to mind and body', but from the 1930s the word became commonly employed to refer to a cluster of disorders such as asthma, peptic ulcer, and migraine in which the emotions play a recognizable role and the involved organ is usually under autonomic nervous system innervation (Kollar & Alcalay, 1967). In practice, it can be argued that all diseases are psychosomatic in the original meaning of the word and that any good clinician is a 'psychosomaticist' (Ackerknecht, 1968). Our need for the word derives largely from the power acquired by somatic pathology since the seventeenth-century mechanization of the world picture (Dijksterhuis, 1961). The word 'psychosomatic' attempts to circumvent certain polarities – mind–body, spirit–matter, subjective–objective – which are firmly enshrined in modern scientific thought. Two particular issues punctuate the pre-history of this hybrid word: the mind–body relationship and the nature of psychic causation (Lewis, 1967; Brain, 1964; Walker, 1956).

The word's Greek roots recall that the Greeks, like many other ancient cultures, developed separate notions for soul (or mind) and body. Although the Hippocratics (fifth–fourth century B.C.) described various conditions in which disturbances of mental state predominate, their principal explanatory system (of humoral imbalance) did not require them to distinguish between psychic and somatic components of an illness. Their holistic 'medical materialism' was codified by Galen (A.D. 129–c. 200), who nevertheless prided himself on his capacity to diagnose emotional disturbance, as in a case of love sickness. This tradition dominated medical thinking for centuries, but Greek poets and philosophers developed alternative ways of conceiving the mind–body relationship. Plato (427–347 B.C.) spoke of a tripartite soul ('appetitive', 'spirited' and 'rational'), hierarchically arranged, separate from the body but influencing and influenced by it. Aristotle's (384–322 B.C.) hylomorphism viewed body and soul (like matter and form) as inseparable parts of a unified whole. Early Christian thinkers grafted these strands on to Biblical formulations of soul and body, sin and suffering (Entralgo, 1955). Although healing could be seen as essentially a spiritual matter, God's status as Creator of both soul and body made a two-way road between them.

These issues were thrown into stark relief by the *locus classicus* of modern physical science, René Descartes' (1596–1650) attempt to construct a comprehensive, objective science of matter and motion (Burtt, 1932). Descartes, a devout Christian, sharply demarcated the immaterial, immortal soul (or mind) from substantial, extended matter, the latter being the proper subject of science. His considerable influence extended to eighteenth-century mechanists and materialists like D'Holbach (1723–89) and La Mettrie (1709–51) who retained Descartes' matter-based physiology but discarded his notion of an immaterial thinking principle. Solidist pathology refined the site of disease and disease processes from the organ (G. B. Morgagni, 1682–1771) to the tissues (F. M. X. Bichat, 1771–1802) to the cell (R. Virchow, 1821–1902). The powerful persuasiveness of pathology encouraged eighteenth- and nineteenth-century alienists to posit physical models to explain mental disturbances.

At the same time, ordinary human and sick-room experience underscored the mutual influence of mind and body, and even Descartes, especially in his discussion of the passions (a word earlier used in roughly the same sense as we now use 'emotions') sought to relate strong feelings like jealousy or love to physiological changes. Doctors were perennially exposed to this phenomenologically two-way traffic: 'the reason why a sound body becomes ill or an ailing body recovers may lie in the mind. Contrariwise the body frequently both begets mental illness and heals its offspring' (Jerome Gaub, 1705–80). 'How can [the medical man] restore calm to the disturbed spirit, to the mind consumed by persistent melancholy if he ignores those organic lesions which such moral disorders can cause and the functional disorders with which they are connected? (P. J. G. Cabanis, 1757–1808; Rather, 1965). These sentiments were often repeated during the nineteenth century, although not until J. M. Charcot (1825–93) was the notion popularized that ideas can cause hysteria and other neurotic disorders (Havens, 1973). Contemporaneously, independent psychological studies by William James (1842–1910) and Carl Lange (1834–1900) established a theory of the relationship between the external precipitating event, physiological reaction, and subjective feeling state that eventually became the starting point for twentieth-century conceptions of psychosomatic disorders (James, 1884; Lange, 1887; Titchener, 1914). W. B. Cannon's (1871–1945) researches implicated the thalamus and autonomic nervous system (Cannon, 1915). 'Stress' and the 'emotions' have been the most commonly studied factors in psychosomatic investigations, which have used multiple methods, including psycho-analytical, individual life histories, physiological, psychological, anthropological, and epidemiological (Wolff, 1953; Cobb, Miles, & Shands, 1952; Seyle, 1950). More recently, the development of 'biopsychosocial' models of disease has further extended the elasticity of the term psychosomatic (Lipowski, Lipsitt & Whybrow, 1977). (For further discussion see also vols. 2 and 4.)

PART II

The clinical phenomena of mental disorders

3
Descriptive and developmental phenomena

F. KRÄUPL TAYLOR

Morbidity

The phenomena which distinguish psychiatric patients from psychologically healthy persons must have special characteristics so that one can say of most people and with sufficient confidence whether they have a psychiatric illness or not. This statement seems obvious for, if it were not true, the identification of psychiatric patients would not be possible. Indeed, in many respects, it holds good for all patients, whether psychiatric or not. Yet when the question is put: What are these special characteristics?, different answers are given and no consensus of opinion emerges.

There was a time when the mark of psychological health in a mature person was rationality. Echoes of this view still linger in legal corridors. It is expected of a responsible person that his behaviour is regulated by reflection and thought without giving rein to the quirks of emotion and temper. Yet by this high-minded yardstick, we all fall short of psychological health in our carefree, and perhaps careless, moments. Psycho-analysts have driven this lesson home. We all harbour in our unconscious minds, they maintain, active infantile complexes which can play havoc with our best intentions and have embarrassing consequences. Our sanity is thus no more than an assumed mask which barely and poorly conceals the psycho-pathological imbroglio beneath it. We are all tinged with mental ill-health and in need of psycho-analytic help.

However, such generalizations are self-defeating. They make nonsense of any distinction between health and disease. In practice, a line, however blurred and arbitrary, has to be drawn between the class of patients and its complementary class of healthy persons. In that case, there must be special characteristics which distinguish the class of patients from its complementary class. We are faced again by the question: What are these special characteristics?

It is generally accepted that one of the features of these special characteristics is their abnormality. There has been some controversy about the kind of abnormality involved and about its assessment in practice. We need not concern ourselves here with these controversies, for abnormality cannot be the decisive feature of the special characteristics. Even if we accept the proposition that they are always abnormal in some way, we still could not assign a person to the class of patients and diagnose him as ill, merely because he has abnormal characteristics. Abnormalities need not be liabilities; they can be assets. There are, for instance, many healthy people with abnormal psychological characteristics that are of social value to them, e.g. abnormally high intelligence or athletic prowess, eidetic imagery in an adult, absolute pitch for musical notes, mnemonist ability (see Luria, 1969), and the like.

It is thus not enough for the special characteristics of the class of patients to be abnormal in some ways, they must also have other and diagnostically more decisive features. Such features would be *morbid* in the sense that they are pathognomonic of the class of patients in general.

Doctors have rarely paused to consider the nature of such morbid features. One suggestion has come from Scadding (1967), which was that they consisted of a 'characteristic or set of characteristics by which [diseased living organisms] differ from the norm for a species in such a way as to place them at a biological disadvantage'. He was aware of the vagueness of the concept of biological disadvantage and did not try to clarify it, indicating that his proposition 'is as precise a statement as can be made about the criteria on which it is generally decided whether deviation from a norm is to be regarded as associated with disease or not'.

Kendell (1975) attempted to make the meaning of biological disadvantage less vague by stipulating that the disadvantage must be innate and not due to reactions by the social environment and that 'it must embrace both increased mortality and reduced fertil-

ity'. These stipulations, and especially the second, led to undesirable consequences. They cast doubt on the usually accepted view that people with neuroses or personality disorders are patients. On the other hand, homosexuals and people leading a life of chastity would be patients, for their sex life would be abnormal in the sense of unusual by population standards and their fertility would be reduced.

It is not only the vagueness of the concept of biological disadvantage which hampers its usefulness as a criterion of morbidity; even its general validity can be queried. There certainly are some abnormalities, usually regarded as morbid, whose biological disadvantages are outweighed by their biological merits. The most obvious examples are the health-promoting immunities that follow mild infections and deliberate vaccinations. Not too disabling wounds sustained in war combat and the symptoms of war neuroses may perhaps also be considered here for their potential life-prolonging qualities.

I have proposed another criterion of morbidity (Taylor, 1971, 1976), which is not as general as biological disadvantage since it applies only to human patients. It could, however, be easily amplified to apply also to animals tended by human beings. The original formulation has since been amended by adding a condition which underlines the special role played by doctors in the diagnosis of morbidity. The suggestion now is that abnormal phenomena in persons should be regarded as morbid, if one or several of three conditions hold:

(1) the phenomena arouse therapeutic concern in the persons affected by them;
(2) the phenomena arouse therapeutic concern in the social environment of such persons; and
(3) the phenomena arouse medical concern which is not just therapeutic, but also diagnostic and possibly prophylactic.

This criterion has the merit of corresponding to actual practice. Morbidity happens to be diagnosed in this way. It may seem to have the disadvantage of relying too heavily on subjective reactions and decisions. But this impression is only partly justified, since medical concern depends to a large extent on an objective evaluation of the diagnostic significance of observed abnormal phenomena.

Morbid perceptions
Perceptions are conscious experiences of phenomena which appear to be located in our environ-

ment (*exteroceptions*), in our bodies (*interoceptions*), or on a poorly located mental stage (*introspections*).

In the waking individual, the phenomena of *exteroception* convey some of the attributes of the physical events which give rise to them. We can see, in favourable circumstances, the location of visible physical events in our environment as well as their movements, sizes, shapes, and colours; we can hear the direction, volume, and musicality of audible physical events; we can have a tactile and thermal awareness of the size, form, pressure, and temperature of physical events which impinge on our skin; and we can taste and smell physical events which stimulate our taste buds and olfactory cells.

The phenomena of *interoception* are divided into proprioceptive and nociceptive ones. In the waking individual, the phenomena of *proprioception* (especially those due to kinaesthetic and labyrinthine sensations) convey information about their origin in the physical events which give rise to them. They are events affecting our body as a whole or in part. We can thus sense the position and movement of our body in a gravitational field; we can become aware of the relative positions of our head, trunk, and limbs; we can monitor the accuracy of aimed movements; we can feel the raised tension in our voluntary muscles during isometric contractions and in some involuntary muscles, especially those of the rectum and bladder (and not only in the waking state). The phenomena of *nociception*, unlike those of proprioception, are often poor and unreliable indicators of the physical events in our body which give rise to them. It is the purpose of clinical investigations to make up for these nociceptive deficiencies.

The phenomena of *introspection* differ in origin from those of exteroception and interoception in that they are not mediated by sensory organs and pathways. Moreover, they convey absolutely no information about the physical events in our brain associated with them. They present themselves as degrees of wakefulness and as a variety of mental act-phenomena (process-phenomena) and mental object-phenomena (content-phenomena). This distinction between act-phenomena and object-phenomena is based on the psychological theories of Franz Brentano (1874; See also Rancurello, 1968). Act-phenomena are such experiences as perceiving, thinking, understanding, feeling, desiring, willing, remembering, recognizing, and the like; object-phenomena are such experiences as an object, event, or image perceived, a concept thought, a meaning under-

stood, a mood felt, a satisfaction desired, an act willed, a name or event remembered, an object recognized, and the like. Act-phenomena are thus like transitive verbs; they need an object for their completion.

Introspective phenomena have close links with those of exteroception and interoception. Most of these links are acquired through learning. Yet, contrary to the past beliefs and teachings of psychologists and philosophers, some links are innate. Bower (1966, 1971), for instance, found to his surprise that babies of only 4 to 6 weeks of age responded to a seen object in ways which indicated that they understood the meaning of some of its attributes, such as its real size, real shape, and real distance in spite of the changes in the appearance of the seen object, when viewed from different angles and different distances.

Morbid abnormalities can occur in all the different kinds of perceptual experience.

Morbid abnormalities of exteroception and interoception
Sensations

Morbid hypersensitivity (hyperaesthesia). Dim lights may then be seen as glaring and dazzling, colours as excessively bright; soft noises may be heard as loud and jarring; average room temperatures may be felt as too hot or too cold; clothes and bed blankets may be felt as unbearably heavy; mild interocepted sensations may be experienced as aches and pains.

Morbid hyposensitivity (hypoaesthesia, anaesthesia). The world is experienced as dulled and muted in all sensory areas; excessive temperatures, burns, open wounds, or sores seem to cause little or no distress (*analgesia*); fractures and acute appendicitis have been overlooked in patients who did not complain and did not manifest objective signs of pain; dark vision is diminished (especially in vitamin-A deficiency) so that night blindness ensues.

Morbidly changed sensations. Visual sensations may be tinged with red (*erythropsia*) e.g. in snow blindness, with blue (*cyanopsia*) e.g. after removal of a 'brown cataract', with yellow (*xanthopsia*) e.g. after poisoning with santonin, phenacetin, sulphonamides, digitalis, and other drugs. Quiet skin sensations may turn into *paraesthesiae*. Sensations in one sensory channel may be accompanied by sensations in another (*synaesthesia*). The most common example is colour hearing, i.e. the appearance of visual sensations and images, when listening to music. But this is not always a morbid phenomenon. Neither are the unpleasant kinaesthetic sensations (shivers down the spine, teeth set on edge) caused by a high-pitched screeching sound such as chalk can make on a blackboard. These and other synaesthesias between various sensory combinations have a morbid significance, when they are produced by psychotomimetic drugs such as mescaline, LSD (lysergic acid diethylamide), psilocybin (Simpson & McKellar, 1955; Shepherd *et al.*, 1968, p. 181).

Agnosias

Meaningless percepts. The phenomena of exteroception and interoception are, for the most part, not just experienced as sensations jumbled together chaotically, but as organized in space and time to form configurations known as *percepts*. In their most primitive form, percepts are predominantly sensory. But learning, experience, and memory link such sensory percepts with the introspective phenomena of meanings, affects, and urges. Of special significance among the latter are meanings. They transform mainly sensory percepts into richly *meaningful percepts*. As a result, percepts, and especially the exterocepted percepts of objects and events in our environment, can be identified as belonging to particular classes whose members are known by their general names and by their class characteristics. Thus when we see the percept of a sudden forked streak of bright light among storm clouds, we identify it as belonging to the class of events known by the general name of 'lightning' and characterized by the special attributes of high-voltage electric discharges. When we then hear the subsequent percept of a loud clap or rumbling noise, we identify it as belonging to the class of events known by the general name of 'thunder' and characterized by its association with lightning events.

The acquired linkage between a percept and its introspective meanings can be disrupted, usually by organic brain lesions. The disruption occurs characteristically in just one particular sensory channel. As a result, the patient concerned has only sensory and therefore almost *meaningless percepts* in that sensory modality. This clinical symptom was named '*imperception*' by Hughlings Jackson (1876). Freud (1891) later renamed it '*agnosia*' and this has become the preferred term today.

A patient with *visual agnosia* can see an object shown to him and may be able to draw it schematically, but he fails to recognize its meaning, i.e. he fails to assign it to its most relevant class of objects. He is therefore unable to give its general name or to indicate its practical significance. (The opposite

response occurs in patients with nominal aphasia who cannot name an exterocepted object, but can indicate that they are aware of its practical significance.) Since in visual agnosia only visual percepts are deprived of meaning, patients can identify the class membership and general name of an object as soon as they explore it by touch. Patients with *prosopagnosia* (Bodamer, 1947) can identify a face as a face, but not as the face of a particular person. They even have difficulty in recognizing their own face in a mirror or a group photograph, or in distinguishing between an obviously male and an obviously female face. The smile or anger expressed in a face may remain equally meaningless to them. In *visuo-spatial agnosia (space blindness)*, individual objects are recognized, but not their correct spatial relationships to other objects and to such body-related standards as up–down, right–left, clockwise–anticlockwise, near–distant. As a result, patients cannot orient themselves correctly in familiar surroundings, have difficulty in drawing a schematic house, a clock face, a simple map of a well-known route, and they fail in attempts to copy simple geometrical shapes on paper or with the help of match sticks or wooden blocks (*constructional apraxia*). In *picture agnosia (simultanagnosia)*, the individual objects in a picture are recognized separately, but not all of them together (simultaneously) so that the semantic relations between them and thus the meaning of the picture as a whole are missed. In *acquired colour agnosia (achromatopsia)*, patients can correctly match objects of the same colour, thus proving that they have colour vision, but they fail in the visual-visual task of sorting differently coloured skeins of wool or in arranging them correctly in sequence (Critchley, 1965). They also make mistakes in the verbal-visual tasks of naming a colour shown, of pointing to a colour named, or of naming from memory the colours of such objects as blood, sky, lawn (*colour anomia*). In typical cases, there are no naming mistakes in other sensory modalities, but there are reading difficulties (Oxbury *et al.*, 1969). In *acquired colour blindness*, patients lose all appreciation of colours and live in a world that is black, white and grey. Their condition is, however, different from the various kinds of *congenital colour blindness* which are not usually regarded as morbid conditions. Indeed they confer the advantage of facilitating the detection of camouflaged animals and objects in game hunting and modern warfare.

In *tactile agnosia (astereognosis, stereoagnosia)*, the patient has only a meaningless sensory percept, when an object is put into his affected hand (or hands), while his eyes are closed. He may describe some of the features of the object, e.g. that it is hard, heavy, cold, wet, and the like, but he fails to recognize what it is, i.e. its meaning. Yet this recognition is immediate, when he opens his eyes and looks at the object.

Patients with *auditory agnosia* cannot recognize familiar sound patterns, such as the jingling of coins, the rustling or tearing of paper, the ringing of a bell, the running and splashing of water, or a previously familiar tune (e.g. the national anthem).

Among the objects and events that can be exterocepted, there is a special variety of great social significance. These are the linguistic and numeral objects and events which not only have their purely linguistic or numeral meanings as letters, phonemes, words, sentences, digits, or numbers, but have, in addition, a *designative meaning* in that they indicate semantic (i.e. non-linguistic) concepts. Patients who lose their previous capacity of understanding these designative meanings are severely handicapped in our literate and numerate society. If this handicap is not due to a clouding of consciousness or some defect in sense organs, it constitutes a special kind of acquired agnosia. It could be called a *'designative agnosia'* and it particularly affects visual and auditory percepts.

When the designative agnosia is visual, it manifests itself clinically as *acquired dyslexia* (*word-blindness*). Severely affected patients no longer recognize script as script or print as print (*word-sight-blindness*). Other patients still recognize script and print, but cannot read correctly because they make mistakes with some individual letters or digits (*literal* or *digital dyslexia*), because they stumble over the order of the letters in a word or the order of digits in a composite number (*verbal* or *numeral dyslexia*). Those dyslexic patients who succeed in reading a word or a sentence correctly are yet unable to appreciate its designative meaning, i.e. the object, event, concept or proposition signified by it (*word-meaning-blindness*).

Acquired dyslexia is usually found combined with colour agnosia. Patients with literal dyslexia can sometimes circumvent the symptom with the help of proprioceptive sensations of a kinaesthetic kind; they trace the outline of a letter with their finger tips or with eye movement. Verbal dyslexia need not be associated with numeral dyslexia, so that patients who falter with simple words may read quite large num-

bers in decimal notation (see Stengel, 1948). The ability to write remains undisturbed in many patients with acquired dyslexia. However, such patients cannot read what they themselves have written either spontaneously or to dictation, once their memory of the written content has gone. Moreover, because they are unable to check their own writing, it will tend to have a variety of mistakes.

When the designative agnosia is of an auditory kind, it constitutes an *acquired sensory* (or *receptive*) *aphasia*. Severely handicapped patients cannot distinguish speech sounds from other sounds (*word-sound-deafness*). Less severely handicapped patients have meaningful percepts of speech sounds in that they recognize them as belonging to the class of speech sounds. They may even succeed in repeating a spoken word correctly, but they would be unable to understand its designative meaning (*word-meaning-deafness*). Thus the speech of other people would be to them no more than a babble of talk that is as unintelligible as any unfamiliar foreign tongue. If their aphasia is only sensory, they can still express themselves in words, but they may have difficulties in monitoring them so that mistakes remain uncorrected, wrong words appear (*paraphasia*), sentence construction becomes faulty (*paragrammatism*), and occasionally speech deteriorates into gibberish (*jargon aphasia*).

Musically accomplished persons may lose their recognition of musical intervals, patterns and rhythms (*sensory amusia*). They then fail to distinguish different notes, to notice a difference in melodies, or to identify a particular and previously familiar melody (Révész, 1953; Benton, 1977). The symptom is often, but not always associated with sensory aphasia.

Neither dyslexia nor sensory aphasia is invariably acquired. You cannot acquire dyslexia, unless you have first learned to read. Unfortunately, there are many children whose ability to learn to read is inadequate. Most of these children manifest a *general developmental dyslexia* (or *general reading retardation*). This backwardness is associated with such factors as low intelligence, educational disadvantage, emotional disturbance, or some personality disorder. Yet among the large number of backward readers, there is a small proportion whose disability is specific and not the result of a generally low mental capacity. As Rutter and Yule (1976) have emphasized, the disability of these children 'arises on the basis of a developmental impairment (often involving speech, language or sequencing functions)' (p. 571). It is not due to a low IQ, though adverse circumstances may aggravate the disability. This special handicap is known as *'specific developmental dyslexia'* (or *'specific reading retardation'*). It has been defined as 'a disorder manifested by difficulty in learning to read despite conventional instruction, adequate intelligence, and socio-cultural opportunity. It is dependent upon fundamental cognitive disabilities which are frequently of constitutional origin' (Critchley, 1970, p. 26). It occurs about four times as often in boys as in girls. There may be some improvement with age and remedial teaching, but children of this kind tend to grow into adults whose reading abilities are below par and whose spelling remains highly erratic.

There is a symptom of sensory aphasia which is not acquired but occurs in children, especially boys, as an inherited handicap *(infantile word deafness)*. Affected children have normal hearing, but they cannot understand the speech of others. Their own speech, having no models and being unmonitored, consists of idiosyncratic utterances *(idioglossia, lalling)* which makes sense only to those in close contact with them. They have to be educated by the same visual and tactile methods as deaf children.

Children with high-tone deafness also have trouble in understanding the speech of other people and in learning to talk intelligibly. Their difficulties may be gathered from experiments with adults. When these were presented with the sounds of nonsense syllables from which all frequencies above 1000 Hz had been removed, only 27 per cent of the syllables were correctly heard (French & Steinberg, 1947).

It is not only true of exteroceptive percepts that they can be meaningless. The same can happen to proprioceptive percepts. It occurs most commonly in patients with threatened or actual left-sided hemiplegia. The result is the symptom of *hemisomatagnosia*. The patients tend to neglect the affected (and usually left) side of their body. They under-use the hand of that side in bimanual activities; they forget to deal with that side of their body, when they wash, dress, comb their hair, or shave. They may even complain that the affected limbs are missing. Yet they can correct this proprioceptive mistake by visual and tactile checks, unless a clouded sensorium interferes with these exteroceptive corrections.

The various proprioceptive percepts a person experiences during his life give rise in his mind to a general concept of the form and proportions of his body. Head (1920, p. 605) called this general body concept a 'schema' against which all changes of position and posture are measured. Schilder (1935) expanded this view and introduced the term *'body image'* which is now in common usage. It designates a comprehensive body concept which is not only built up from proprioceptive percepts but also from exteroceptive and introspective body experiences. The body image is thus, when consciously experienced, a meaningful phenomenon which contains an accumulated store of knowledge, belief, and emotion about the appearance and capacities of one's own body.

This body image can be morbidly changed in many ways (Critchley, 1950, 1953). One of them consists in depriving some parts of the total body image of their topographical meaning so that patients have difficulties in identifying parts of their body and relating them to each other. This represents a special kind of agnosia which is not confined to just one sensory channel. It is known as *'autotopagnosia'*, though it can also be a *heterotopagnosia*, when patients also make mistakes in identifying or naming parts of other people's bodies. The identification of the parts of environmental objects which are not human bodies need not be disturbed as well. A spatial disorientation between parts of his body image can severely handicap a patient, when he tries to put on his clothes. He can then get into absurd contortionist tangles *(dressing apraxia)*. Autotopagnosia can be confined to the fingers only *(finger agnosia)*. In the so-called *'Gerstmann's syndrome'*, finger agnosia tends to be combined with right-left disorientation and difficulty in writing, in doing simple sums and in copying easy patterns and designs.

In nociceptive agnosia (pain asymbolia), patients are able to perceive painful stimuli, but they do not seem to appreciate their potentially noxious meaning and therefore do not respond adequately or defend themselves from a repetition of such stimuli. Once burnt, they are not twice shy.

Illusions

The term 'illusion' is often very loosely applied. In fact, it is often quite inadequately defined as a 'false percept'. We shall here use the term in its technical sense as a false percept of a very special kind. In agnosias, as we have pointed out, the percepts of objects and events are meaningless in the sense that they are not identified as members of their most relevant classes. In illusions, on the other hand, the percepts of objects and events are meaningful in that they are correctly identified as far as their most relevant class membership is concerned. However, they are not quite correctly identified in one or both of two additional senses. The percepts are experienced as having attributes which are not actually present in the objects and events to which they refer and/or they are endowed with an interpreted meaning which does not correspond to reality. The falsity of illusions derives from this discrepancy between the experienced percepts and the real state of affairs. As there are two kinds of discrepancies, we must make a distinction to which insufficient attention has been paid so far. We must distinguish between two kinds of illusions: *attribute illusions* and *interpretive illusions*.

The two kinds of illusions are not independent because there can be no attribute illusions of sensory percepts, unless an illusory interpretation of the percepts had taken place. This psychological fact was emphasized by the Gestalt psychologists who demonstrated our automatic tendency to transform incomplete percepts into whole ones. Gregory (1974) has also come to the conclusion that what we perceive depends on the 'perceptual hypotheses or models' evoked by sensory information. 'A wrong model – or the right model wrongly scaled – gives corresponding illusions' (p. 379). In spite of this, the distinction between attribute illusions and interpretive illusions has practical significance because, when we experience attribute illusions, we are not aware of the false perceptual meanings which are responsible for them. It needs indeed much experimental ingenuity to unearth them. On the other hand, persons experiencing interpretive illusions are fully aware of the meaning of their percepts, though not necessarily aware that the meaning is an illusory interpretation.

There are many attribute illusions which are normal by population standards since they are experienced by almost everybody. They occur in all sensory channels, but those occurring visually have attracted most attention because we usually rely on vision to provide us with the most accurate and detailed information about out environment. The Müller-Lyer arrow figures and the Necker depth-reversal cube are two of the best known of these visual attribute illusions.

Morbid attribute illusions distort the appearance of objects (or events) in a way which patients recognize as wrong so that they complain about them. Objects look abnormally large (*macropsia, megalopsia*) or abnormally small (*micropsia*) or larger on one side than the other (*dysmegalopsia*) or their shape is changed in more complex ways (*metamorphopsia*). Single objects are seen double (*diplopia*) or multiple (*polyopia*). Very occasionally, an object is seen extended beyond its known boundaries (*illusory visual spread*) so that the pattern of a tie extends to the face of the wearer or iron railings jut out into the street. This has been regarded as a visual perseveration in space (Critchley, 1951). Stationary objects are seen as approaching, receding, rotating, tilting, or moving in some other ways. The speed of events is experienced as accelerated or slowed down. The environment appears to move around a dizzy person. The world can look flat and without depth to some patients. Rooms and corridors can look uncomfortably narrow and open spaces uncomfortably vast.

Illusions of this kind can also affect proprioceptive percepts so that patients experience changes in the size, shape, position, or movement of their body, or of part of it, which they know to be unreal or can easily correct from the evidence of exteroceptive senses. They may wrongly feel that their body is rotating, tilting, floating, or falling, that their body, or some part of it, is expanding and swelling (*macrosomatognosia*) or shrinking to a small size (*microsomatognosia*), that they are hollow and excessively weightless or massive and excessively heavy, that their head is nodding or shaking (and they may seek reassurance by resting it on a hand), that their hands and knees are trembling, that their face is blushing, that their body merges with the world around them in a mystical experience, and so on.

Morbid interpretive illusions: Whereas patients with morbid attribute illusions are always aware of the abnormality and unreality of their experiences, patients with interpretive illusions do not always have this insight and may accept their experiences as real.

Events may acquire the meaning of being familiar, of having occurred before so that one has a specious premonition of what is going to happen next (*déjà vu illusion, illusion of familiarity*). It is a phenomenon that is morbid only when it occurs so often that it is complained about or when it is accepted as signifying a true reminiscence. The contrary phenomenon is the experience that the particular events perceived are entirely new and had never happened before (*jamais vu illusion, illusion of unfamiliarity*). The environment can appear unreal, strange, dreamlike, or like a stage set (*derealization*); it may also become sinister and threatening, sometimes with such impressiveness that patients become convinced with absolute delusional certainty that the change in the environment is genuine (*delusional atmosphere*). Delusions are, of course, very often the source of morbid interpretive illusions (*delusional illusions*). For example, the whole world can appear dead, empty, and standing still to a deluded depressive; it can appear full of personal messages, innuendoes, and influences to a deluded schizophrenic. Occasionally delusions convince a patient that the people around him are impostors who are out to befool and harm him; he may even reject his closest relatives because he is delusionally certain that they are deceiving doubles of his real relatives (*Capgras syndrome*). Frightened and anxious patients may misidentify shadows, glimmers, or creaking noises as possible or certain signs of lurking evil-doers; and if their sensorium is clouded (e.g. in delirium tremens), these misidentifications can assume nightmarish and grotesque proportions. There are schizophrenic patients who listen to their hallucinated voices only, or mainly, when there is a conspicuous external noise, e.g. an aeroplane or a running tap. Such patients are usually said to have *'functional hallucinations'*. But it is equally possible that they did no more than misinterpret their auditory percepts. When paranoid schizophrenics hear that people in their environment make personal remarks about them, it is often more plausible to assume that they are not really hallucinated but have auditory interpretive illusions of verbal sounds actually overheard. Indeed it is quite probable that many hallucinations are no more than interpretive illusions of sensory percepts. Delirious patients, for instance, have fewer visual hallucinations in an unpatterned environment of white walls and plain curtains. Harris (1959) has shown that, under conditions of perceptual deprivation in which visual, auditory, and tactile stimulations are kept monotonously uniform, the visual, auditory, and tactile hallucinations of schizophrenic patients tended to be less vivid and troublesome or to disappear entirely. This is in contrast to the response of normal persons who tend to experience pseudo-hallucinations under these conditions.

The clinical symptom known as a *'negative hallucination'* is a special kind of interpretive illusion. The symptom can occur in all sensory modalities and is due to hysterical (i.e. autosuggestive), hypnotic or post-hypnotic (i.e. heterosuggestive) influences. Such patients, though subjectively blind, do not bump into physical objects which should be invisible to them. Similarly, when they are subjectively deaf, they raise their voice like a person with normal hearing, when a Bárány noise box is put into their ear. Patients of this kind who are subjectively without touch, heat or pain sensations in some skin areas may respond with 'No', when that area is stimulated without their knowledge after having responded with 'Yes', when so stimulated in other skin areas. They thus demonstrate that they experience a sensory percept, but interpret it as non-existent.

When morbid interpretive illusions affect proprioceptive percepts, one of the clinical consequences can be *hypochondriacal* symptoms. Normal bodily sensations are interpreted as morbidly disordered or inadequate. Among common hypochondriacal complaints are an inability to breathe deeply enough; a constricting lump in the throat (known misleadingly as 'globus hystericus'); palpitations, irregularities, and other presumed anomalies of the heart beat; insufficient elimination of bowel contents; weakening seminal losses; sleep inadequacies; fatigue; inability to concentrate; aches, pains, discomforts and many other unpleasant bodily sensations. The driving force of hypochondriacal misinterpretations can be a morbid fear of ill-health. It can also be a morbid conviction of ill-health in situations, such as battle stress or financial compensation claims, which are disease-rewarding (F. Kräupl Taylor, 1979b, pp. 254ff.). In either case, hypochondriacal misinterpretations cannot be readily corrected by the reassurance of normal findings on clinical investigation. On the contrary, such reassurance can aggravate the clinical picture and induce the patient to seek medical or paramedical help elsewhere.

The opposite of hypochondriacal symptoms is the symptom of illness denial (*anosognosia, nosoagnosia*). This is not an agnosia at all and is not limited to just one sensory channel. It is an interpretive illusion which derives from a cherished body image of somatic integrity and functional health. The perception of any possible manifestation of ill-health is then misinterpreted as non-existent or as having a nonmorbid background. The term 'anosognosia' was coined by Babinski (1914) to designate the behaviour of some brain-damaged patients with (usually) left-sided hemiplegia who, against all objective evidence, refuse to admit that they are paralysed. Denials of this kind are not uncommon in brain-damaged patients with a variety of symptoms (cf. Brain, 1961, pp. 168f.), such as paraplegias and other paralyses, involuntary movements, sensory aphasia, acquired dyslexia, urinary and faecal incontinence, vomiting, blindness, deafness, loss of memory, and so on. Such physical handicaps are so much at variance with a patient's flawless body image of himself that he may go to the length of disowning his paralysed limbs and perhaps attribute them to someone else. He may get very upset, if his protestations of intact health are too persistently challenged and then show what Goldstein (1942) has called a *'catastrophic reaction'*.

Anosognosia is, however, not a symptom that is exclusive to brain-damaged patients. It occurs in a most flamboyant form in manic patients who reject the idea of their being ill with a roar of laughter or an angry outburst. Anosognosia is also common in otherwise healthy persons who gradually become hard of hearing. Moreover an anosognosic tendency can be a personality trait. Such persons play down or disregard completely the possible health hazard of incidental bodily and functional changes in themselves which come to their notice. This may be an ostrich response evoked by a fear of illness, of doctors, or of hospitals; it may also be a self-deceptive conceit of having an iron constitution which shakes off all ills. Such anosognosic tendencies can have disastrous consequences, for example when a woman disregards a growing lump in one of her breasts.

A related phenomenon which is so common as to be normal by population standards is the persistence of a body image that is many years younger than the actual body of the person concerned. This illusory youthfulness can have certain morbid implication, for example when it leads to a damaging physical overtaxing of an aging body or when the discrepancy between illusion and reality is brutally brought home to a narcissistic woman past her prime. It is this same resistance of the body image to change that gives rise to the phenomenon of phantom limbs in amputees.

However, the body image is not totally resistant to any change. Changes can occur of which the patient becomes aware as something odd and unpleasant. Most commonly the changes are those which belong to the syndrome of *depersonalization*. They may be of only short duration (minutes, hours) or last for several months. It is usually hard for patients to convey the true tenor of their experiences which, incidentally, do not always have a morbid import. Their descriptions are thus replete with metaphors and 'as if' clauses. They feel strange and unreal, as if they were mere robots, automata, puppets, mere bystanders observing how their body acted and their mind thought and felt. The syndrome is not often experienced on its own, but more usually com-

bined with such phenomena as derealization, anxiety, depressive mood, uncertainties of identity, or altered sensorium (see Mayer-Gross, 1935; Ackner, 1954).

In psychotic conditions, delusions can bring about changes in the body image which are of a bizarre hypochondriacal kind. Such patients may have *Cotard's* (1882) *syndrome of nihilistic delusions* in that they are convinced that they no longer have a body or that the body they have is dead and decaying. Other patients have the delusion that they have changed their sex or been transformed into another person or an animal; that there are foreign objects, people, animals, or demons inside them; or that there are various ominous pathological changes in some or all of their organs (Lukianowicz, 1967).

More common are changes in the body image which originate in anxieties. When such changes are objectively unjustified, they can yet be perpetuated by a vicious circle, if they cause the patients to perceive confirmatory attribute illusions on examining their body or confirmatory interpretive illusions on watching the behaviour of other people towards them. There are unwarranted anxieties about body odour, halitosis, too dry or too greasy hair, dandruff, hair in unwanted places or loss of hair, skin blemishes, plumpness or thinness, the proper formation of sexual organs, breasts, muscles, and so on. Commercial interests exploit the high prevalence of these anxieties in our society and foster them for their own gain. However, they also provide a therapeutic service, even if it has often only a placebo effect. Yet this may explain why only a small number of patients with moderate anxieties of this kind come to the notice of doctors.

These mild changes of the body image occasionally attract attention, when they are combined with a serious clinical condition. For example, Slade and Russell (1973) noticed that patients with anorexia nervosa had a tendency to over-estimate the width of their body. Crisp and Kalucy (1974) confirmed this but found similar tendencies in their normal control group. Halmi and colleagues (1977) established that the over-estimation of body width is, in our western culture at least, a normal phenomenon among adolescent girls of quite normal weight. It seems, however, that the over-estimation is significantly larger and also more variable in patients with anorexia nervosa than in normal persons (Pierloot & Houben, 1978).

Anxieties, whether justified or not, about body

image changes can engender obsessional preoccupations with certain attributes and parts of the body. Patients will then clamour with more or less importunity for medical attention or for surgical help, if that is possible. Their whole life may be governed and ruined by nagging fears of being disfigured (*dysmorphophobia*). Among the attributes and parts of the body involved are the nose, chin, ears, mouth, teeth, breasts, penis, wrinkles, facial hair, baldness, height, weight, and so on. When cosmetic operations are available, their success (especially as far as rhinoplasty is concerned) does not appear to depend on the objective degree of deformity, though psychological factors have to be considered before recommending operation (see Hay, 1970a, 1970b; Hay & Heather, 1973). Past assumptions that minimal degrees of objective deformity have a bad post-operative prognosis have not been borne out by follow-up investigations.

Hallucinations and allied phenomena.

Hallucinations belong to a class of exterocepted or interocepted phenomena which falsely indicate the presence of objects in one's environment or one's body. We need a generic name for the diverse phenomena in this class and the term *'para-percepts'* is proposed for this purpose. Para-percepts differ from illusions in that the latter correctly indicate the presence of such objects, but falsely indicate their attributes or meaning. Para-percepts also differ from memory images, since these are not exterocepted or interocepted at all, but are introspected in an inner subjective space.

Among exterocepted para-percepts are certain visual phenomena known as *'phosphenes'* (shining lights). They make their appearance in dark visual fields or interfere as *positive scotomata* with normal vision. Phosphenes may be no more than simple round or stellar shapes; they may be scintillating specks of coloured light, arranged in lattice or chessboard form; they may appear as filigree patterns, as lines resembling a network of blood vessels, and the like.

They may be ocular in origin. Pressure on the eyelids brings them about and some people are excessively sensitive in this respect. Oster (1970), for instance, in a well-illustrated article on phosphenes, mentions a woman 'who, if she inadvertently rubs her eyes with a towel in the morning, provokes such intense phosphenes that they are superposed on her normal vision for hours afterwards'. Other phosphenes of ocular origin are the well-known *visual after-images,* whether positive or negative, and the phenomena experienced in *photopsia* due to a detached retina.

Phosphenes due to ocular processes move in the visual field with the gaze. Those of a more central origin do not. The latter can be caused by a blow on the head (seeing stars), by electric stimulation of the visual cortex (Brindley & Lewin, 1968), by the toxic substances known as 'hallucinogenic', 'psychotomimetic' or 'psychedelic' (Klüver, 1966; Siegel, 1977), and other cerebral disturbances. Among centrally caused morbid phosphenes are the scintillating hexagonal designs seen in migraine attacks (Richards, 1971). These are known as *'fortification spectra'* and the seeing of them as *'teichopsia'* (seeing walls with hexagonal fortification towers). Critchley (1951) has described *perseverated visual after-images* as rare morbid symptoms of central origin. The perseveration can occur in temporal or spatial dimensions. The former present themselves as intrusive repetitions of scenes just seen, an experience with Critchley called *'paliopsia'*. A similar, though non-morbid, experience can occur after a day's motoring, skiing or sailing in bright sunshine. When the morbid perseveration of after-images takes place in space, while the object concerned is still in view, it seems to extend itself into its environment. It is thus an attribute illusion in the sense that the object's spatial characteristics are falsely perceived; at the same time it is also a para-percept in the sense that the presence of the extended part of the object is falsely indicated. Critchley spoke of an *'illusory visual spread'*.

When there is no patterned visual field with which phosphenes of whatever origin can interfere, they are then seen against the blackness of closed lids, totally dark environments or complete blindness. Such phosphenes are para-percepts which belong to the category of visual hallucinations and allied phenomena. It is a category that is surrounded by conceptual and terminological uncertainties.

Through the investigations of Kandinsky (1885) and the very influential writings of Karl Jaspers (1948, orig. 1913) a distinction was drawn between visual hallucinations and visual pseudo-hallucinations. Yet this distinction was in many ways inconsistent and perplexing as Hare (1973) pointed out. Judging by the characteristics attributed to visual pseudo-hallucinations by Kandinsky and Jaspers, one gets the impression that they were regarded as truly 'pseudo-'

in that they were not hallucinated para-percepts at all. They were merely introspected visual images which were experienced in a subjective inner space and not in the physical environment in which genuine visual hallucinations were seen.

When Sedman (1966) examined the concept of visual and other pseudo-hallucinations and introduced it into British psychiatry, he came to the conclusion that there are phenomena to which the term 'pseudo-hallucination' can be justifiably applied. These phenomena, however, are genuine hallucinations of a special kind in that they are 'recognized by the patient as not being veridical'. The prefix 'pseudo-' is thus no longer merited, though it has not been replaced. Hare (1973) gave Sedman's views some qualified approval and so did Hamilton (1974). However, they continued to regard pseudo-hallucinations as exclusively morbid para-percepts. This does not seem to be justified. There are perfectly normal and healthy pseudo-hallucinations. Remembered dreams are the most obvious examples. It therefore seems best to adopt the following definitions:

Hallucinations are para-percepts which are falsely experienced as veridical at the time of their occurrence.

Pseudo-hallucinations are para-percepts which are correctly experienced as non-veridical at the time of their occurrence or when viewed in retrospect.

Pseudo-hallucinations. Dreams are pseudo-hallucinations, when remembered as dreams in the waking state. They are hallucinations, when experienced during sleep, except on the rare occasions when the sleeper is aware that he is dreaming. Visual and auditory pseudo-hallucinations are fairly common, though usually quickly forgotten, para-percepts, when falling asleep or waking up (*hypnagogic* or *hypnopompic* pseudo-hallucinations).

Phosphenes seen in a totally dark visual field are visual pseudo-hallucinations. In persons with acquired blindness, they can be a source of diversion or annoyance. Critchley (1965) reported a woman of 60, blind from cataracts, who saw an incessant golden rain pouring down in the darkness of her eyes. She was so distressed by it that she submitted to two leucotomies.

In experiments with perceptual deprivation in which people are kept for hours in an environment where the patterning of visual, auditory and tactile sensations is drastically reduced to a uniform monotony (Bexton *et al.*, 1954), the subjects are liable to experience visual, auditory, and proprioceptive para-percepts which have often been called 'hallucinations', though most of them are in fact pseudo-hallucinations (Leff, 1968).

Prolonged activities in a monotonously uniform environment may give rise to similar para-percepts of an hallucinatory or pseudo-hallucinatory kind. These may have a morbid significance in that they can cause accidents to motorists driving long distances at night, in fog or on tedious motorways, or to pilots flying in the cloudless sky of high altitudes. McFarland and Moore (1957) found that 30 among 50 American long-haul truck drivers had experienced such para-percepts. They had suddenly braked at the sight of non-existent red lights at a crossroad or swerved at the sight of non-existent obstacles in their path.

A striking, though uncommon, visual pseudo-hallucination is the deceptive sight of oneself (usually only head and shoulders) in the environment. This experience of *autoscopy* (of one's double or *Doppelgänger*) is not necessarily morbid as it has been reported by healthy people in times of stress or fatigue. It is not restricted to the visual modality either, but may have auditory and tactile components (Lhermitte, 1951; Lukianowicz, 1958). Autoscopic visions are usually only short-lived, but they can be prolonged in some patients with recent brain damage (Dewhurst & Pearson, 1955). Such patients may even see their pseudo-hallucinated double outside their field of vision, standing behind them or moving about in another room (*extracampine pseudo-hallucinations*).

Social isolation among polar explorers and solitary sailors may give rise to pseudo-hallucinations or interpretive illusions of a visual, auditory, olfactory, or tactile kind (Ritter, 1900; Lewis *et al.*, 1964; Bennet, 1973). The social deprivation of recent bereavement may also cause such transiently deceptive sensory percepts of the deceased person.

The pseudo-hallucinations mentioned so far are autonomous and intrusive para-percepts which come and go of their own accord. There is, however, a special visual variety which depends on a deliberate mnestic intention. These pseudo-hallucinations are known as '*eidetic images* (or *memories*)'. They differ from the usual rather shadowy memory images which are introspected in an inner subjective space – on a mental stage, as it were. Eidetic images are visually exterocepted, they are actually seen, especially against an unpatterned background, with great clarity and detail. They thus come close to the notion of a photographic memory in that previously unnoticed details may be searched for in them. In investigations before 1935 (e.g. Allport, 1925; Jaensch, 1930; Klüver, 1931), eidetic imagery was reported to be present in about half the children in elementary schools, but it disappeared almost invariably after puberty. However, the diagnoses of eidetic imagery seem to have been made on too slender and unreliable evidence. When Haber (1969) examined elementary school children more recently, he found that only 5 to 10 per cent of them had some eidetic ability, though their images lasted only a few minutes and then faded in uneven patches. Yet there seem to be occasional adults who retain their eidetic capacities to some extent. The investigation by Luria (1960, 1969) of the mnemonist Shereshevski revealed that he could revive eidetic memories even after an interval of over fifteen years. His difficulty was not the act of remembering, but the ability to forget unwanted information. As Luria reported: 'S. frequently gave several performances an evening, sometimes in the same hall, where the charts of numbers he had to recall were written on the one blackboard there and then erased before the next performance'. S. had to learn special techniques to prevent the appearance of eidetic images belonging to a previous performance.

Pseudo-hallucinations can also be of an interoceptive (proprioceptive, kinaesthetic) kind. Among these, the most common are those that give rise to the experience of *phantom limbs* which can be moved intentionally in an imaginary space that takes no account of obstacles in real space. Proprioceptive pseudo-hallucinations can also be experienced after the removal of breasts, eyes, nose, penis, or rectum. They can occur as well in patients whose limbs are still physically present, though completely paralysed. This leads to *pseudo-hallucinatory reduplications* of the limb or limbs concerned. They can cause much distress to a patient, especially when the position of the reduplicated limb is at variance with that of the actual limb (Brain, 1956). Such reduplications of parts of the body or of the whole of it are also sometimes experienced by patients who have no motor paralyses (Lukianowicz, 1967). However, not all reports of reduplicative experiences are due to proprioceptive pseudo-hallucinations, they may instead be of delusional origin (Weinstein *et al.*, 1954).

Hallucinations proper are exterocepted or inter-

ocepted para-percepts which are falsely experienced as veridical at the time of their occurrence, i.e. they are experienced as corresponding to objects or events which actually exist in physical reality. Hallucinations proper thus differ from pseudo-hallucinations in that they are accompanied by an experience of their reality instead of a realization of their unreality. Aggernaes (1972a) has enumerated seven characteristics which are implied by the reality experience of exterocepted hallucinations. Among them are the immediate awareness that the phenomena experienced are not just introspected thoughts or memory images but are exterocepted percepts of environmental objects or events; that one could obtain confirmation of their reality through other sensory channels oneself or through the exteroception of them independently by other people; that they exist quite apart from any one experiencing them; that they cannot be altered merely by willing them to be altered; and that they are not experienced on account of some morbid changes in oneself. Using these characteristics as criteria, Aggernaes (1972b) showed that the exterocepted pseudo-hallucinations of young drug abusers convey less reality experience than the exterocepted hallucinations proper of schizophrenic patients.

Patients can be hallucinated in several sensory modalities at the same time, but one or the other modality generally predominates. Exterocepted hallucinations which occur in clear consciousness and are frequent and persistent set special problems for the patients who are bound to realize that other people do not share those exteroceptions. The problems can be solved in different ways: some patients eventually learn to keep their hallucinatory experiences to themselves; some find delusional explanations, for example that there is a conspiracy among people to deny sharing the patients' experiences or that malevolent influences are brought to bear on the patients so that they alone have those experiences or that the patients have been chosen by divine authority to witness supernatural phenomena; some patients try to convince others, and especially cohabiting relatives or associates, that they too must experience the hallucinated events because they are undeniably real and if those others are suggestible, the patients may succeed and bring about *induced hallucinations*.

Visual hallucinations which occur in a clouded sensorium are often fantastic and frightening. Many are of small animals, such as mice, spiders, or insects. It is possible that the basis of such hallucinations are phosphenes which are not recognized as para-percepts but interpreted as real events in the environment. In some patients, such as those with delirium tremens, those interpretations can be changed in obedience to hetero-suggestions so that the patient will describe some specified scenes or read from a blank sheet of paper, when he is told it is a letter. In clear consciousness, visual hallucinations may be merely indistinct and blurred manifestations which, though accepted as genuine percepts, differ in character from the rest of the visible environment. They may, however, also be very detailed, clear, and definite so that they are indistinguishable from other objects and events in the environment. A rare phenomenon are *Lilliputian hallucinations* of tiny animals and people that are vividly coloured, rapidly moving, and enjoyable to watch.

Auditory hallucinations vary from vague phenomena (bangs, whistles, rushing sounds, verbal mumbles) to quite distinctly heard animal noises, cries of tortured people, music, or speech. When speech is heard, patients may understand only its meaning and not the actual words. On the other hand, they may clearly hear the voices involved and know whether they come from men or women, children or adults, foreigners or natives. The voice, or voices, may comment on the patient's thought or behaviour, mock him, command him, question him. The voices may talk among themselves, mentioning the patient in the third person. The hallucinated speech sounds, whether mumbled or distinct, can be clearly located in a space that is not just environmental but includes the interior of the patient's body. He may thus hear speech sounds emanating from various parts of his anatomy. Such speech sounds, or 'inner voices', are not always interpreted as the ego-alien utterances of known or unknown beings that somehow dwell inside him, but as having their origin in his own mind, as being perhaps the voice of his conscience or the sound of his thoughts (*thought hearing, Gedankenlautwerden, écho de pensée*). Such thought hearing may cause fears that strangers will be privy to the most intimate workings of his mind.

Gustatory and *olfactory hallucinations* are common in patients with temporal lobe epilepsy. They also occur in patients with delusions of being poisoned.

In the interoceptive field *motor hallucinations* occur and may plague schizophrenic patients. They usually have the kinaesthetic experience that some of their facial muscles move spontaneously. They may respond by spending a long time in front of a mirror searching for the hallucinated movements and imitating them through grimaces.

Morbid abnormalities of introspection
Intellectual subnormalities.

Among introspective phenomena, thoughts and reasoning take pride of place. A person's capacity to deal with the manifold problems of daily life in a reasonable manner unhampered by emotional twists constitutes his *intelligence (intellect)*. It can be measured by specially devised and standardized tests and expressed as an intelligence quotient (IQ), namely 100 times the quotient between the test result and the average test result of his peers. Like all human capacities, intelligence is partly genetically determined and partly modified during ante- and post-natal life through contingent influences. The distribution of intelligence quotients in a human population is by and large statistically normal with a mean IQ of 100 and an approximate standard deviation of 15.

A person's degree of intelligence can have morbid consequences in two main ways. He may introspectively realize that his ability to solve the problem of acquiring educationally prescribed knowledge falls short of his ambitions or the expectations of his environment. This subjective realization of a relative intellectual inadequacy can give rise to morbid emotional reactions in him or others.

A person's degree of intelligence can also be objectively inadequate, whether this is subjectively realized by him or not. If his IQ is below 70 (i.e. two standard deviations below the mean of his peers), his degree of intelligence is statistically subnormal by the standards of his peer population. This in itself is not a morbid phenomenon. Yet whenever it leads to such a degree of social incompetence that it arouses therapeutic and medical concern in the community in which he lives, then it has acquired morbid significance (O'Connor & Tizard, 1956). Persons, or patients, with an IQ below 70 are said to manifest '*mental (intellectual, social) subnormality (deficiency, retardation) or oligophrenia*'. All these terms are used in a narrow technical sense indicating only innate intellectual shortcomings and not any intellectual deteriorations of later onset. Persons with an IQ between 45 and 70 are regarded as belonging to the *subcultural* (or *multifactorial*) *section* of people with mental subnormality and those with an IQ below 45 as belonging to a *specific* (or *pathological*) *section* of such people. In the last-named section, there are more members than expected in a statistically normal distribution of values or in an attribute of multifactorial origin. The numbers in that section are increased by specific influences deriving usually from pathological genes or chromosomal karyotypes rather than some cerebral pathology of later onset (Penrose, 1963, 1970).

Dementias and pseudo-dementias.

When there is a global deterioration of the intellectual functions of a fully conscious person so that his cognitive processes fall significantly below his previous standards, he manifests the clinical phenomenon of dementia. Unfortunately, the concept of dementia has been given incompatible meanings in different contexts. It seems that it was originally assumed that dementia always indicates an *irretrievable* impairment of a person's previous level of intelligence so that there was no chance of a substantial recovery. This assumption was, for instance, one of the reasons why Kraepelin's term 'dementia praecox' gave way to E. Bleuler's term 'schizophrenia', since there was no doubt that the patients in question can recover. The concept of an irrecoverable dementia presupposed a widespread and irreversible loss of brain tissue. It has, however, been realized by now that there are forms of obvious clinical dementia in which no brain tissue is irreversibly lost. Such patients retain their previous level of intelligence, but this cannot manifest itself on account of influences which globally interfere with the normal biochemical functions of the brain – an interference that is reversible, at least in theory and quite often today also in practice.

Dementia shows itself not only in a deterioration of intellectual functions. Since it is due to a global reduction of brain functions either on a structural (organic) or a biochemical (functional) basis, there is also a global impairment of memory and a deterioration of personality through untempered emotions and an autistic retreat from social contact and conformity. Dementia is thus a syndrome. Lishman (1978, p. 9), for example, defines it as 'an acquired global impairment of intellect, memory and personality, but without impairment of consciousness'. He is at pains to point out that the syndrome is defined 'in terms of global impairment of *functions,* and not in terms of diffuse cerebral damage' or in terms of irreversibility. (Italics in the original.) Diffuse and irreparable organic brain damage is only one of the causes of this syndrome. Others are potentially remediable disorders of brain functions through biochemical anoma-

lies, such as in hypothyroidism or in deficiencies of such vitamins as cobalamin (B_{12}) or folic acid.

Mild degrees of the dementia syndrome are not usually regarded as morbid, but are accepted as signs of the *normal senescence* of advanced age. This weakens a person's ability to tackle unaccustomed problems, blunts his judgement and renders his memory unreliable. He may, or may not, have insight into these shortcomings. As long as he can circumvent them and can continue to lead an adequate life, though perhaps within a narrowed sphere of largely routine activities, he is likely to reject any therapeutic concerns of others (Allison, 1962; Post, 1965).

When the syndrome of dementia becomes disabling, it has turned into a morbid phenomenon. Persons over the age of 65 are then regarded as suffering from *senile dementia* and younger persons as having one of the various kinds of *pre-senile dementia.* The earliest of these is the *infantile dementia* described by Heller (1930) in children of the age of 3 to 4 years whose ability to speak and understand language deteriorates, who lose interest in their environment and withdraw into a solitary world of stereotyped and manneristic behaviour. Adult or old patients with pre-senile or senile dementia usually first arouse therapeutic concern because of a deterioration of their memory. Since this is generally concomitant with intellectual decline and poor judgement, the patients have no insight into being ill (anosognosia) and may obstinately reject well-meaning offers of help. Their forgetfulness can spell hazard, when open gas taps remain unlit, wash basins overflow, food rots, waste accumulates, dirt spreads, and there is muddle everywhere. The patient's world narrows to an egocentric circle, his thoughts lose abstract generality and are hemmed in by a 'concrete attitude' (Goldstein, 1942, pp. 89f.) which ties them to particular aspects of their immediate environment. The normal rational control of emotional urges is weakened so that troublesome anxieties, depressions, suspicions, hypochondriacal fears, peevishness, bursts of weeping and laughing, or a fatuous euphoria become prominent. Delusions and hallucinations can emerge and some clouding of consciousness can occur, especially at night. Manners become uncouth, churlish, and tactless. Morals crumble in the face of temptations to steal or to misbehave sexually.

Eventually memories of past events, whether recent or remote, vanish more or less completely, and so does the remembering of new experiences. Patients are disoriented for time, place, and person, and lose their way in unaccustomed surroundings. Behaviour dwindles to indolence and becomes entangled in purposeless activities or the senseless hoarding of trifles. What amount of speech is left consists in fragmented, disorganized, or perseverative utterances of little or no meaning. Personal appearance and hygiene are neglected. When incontinence occurs, it rouses hardly a response in the patient. In the terminal stages, there is only mental vegetation and physical marasmus.

Severe depressions in elderly patients can masquerade clinically as dementias. The patients manifest an apparently gross impairment of general knowledge, memory, and orientation. Their appearance can be as unkempt and their physical state as decrepit as many a truly senile dement. Post (1965, p. 88) remarks that the diagnosis of a depressive illness in such patients is helped by two observations: (1) the patients' intellectual abilities and memory functions had shown no decline before the appearance of depressive symptoms, and (2) the patients make no facile excuses, when they fail to answer questions correctly, but stoically accept their inadequacy and simply repeat that they do not know. Such patients may also show some uncertain neurological signs, such as a shuffling gait, a coarse tremor, and various rigidities. Such signs cannot be taken, however, as foreshadowing the onset of an organic dementia.

These *depressive dementias* are still usually regarded as *pseudo-dementias*, perhaps because a psychological pathology is presumed instead of a biochemical one or because the clinical symptoms can so often be easily removed by electric shock treatment or antidepressant medication. Yet depressive dementias are on a par with other functional dementias which are accessible to appropriate treatment, such as those due to hormone or vitamin deficiencies. They are even comparable to those organic dementias that can be remedied by suitable measures, such as the surgical removal of dementia-causing brain tumours, a shunt operation in normal-pressure hydrocephalus, or antibiotic treatment in certain cerebral infections.

The nosological status of pseudo-dementias is still a very precarious one. Their diagnosis rests on rather fallible clinical guesses of a psychological origin. All too often the diagnosed pseudo-dementias turn out in the end not to have been 'pseudo-' at all. The classical, though admittedly rare, example of a pseudo-dementia is a clinical condition described originally by Ganser (1898) and regarded by him as hysterical in origin. It has since become known as *'Ganser syndrome'* (to characterize in clinical colloquialism 'Ganser' patients or patients who 'ganser'). Its core symptom is a fluctuating tendency to respond to questions with *approximate answers* ('*vorbeireden*', *talking past the point*) and those answers also are, as Whitlock (1967) pointed out, quite obviously absurd. The patients seem deliberately to act like fools in an unconvincing charade of fatuous buffoonery. In addition, typical Ganser patients have a changeable clouding of consciousness, seem disoriented, and report hallucinations. The tomfoolery of their behaviour which is riddled with glaring inconsistencies and contradictions always rouses the suspicion of barefaced malingering, especially since the silliness of their conduct during clinical observation is not carried over into all the activities of their daily life, so that they come to no harm and suffer no hardships. Ganser patients can recover abruptly and are then left with an amnesia for the duration of their illness. In many patients, however, the syndrome turns out to be the unsuspected forerunner of a schizophrenic or epileptic disease or of a pre-senile dementia.

The core symptom of approximate answers often occurs by itself in psychiatric patients who have nothing else in common. It therefore has no diagnostic significance. For that reason, this *Ganser symptom* should be distinguished from the fully blown and uncommon Ganser *syndrome* (Scott, 1965).

There are patients who are motivated by a conscious or unconscious desire to appear mad in order to escape from some intolerable social situation. The lay image of madness often comes close to the clinical picture of pseudo-dementia. The patients lose their ability to read, write, or do simple arithmetic. Their knowledge of public personages, places, and events, as well as of important happenings in their own life, becomes hazy or absurdly false. They do not recognize where they are, misidentify people in role-indicating attire (doctors, nurses, policemen), fumble ludicrously when asked to perform accustomed tasks, such as striking a match, using a key or scissors, and the like.

Depending on the clinician's opinion of the consciousness or unconsciousness of the patients' pathological motivations, the diagnosis of the clinical condition observed will be either *malingered pseudo-dementia* or *hysterical pseudo-dementia*. When patients regress to an infantile state so that they can only crawl on all fours, make inarticulate noises, suck their thumbs, smear their food, and wet their bed, the diagnosis is one of *hysterical infantilism*. Yet the confidence with which such diagnoses are made after a short-term clinical observation often turns out to be ill-founded, when the patients are followed up for some time. Even when the confidence is later proved to have been justified, we may still be left in the dark as to whether the clinical picture of pseudo-dementia was hysterical or simulated. Retrospective admission of simulation, as in the case of Rudolf Hess (Rees, 1947), can only be taken with a pinch of salt as the patient may unknowingly deceive himself. Indeed it is quite likely that the clinical picture of this kind of pseudo-dementia is often compounded of hysterical and malingered components, though perhaps in unequal proportions. There is, however, one differential-diagnostic hint to which I drew attention (1979b, p. 265). Patients whose pseudo-dementia is of mainly hysterical derivation remain surprisingly unmoved, when the convenient inconsistencies of their behaviour are pointed out to them. Not so the patients who are conscious of malingering. They become flustered, try to find excuses and explanations, and subsequently do their utmost to be more consistent and convincing in their simulations. Yet this is a task that cannot be kept up for any length of time as Anderson and colleagues (1959) have shown.

Schizophrenic impairment of thought and talk.

Young schizophrenics can become introspectively aware that their thought processes are falling off (Hoffer, 1946; Chapman, 1966). They may experience blank spells, when their minds seem to stop; they may feel that their thoughts become unbridled or that they cannot express them in suitable words, because no words will come or unwanted words intrude; they may realize that single-minded concentration is no longer possible for them. Objectively, such introspected experiences manifest themselves in the patients' behaviour. Their talk may trail off and stop in mid-sentence or mid-thought (*thought blocking*) to be followed without embarrassment by a self-absorbed silence or an unexpected turn to a new topic; their sentences may become so ill-constructed and their ideas so vague, dissociated, and incoherent that they fail to convey any sense. For the most part, schizophrenic patients are too apathetic to complain about the disarray and poverty of their thoughts, if they notice this at all. They become socially isolated and phlegmatically retreat into autistic reveries or sink into an empty-headed indolence.

In *infantile autism*, which may be the earliest manifestation of a schizophrenic disease (though this has been disputed, e.g. Rutter, 1976), symptoms appear before the age of 30 months and are characterized by difficulties in expressing or understanding speech, by social isolation, self-absorbed rituals and a desperate clinging to sameness and routines.

In *childhood, adolescent or early adult schizophrenia*, muddled thinking halts educational progress and muddled speaking puts a bar to emotional and sexual companionship. The linguistic handicap of these patients is accessible to quantitative evaluations based on concepts and methods elaborated by the 'information' theories of communication engineers (Maher, 1972; Silverman, 1972, 1973). The upshot of these investigations seems to be that the choice of words by thought-disturbed schizophrenics cannot be adequately predicted, because the patients have fewer word types introspectively available than healthy persons and therefore repeat them, even when they are inappropriate.

There are, of course, many abnormalities of talk in schizophrenic patients which are clinically conspicuous. Patients can be mute, they may talk to extrasensibly perceived presences, converse with their hallucinatory voices, or shout at them in anger. Their answers to questions can be short and telegrammatic; they can also be diffuse, though empty of content – a symptom that must be gross to be marked as morbid for, in a milder form, it 'may appear to be readily recognizable in some of one's colleagues' as Wing and colleagues (1974, p. 186) lament. Words may acquire a private meaning that is lexically unknown, phrases and phrasing may become stilted to the point of caricature, and verbal novelties and monstrosities (*neologisms*) can make their appearance.

Delusions.

Delusions are not simply false beliefs. Such a naive notion might justify us in regarding as deluded the followers of religious, political, or scientific creeds and doctrines which are alien to the system of beliefs we hold to be true. Beliefs which are collectively held, however absurd they may appear to the outsider, are not morbid phenomena; they are not delusions in a psychiatric sense.

The delusions of psychiatric patients are not just strong beliefs; they are convictions of absolute certainty. They are, for the most part, unshared. Only occasionally are they shared with one or the other close associate who then exhibits *induced delusions* so that clinically a *'folie à deux* or *à trois,* etc.' exists (see Gralnick, 1942). Delusions are the hallmark of most psychotic diseases whether due to schizophrenic, manic-depressive, dementing, or other pathological processes. I propose to characterize delusions as convictions of the truth of a proposition which are *absolute, idiosyncratic, ego-involved, incorrigible,* and often *preoccupying.* They are absolute because they are beyond any shadow of doubt; they are idiosyncratic because they are unshared; they are ego-involved because they are of sensitive personal significance to the patient; they are incorrigible because they resist all powers of persuasion, coercion, or brain washing (though they are amenable to electric shock treatment or psychotropic drugs); they are preoccupying during the active phase of a psychosis, when they almost totally monopolize a patient's mind.

Delusions are not always without factual justification. There are some which happen to be *self-verifying delusions,* especially in a social context. This applies chiefly to paranoid patients whose delusions convince them that their health, reputation or property is damaged by the underhand malevolence of relatives or neighbours. If they then harass those involved through accusations or chicanery, they may provoke the very signs of enmity they had delusionally anticipated.

Some delusions arise without apparent precipitation as happens, for instance, when a patient is suddenly gripped by a *delusional mood* which creates an eerie *delusional atmosphere* in the world around him so that it becomes pregnant with new meanings which the patient may be unable to decipher. Sometimes a dubious distinction is made between such 'primary' delusions which seem to occur *de novo* and 'secondary' delusions which are credited with causal precursors. Certainly delusions can be associated with other mental phenomena, though which comes first is often mere guesswork. Many delusions are, for example, associated with a morbidly altered mood, either emerging from it or responsible for it. There are *grandiose delusions* (being of royal connection, exceptional wealth or genius, having a religious or political mission); *delusions of unworthiness* (having lost one's fortune, reputation or ability, being guilty, culpable or condemned); *hypochondriacal delusions* (having organic lesions and deformities, often of a bizarre nature); *delusions of persecution* (being victimized, harassed, or poisoned by anonymous or known persons or by scapegoat groups such as the Government, Communists, Jews, Freemasons, etc.); *delusions of reference* (seeing ego-involved meanings of a sinister or helpful kind in the most ordinary events in the environment, newspapers, radio, etc.); *delusions of jealousy* (searching for evidence and confession of a tormenting foregone conviction of infidelity, and twisting trivial findings into incontestable proofs); *erotic delusions* (of being passionately loved by a person of social standing or some frequently encountered stranger – with embarrassing consequences, when the unsuspecting fantasy lover is assured that his feelings are reciprocated – *'de Clérambault syndrome'* (Clérambault, 1942)).

Some delusions seem to originate in self-deceptive efforts to explain certain morbid experiences: delusions of *thought insertion* (to explain thoughts the patient rejects as alien); delusions of *thought withdrawal* (to explain poverty of thought or thought blocking); delusions of *influence* (or *control* or *passivity*) (to explain the patient's feeling that he is no longer fully master of his thoughts and actions); delusions of *thought dissemination* (to explain the patient's delusion that his thoughts are somehow known to others).

The various delusions that are held by a patient may be inconsistent and contradictory or they may be built up into a logically coherent system (*systematized delusions*). They may interfere with many aspects of his life and make him difficult, combative, contentious, and sometimes tenaciously litigious. Yet eventually, when a chronic phase of the illness is reached, delusions may become dormant so that they come to light only on special enquiries.

Morbid disorders of affect.

In normal circumstances, emotional reactions to particular experiences are understandable to people sharing the same cultural background. In our culture it is understandable that people feel grief and sorrow on bereavement, joy after a happy event or windfall, anger at insults, fear in danger situations, and so on. Yet even understandable emotions can have a morbid significance. They can be too *explosive* or *dramatic* in persons with an uninhibited or histrionic bent; they can be too *labile* in patients with organic dementia so that they vacillate between tears, laughter, and annoyance in response to changing thoughts and circumstances; they can be *perplexed* and *bewildered,* when demented patients cannot orient themselves in their environment and when schizophrenic patients in the early phases of their illness are overwhelmed by puzzling new experiences.

When emotional reactions to the brutalities of combat are blunted in battle-hardened troops, we can to some extent understand this, considering their training and habituation. But understanding and empathy boggle in the case of *affectionless psychopaths* who remain unmoved by the havoc and suffering they inflict in their uncaring pursuit of selfish desires or in the case of schizophrenics with such *poverty of emotions* that they remain stolidly apathetic to discomfort, hardship, incontinence, and filth. More circumscribed forms of emotional non-response occur in patients with hysterical symptoms from which some real or imagined gain is derived. They accept their often considerable handicaps with bland equanimity (*'belle indifférence'*).

Our understanding of emotional reactions fails completely, when they occur without apparent reason or incitement, are at variance with those normally expected in the circumstances, or arise from a groundswell of morbid mood. There are no apparent reasons for the *mirthless giggles* of socially withdrawn schizophrenics, for the *foolish cheerfulness* or *senseless spite* of some of them, or the unexpected outbursts of violence and destructiveness in catatonic and epileptic patients (*catatonic hyperkinesis, epileptic furor*).

Emotional reactions which are at variance with normal expectations occur in many psychiatric illnesses. For instance, patients with phobias of objectively and culturally harmless objects and events are shaken by an incapacitating fear on exterocepting them and yet they know that fear to be contrary to normal expectations, to be so senseless and often so ridiculous that they try to hide or camouflage it, unless it happens to be widely shared, such as the fear of heights, mice, or spiders. Patients with intense depressions or elations of mood may similarly react abnormally to events in their surroundings, because their feelings follow their moods. Yet this is not invariably so. Lewis (1934), for example, found that 'twenty-four [of his sixty-one depressed] patients seemed to show almost average or normal adaptation to their surroundings'. An unexpected *incongruity of affect* of a shallow and half-hearted kind is sometimes seen in young schizophrenics who smirk on receiving sad news or look dejected on learning of something cheerful and heartening. Another paradoxical emotional reaction which should be more widely known and respected, as this can save clinicians many an unpleasant experience, is the explo-sive response of paranoid patients to an encouraging and friendly smile which they suspect to be a sign of ridicule and derision.

Morbid moods differ from morbid emotional reactions in that they are not evoked by overtly observable events, but have an endogenous biochemical origin. This limits the extent to which they can be psychologically understood, though attempts at such an understanding are always made since they satisfy a human need. Morbid moods can occur in schizophrenic patients and obscure the clinical picture, but most schizophrenic moods have a different derivation because they arise in association with prevailing delusions or hallucinations. In epileptic patients, and especially those with temporal-lobe lesions, moods can make their appearance and range from depressions of potentially suicidal intensity, rage of potentially homicidal violence, through irritability and anxiety to feelings of ecstatic happiness and mystic joy. Morbid moods which can be diagnostically misleading, running the gamut from depression, anxiety, hypochondriacal worry, and anger to elation, occur also in diseases whose primary pathological basis is not an endogenous biochemical disturbance in the brain, e.g. in hypo- or hyperthyroidism, general paralysis of the insane, multiple sclerosis, brain tumours, and so on.

In the group of *manic-depressive diseases*, morbid moods of an endogenous biochemical origin in the brain make up the pathological core.

In *severe depressions*, patients are engulfed by a mood of gloom, despair, and dejection. There are those who sit quietly and silently in their hopeless misery (*retarded depressions*) and others who are continually distraught, loud in their moans, and importunate in their urge to give voice to their worries and terrors (*agitated depressions*). Their delusions and hallucinations harp on their many acts of wickedness and depravity, and they portray vividly the irrevocable doom and lingering horror that is in store for them and their families so that only suicide, coupled perhaps with the murder of those dear to them, seems to offer a merciful way out. But *delusions and hallucinations of guilt and deserved punishment* are not the only psychotic manifestations in severe depressions. In Lewis's (1934) sample of patients, for instance, the majority also showed *delusions of reference* (people showing their contempt of them, jeering at them, avoiding them) and *of persecution* (being spied upon, poisoned, harassed). Certainly critical denouncement is not always exclusively self-directed, but can spill over into querulous and abusive attitudes towards others. Even elements of cheerfulness need not be totally absent in severe depressions, though it is usually of the gallow's-humour kind and any smile connected with it does not hide the sadness of the eyes. Patients who do not respond to treatment and are determined on suicide may even succeed in completely dissimulating their real mood and adopting instead a deceptive air of genial normality. For the most part, however, when a depression is of psychotic severity, the correct diagnosis can hardly be missed, though this sometimes happens in elderly patients, if their clinical manifestations of retardation and self-neglect resemble superficially those of senile dementia.

In *mild depressions,* the correct diagnosis can be easily overlooked, when the fundamental mood disturbance is masked by more prominent symptoms. Many patients may then be regarded as having a personality defect, a neurotic illness, or some obscure non-psychiatric ailment whose identification defies the diagnostic efforts of a great many specialists consulted. Yet diagnostic mistakes in these patients can be fatal because of the everpresent risk of suicide. Sainsbury (1968) examined the literature on suicide in affective disorders and found that reliable follow-up studies agreed in indicating an average suicide incidence of 15 per cent; that is, every sixth patient with a diagnosis of depression will thus end his life. The incidence is likely to be smaller in undiagnosed depressives, but it can certainly not be regarded as negligible. As one of the measures of suicide prevention, Sainsbury stressed the importance of recognizing and adequately treating depressions.

Among the main features of mildly or moderately depressed patients is their inability to enjoy anything either all day and every day or only in the mornings or evenings, because there is a marked diurnal variation of mood. Interest in work and hobbies flags. Energy, concentration, and initiative is at a low ebb so that the patients cannot bring themselves to carry on with a job that has come to overtax them, even if it is a familiar routine job or the daily round of housework and caring for children. They lack self-confidence, feel criticized, and are indecisive, pessimistic, and often full of hypochondriacal complaints (Kenyon, 1976). They tend to be indolent and self-centred at home, as well as ill-tempered and irritable so that they are difficult to live with. The tolerance of their spouses and other home companions is furthermore sorely tried, when the patients get animated and genial with visitors or at evening parties. Their sleep patterns are usually disturbed in one way or another by wakeful interruptions of sleep or anxiety dreams, early arousal in the morning, somnolence or naps during the day, or difficulty in falling asleep at night. Their appetite tends to recede, though some overeat for comfort; their bowels may become sluggish, and occasionally an irritable bowel syndrome develops with abdominal pain and distension which are relieved by a bowel motion.

Feelings of depersonalization and derealization can be very troublesome. Even more disturbing can be attacks of anxiety which are sometimes no more than vague feelings of apprehension, but they can swell to an onslaught of terror-stricken panic. There may be no obvious reason for these emotions or they may be precipitated by particular situations or the anticipation of them so that the clinical picture is dominated by such phobias as leaving home, going to school, meeting people, and the like. But the converse of anxiety is also often noticeable, namely a foolhardy search for hazards and risks. Children may engage in antisocial activities (Rutter, 1966; Shaffer, 1974), middle-aged women go on shoplifting expeditions (Gibbens & Prince, 1962; Gibbens *et al.*, 1971), and car drivers get involved in reckless accidents (Eelkema *et al.*, 1970).

The libido of mildly depressed patients is usually low or absent. In that case, the sex life of men comes to a halt, whereas women tend to show signs of sexual aversion and avoidance or only submit passively to the demands of a sexual partner out of duty or to avoid scenes. Sometimes, however, such passive submission is made impossible through the development of an over-powering phobia of the sexual advances of the partner (Taylor, 1978). It can also happen that libido which has been dormant towards a routine partner is roused by a stranger perhaps through the spice of novelty or the comfort of finding warmth and understanding in a person in contrast to the animosity of a sexually frustrated partner. Sometimes the newly roused libido kindles an intense infatuation which persists, even if the sexual attachment is only one-sided and therefore a source of great torment. One is then reminded of the imprinting processes that have been described in birds by Lorenz (1935, 1958) and other ethologists. All these complications in the love and sex life of mild depressives deserve more attention than they have so far received, for their consequences can be disastrous to the stability of a patient's marriage or marriages.

In *severe manic moods,* a turmoil of ideo-motor activity overwhelms the patients and shakes their environment. They are on the go without pause, flitting from one task to another without completing any, continually disrupting even their meals and toilet. All this is accompanied by incessant talk that is loud and boisterous, showing flights of ideas and such pressure of vocalization that words may be strung together without reason, though perhaps with rhyme and punning, interspersed with laughter, singing, or just roaring. But voice alone has not enough decibels for the patients. They must also create a cacophonous din by banging, clapping, stamping, and other hullabaloo. They address all and sundry, interfering with them, usually in an infectious spirit of jovial hilarity. They can, however, also be domineering and demanding, pushing and ordering people about, flaring up in anger when thwarted or contradicted, and hurling insults, curses, blows, and missiles at their opponents. But these outbursts are short-lived, leaving no resentment behind, at least in the patients whose attention veers away to new targets and some new emotion, perhaps even an occasional maudlin sob. They need little sleep so that their nights are as restless and disturbing as their days. Their self-confidence and conceit knows no bounds, they feel supreme physically and mentally, and are full of wild and grandiose ideas which have a delusional flair, but for the fact that they are neither incorrigible nor preoccupying because they are too ephemeral to become fixed. Their energy seems inexhaustible but, without proper treatment, they eventually exhaust themselves through lack of sufficient food, rest, and sleep, and sink into an emaciated, enfeebled, and confused state that is life-threatening.

Hypomanic moods may cause great havoc to the reputation of patients who may be mistakenly denounced as having character defects of irresponsibility, dissipation, recklessness, and trickery. Even when the correct diagnosis has been made, there will be great difficulties in persuading the patients to accept the medical and legal measures needed to save what is left of their financial resources and their standing as reliable and sensible citizens. The patients are bubbling over with enterprise and new ideas, they need only a few hours of sleep so that they can extend their days into late-night activities. They rush into risky ventures, bypassing any irksome restraints of law and custom. They waste money on extravagant purchases and generous gifts. They are sure they know the answer to all social problems and often send reams of advice to the powers that be. They enjoy life in a spirit of self-confident good humour, they are expansive in their gestures and conversation, and often eccentric and even grotesque in their dress and adornments. They are forward in their approach to strangers, radiating *bonhomie,* but their remarks are often so personal as to give offence and their wit can be biting. Often they are overbearing and inconsiderate. They blunder into legal, social, and financial troubles which they disregard or disavow. Their appetites are keen, including their libido, so that sexual licence and promiscuity add their share to a prodigal life.

When an euphoric mood remains within the limits of normality by population standards (*hyperthymic mood*) and does not override the counsels of caution and judgment, we are not dealing with a morbid state, but with a fortunate condition that enhances a person's vivacity, creativity, and aesthetic sensitivity. As a result, his fortunes flourish and his achievements can be high, especially in the spheres of business enterprise, music, literature, and other artistic pursuits. Many people whose later mood swings reach morbid dimensions have laid sound foundations of prosperity and repute in their own circles or the wider world during preceding hyperthymic periods.

Neurotic anxieties are often defined as anxieties which are objectively unjustified. This would, however, include anxieties aroused by a false alarm, such as a bomb hoax, or by the infringement of some culturally or religiously prescribed taboo (Steiner, 1956). It therefore seems preferable to stipulate that anxieties should be regarded as neurotic only when patients are subjectively aware that their feelings are totally or largely unjustified and would be ridiculed or denounced as senseless by other people. For this reason it is an almost invariable feature of neurotic anxieties that patients do their utmost to hide them from strangers.

Neurotic anxieties vary in intensity from mild unease to terror-stricken panic. There is also a wide variation in the stimuli precipitating them in different patients. In some patients, there are no subjectively perceived precipitating stimuli. Their anxieties well up out of the blue; they are *free-floating* in the sense that the patients are not anxious of anything in particular. They are, in Brentano's (1874) terminology, act-phenomena without any object-phenomena. Such anxieties give rise either to a persistent *anxiety state* or to *anxiety attacks* which afflict a patient unexpectedly and then die away gradually (Walker, 1959). Illnesses characterized by free-floating anxieties are usually self-limiting, but may recur. Most of the patients concerned also show signs of a depressive mood swing and are usually amenable to antidepressant medication.

Neurotic anxieties which are precipitated by particular stimuli are known as *'phobias'* and the stimuli (objects, events, situations) precipitating them have the epithet 'phobic'. The clinical manifestations of phobias are manifold, depending on their development, the particular phobic stimuli involved, and their complexity (Marks & Gelder, 1966; Marks, 1969, 1970). There are phobias which are precipitated by only one or two specific stimuli (*specific phobias*), leaving the patient symptom-free in their absence. Such phobias usually make their first appearance in childhood before the age of eight. Examples are phobias of certain animals or insects, of heights, thunder, or darkness. Many of these continue into adulthood, especially in urban women. Yet they need occasion little inconvenience, even if they are of common occurrence, such as the phobias of mice, spiders, or harmless snakes. Less common specific phobias can, however, cause considerable embarrassment to patients who, for instance, find themselves obliged to cross a busy road rather than pass a pigeon in their path or to run from a room, because there is a moth in it. There are occasional specific phobias which do not date back to childhood. They may emerge after a traumatic experience in adult life (e.g. being bitten by a dog or scratched by a cat) or when a free-floating panic attack happens to overwhelm a patient in an unusual environment which thereafter has to be avoided.

Specific phobias behave clinically like ingrained habits of behaviour and emotional response which had been established through classical or operant conditioning procedures (Pavlov, 1927; Skinner, 1938, 1953). They are immune to exhortation or an appeal to reason and will-power. Yet they are often amenable to deconditioning procedures, such as systematic forms of desensitization (Gelder & Marks, 1966; Gelder *et al.*, 1973).

Phobias of a clinically different kind occur in patients who are sensitive to constellations of several phobic stimuli (Snaith, 1968). Such *multiple phobias* constitute illnesses which have a different pathological background from that of specific phobias. The illnesses have their onset after puberty and tend to run a recurrent or fluctuating course. Among their symptoms are not only phobias but also depressive moods, obsessions, and feelings of depersonalization and derealization. The phobic constellations in these illnesses are of two overlapping kinds which are distinguished as agoraphobias and social phobias.

The term *'agoraphobia'* is misleading. It means literally a fear of the market place or open spaces. But this is merely one facet of a phobic constellation which can include several other fears, such as of crowds, shop assistants, bridges, enclosed spaces (lifts, tubes, locked bathroom doors, closed bedroom windows), the sight of blood or vomit, being unable to escape easily from a situation (a moving train, having to wait in queues or waiting rooms, sitting still at the hairdresser's or dentist's, having a seat in the middle of a row in a theatre or similar public gathering), being overcome in inconvenient situations by a compelling urge to urinate or defaecate (a fear which may become self-verifying), or having to admit and confide these and similar phobias to strangers, and these may include psychiatrists with whom no close psychotherapeutic relationship has been formed. The majority of agoraphobic patients are women and there are some who become totally housebound. Their condition may be aggravated, if they also have a fear of being alone in their home. In the company of trusted persons, agoraphobic patients may be able to set out on short expeditions. Some patients are enabled to sidestep their fear of walking in the street, if they can push a bicycle, pram, or shopping trolley. Even longer excursions are possible, when no walking is involved, but only a ride on a bicycle or a drive in a car with the patients in the driving seat, feeling reassured that they can quickly return to the safety of their homes in case of need.

Social phobias urge patients to avoid, if at all possible, any situation which causes them to believe without objective evidence that they have become conspicuous, have attracted criticism, or have invited ridicule and contempt. There may be a fear of making a spectacle of themselves in public, perhaps through fainting, vomiting, or committing some social gaffe. Even signing their signature in the presence of possible watchers can be an ordeal, and the same may be the case with any other skilled performance in similar circumstances (e.g. walking, singing, or playing a game). Entering a well-lit public place (restaurant, bar, theatre) or just going out during daylight may be difficult or impossible. Passing a queue of people can cause acute embarrassment and sitting opposite other persons (e.g. on tubes or buses) may be studiously avoided, unless it is possible to hide behind a newspaper. Patients may even shy away from their own reflections in a mirror or shop window. If the phobia is one of eye contact with other people, patients may take to wearing dark glasses. Stage fright, which to a minor degree is normal in public performers, may become so overwhelming as to cut short or temporarily interrupt a stage career. Similarly, a phobia of examinations may ruin promising academic prospects. Fear of speaking in public is a very common social phobia, but there are also patients whose main or sole difficulty lies in talking to individuals. Such patients also often have a fear of blushing, trembling, behaving awkwardly, or making inept remarks and such fear may well be self-verifying.

There is some association between multiple phobias and depressive illness (Schapira *et al.*, 1970). This may explain why patients tend to respond favourably to an antidepressant medication consisting of a monoamine oxidase inhibitor, perhaps combined with a benzodiazepine, during the day and, if necessary, amitriptyline or trimipramine up to 150 mg at night (Sargant, 1969; Kelly *et al.*, 1970).

Psychological approaches have, of course, also an effect. However, systematic desensitization is certainly of much less avail in multiple phobias than in specific ones (Gelder & Marks, 1966; Gelder *et al.*, 1973). Yet the psychotherapeutic (or 'behavioural') method known as 'flooding' or 'implosion' has a fair chance of achieving results despite the distress it causes the patient (Boulougouris *et al.*, 1971). Other distressing situations in which the patients suffer humiliation and intimidation without respite have also shown themselves capable of removing or greatly alleviating multiple phobias. This was noticed in Nazi concentration camps. Kral (1952), for instance, reported from one such camp in Theresienstadt in which there were only 20 000 survivors among 140 000 inmates that phobic symptoms 'either disappeared completely or improved to such a degree that the patients could work', though the incidence of psychoses seemed unchanged. After the war, 'some of the old neurotics who had been free of complaints during their stay in the camp again developed their former symptoms'. On the other hand, when agoraphobic patients are not continually terrorized, the fear of a panic attack can prove stronger than the fear of some real danger. This was shown during the bombardment of cities in the Second World War, when agoraphobic patients often preferred the danger of being killed in their homes to their suffering phobic agonies in the relative safety of overcrowded public shelters.

Not all phobic stimuli exist in the environment and elicit fear reactions on being exterocepted. There are also phobic stimuli that exist in the mind as introspected phenomena. These can, however, become phobic stimuli only if their contemplation cannot be avoided or evaded; that is, if they cannot be banished from consciousness, but force themselves upon a patient's attention so that he is obsessed by them against his will and striving. Introspected phobic stimuli are therefore *obsessional* (or *obsessive*) *symptoms*. Since this can only happen when the introspected stimuli have an overwhelming intrusive compulsion to be contemplated, the symptoms are often also termed '*obsessive-compulsive*'.

Anticipatory obsessional symptoms occur in phobic patients as a reaction to the realization that they will have to face a phobic situation. Amateur actors, for instance, with a moderate social phobia in the form of a manageable stage fright know such anticipatory obsessions only too well. Days before the date of their performance, they are in the grip of anxious persistent thoughts and images of the anticipated event of their appearing on the stage. Similarly, an agoraphobic patient who knows he will have to leave his home, perhaps for an urgent visit to his dentist, will be obsessed for hours beforehand by fearful imaginings of the dreaded excursion. Anticipatory obsessive symptoms are thus reactive phenomena which are limited in time, as they vanish when there is no longer the prospect of encountering an environmental phobic stimulus.

Primary obsessional symptoms are of much graver clinical import. They are not dependent on environmental precipitations, though they can be aggravated by feared environmental situations. They invade a patient's mental life unbidden and unwanted, to monopolize it stubbornly for many months and often years. They may be thoughts, images, or impulses of a trivial and futile kind which are exasperating only through their nagging and time-wasting persistence. They may, however, also be of an objectionable and repulsive kind, running counter to a patient's strict moral and religious principles. Such obsessional preoccupations function as phobic stimuli, rousing obstinate and merciless fears in a patient that he may somehow divulge them in word or overt action.

The compulsion exerted by obsessional preoccupations is recognized by the patients as a product of some unwelcome part of their own minds. This distinguishes obsessional compulsions from the compulsions experienced by schizophrenic patients with delusions of influence and passivity, because those compulsions are attributed to the malevolent machinations of external agencies. An obsessional compulsion is also known as 'anankastic', a term borrowed from German psychiatric literature where it was originally introduced by Donath (1897), because the German word for 'compulsion' ('Zwang') has no suitable adjective. For a feeling of compulsion, an anankastic feeling, to be obsessional in a psychiatric sense three criteria are required: (1) it must be a compulsion to introspect thoughts, images or impulses – or at least associated with such a compulsion; (2) it must be a distressing compulsion; and (3) there must be a genuine effort to resist the compulsion, however ineffectual the effort turns out to be.

If any one of these criteria is absent in a clinical manifestation, then it is not an obsessional psychiatric symptom. (1) There are compulsive automatic activities which are not associated with any conscious compulsion to enact them. Examples are such non-obsessional symptoms as tics, spasmodic torticollis, dystonia, dyskinesia, akathisia, mannerisms, perseverations, and the like. (2) There are compulsive introspective activities which are not distressing. Examples are such non-obsessional manifestations as the melodies, rhymes, or sayings which harmlessly monopolize a person's mind for a while, or the incessant thoughts and fantasies about a passionately loved person or a fanatically espoused cause. (3) There are compulsive preoccupations which are not, or hardly, resisted because they satisfy an overriding urge. Examples are found among sexual offenders, alcoholics, gamblers, among patients with forceful delusions of a depressive, paranoid or jealous kind, or among people with the self-absorbing interests of ardent collectors, scientists, inventors, or problem solvers of any sort.

The three criteria mentioned, however, characterize only morbid obsessional *symptoms*, they do not characterize non-morbid obsessional *traits*. These are not compulsive; they are *prescriptive* in the sense that they oblige a person to conduct himself rigidly within the confines of the moral and legal standards collectively sanctioned by his society, or rather the society of his choice. The enforced compliance with these standards is not distressing; on the contrary, it conveys a feeling of righteous satisfaction. Nor is there a resistance against the compliance, only against any deviation from it, and this resistance is coupled with narrow-minded condemnations of any deviant and an urge to subject him to punitive methods of correction.

There are two kinds of persons in whom obsessional traits predominate, two kinds of *obsessional personalities*. There are those who are *extrapunitive*; they are stern and inflexible task masters who feel bound to model others into copies of their own law-abiding self-assurance. There are others who are *intrapunitive*; they are self-critical in their constant urge always to find the best choice among alternative possibilities and they become indecisive and unsure of themselves. Among the traits that can be found additionally in both kinds of obsessional personalities are those of orderliness and tidiness (at least in some areas of their lives), precision, pedantry, punctuality, diligence, perseverance, caution, and other characteristics of a disciplined and upright citizen. In practice, of course, there are no such paragons of all social virtues, since even the most obsessional of persons is bound to have his aberrations from immaculate grace.

Obsessional symptoms can occur in persons who had no obsessional traits beforehand. They are, however, often associated with such traits. In that case, obsessional symptoms which are not just trivial and futile, but are of an objectionable nature are doubly distressing, because they run counter to the strict principles of an obsessional personality, forcing on him the contemplation of mental phenomena which are not just introspected phobic stimuli but also arouse feelings of deep guilt, disgust, and revulsion. They infringe his rigid canons of religion, morality, hygiene, and modesty. Examples are blasphemous thoughts, obscene images, impulses to steal, to harm people, to engage in sexual transgressions, to make contact with dirty and germ-carrying articles, to shout aloud to the world at large the wicked thoughts he entertains or to reveal them more stealthily, perhaps in a forgotten whisper to a stranger or through some absent-mindedly scribbled note. The patients' helpless subjection to the compulsive sway of their obsessions awakens in them superstitious beliefs in the magic power of thoughts which may come true, like evil charms and spells. The patients may thus be racked by interminable doubts about the consequences of their sinister mental experiences. Have they betrayed them? Have they given in to them in an unguarded moment? Have the thoughts worked a wicked magic? The patients may be driven to ransack their memories of every moment of their waking day. But can they be sure they have not committed a somnambulistic crime?

Obsessive symptoms are not entirely independent of environmental conditions. They can be aggravated by particular situations and observations. A church service may give rise to a plague of blasphemous thoughts, the sight of a baby in a pram evoke the idea of strangling it, pins on the floor or some sharp instrument in the neighbourhood can suggest the thought of injuring people with them, writing material on a desk can rouse the impulse to pen a scurrilous or libellous message, passing an unkempt stranger may excite fears of having been soiled and contaminated, and there are endless other environmental sources of obsessional torment. Patients with phobias of a particular environmental situation can allay their fears, if they can get away from it. This expedient is, however, not open to obsessional patients. Even when they remove themselves from an obsession-rousing situation, they remain prey to the fears and doubts in their minds.

Lewis (1957) has suggested that obsessional symptoms should be divided into primary and secondary phenomena, the latter being of a defensive nature aimed at preventing or relieving the distress suffered. 'An example', he said, 'would be first the insistent feeling that one is dirty – that is the primary phenomenon; and then there is the impulse to wash – the secondary phenomenon in order to obtain relief from the primary disturbance'. These secondary phenomena usually have their origin in a superstitious pact made by the patients with themselves to outwit their obsessions which they cannot fight directly. The pact involves the performance of some mental or physical activity endowed with the good-luck hope of a gambler's wishful thinking. This may work at first and then it turns into a ritual which has to be enacted, even if its success becomes variable. Failures are blamed on inaccuracies and flaws in the performance of the ritual. As a result, rituals have to be repeated again and again until a 'lucky' number has been reached or they have finally been cleared of imperfections. Thus they become time-consuming, strenuous, and even desperate compulsions which can be greater ordeals than the original obsessions which they had been designed to combat.

Some rituals are purely mental performances. Prayers, phrases, or words of purely private meaning may have to be repeated a prescribed number of times in flawless forms, images may have to be conjured to a specified degree of clarity, events of the day may have to pass a searching review, futile questions (e.g. about the meaning of life or the nature of nothingness) may have to be revolved in the mind interminably, and there are many other compulsive ruminations and preoccupations. Many of these mental rituals have to be performed in absolute privacy, because any interruption or distraction might spoil their superstitious spell so that the despairing patient has to begin the exasperating ritual task all over again.

There are also many motor rituals. Some consist in repetitive doing–undoing activities, such as putting on and taking off a garment several times. The routine activities of daily life thus take an inordinately long time. Patients may have to get up in the early hours of the morning to meet some deadline during the day. It may literally take hours before they can emerge from the lavatory or their bedrooms and it can take hours again before they reach their beds in the evening after a prolonged ritual of undressing and of arranging their clothes in some strictly prescribed order. For most of these motor rituals, the patients seek privacy and some of them can be completely hidden from other household members, such as their often complicated and embarrassing lavatory antics. Motor rituals which are performed in public view are usually camouflaged so that they can escape the notice of casual onlookers. A patient, for instance, who has to walk three times through an entrance will take good care to remain inconspicuous. Patients with a compulsion to touch, say, every lamp post they pass are generally not quite as successful in escaping attention. It was, for example, widely known that Dr Samuel Johnson had to touch every post on his way and was forced to retrace his steps if a post had been missed.

Among the most common and the most harassing rituals are those of compulsive washing which leave their victims with permanently chapped and sore hands, and the rituals of compulsive checking which (to give just two examples) enforce endless scrutinies of letters written to ensure the absence of howlers or forbidden material, or drive patients on endless errands every night to ensure that everything is safely locked, closed, and turned off, to be followed perhaps by a compulsive mental recall of everything done on the errand and a repetition of the errand should the mental recall raise doubts about its fullest adequacy. There are also checking procedures which involve the co-operation of another person who may have to reassure the patient that sharp instruments are inaccessible to him or that there is no contraband in his pockets, such as perhaps pen or paper or stolen goods. The rituals of children may have to be carried out with the active participation of one or both parents, even when there is no checking needed.

Compulsive rituals remain, for the most part, within the limits of propriety and can therefore be performed without risk to the patients' health and reputation. But there are rare exceptions, when motor compulsions carry such risks. Examples are the licking of bathroom floors, tasting one's urine, touching a stranger's bottom, lifting a girl's skirts, or stealing some article from a shop and then perhaps returning it by post. Motor compulsions of this kind are strongly resisted by patients until they are occasionally forced to submit.

It would be a mistake to regard all repetitive activities as obsessive-compulsive rituals. They may be no more than signs of boredom or institutionalization. The rituals of children are often only playful games indulged in and repeated for their very pleasure. There is, however, one variety of childhood rituals that deserves special mention. These rituals are those associated with *imaginary companions* (Svendsen, 1934; Bender & Vogel, 1941) with whom children enter into repetitive make-belief plays. There certainly is a general tendency for the games of children to become ritualized, as the researches of Opie and Opie (1959) into childhood lore and language have shown.

It happens occasionally that the anticipatory obsessional symptoms of a phobic patient become independent of the anticipation of the external phobic situation. The patient then feels compelled, irrespective of circumstances, to contemplate encountering the external phobic situation, is distressed by this compulsion, and tries ineffectually to resist it. In other words, the compulsion has all the three criteria of an obsessional one. The anticipatory obsessional symptom has turned into a primary obsessional symptom. It can then also happen that the patient develops a defensive ritual against this obsession. In some instances, this ritual consists in a self-daring compulsion to approach the external phobic situation as closely as possible. Such a *counterphobic compulsion* may lead to a prolonged to-and-fro ritual of approach and retreat with the result that the patient spends a great deal of his time in the vicinity of the external phobic situation. On rare occasions, such compul-

sions have a therapeutic outcome through a gradual desensitization against the phobia. A patient with a past phobia of deep water may then turn into an accomplished (and perhaps even enthusiastic) swimmer or sailor, and a patient with a past phobia of public speaking may eventually grasp every opportunity of addressing an audience.

Patients with self-damaging addictions are the victims of compulsions which are not obsessional because they are more self-indulgent than distressing and because resistance against them is either absent or weak-willed. Such *compulsive addictions* are liable to play havoc with a patient's life. In his soberminded moments, he may recoil from the dismal prospect of remaining helplessly and hopelessly subservient to his cravings. He may then firmly resolve to renounce them utterly in future. Such resolve is unfortunately only too likely to falter and fail. Yet its existence lends an air of resemblance to the quandaries of patients fighting addictive cravings unsuccessfully or obsessional compulsions equally unsuccessfully. Yet the resemblance is misleading and may be overstressed. For example, in describing the syndrome of *alcohol dependence*, Edwards and Gross (1976) state that 'the subjective experience of dependence may come close to fulfilling the classic conditions for a diagnosis of compulsion. The desire for a further drink is seen as irrational, the desire is resisted, but the further drink is taken'. The difference is that the compulsion of alcohol dependence is not obsessional; it is not sufficiently distressing and anxiety-dominated to oust the lure of the addiction and the craving for self-indulgence. There is also the difference that alcohol dependence does not give rise to secondary obsessional phenomena in the form of superstitious and compulsive rituals to combat a craving that is in due course more desired than dreaded.

The same irresolute and weak-willed form of resistance occurs in other addictions which have a compulsive, though non-obsessional, element. In the addiction of *compulsive* (or *pathological*) *gambling,* there is a further similarity with obsessional symptoms in that superstitious rituals can occur. But these rituals are performed to invoke good luck rather than to obviate bad thoughts. Moran (1970a,b) mentions as one indicator that gambling has become pathological the realization by the patient of his ambivalent attitude towards it 'so that whilst being longed for, it was also dreaded, since it had become irresistible'. Other indicators were an intermittent or continuous preoccupation with the thought of gambling; loss of control once gambling had started; economic, social, and psychological difficulties caused by gambling, such as debts, loss of employment, social uprooting, criminality, imprisonment, marital problems, depressions, suicidal attempts, and the like.

Similar remarks with appropriate modifications apply to other kinds of compulsive addictions, such as addictions to drugs, food, and sexual objects and practices.

In most drug addictions (including that to alcohol), a physical dependence on the drug develops (in addition to the psychological one), because biochemical changes arise which make abstinence unbearable and even a potential danger to life. In such circumstances, any psychological resistance against the addictive compulsion is a forlorn hope from the start. Only a gradual and carefully controlled regime of withdrawal is possible and has a chance to succeed, if a patient can muster a sufficiently determined resistance. Glatt (1974) has reviewed addictive drugs and the kinds of dependence they engender. Among those which induce no physical dependence are cocaine, cannabis, LSD, amphetamine, and perhaps nicotine.

Glatt (1974) has also considered addictions which do not involve drugs. Among these was *food addiction* (or *compulsive overeating*). It differs from the habitual overeating of obese persons. Genuine food addicts are in some respects similar to alcohol addicts. They are both past masters in deceiving themselves and others with regard to the amounts they consume; they hide food and sweets in secret places and indulge in clandestine eating binges. When a compulsive eater is put on a strict slimming diet, he suffers withdrawal symptoms with obsessional images of meals, irritability, anxiety, tension, fatigue, and other signs of deprived cravings.

Sexual cravings are not usually classified among addictions. Yet they can arouse the same compulsive preoccupations as are found in other addictive conditions. The power of such sexual cravings (infatuations, 'crushes', feelings of passionate love) is revealed by the hours spent in thinking and dreaming of the loved one, the signs of genital arousal, and the stratagems devised to be near him or her. When there are no prohibitions of conscience or social code against such cravings, there need be no resistance against them apart from restraining their too overt display. When there are such prohibitions, there will be resistances of the same irresolute and vacillating kind

as are present in other addictions. If there are insurmountable obstacles to the gratifications of sexual cravings, the patients will suffer the same torments as any other psychologically dependent and frustrated addicts. As these conditions have not received special mention in modern psychiatric treatises, though they fill pages in many novels, let me quote the rather hyperbolic remarks of Robert Burton in his *Anatomy of Melancholy* (1641): 'The symptoms of the mind in lovers are almost infinite; ... love is a plague, a torture, an hell, a bitter sweet passion at last; ... the Spanish Inquisition is not comparable to it'. When there are obstacles of social propriety which are overcome by hook or crook, the consequences can be disastrous to health, marital stability, or personal reputation and fortune.

The sexual urges of human beings have many interwoven aspects and something often goes wrong with them. They may not be in harmony with each other or some aspect may assume a form that is unusual by population standards, though not necessarily morbid. Yet *unusual sexual cravings* pose many medical, social, and legal problems. In considering them, three main components and their interrelations have to be taken into account: gender role, sexually stimulating objects, and sexual practices.

A child's *gender role* is almost invariably decided at birth by the appearance of its external genitalia. In intersexual states (Bishop, 1966), however, mistakes can be made in diagnosing a child's actual sex, i.e. the sex of its gonads and/or chromosomal karyotype. The gender role assigned to such a child usually determines its later sexual preferences. They will, in all probability, be in accordance with its gender role rather than its actual sex, if there is a discrepancy between the two. In that case, the erotic partners chosen later in life will tend to be of opposite gender but of the same sex. A sexual male, for instance, brought up as a girl will be drawn towards male partners. But the wrong gender role can cause trouble at puberty, when an apparent girl acquires a male voice and grows a beard, and an apparent boy begins to menstruate and grows breasts. Such embarrassing developments call for medical intervention. For the most part, this will be such that the patient can continue in the same gender role as far as possible. Occasionally, however, a change of gender role (i.e. a change of social sex) is needed, perhaps combined with some surgical improvement of the genital apparatus.

The original investigators at Johns Hopkins

(e.g. Money *et al.*, 1955, 1956) into the consequences of such medical interventions came to the conclusion that a change of social sex should not be undertaken after the age of eighteen months, because the psychological difficulties caused would be too great. It has since been reported, however, that sex-change operations have been successfully performed in older children, adolescents, and even adults. Dewhurst and Gordon (1963), for example, reported on 17 such operations of which all but four had a favourable outcome. They concluded: 'Although we agree that the sex of rearing is very important in this respect [i.e. establishing a gender role], some of these cases do suggest that the children had an affinity to the sex opposite to that in which they were being brought up. . . . [We] believe that the child's natural tendency to the gonadal sex will *sometimes* militate against the sex of rearing and may even overcome it'. (Italics in the original.)

However, even when a child's external genitals are normally formed and its sex therefore correctly diagnosed at birth, the gender role assigned to it can meet with increasing psychological resistance. Such children grow into persons with an addictive compulsion to adopt the role of the opposite gender in some respects or even fully and wholeheartedly. The clinical manifestations in these patients vary from some form of *transvestism* to *trans-sexualist* urges that can be assuaged only at the cost of painful and complicated sex-change operations. Randell (1959) noticed that 60 per cent of his 25 non-homosexual male transvestites were steadily 'preoccupied with thoughts of cross-dressing, of feminine activity, and fantasy of transvestite acts and opportunities. . . . Suffering, instead of gratification in the transvestite compulsion, is often experienced in these patients who live the whole of their lives in the shadow of the impulse and in whom suicide may occur'. Similar observations were made by Benjamin (1966).

Sexually stimulating objects are of many different kinds. The majority of people are heterosexual in their inclinations so that persons of the opposite sex and of suitable age can arouse erotic feelings and sexual desires in them. Even most transvestites, and especially those of male sex, are predominantly heterosexual in their choice of partners, and may be married and have children. Yet the closer transvestites come to being trans-sexualists, the more homosexual they are in their orientation. West (1977), in his comprehensive survey of homosexuality, remarks on the 'gender discontent which in varying degrees,

afflicts many homosexuals' (p. 56). At the end of his book, he thoughtfully points out: 'Most people discover their sexual inclinations, they do not choose them' (p. 322). Some unfortunate people discover to their discomfiture that their sexually stimulating objects are of such an unusual kind that they can find gratification only at the risk of attracting censure and even legal prosecution (Gunn, 1976). There are persons with an urge for novelty in their sexual partners so that they become promiscuous and risk the dissolution of a stable union, if they have ever been able to form any; there are persons who are sexually aroused by garments of rubber or leather, other articles of clothing, or erotically quite neutral objects which have turned into sexual fetishes; there are those who need the sight of sadistically inflicted fear and suffering or who need to feel the pain and humiliation of masochistic practices; there are paedophiles, gerontophiles, necrophiles, those drawn to statues (Pygmalionism), animals (bestialism), the sight of raging fires (pyromania), the clandestine observation of undressed women or copulating couples (voyeurism), rape, sexual murder, incest, exhibitionism, and so on. Obviously, many persons will be successful in their resistance to such urges, especially if they have other sexual outlets, but those who succumb run the gauntlet of many risks and penalties.

Addictions to *special sexual practices* which differed from sanctimoniously narrow norms used to be condemned as perversions. In the more permissive climate of today's western culture, many of them have been accepted as being normal variations on individual themes of love-making. Examples are mutual masturbation, oral sex, and many deviations from the 'missionary position'. Objections can still be raised at times against the performance of anal intercourse and against the commercial provision of lust without love by prostitutes. The clients of prostitutes are driven by many motivations. Among them is the search for unusual sexual services or the desire for sexual gratifications which are free of any commitments to form affectionate bonds (Gibbens & Silberman, 1960).

Not all persons are so constituted that impulses which are objectively obnoxious are resisted by them. Such persons are not troubled by obsessional doubts and ruminations; they simply act impulsively on the spur of the moment. Such *impulsive persons* are at the mercy of all temptations or merely of certain overpowering drives, giving no thought, at least at the time, to any harm that may befall them or others. As a result, some of them are shiftless and unreliable in their social conduct, while others are given to occasional outbursts of excessive aggression. They are thus liable to fall foul of the law by antisocial, delinquent, or criminal actions. Patients of this kind fall into the poorly definable class of *psychopaths*. It is a class that has to be distinguished, on the one hand, from the class of patients with definite psychiatric and organic diseases, and, on the other hand, from the class of culpable rogues. Yet all such distinctions are bound to be controversial, since they depend on the subjective criterion of therapeutic concern. Persons who arouse sufficiently strong therapeutic concern for themselves in medical and judicial authorities will be deemed to be psychopaths, whereas persons who fail to arouse such therapeutic concern will be held to be fully or partly responsible for their actions and therefore culpable. That this is so can be gleaned from some definitions of psychopathy. For example, the Mental Health Act, 1959, defined 'psychopathic disorders' as a 'persistent disorder or disability of mind . . . which results in abnormally aggressive or seriously irresponsible conduct on the part of the patient and *requires or is susceptible to* medical treatment'. (Italics added.) Scott (1960), after considering this and two other definitions of psychopathy, came to the conclusion that a psychopath is a person 'who does not fit readily into other psychiatric categories, who is persistently antisocial or asocial, and who *needs specialized treatment'*. (Italics added.) He classified psychopaths into four categories. Two of these do not contain impulsive persons, but persons who deliberately engage in antisocial behaviour in accordance either with the standards of a delinquent subculture to which they belong or with a personal standard of misbehaviour which overcompensates for real or imagined handicaps, a standard with which they are identified, and of which they are proud. Scott's other two categories contain impulsive persons. These are either people who from early childhood had conduct difficulties, because they had no guiding standards of behaviour and thus fell prey to any tempting impulses that promised pleasure or gain. Alternatively, they are people who, at an early age, had acquired the habit of responding to any frustrating situation with an impulsive outburst of a stereotyped kind which took no account of the kind of frustrating situation experienced. An offender of this type, according to Scott, 'often helplessly dissociates himself from his behaviour, but may be genuinely remorseful and anxious about it [afterwards].

. . . The observer cannot feel sympathy with the offender or the offence. . . . The behaviour appears to be compulsive but it is not so, for it is not resisted'.

Morbid disorders of memory.

All conscious experiences leave behind some changes in psychological reactivity which constitute *mnestic dispositions*. Most of them are ephemeral, but some are more or less enduring. Their neurophysiological basis is still an almost total mystery. They can be activated in two ways which make them more or less introspectible. The activating processes are known as 'recall' and 'recognition'.

Recall is not always a conscious process, but may become active on its own, for instance, during dreams, automatisms, or mannerisms. Psychoanalytic theories also postulate the activation of certain mnestic dispositions (the so-called 'unconscious memories, or complexes') by processes which are not those of recall so that the mnestic dispositions do not become introspectible, but have to be intuitively inferred from other consequences.

Mnestic dispositions which can be recalled are of three kinds: (1) rote memories, (2) personal memories (or reminiscences), and (3) impersonal memories.

The recall of *rote memories* leads to semiautomatic mental or motor activities (habits, skills) which, once initiated, proceed with little introspection. Too much introspection may indeed disrupt the recalls. They may also suffer disorder through many fortuitous influences which give rise to such usually harmless derangements as slips of the tongue, Spoonerisms, spelling mishaps, and such examples of skill fatigue as the double faults of professional tennis players and similar errors in other sports. There are also morbid derangements such as those of *motor aphasia, agraphia, acalculia, ideomotor apraxia*, and the like.

The recall of *personal memories (or reminiscences)* gives rise to the introspection of personal experiences. Among the data contained in these experiences, especially when recent, are spatio-temporal indications of where and when they had occurred to one. The veridicality of these spatio-temporal indications generally diminishes with time.

Hebb (1949, p. 61) advanced the hypothesis that there are two kinds of memory stores, a short-term and a long-term one, and that each may have a different neurophysiological basis. The activation through recall of the short-term memory store would give rise to the introspection of a phenomenon that may be called a *'short-term reminiscence'*. Similarly, activation through recall of the long-term memory store would give rise to the introspection of a *long-term reminiscence*. Psychological experiments on the forgetting of memorized information has since given qualified support to this hypothesis (e.g. Brown, 1964; McGaugh, 1966; Peterson, 1966).

Long-term reminiscences progressively lose many of the data originally contained in them. Moreover, the reminiscences of relatively recent experiences are more veridical than the reminiscences of experiences dating from a more distant past. The reliability of reminiscences of the latter kind are therefore always suspect to some extent. They are liable to contain unwitting falsifications of memory (*paramnesias*). There is a good deal of evidence for this in investigations of the testimony of witnesses and the anamnestic accounts of patients (e.g. Bartlett, 1932; Stern, 1939; Belbin, 1950; Hunter, 1957; Haggard *et al.*, 1960).

The recall of long-term reminiscences can be morbidly reduced through injuries to the brain or other interference with its adequate functioning. Experiences made during a confusional state or some other clouding (*obfuscation*) of consciousness (e.g. after a concussion or other cerebral trauma) cannot be subsequently recalled, when clear consciousness has been regained. Such patients have a *post-confusional* (*post-concussional, post-traumatic*) *amnesia* and they are usually subjectively aware of this disability. The amnesia, moreover, is not limited to the experiences made during the state of clouded consciousness. There is also a *retrograde amnesia*, i.e. the reminiscences of events occurring during a period antedating the state of clouded consciousness cannot be activated through recall either. This retrograde amnesia may cover a period of only a few seconds, but it can be very much longer. It tends to shrink as the patients' clinical condition improves.

Gaps in reminiscences may occur not only after a period of organically determined obfuscation but also after some other states of altered consciousness, e.g. a state of partial sleep (sleep walking or other 'oneiroid' activities) or a state of hypnotic trance. During such states a patient may be in sufficient touch with his surroundings for his behaviour to seem fairly normal, though perhaps somewhat absentminded and bemused. The reminiscence of events encountered during that time may be 'state-dependent', i.e. available only during the state of altered sensorium and even then merely in part and mingled with

interloping paramnesias. That is why, for example, a patient who is still in a state of obfuscation after a head injury may be able to report on experiences which happened immediately after the trauma, but has no reminiscence of them on returning to the state of normal consciousness.

The state-dependence of reminiscences can sometimes be demonstrated by a return to the same altered state of consciousness in which their long-term memory stores had originally been established. The reminiscences may, however, not be quite veridical because of paramnesias. For example, events during a deep trance leave reminiscences which may not be remembered when the sensorium is normal, but may become accessible to recall again on induction of another deep trance. Similarly, there may be a 'black-out' of reminiscences the day after a heavy bout of alcohol intoxication, though at the time the patient may have behaved quite adequately and may even have given some correct and quite complicated professional advice. Yet some of the blacked-out reminiscences may become recallable in another state of alcohol intoxication (Goodwin *et al.*, 1969, a,b,c).

In an altered state of consciousness, there can be evidence of a retrograde amnesia. This may change a patient's *sense of personal identity* so that it no longer squares with his present life situation, but is dominated by misleading reminiscences of some earlier period in his life and perhaps also by emotionally toned paramnesias. The alteration of consciousness can have a physical or psychological basis, and very often both. Whatever the basis, it can enable patients to remove themselves from a life situation that is charged with stress and threat, such as a battle area, impending criminal proceedings, or family tensions. They thus escape from themselves and the consciousness of their failure. This clinical picture of a *fugue* can last for hours, days, or weeks. Some patients wander about aimlessly, others seem to have a definite target. Some live a rough and unkempt existence, others move about in relative comfort as long as their money lasts. Depressive moods also can play their part in originating a fugue in a vain attempt to escape from misery (Stengel, 1941, 1943; Berrington *et al.*, 1956).

Patients with a tendency to repeated fugue states often show other signs of a disorder of mnestic functioning. In particular, they may experience confabulatory paramnesias which earn them a reputation as *pathological liars*. Stengel (1941) remarked that 'a considerable proportion of the patients showed the tendency to habitual lying, which in the majority amounted to pseudologia fantastica'. Berrington and colleagues (1956) also found that there was an association between lying and fugue states which was significant at the 5 per cent level of confidence. (They obtained similarly significant associations between fugue states and depressions, frequent drunkenness, and a history of severe head injuries.) *Pseudologia fantastica* is a memory disorder that is, of course, not restricted solely to patients with repeated fugues.

A patient who recovers from a fugue state usually regains his correct sense of personal identity. He then has a more or less total amnesia for his personal experiences during the fugue and perhaps also a retrograde amnesia for some period antedating the fugue. In that case, he has no difficulty in finding his way back to his home and in taking up the threads of his former life. Yet if, on coming out of the fugue, a patient does not regain his correct sense of personal identity, all the reminiscences available to him date only from the moment when his fugue had come to an end. A retrograde amnesia covers all the personal experiences of his earlier life. He has 'lost his memory', as the saying goes. He does not know his name, occupation, or whence he came, nor does he recognize his relatives, when he meets them. Yet some unexpected recognitions of certain persons and of the location of certain places may turn up. Such inconsistencies are accepted with equanimity by genuine patients who, in this respect, differ from people who simulate a loss of memory. Since the patients' impersonal memories are in order and there is no anterograde amnesia to hinder them, they slip back easily into the routine of their lives.

There have been two well-authenticated patients who, after a fugue, assumed a new identity with a new name and a partly confabulated, but mostly blank, past. The first was the carpenter and itinerant preacher Ansel Bourne who, after having withdrawn a fairly large sum from his bank, disappeared from his home town and a nagging wife to start a new life two weeks later in a different town as the shopkeeper Albert Brown (having kept his initials) until he woke up one day as Ansel Bourne again, who knew nothing of Albert Brown and his shop. His story was examined and checked by William James (1890). The second patient was Charles Poultney from Dublin, who became for a while Charles Poulting from Florida. His case was reported by Franz (1933).

A number of patients have also been described who did not change their social identities, only their personalities, and this without an intervening fugue. Each of these different personalities had its own set of reminiscences which was inaccessible to the others. Before 1910, there used to be much interest in these *dual or multiple personalities*. Since then there has been a tendency largely to discount these clinical observations as artefacts caused in suggestible and obliging patients by doctors with an obvious interest in clinical manifestations of this kind. Yet, since the last war, some new patients with multiple personalities have turned up. The best known of these is perhaps the patient described under the pseudonym of Mrs. Eve White. Her story reached a wide public through the book *The Three Faces of Eve* (Thipgen & Cleckley, 1957) and the film based on it. Ellenberger (1970, pp. 126–41) presents some further details about these rare and striking disorders of reminiscences.

When bilateral lesions in the hippocampal zones of the brain are surgically produced (see Milner, 1966), patients do not only show the signs of retrograde amnesia for events prior to the operation, they have also become unable to recall the long-term reminiscences of events they had experienced fairly recently. All the reminiscences they can recall at any one time are long-term reminiscences of remote experiences in their younger years and of some very recent experiences in the last few minutes. This kind of ongoing forgetting of personal memories, together with any new information contained in them, is known as *'anterograde amnesia'*. The combination of retrograde and anterograde amnesia constitutes a *dysmnesic (amnesic, Korsakow) syndrome*.

This syndrome is only very rarely the result of surgical interference with the hippocampal zones, but is due to brain damage in many areas caused by vascular accidents, tumours, or an accumulation of many minor physical traumas. When an amnesic syndrome is not associated with the signs of other organic brain lesions and a conspicuous lack of initiative, patients can appear fairly normal to a casual observer, since only the recall of reminiscences has been disrupted, but not the recall of rote and impersonal memories. They are thus in command of their previous motor skills and habits, their linguistic and general knowledge, and their ability to reason from premises which are unrelated to their recent past. Yet they have obvious difficulties in adjusting to unaccustomed surroundings and the present date, since they can no longer learn from new experiences and live for the most part with memories of a long lost past. They may not even be aware of their memory deficits or seem to care little about them. Some are given to *con-*

fabulations in that they fill in memory gaps with imaginary reminiscences, especially when they are asked to give an account of their recent activities. The confabulations are usually derived from actual experiences in the past, but they may be mere fantasies of a wishful kind (Bonhoeffer, 1904; Berlyne, 1972).

From clinical and experimental studies, Weiskrantz (1966) has developed hypothetical models of the time span of short-term and long-term reminiscences in patients with a dysmnesic syndrome. He has postulated that the data in short-term reminiscences vanish exponentially in time so that about half of them are patchily lost in about twenty seconds, unless they are deliberately kept accessible by constant recall. Long-term reminiscences also escape recall fairly quickly and patchily, though their life span is measured in minutes rather than seconds. If long-term reminiscences did not function at all, patients would have only staccato experiences, changing every few seconds. It is, however, doubtful whether such a mnestic disorder occurs. Only one patient has been described with a so-called 'one-second memory' ascribed to an organic brain damage (Grünthal & Störring, 1930a,b), but it turned out eventually that the clinical picture of this patient largely derived from hysterical and malingered motivations (see Zangwill, 1967).

The individual data contained in a reminiscence are composed of basic *impersonal memories* and their familiar or unfamiliar constellations. Basic impersonal memories and their familiar constellations have been abstracted from the experiences of many previous occasions. They can be recalled as thoughts (meanings, concepts) or as sensory or verbal images which need have no particular spatio-temporal indications. Morbid disturbances of the recall of impersonal memories give rise to such symptoms as *poverty of thought* or *nominal aphasia*. Unfamiliar constellations of impersonal memories contained in a reminiscence (e.g. strange foreign words or new phone numbers) tend to be quickly forgotten; they have to be memorized before they become accessible to recall. Normally, even familiar data in a particular reminiscence are gradually forgotten for the most part so that only the occurrence of the experience and some of the familiar data in it remain accessible to recall after some time. This process of forgetting becomes accentuated in old age, giving rise to what Kral (1962) called *'benign senescent forgetfulness'*. It totally erases some of the personal memories of an earlier age and renders inaccessible to recall, at least at times, certain impersonal memories contained in recent experiences, such as names, locations, times of occurrence, or social circumstances. When senescent forgetfulness grows to morbid proportions, it has turned into the dysmnesic syndrome of senile dementia.

Some exceptional persons have been reported for whom the forgetting of personal experiences hardly existed. One person with such *hypermnesia* was the stage mnemonist, S. V. Shereshevski, whom Luria (1960, 1969) investigated in great detail over many years. He memorized abstract data by turning them into sensory images grouped around a central and emotionally coloured theme. The reminiscence of the memorizing occasion and of the data then memorized remained accessible to his recall through eidetic imagery over a time span that could exceed fifteen years. He made only minor mistakes at times. His mental life was, however, so dominated by his concrete imagery that he had difficulty in forming abstract generalizations.

A more circumscribed hypermnesic ability is occasionally found as an isolated talent in patients who are otherwise educationally backward. The talent becomes noticeable at an early age, because the patients are eager to display their one exceptional achievement. But it is a very limited talent. Often their forte is calendar dating in that they can quickly fit the correct weekday to a past or future date, and this without any knowledge of the formulas available for that purpose. In addition, they may have detailed reminiscences of the events that had happened to them on a particular day, including the names of people, streets, and places encountered. Some of them have also shown a surprising musical ability which resists, however, any attempt to develop it by tuition. Such patients have sometimes been called *'idiots savants'*, though they are neither idiots nor savants. It is possible that their educational backwardness is due to some extent to their hypermnesia which is so concrete, personal, and situational that they cannot readily form abstract concepts which transcend the spatio-temporal connotations of reminiscences (Rothstein, 1941; Scheerer *et al.*, 1945; Hill, 1975).

Mnestic dispositions are not only activated by processes of recall, but also by the exteroception of objects (events, scenes). Such activation constitutes the phenomenon of *recognition*. It endows the exterocepted object with meaning and other attributes.

In principle, the acquisition of meaning by an exterocepted object corresponds to the realization that the object in question is a member of a particular class of objects and therefore shares their defining characteristics. The concept of a particular class of objects is linked to a particular mnestic disposition, a particular personal or impersonal memory. For example, if the sight, taste, smell, and feel of an object evokes the recognition that it belongs to the class of apples, it has activated the impersonal memory of that class and thus endowed the object with the meaning of having the defining characteristics of apples. In addition, since the recognition depends on the activation of the memory of a class concept with many individual members, the object acquires the attribute of having been perceived before and of being one of many. When recognition of this kind is morbidly affected, it can give rise to the symptoms of *sensory agnosia* which have already been considered as examples of meaningless percepts.

In the recognition of unique objects, the mnestic disposition activated is linked to the concept of a known unit class of which the object in question is the sole member. The recognition of the object thus endows it with the meaning of having been perceived before and of being unique. This kind of recognition usually goes astray in dysmnesic patients. If they meet a unique object, say a particular person, the reminiscence of this meeting and the impersonal memory of the person are short-lived. If the person is perceived again by the patient a short while later, he is only recognized as a stranger, i.e. as belonging to the large class of strangers. Sometimes, however, the impersonal memory of the person previously met can still linger sufficiently to make the stranger vaguely familiar. The result can be the assumption by the dysmnesic patient that someone resembling the stranger had somewhere and somewhen been met in the past. The stranger is then recognized as a member of a particular pair class consisting of him and a known person like him. This symptom has been termed '*reduplicative paramnesia*' (Pick, 1903; Zangwill, 1941).

It can also happen that the reminiscence of the occasion is forgotten, when some still remembered event has last been encountered. This can turn some persons with benign senescent forgetfulness into tedious bores, when they quickly forget the last occasion of their recounting some particular news or anecdote. They may then regale the same companions with the same conversational piece at short intervals again and again. A related and sometimes very embarrassing shortcoming of this kind is not limited to senescent forgetfulness. It consists in the persistence of an impersonal memory of recent origin, though the reminiscence of its acquisition has been lost. In that case, the impersonal memory may be recalled without being recognized as belonging to the class of memories. This lack of recognition is known as '*cryptomnesia*'. The unrecognized memory appears to be something one has newly thought of. If it happens to be an idea, invention, poem, or musical motive which is the original creation of someone else, an act of *unconscious plagiarism* has been committed. Jung (1902) examined cryptomnesic phenomena in his doctoral dissertation and reported (1905) a possible example of unconscious plagiarism in Nietzsche's *Thus Spake Zarathustra*. Other possible examples have been examined by Taylor (1965).

The experience of a commonplace situation activates a mnestic disposition which is linked to the concept of a class of similar reminiscences of such a situation. The newly experienced commonplace situation is thus recognized as being similar to others and being one of many. Occasionally, this recognition fails to work adequately. There may be, in addition, an activation of the concept of a unit class whose sole member is the reminiscence of a particular past situation. This gives rise to conflicting recognitions of the newly experienced situation as being both similar to situations previously experienced and also a replication of a particular past situation. An analogous conflict of recognition occurs, when a newly experienced situation activates not only the usual concept of a class of similar reminiscences, but also the concept of a completely novel situation for which no reminiscence exists. Then the newly experienced commonplace situation is recognized both as familiar and as completely unfamiliar. In either case, the patient is aware of the conflict of recognitions and experiences an *illusion of familiarity* (*déjà vu*) or *unfamiliarity* (*jamais vu*), symptoms which have already been considered as examples of morbid interpretive illusions.

Morbid disorders of muscular action.

The disorders are characterized by abnormalities in several dimensions: (1) quantitative–qualitative, (2) generalized–localized, (3) continuous–episodic, and (4) purposive–purposeless.

An excess of muscular action manifests itself in two overlapping forms: as hyperkinesis or raised muscular tension (hypertonicity).

Hyperkinesis constitutes motor over-activity. It occurs in a generalized, continuous and purposive form in the so-called 'hyperkinetic syndrome of children' (see Cantwell, 1976). It is then combined with distractibility and impulsive reactions. There can be a significant genetic determination and a tendency to antisocial behaviour that may continue into adulthood. The syndrome can also have its origin in brain injuries (see Black *et al.*, 1969) and was one of the troublesome consequences of the epidemic encephalitis after the First World War. Autistic and mentally retarded children may show ritualistic forms of hyperkinesis which can result in self-injuries.

In adult patients, such a continuous and purposive form of hyperkinesis was displayed by some catatonic schizophrenic patients before the days of neuroleptic drugs. The patients spent their waking days in endlessly reiterated stereotyped behaviour.

Episodic hyperkinesis of a generalized and purposive kind makes its appearance in some psychiatric diseases. It is an understandable consequence of the bustling exuberance of manic patients and of the terror-stricken despair of agitated depressives. It is an inexplicable event, when it occurs as a sudden outburst of senseless violence and destruction in patients with catatonic schizophrenia or an epileptic predisposition. Running amok is a homicidal variant of such outbursts in people whose mental explosiveness may not have been apparent before. It used to be regarded as an ethnic peculiarity of Malay people, but this is not justified, as Yap (1951) has pointed out. Amok-like attacks certainly occur among all races and all cultures, though they are likely to be called by other names, such as 'going berserk' which has a Scandinavian etymology.

Among *episodic and purposeless forms of hyperkinesis* are epileptic seizures. In grand mal, the hyperkinesis is generalized in the clonic phase; in focal epilepsy, it can remain localized; in myoclonic epilepsy, it is localized and usually episodic. Nocturnal myoclonic jerks are quite common among healthy persons and thus have usually no morbid significance. The purposeless and localized hyperkinetic movements in choreic diseases can be combined with purposive and generalized hyperkinesis. Tics (habit spasms) may begin as episodic symptoms, but have a tendency to become continuous manifestations, especially in adults, affecting particular muscle groups (eye blinking, head shaking, shoulder rolling or shrugging, sudden gestures, or facial movements). When the muscles of vocalization are involved, noises are produced (hiccups, coughs, barks, grunts). In the Gilles de la Tourette syndrome, vocal tics turn into barked obscenities (coprolalia) and other tics may become indecent gestures (copropraxia). Some forms of purposeless hyperkinesis have recently acquired special significance in psychiatry, because they can be induced by tranquillizers and do not always disappear when medication is stopped. The most troublesome form are writhing movements in the orofacial region which have become known as 'tardive dyskinesia' (see Crane, 1973). A generalized and purposive form which is not always due to tranquillizers is known as 'akathisia' (Haškovec, 1901, 1904; Bing, 1923) or 'restless legs' (Ekbom, 1945, 1950). Episodic hyperkinesis of the respiratory muscles in the form of tachypnoea can occur during panic attacks. The resulting hyperventilation can give rise to tetanic symptoms with increased muscular excitability and the hypertonicity of carpo-pedal spasms. Tremors are purposeless forms of hyperkinesis which may be episodic or continuous. Many of them have an organic or toxic origin. Another common source is anxiety. It can give rise to tremulous legs, hands or voice, and patients can become acutely self-conscious about these symptoms. Moreover, the symptoms can be considerable handicaps in the careers of professional actors and musicians. Dramatically disabling and very coarse tremors characterized the hysterical shell-shock symptoms of the First World War.

Muscular hypertonicity affects only particular muscle groups and thus leads to distortions of posture (dystonia). It often has an organic pathology, but can also have a functional or psychological origin. Catatonic schizophrenics may adopt and maintain bizarre positions, lie in bed with their heads lifted off the pillow, or hold their lips in a constant pout (*Schnauzkrampf*, snout cramp). Indian Yogis train themselves to twist their bodies into abstruse distortions (see Hoenig, 1968), and in hypnotic trances rigidly held positions may be induced. Abnormal postures also result from the irregular distribution of muscular hypertonicity in the so-called 'stiff-man syndrome' (Moersch & Woltman, 1956; Gordon *et al.*, 1967).

Episodic muscular spasms are symptoms in which hyperkinesis and hypertonicity of muscles are combined. They may be due to serum electrolyte abnormalities (e.g. in tetany) or occur without known pathology. The latter is the case in the common complaint of nocturnal cramps which respond well to prophylactic quinine medication. A more persistent and potentially crippling variety occurs also diurnally. In writer's cramp and similar 'occupational neuroses', muscular spasms and jerks bring to a painful and embarrassing halt some well-practised vocational activity. Conditioned reflex spasms in response to particular situations can occur in certain muscle groups, e.g. in the muscles around the vaginal entrance in the disorder known as 'vaginismus' or in the detrusor muscles of the bladder in the disorder known as 'pollakiuria' which consists of frequency and urgency of micturition and can be a source of constant worry in many over-anxious female patients.

A reduction of muscular action also manifests itself in two overlapping forms: as hypokinesis or hypotonicity.

Hypokinesis constitutes muscular underactivity on account of diminished or absent motor initiative. It happens in a generalized form in patients with retarded depression or catatonic schizophrenia. A complete cessation of motor activity, with the exception of ocular movements, occurs in the clinical condition known as 'akinetic stupor'. In Parkinsonian patients, hypokinesis is responsible for the general poverty and slowness of their movements (bradykinesis). Lishman (1978, p. 748) suggests that 'hypokinesia probably accounts for many of the classical features of parkinsonism – the mask-like face, infrequent blinking, clumsiness of fine finger movement, crabbed writing and monotonous speech'. It may also account for the slow, shuffling gait of these patients which can, however, end in a 'festinant' acceleration, when the body has moved further than the feet and a fall threatens. Localized forms of hypokinesis manifest themselves as hysterical paralyses. When hypokinesis affects the muscles of vocalization, aphonia or mutism results. In children, there can be 'elective' mutism which appears only in special social situations (Tramer, 1934).

Muscular hypotonicity in the form of muscular weakness accompanies many systemic and neurological diseases. It presents as a possible autoimmune disorder in myasthenia gravis and, in connection with serum potassium levels, in periodic paralyses of a familial or acquired kind. When the onset of muscular hypotonicity is sudden and results in a general flaccidity of muscles, the patient's body slumps. This happens in narcoleptic attacks of cataplexy, interictally in epileptic conditions, and in senile drop attacks.

Qualitative disorders of muscular action disorganize purposive activities. Examples are stammering, dysarthria, dysphasia, apraxia, and gait disturbances. In catatonic schizophrenics, disordered forms of behaviour arise through either negativism or automatic obedience. The negativistic patient performs actions which are contrary to those expected or requested of him so that he may, for instance, respond to a question with silence, but begin to answer it when the questioner acknowledges failure and turns away. Automatic obedience allows one to arrange a patient's body in peculiar postures which are maintained afterwards for quite a while (*flexibilitas cerea*). A culture-dependent, but now probably obsolete, form of automatic obedience has been described, e.g. as 'latah' in Malaya or 'arctic hysteria' in Siberia (see Yap, 1951, 1952). Allied manifestations are echoreactions, such as echopraxia and echolalia (Stengel, 1947; Chapman & McGhie, 1964). Schizophrenics often perform ambivalent movements in which some purposive action is reversed mid-way so that, for example, a handshake never quite materializes.

Morbid disorders of consciousness.

Consciousness (or sensorium) can be altered along three dimensions which are not independent: (a) wakefulness–sleep, (b) lucidity–obfuscation, and (c) vigilance–absorption.

Wakefulness–sleep. Wakefulness and sleep alternate regularly as both modes of consciousness are needed for the maintenance of normal mental functions. The approximate 2:1 ratio between the hours of wakefulness and sleep in 24 hours in adult persons can be altered for many reasons. When the ratio is increased, it indicates insomnia. This occurs as a clinical symptom in many stressful conditions, but there is increasing evidence that it can occur on its own as a primary disturbance (Fenton, 1975). Yet, very occasionally, it can also be a perfectly normal characteristic by the individual standards of some exceptional persons. Jones and Oswald (1968), for instance, reported two men who were healthy and energetic, though certainly not hypomanic, yet needed no more than three hours of sleep a day. It is of interest that in these men REM sleep occurred in less than 45 minutes after the first onset of sleep spindles in the EEG – an occurence that has been regarded as pathognomonic of the narcoleptic syndrome (Rechtschaffen *et al.*, 1963).

It is often assumed that increasing age reduces the hours of sleep needed, but the findings of Tune (1968) have thrown doubt on this assumption. He noticed that, despite the high incidence of nocturnal awakening in older people, they managed to get at least as much sleep as their juniors by falling asleep earlier in the evening, waking up later in the morning, or taking naps during the day. Yet the prevalence of insomnia seems to increase with age. McGhie and Russell (1962), in their investigation of two Scottish areas, found that the use of sleeping tablets rose with age in both men and women, but significantly more so in the latter.

An enforced change of the normal sleep rhythm is, at least partly, responsible for the so-called 'jet-lag symptoms' of long-distance air travellers. Prolonged sleep deprivation eventually produces signs of obfuscation in the form of disorientation, hallucinations, delusions, and epileptic phenomena. It has become one of the torture methods used by unscrupulous investigators in police states to dehumanize their victims and undermine their self-determination.

Overpowering episodes of sleep are among the characteristics of the narcoleptic syndrome in which patients are irresistibly drowned by sleep in the midst of everyday activities. In hypersomnia, the hours of sleep overflow into the day. The combination can be combined with 'sleep drunkenness' (Roth *et al.*, 1972), when some semblance of wakefulness is finally achieved. Episodes of hypersomnia associated with over-eating characterize the Kleine-Levin syndrome (Kleine, 1925; Levin, 1936). In the Pickwickian syndrome, hypersomnia is combined with extreme obesity and interrupted breathing (Burwell *et al.*, 1956).

One may speak of 'partial sleep', when phenomena of sleep and wakefulness are intermingled. Sleep phenomena can encroach on wakefulness in hypnagogic or hypnopompic states. Examples are brief pseudo-hallucinations, usually of an auditory kind, or short periods of sleep paralysis in a person consciously aware of an environment in which he cannot move and which may have acquired an eerie connotation (a condition known as 'night nurses' paralysis'). Such manifestations of partial sleep are exaggerated and more frequent in patients with narcolepsy.

Phenomena of wakefulness can also intrude into the sleeping state. Sleepwalking (somnambulism) occurs at least once in 15 per cent of children, mostly male, and then has a good prognosis (Fenton, 1975). It does not seem to be an acting out of dreams. It is often associated with enuresis and night terrors. Somnambulism occurs rarely in adults and then tends to be linked to emotional psychopathy (Sours *et al.*,

1963). In some senile patients, confused nocturnal behaviour and wandering can be due to the half-conscious acting out of dreams. Sleep-talking (somniloquy) (Rechtschaffen *et al.*, 1962; Arkin *et al.*, 1970) and nocturnal teeth-grinding (bruxism) (Reding *et al.*, 1968; Satoh & Harada, 1971) occur usually in superficial phases of sleep.

Lucidity–obfuscation. Whereas wakefulness and sleep are basically physiological phenomena, though they may be affected by morbid conditions, obfuscation (or mental clouding) always has a pathological origin. Lucidity of consciousness is no more than absence of obfuscation. Mild forms of mental clouding produce a sleep-like (oneiroid) clinical picture and may indeed be combined with sleep phenomena as evidenced by the EEG. When the obfuscation deepens, organic confusional states make their appearance. The patient is then only vaguely and precariously in touch with the environment, is disoriented in time, place and person, and is dysmnesic (cf. Lishman, 1978, pp. 11–23). When hallucinations, usually of a visual kind, occur, the patient is regarded as delirious and may be fussily over-active in this state. When obfuscation deepens further, the patient sinks into an unconscious stupor in which he exhibits only some reflex or semi-purposive actions. Further deepening leads to coma in which the patient is unresponsive to any stimuli.

Vigilance–absorption. This is the vaguest of the three dimensions of consciousness. A wakeful person is vigilant, when his attention can move freely from one to another phenomenon. Manic patients are morbidly vigilant, because their attention mobility is vastly exaggerated. When people are mentally absorbed by some thought or emotion, their attention mobility is reduced so that they are absent-minded in all other respects. The ability to become mentally absorbed is normal by population standards, when the content of the mental absorption is remembered afterwards. It is abnormal by population standards, when there is no such memory after attention has returned to its usual mobility, since this ability is limited to a minority of people who can achieve the special state of consciousness required for such mental absorption. Such persons may have a state-dependent memory for the content of their mental absorption during their unusual state of consciousness. It seems that these unusual states of consciousness can be of two kinds which may be distinguished as states of 'transcendental meditation' and states of 'trance'.

In *transcendental meditation* as practised in the Far East by adherents of Raja Yoga or Zen Buddhism or, more recently, in the Western World, especially by followers of the Maharishi Mahesh Yogi, it appears that the mind is allowed to become absorbed by the kind of experience that has as its EEG correlate an increase of slow alpha waves of 8 or 9 cycles per second in the frontal and central regions of the brain (Anand *et al.*, 1961; Hoenig, 1968; Wallace & Benson, 1972). This state of consciousness is also associated with a reduction of metabolism as was definitely demonstrated by the last-mentioned authors on American subjects with relatively limited experience of transcendental meditation.

In *trance* states, the mental absorption is not necessarily associated with the physiological changes found in transcendental meditation. In a superficial trance, a person appears to be in only absent-minded contact with his environment. In a deep trance, the behaviour of a person varies with the experiences that absorb him. He may be in an 'entranced' akinesis, perform some purposeful actions, or enact ecstatic and rapturous emotions. Trance states can be induced by hypnosis, revivalist meetings, and rhythmic or abandoned dancing (Backman, 1952; Taylor, 1956; Sargant, 1957). They can also be induced in highly autosuggestible persons by convictions of a morbid or zealously religious kind. The result may be the occurrence of so-called 'conversion-hysterical' symptoms in the form of seizures, gait disturbances, paralyses, tremors, anaesthesias, analgesias, blindness, deafness, the signs of pregnancy (pseudocyesis) (Bivin & Klinger, 1937), and changes in neurovascular functions. The last-named are responsible for the ability of persons in trance, such as dervishes, to pierce their tongues and cheeks without shedding blood. They can also lead, through local suffusions of plasma and blood from capillary vessels, to striking skin manifestations, such as weals and petechiae (Moody, 1946), blisters, and blood-stained erosions. Trance states induced by evangelical fervour are also the most likely source of the stigmata of Christ which have occurred in more than 300 'stigmatists' since their first manifestation in St. Francis of Assisi in 1224 (Biot, 1962; Whitlock & Hynes, 1978).

4
The neuropsychology of mental disorders

4.1
Introduction

O. L. ZANGWILL

Neuropsychology may be said to owe its origins largely to the American psychologists, S. I. Franz (1874–1933) and K. S. Lashley (1890–1959), whose studies on brain mechanisms and learning in the rat and monkey, begun jointly but continued over many years by Lashley alone, set the stage for the modern study of the brain as the instrument of behaviour. It should be noted that although much of their work was carried out with animals, its significance was general rather than comparative and both men were convinced that their experimental results could be generalized to the human brain and the changes which it might undergo in consequence of injury or disease. Indeed, Franz might be described as the first clinical neuropsychologist in so far as, in addition to his experimental work with Lashley, he had contributed important studies on aphasia and the effects of frontal lobe lesions in man. Equally, Lashley, while not working to any extent with human subjects, had little doubt that his concepts of cerebral equipotentiality and mass action were applicable to man no less than to animals, and might well bear upon clinical issues of real importance, in particular, dementia. Although the concept of mass-action is out of favour today, it was of great importance in bringing out the limitations of conventional localization theory and as providing the first modern blueprint of the cerebral organization of behaviour.

While the work of Lashley and several of his younger associates, in particular Donald Hebb and

Karl Pribram, has done much to further both experimental and clinical neuropsychology, it must not be supposed that its development has been centred wholly within the framework of the behavioural sciences. Neuropsychology has from the start regarded itself as multidisciplinary and has been much influenced by the long tradition of interest within clinical neurology in the problems of aphasia, apraxia and agnosia, and by the opportunities created by modern neurosurgery to correlate the effects of cerebral excisions in man with more objective assessments of intellectual loss. In this connection, the work of Brenda Milner, originally a pupil of Donald Hebb, provides an outstanding example. The work of the late Lukas Teuber and his colleagues on the psychological sequelae of focal war wounds of the brain might likewise be said to reflect clinical neuropsychology at its most promising. Mention should also be made of the outstanding Soviet neuropsychologist Alexander Luria, (1902–77), whose wide activities in research, genial personality, and prolific writings added a truly international dimension to the neuropsychological scene.

There are two recent lines of development in clinical neuropsychology which might be thought to possess high potential relevance to issues in clinical psychiatry. The first is the study of disorders of memory, which has escalated with astonishing rapidity during the past ten years or so; the second is research within the general field of inter-hemispheric relations and cerebral dominance. Whereas the study of memory disorders finds its origin in the field of clinical psychiatry, more especially that of the organic psychoses, the study of functional lateralization and cerebral dominance has grown out of the neurology of language from Broca and Hughlings Jackson to the present day. In this latter field, the work of Roger W. Sperry on the effects of commissurotomy in animals and man has deservedly won the highest praise. The elegance and ingenuity of his experiments are matched by the simplicity and modesty of his theoretical contribution. True, his work has indirectly contributed to the proliferation of some theoretical models of dubious validity and to the popularity of certain ill-founded hypotheses that do no credit to serious science. But the blame for these certainly cannot be laid at Sperry's door and it may be hoped that neuropsychology will soon outgrow such immature enthusiasms.

In the view of the editors of this volume, the contribution of neuropsychology to clinical psychiatry is indirect rather than direct, potential rather than actual. Accordingly, it was suggested to the authors of this chapter that they should select limited areas of indisputable relevance to psychiatry rather than to try and outline the whole field of modern neuropsychological inquiry. After careful consideration, the areas formally chosen were intellectual function and its disorders, memory defect, disorders of language, and the neuropsychology of emotion. While being given complete freedom to plan and write their respective sections in their own way, the contributors were asked to regard actual or potential relevance to psychiatry as the main consideration to bear in mind in selecting and organizing their material. It is hoped that the outcome of their labours will prove acceptable within these terms of reference and contribute to the growth of neuropsychological inquiry within the framework of psychological medicine.

4.2
Disorders of memory

O. L. ZANGWILL

Although disorders of memory, more especially those arising from head injury or stroke, find mention in numerous nineteen-century psychiatric writings, (Brodie, 1856; Winslow, 1860; Abercrombie, 1867), it was not until the closing years of the century that the subject began to attract serious scientific attention. This was due to the increasing recognition of memory as a basic biological fact (Hering, 1870), and more particularly to the publication of Ribot's well-known book on *Diseases of Memory* (Ribot, 1881; English translation, 1882) in which the author, himself an academic psychologist, made a sustained attempt to explain derangements of memory in the light of Hughlings Jackson's principles of the evolution and dissolution of the nervous system (Jackson, 1931). This was followed a few years later by the appearance, first in Russian but later in French and German, of several papers by S. S. Korsakoff (1889, 1890; see also Victor & Yakovlev, 1955) describing the syndrome which later came to bear his name. Although Korsakoff's belief that he had discovered a new disease entity ('cerebropathia psychica toxaemica') having both central and peripheral nervous manifestations failed to gain general acceptance, his description of a severe disorder of memory not apparently associated with gross confusion or dementia aroused widespread interest. While recognition of the focal basis of this syndrome came only much later, Korsakoff's work illustrated convincingly that memory, like language, might undergo dissolution in patients who failed to exhibit obvious deterioration in intelligence and judgement. In this respect, Korsakoff paved the way for the modern study of amnesia as a circumscribed cerebral syndrome.

The first to suggest that experimental psychology might find application to psychiatric issues was Emil Kraepelin, who had himself studied under Wundt at Leipzig and published several papers (e.g. 1886, 1900) on the psychology of memory. In 1904, his pupil R. Krauss, communicated an experimental study of perception and registration in the Korsakoff syndrome; several other papers concerned with measurements of the span of apprehension, reaction time, and residual learning capacity in organic amnesic states appeared in Germany at much the same time (Brodmann, 1902, 1904; Gregor & Römer, 1906; Gregor, 1909). English summaries of these papers were produced by Wechsler (1917), who himself carried out an investigation of Korsakoff patients along similar lines, and many years later by Talland (1965). Otherwise, there was virtually no experimental work on deranged memory carried out in English-speaking countries until quite recent years.

Although much of this early German work might nowadays appear very dated, it must be borne in mind that Kraepelin and his pupils were the first to demonstrate that immediate (or short-term) memory as tested by digit-span and similar tests typically remains intact in Korsakoff patients and that appreciable residual learning and memory-retention can be demonstrated in such patients using the 'savings' method of Ebbinghaus (1885). This latter finding has been extensively replicated by other methods in recent years, particularly in the sphere of perceptual learning, using the 'partial information method' introduced by Warrington and Weiskrantz (1968, 1970; see also Warrington, 1971), and the learning of motor skills (Milner, Corkin & Teuber, 1968; Starr & Phillips, 1970; Milner, 1972). Some more general aspects of this phenomenon are touched upon later in this chapter (pp. 101–3).

The development of a more sophisticated neuropsychology of memory may be said to date from the publication of G. Talland's study, *Deranged Memory*, in 1965. Apart from providing a detailed review of both clinical and experimental work on the Korsakoff syndrome, Talland recognized the need to explain it within the context of contemporary theories of memory. Although his own theory was not worked out in any detail, Talland's book contributed in an important way to the remarkable growth of interest among psychologists in the study and analysis of amnesic states. While this has resulted in a marked increase in our understanding of organic amnesia and its relations to cerebral pathology, it has also generated a great deal of controversy. This centres principally on the relations between defect in short-term and in long-term memory, the extent to which impairment of memory function may be due to either defective encoding or failure to retrieve recently stored material, the nature and role of consolidation in long-term memory, and the scope of retrograde amnesia. These controversies have been ably reviewed by Piercy (1977) and it is not proposed to dwell upon them in any detail here. Instead, an attempt will be made to specify certain current issues in the study of memory disorder which might be thought to possess relevance to clinical psychiatry. A similar, though somewhat briefer, account has recently been presented by Lishman (1978, pp. 34–48).

Amnesia or amnesias?

This question is the title given by Piercy (1977) to the penultimate section of his recent substantial review of experimental studies of the organic amnesic syndrome. As he rightly states, the fact that different workers have used quite different criteria for the selection of patients for study could be a source of some of the conflicting findings that occur in the literature of amnesia. In particular, he suggests, disagreements of this kind may well arise because different kinds of memory impairment are associated with cerebral lesions differing in nature or location, or in both. It is proposed to explore this issue further in the present section.

In an account of the Korsakoff syndrome originally published in 1966 and reprinted with a short postscript in 1977, the present writer laid stress on certain features which appear to differentiate this syndrome from the amnesic states that not infrequently occur after encephalitis or meningitis or operations (especially when bilateral) on the temporal lobes. In such cases, of which the best known is the famous patient H.M., originally communicated by Scoville and Milner (1957) and followed up by Milner and her associates over many years (see Milner, Corkin & Teuber, 1968), the amnesic state appears to differ from the familiar Korsakoff syndrome in that the patient has full insight into his loss of memory and seldom, if ever, confabulates. Although wholly unable to maintain any continuous memory of his activities, he is none the less seldom disoriented in a systematic fashion and, unlike the typical Korsakoff patient, rarely displays gross and insightless loss of judgement, as was described many years ago by Pick (1915). Zangwill (1977) was therefore led to conclude that, along with the amnesic syndrome, the Korsakoff presents a superadded syndrome of 'denial of illness' (anosognosia) of the kind described by Weinstein and Kahn (1951, 1955). According to these authors, this syndrome not infrequently comprises confabulation, disorientation, reduplication, and occasionally paraphasia in addition to denial of illness and is thought to result from acute lesions involving the third and lateral ventricles, the diencephalon, and the midbrain.

The contrast between these two conditions, which are nowadays often referred to as 'hippocampal' and 'diencephalic' amnesia respectively, was well brought out by Zangwill (1977) in the comparison he drew between the clinical picture in two cases of amnesic syndrome, in one of which the memory defect was secondary to meningitis and in the other a classical alcoholic Korsakoff case. Whereas the first patient retained almost perfect awareness of his memory deficit, the second showed marked confabulation, incorrigible disorientation, and total denial of illness. He also directed attention to four cases of post-encephalitic amnesia communicated by Rose and Symonds (1960), three of which he had himself studied, in which confabulation and denial of illness were likewise absent despite severe and persistent memory loss. He also directed attention to occasional reports of similar conditions in the earlier literature (Ewald, 1940; Conrad, 1953). It was suggested that whereas 'pure' amnesic syndromes, without either confabulation or denial of illness, appear to owe their origin to bilateral lesions involving the hippocampal region, the Korsakoff syndrome is most commonly associated with lesions involving the terminal portion of the fornices, the mamillary bodies, and the dorso-medial nucleus of the thalamus (Victor, Adams & Collins, 1971; Brierley, 1977; Mair, Warrington & Weiskrantz, 1979). Ultimately, therefore, the special features of the Korsakoff syndrome may well turn out to be bound up with the nature and localization of the underlying pathology.

In 1972, Lhermitte and Signoret drew a very similar comparison between the psychiatric picture in a patient who exhibited a severe post-encephalitic syndrome and a typical case of alcoholic Korsakoff syndrome. The post-encephalitic patient had previously been reported by Delay and Brion (1954). Whereas the Korsakoff patient was insightless, confabulatory, and disorientated in all spheres, the post-encephalitic patient exhibited an acute awareness of his amnesia. In the former, there had been appreciable involvement of thalamic structures verified at necropsy, whereas in the post-encephalitic patient air-encephalography disclosed elective dilatation of both temporal lobes. To this extent, the findings would seem fully compatible with Zangwill's contentions.

Lhermitte and Signoret were not, however, content with these purely clinical and anatomical considerations. They enquired further whether a careful study of the finer properties of the amnesic state in these two types of patient might not reveal further differences between 'hippocampal' and 'diencephalic' amnesic syndromes. To throw light on this issue, they were led to compare the performance of ten Korsakoff patients, four of whom were judged clinically to be completely lacking in insight, with that of three post-encephalitic patients (one of whom was the patient already referred to) on a novel battery of psychometric tests. Of these, the most revealing was one of learning and retaining the spatial position of each of nine pictures of familiar objects simultaneously displayed. The criterion of learning was three consecutive correct performances and subjects who attained this criterion were re-tested by various methods at intervals varying from three minutes to six days. It was found that all ten Korsakoffs and one of the three post-encephalitic patients duly learned the task, though requiring significantly more trials than the control subjects. Evidence of retention of what had been learned for up to four days was apparent in all Korsakoff patients but the one successful post-encephalitic patient scored at chance level even after an interval as short as three minutes. On the other hand, the performance of the three post-encephalitic patients was superior to that of the Korsakoffs on certain other tests in this battery which called for an understanding of simple codes and logical relationships. Although the methodology of Lhermitte and Signoret's experimental work is far from wholly satisfactory (Huppert & Piercy, 1979), it does seem that when Korsakoff patients and those with amnesia resulting from encephalitis are brought to the same criterion of memory performance, the Korsakoff patients retain the material more or less normally while the patients with presumed hippocampal damage fail to do so.

This suggestion that the rate of forgetting is markedly accelerated in post-encephalitic as compared with Korsakoff patients gains further credence in the light of two studies carried out with Scoville and Milner's celebrated amnesic patient, H.M. This patient, it will be remembered, had undergone bilateral medial temporal lobe resection for intractable epilepsy in 1953 and there had been little improvement in his memory when tested by Milner in 1962 or subsequently by Huppert and Piercy in 1978. Milner (1972) attempted to measure the rate of forgetting in short-term memory in this patient using a method of delayed comparison originally devised by Konorski (1959) for use in animal experiments. The method consists in presenting two stimuli, such as clicks or light flashes, in close succession, separated by a variable time interval. The task of the subject is to report whether its second stimulus is the same or different from the first. Its difficulty may be increased either by lengthening the inter-trial interval or by introducing a distraction before the second stimulus is presented. Her findings (as reported by Prisco, 1963) show that, in H.M. there is a sharp deterioration in accuracy of judgement over a delay period of 30 seconds even without distraction; with an inter-trial interval of one minute or more, this patient's performance fell to chance level. This appears to imply that the rate of forgetting even in short-term memory was markedly accelerated.

A more recent study by Huppert and Piercy (1979) points in the same direction. In an earlier study, these authors had demonstrated that Korsakoff patients who had learned after relatively prolonged exposure to recognize pictorial material at a level comparable to that of healthy control subjects did not differ from the latter in their picture recognition performance (Huppert & Piercy, 1978). It might therefore appear that the memory defect in Korsakoff patients is due to slow initial learning rather than to failure of storage or retrieval. In the present study, they report two attempts to equalize the initial scores obtained by H.M. and a group of alcoholic Korsakoff patients on a comparable pictorial recognition test. The second attempt was successful and provided clear evidence that when the opportunity for learning was sufficient to enable H.M. to recognize novel pictures after a ten-minute interval as efficiently as the Korsakoffs, his performance declined more sharply than that of the Korsakoff patients when re-tested after one and 24 days. This suggests that, whereas Korsakoff patients, in spite of their diminished learning capacity, adequately retain what they do succeed in mastering to a degree comparable with that of normal subjects, patients with hippocampal amnesia exhibit in addition to slow learning a marked acceleration in speed of forgetting. Although in need of confirmation, this conclusion would appear to be in line with the present writer's experience of post-encephalitic as opposed to diencephalic amnesic states. In the former, the defect is shown principally in rapid forgetting, which in severe cases takes place as soon as the memory span is exceeded (see also Conrad, 1953), while in the latter, in spite of ostensible forgetting, some retrieval of recent memories can often be elicited by persistent and skilful interrogation (Grünthal, 1923) or by the provision of 'partial information', i.e. a cueing technique (Williams, 1953; Warrington & Weiskrantz, 1968, 1973).

In the light of these various considerations, it might be concluded that two distinct varieties of amnesic syndrome exist. In the first, there is severe amnesia associated with lack of insight, denial of disability, and not infrequently confabulation, at all events in the acute or early stages of the illness. This is the classical Korsakoff syndrome. In the second, there is equally severe amnesia but insight and judgement are well preserved. This is the amnesia associated with medial temporal lobe lesions, almost always bilateral, and is usually associated with hippocampal damage (though this has been questioned by Horel, 1978). Although the amnesia *per se* is otherwise very similar in the two syndromes (in both of which appreciable residual learning capacity may be established under appropriate conditions), there is some evidence that whereas storage capacity is diminished and forgetting is much accelerated in temporal lobe amnesia, in the Korsakoff syndrome the defect seems to bear principally, as Korsakoff (1889) himself supposed, on the retrieval of recently acquired information. The extent to which these two forms or manifestations of amnesia may overlap in patients with the multifocal or diffuse cerebral lesions so commonly encountered in psychiatric practice remains to be ascertained.

Claparède's paradox

In one of his early papers on organic amnesia, Korsakoff remarked that although a patient who sees his doctor every day may say that he has never seen him before and has no idea whom he may be, he none the less does not react to him as a total stranger. Some twenty years later, the Swiss psychologist

E. Claparède (1911) published a paper on recognition which owed much to the study of a patient who had been diagnosed as a case of Korsakoff's psychosis. Although attracting little notice at the time, this paper has had considerable influence on later students of the amnesic syndrome (see MacCurdy, 1928; Zangwill, 1977; Williams, 1979; Warrington & Weiskrantz, 1979) and is extremely relevant to the relations between recognition and recall and to the issue of residual learning capacity in amnesic states.

As Claparède saw it, the experimental work of his graduate student, D. Katzaroff (1911), appeared to have established that the basic factor in recognition is affective rather than cognitive and may be described as the feeling of familiarity. Recognition is in the first instance at least independent of recall, comparison, and judgement, though its justification and contextual reference may call for their exercise. In the language of Hughlings Jackson, the experience of familiarity implies subject consciousness rather than reference to an external event (Jackson, 1931), and Claparède spoke of it as the sense of *moïté* (translated by MacCurdy as 'me-ness'), which implies that the object or situation eliciting it is accepted as falling within the previous experience of the subject. He then cites observations based partly on his case of Korsakoff's psychosis and partly on some observations of post-hypnotic amnesia in support of his contentions.

The Korsakoff patient was a lady, aged 47, who was seen by Claparède several years after the onset of her illness. At this stage, she is stated to have shown good preservation of early memories and general knowledge though gross amnesia for recent and current events. Although she had been confined for the previous five years in the same institution, she was grossly disoriented in all spheres and claimed not to know her doctors or a member of the nursing staff who had been in attendance upon her for the previous six months. She was likewise disorientated for personal age. In all these respects, she presented the typical picture of the Korsakoff syndrome.

Claparède observed that whereas this patient appeared quite unable to initiate recall of recent events or to recognize them should they recur by chance, she none the less could be shown to possess appreciable residual memory capacity. For example, she showed distinct 'savings' on re-learning lists of paired associates – an accomplishment first demonstrated in Korsakoff patients by Brodmann (1902, 1904). While denying that she had ever heard a short story read to her a few minutes earlier, she could none the less give the age of a lady who featured in it, as if by guesswork, in answer to a direct question. Although denying that she had drawn a simple figure ten minutes before, when asked to draw the first figure that came into her head she would draw a figure which evidently derived from one that she had been shown. In short, evidence of memory retention could be elicited in spite of the patient's evident conviction that she had no knowledge of the items to which her attention had been directed.

It was demonstrated by Claparède that the acquisition of simple habits might likewise be within this patient's capacity. For instance, a test not infrequently used by German psychiatrists of this period (Coriat, 1904; Zangwill, 1967) consisted in pricking the patient's hand with a pin concealed in the examiner's hand. When asked a few minutes later, an amnesic patient may deny having felt the prick but none the less exhibits definite withdrawal or avoidance tendencies if the examiner goes through the motions of delivery of a second prick. This effect Claparède was likewise able to demonstrate in his own patient, her avoidance behaviour being justified by facile rationalization. Claparède was further able to show that whereas his patient was unable to describe the lay-out of the hospital in which she had spent many months, she had in fact learned in practice to orientate herself within the building and to ask appropriate questions of those whom she happened to encounter though, to direct questioning, would deny that she had met them before or was aware of their identity.

In Claparède's view, these phenomena of residual learning without acknowledgement of what has been learned or retained find a certain analogy in phenomena of post-hypnotic suggestion, as when a subject successfully carries out an instruction for which amnesia after awakening has been induced but when asked why he did so, justifies it by facile rationalization. In such a case, the deficit in sense of familiarity or 'me-ness' together with a failure of voluntary recall indicates a disconnection between a particular past event and its relation to the continuity of personality. The possible significance of this observation to an understanding of the relationship between organic and psychogenic amnesias is considered below (pp. 111–13).

The Canadian psychiatrist, J. T. MacCurdy, who worked for many years in Cambridge, summarized Claparède's findings in an attempt to delineate common principles in physiology and psychology (MacCurdy, 1928). Previously, he had encouraged D. Wechsler (1917) to undertake one of the earliest experimental studies of short-term memory and associative learning in Korsakoff patients, from which he concluded that the major deficit in the Korsakoff syndrome lies in the learning and retention of novel associations. Like Claparède before him, MacCurdy had been much struck by the discrepancy between the behaviour and the conscious memory of Korsakoff patients and, in addition to confirming a number of his observations, devised a useful informal test, in which he required the patient to 'guess' what the physician's name and address might be shortly after he had been given this information. If he failed, he was then presented with a number of surnames and addresses, including those of the physician, and asked to select those most likely to pertain to him. 'To my surprise', wrote MacCurdy, 'the guesses were nearly as accurate as would be the conscious memory of such data by normal subjects.' (MacCurdy, 1928, p. 121).

The present writer has frequently had occasion to repeat observations substantially similar to those of Claparède and MacCurdy. For instance, one alcoholic Korsakoff patient who invariably claimed that he had been admitted to hospital earlier on the same day (in fact, he had been resident in the same hospital for several months) was none the less able to conduct his examiner to his bed in the ward and evidently recognized it. The same patient was able after several weeks in hospital to give the correct name of the hospital when asked, but the name was given tentatively, as if by guess-work, and justified by facile rationalization. Another Korsakoff patient who invariably denied that he had been twice married, none the less immediately recognized his second wife and introduced her as such on her visits to the hospital. The present writer has also described a young patient with a post-meningitic amnesic syndrome who despite good insight and recognition of his disability was quite unable to recall or describe visits on the same day to different rooms or sections of the hospital complex yet was able in practice to orientate himself satisfactorily within it (Zangwill, 1977). Comparable deficits of conscious or voluntary retrieval in spite of evidence of appreciable retained learning capacity have also been described in a variety of experimental situations (see Warrington & Weiskrantz, 1968, 1979).

This dissociation is brought out exceptionally

well in a recent report by Warrington and Weiskrantz (1979) on eye-blink conditioning in two severely amnesic patients, one a case of Korsakoff's psychosis and the other a post-encephalitic amnesic state. Both subjects were successfully conditioned to a compound visual and auditory signal with retention of the conditioned response over intervals of ten minutes and 24 hours. Although the findings do not permit a definite conclusion as to whether the rates of learning and retention of eyelid conditioning were within normal limits, interrogation of the patients (extracts of which are reproduced in the paper) are remarkably reminiscent of Claparède's original observations. In neither case was the patient able to recall or describe the conditioning procedure or even to remember the delivery of air puffs to the eye. Although the verbal responses of the Korsakoff patient were more discursive than those of the post-encephalitic patient – indeed on occasion frankly confabulatory – neither patient possessed more than a fragmentary recollection of the experiment and its attendant circumstances even ten minutes after the conditioning procedure had been concluded. Although the conditioned response had been acquired, its acquisition had apparently not been recorded at a communicable level. Unfortunately, it is not clear from this brief report whether a 'guessing' or multiple choice recognition technique might have yielded information indicating more extensive registration of the technique and circumstances of the experiment than was forthcoming at interview. It does, however, provide indisputable evidence of a clear dissociation between the subjects' commentaries and their objective procedure.

There is some evidence from studies of animal learning that a dissociation may exist between performances which might appear to depend on the sense of familiarity and those built up on the basis of associative learning. In his studies of fornicectomy, Gaffan (1972, 1974) has reported that rats which have sustained this operation appear defective after it on tasks in which the only clue to correct performance appears to be a sense of familiarity, while remaining unimpaired on performances which necessitate the learning of an association between an object and food reinforcement. This finding led him to set up an experiment in which a severely amnesic patient with presumed involvement of the hippocampal region was required to learn a simple colour discrimination task of a kind much used in studies of associative learning in animals. Gaffan (1972) was able to demonstrate good retention of the discrimination habit after an interval of 24 hours in spite of the fact that the patient categorically denied having seen either the apparatus or the examiner before, thus betraying an apparent loss in sense of familiarity. As it has been alleged that animals with hippocampal lesions can learn and retain only habits that do not presuppose recognition memory, this might suggest, as claimed by Claparède, that a comparable dissociation between recognition and voluntary recall can likewise be demonstrated in man.

As was maintained earlier, the amnesic patients studied by Huppert and Piercy (1976) were found to demonstrate surprisingly good recognition of complex pictorial material in spite of slow initial learning. This might seem to suggest that the sense of familiarity is substantially intact. None the less, it has long been known that amnesic patients, when tested under conditions less stringent than either two-choice or 'yes–no' recognition, often exhibit a striking degree of reduplicative paramnesia. Thus it was shown by Zangwill (1941) that when Korsakoff patients are presented with material, such as pictures or even common objects, that had previously been shown to them, they not infrequently deny that they have seen them before and will concede only that they have seen 'something similar'. In such cases, interrogation often reveals a number of alleged 'points of difference' between the picture now shown and the supposed picture alleged to have been shown previously. Zangwill was therefore led to speak of an incapacity to respond to identity, which although it might depend in part on a defective sense of familiarity, probably involved other factors as well, e.g. partial forgetting and impoverished critique. At the same time, he had no doubt that recognition in such patients as a general rule is vastly superior to voluntary recall.

It is argued by Huppert and Piercy (1976) that these differences between recognition and recall are best interpreted in terms of inability to organize experience in terms of an appropriate spatial or temporal framework. Following the line of thinking adumbrated by van der Horst (1932, 1956) some years ago, they argue that there is typically failure in the amnesic patient to endow successive experiences with a 'time-tag' or to organize them in appropriate temporal sequence. For example, their patients were found to be unable to discriminate between two pictures shown to them on different days (or at different times on the same day) although either picture, when shown alone, was confidently recognized. This might suggest not an uncomplicated deficit in the sense of familiarity but rather a defect in temporal encoding resulting in what Talland (1965) referred to as 'contextual isolation'. This indicates a failure in association which is probably at least as important as the deficit in what Claparède termed familiarity sense or *moïté*. Moreover, it is now well established that amnesic patients are (within limits) well able to improve upon their initial performance on simple sensori-motor tests as a result of practice and it is noteworthy that such tasks presuppose only a gain in skill and do not involve the ordering of items in sequence or their referral to a specific and circumscribed context (Milner, Corkin & Teuber, 1968; Starr & Phillips, 1970). One may conclude that of the many theories which have been put forward to explain anterograde amnesia, that to which Piercy refers (1977, p. 47) as the *contextual memory hypothesis* has evidently much to commend it. At all events, it goes some way to account for the noteworthy difference between recognition and recall in amnesic persons and thereby to resolve in part Claparède's paradox that an amnesic patient in some sense remembers in spite of dense amnesia.

Retrograde amnesia and Ribot's law

According to Ribot's 'Law of Regression', '. . . the progressive destruction of memory follows a logical order – a law. It advances progressively from the unstable to the stable. It begins with the most recent recollections which, being lightly impressed upon the nervous elements, rarely repeated and consequently having no permanent associations, represent organization in its feeblest form. It ends with the sensorial, instinctive memory, which, having become a permanent and integral part of the organism, represents organization in its most highly developed stage.' (Ribot, 1882, p. 121–2). Although Ribot was mainly concerned with the progressive dementia associated with diffuse brain disease, his principle was soon applied to phenomena as diverse as the dissolution of language in aphasic polyglots and the scope and mode of recovery of retrograde amnesia after concussional head injury, in both of which the main emphasis was placed on the relative recency of acquisition in relation to breakdown. It should, however, be borne in mind that he regarded recency as only one of the factors governing the stability of recent memory and its relative vulnerability to the effects of brain injury or disease. Another was fre-

quency of usage or of reproduction, which has since been shown to be of greater importance in governing disorders of object-naming in aphasia than age of acquisition of names (Oldfield, 1966; Newcombe, Oldfield & Wingfield, 1965; Rochford & Williams, 1962–4). It is likewise probable that it is also a factor of some importance in relation to differential impairment of individual languages in aphasia in polyglots.

In the present section, we shall be concerned only with the factor of *recency* in relation to the scope and course of recovery of amnesia after head injury or the onset of focal brain disease. Let us consider first traumatic amnesia. As is well-known, after head injuries of sufficient severity to give rise to loss of consciousness, there is almost invariably a brief period of traumatic amnesia (PTA) usually permanent, together with a retrograde amnesia (RA) which may at first cover a period varying from a few seconds to many minutes, hours or even days preceding the accident. Its duration increases with increasing severity of head injury, and probably also, if less regularly, with increasing age of the patient. (Russell & Smith, 1961; Russell, 1971).

While PTA remains as a permanent gap in memory, RA almost always undergoes some degree of 'shrinkage', and its final duration, as a rule brief, provides a widely accepted index of the severity of the injury, (Russell, 1971). In cases in which the head injury is severe, recovery of consciousness is followed by a confusional state which may at first cover months or years of the patient's life antedating the accident. Indeed, sometimes it persists for a prolonged period (traumatic Korsakoff state), though as a rule it undergoes appreciable shrinkage during and after remission of the confusional state. This situation provides a good opportunity to test the validity of Ribot's law.

In early studies of the recovery of memory of events antedating a head injury, the course of recovery was on occasion found to be much as predicted by Ribot, memory for more remote events being restored before that for those more recent. This was very clear in the case reported by Kömpfen (cited by Ribot, 1882 and later discussed by Janet, 1928). But in another early case reported by Abercrombie (1867), the course of recovery was apparently in the opposite direction, events that took place shortly before the accident being remembered before those of the previous day. In a more systematic study of 'shrinkage' of retrograde amnesia after mild head injuries, Williams (see Zangwill, 1961) found that the first step in the restoration of memory for the recent past is the emergence of an isolated recollection, without temporal context, which was typically of a relatively trivial event which had occurred between 15 or 20 minutes before the accident and which the patient accepts as his 'last' memory before finding himself in hospital. Further memories emerge in the course of the next few hours or days and may relate to events which either preceded or followed the 'last memory'. At this stage of recovery, recollections may appear to possess a curiously remote, even unreal, character and are not uncommonly transposed or mislocalized in time. Although the order of their return may follow a chronological sequence, more commonly their retrieval is apparently haphazard, depending on cues or chance associations provided by conversation with relatives. In essence, however, this process of 'shrinkage' is essentially endogenous (Whitty & Zangwill, 1977), though it may on occasion be slightly accelerated by investigation under barbiturate narcosis (Russell & Nathan, 1946). In accordance with Ribot's law, however, there is some evidence from studies of transient retrograde amnesia following electro-convulsive therapy that the shorter the interval between the presentation of a test item and the delivery of the treatment, the less likely is it to be regarded as familiar on a subsequent recognition test (Mayer-Gross, 1943).

In recovery from more severe head injuries, prolonged retrograde amnesias comparable to those found in the chronic alcoholic Korsakoff syndrome are not uncommonly described, more especially in elderly patients. Initially, these may extend over several years antecedent to the accident, though there are as a rule some (though usually ill-defined and fluctuating) 'islands of memory'. As in the Korsakoff syndrome, the scope of this amnesia is often found to determine, at all events in part, the content of disorientation for time, place, and personal age, and may likewise govern the themes expressed in confabulation. (Paterson & Zangwill, 1944; Benson & Geschwind, 1967). As Benson and Geschwind rightly point out, such extended retrograde amnesias are usually, perhaps invariably, linked with lack of insight and denial of illness and their shrinkage begins only with remission of the post-traumatic confusional state and the restitution of continuous day-to-day memory. It is noteworthy that after shrinkage of amnesia has apparently ceased, interrogation under barbiturate sedation may provoke reinstatement of the amnesia, disorientation, and

denial of illness which marked the earlier confusional state (Zangwill, 1977; Benson & Geschwind, 1967).

It has been shown by Williams and Zangwill (1952) that occasionally after recovery from mild head injuries and frequently after recovery from more severe ones, episodes of retrograde amnesia for incidents in personal experience dating from up to a year before the accident commonly occur. These may be noted with some surprise by the patient long after he has regained continuous memory for day-to-day events and retrograde amnesia as ordinarily assessed has long since 'shrunk' to its final, brief duration. For example, the patient may claim to have completely forgotten how or where he spent his last summer holiday though this information is readily given by his relatives. Williams (1979) has also given examples of dense and apparently extended retrograde amnesias which may remain in evidence indefinitely after full recovery from tuberculous meningitis. These amnesias do not appear to undergo further shrinkage and are apparently permanent. In one of her patients, for example, memory capacity for recent and current events appeared to be fully restored though the patient remained amnesic not only for the period in which he was acutely ill but also for a period of approximately two years preceding the onset of the illness. There were, however, isolated 'islands of memory' though these were lacking in temporal reference. A point of particular interest is that he had apparently lost his ability to type, acquired shortly before the onset of the illness, indicating that recently acquired motor skills are no less subject to retrograde amnesia than personal recollections.

Although Korsakoff himself placed little emphasis on retrograde amnesia in the syndrome that now bears his name, Bonhöffer (1901) accepted it, along with anterograde amnesia, disorientation and confabulation, as a cardinal element in this syndrome. Both he and Liepmann (1910) described cases of retrograde amnesia in cases of alcoholic Korsakoff syndrome extending over ten or twenty years, though memory for childhood and early life apparently remained intact. Although such retrograde amnesias are often less well-defined and may exhibit a good deal of condensation, misdating of recollections, and related inconsistencies, sharply-bounded retrograde amnesias of long duration are far from rare. As Meggendorfer (1928) has pointed out, experiences at the threshold of the amnesic gap may in such cases exert a prepotent influence on the content of disorientation for place, time and personal age (Paterson & Zangwill, 1944; Zangwill, 1953, 1967). Zangwill (1950) has also pointed out that retrograde amnesia of long duration may apparently influence the content of generic mental images. In a case of chronic alcoholic Korsakoff syndrome, for example, he reported that the patient reproduced, as if contemporary, styles of dress out-moded by ten to fifteen years. Drawings of other objects in which there had been clear-cut changes in design, e.g. motor cars or buses, showed comparable regression (Zangwill, 1950).

The reversibility of retrograde amnesias of diverse aetiology, in particular traumatic, strongly suggests that this deficit is due to failure of recall or retrieval rather than to a true abolition of remote memory. Even in Korsakoff patients with prolonged and apparently dense retrograde amnesias, the provision of cues, if sufficiently salient, will often bring about retrieval, at all events temporarily. For example, a patient with a retrograde amnesia of at least 15 years could recall nothing whatsoever of his activities in the year prior to the onset of his illness. None the less, he recognized, if somewhat hesitantly, a workmate with whom he had become acquainted a year or so before the onset of his illness and correctly recalled the name of their place of work, of which he ordinarily denied the slightest knowledge. Again, a patient studied by the writer (Zangwill, 1977) with a dense retrograde amnesia covering approximately five years, completely denied that he had been twice married but at once recognized his present wife and accepted her as such when she visited him in hospital. Although the role of retrieval defect in anterograde amnesia is controversial, in the case of retrograde amnesia it can hardly be doubted that failure to retrieve information recorded and stored at a time when the brain was undamaged is relative rather than absolute, i.e. reflects a failure in the mechanism of retrieval.

The tendency for retrograde amnesia to involve more recent rather than more remote memory, together with the retrogressive amnesias commonly observed as a consequence of progressive brain disease, has for long been accepted by clinicians as broadly true and as providing substantial support for Ribot's generalization. In recent years, however, neuropsychologists have endeavoured to subject Ribot's law to more highly controlled experimental verification. Whereas it is clearly difficult to apply controlled methods to the acquisition of biographical material relevant to a patient's life history, it is by no

means impossible to develop quantitative methods of sampling memory for events of general or public interest and several attempts to achieve this have been attempted in recent years. In view of the long-standing interest in Ribot's law and its bearing on the cerebral organization of memory, this work on 'gradients of recency' may be briefly summarized.

The pioneer study was that of Sanders and Warrington (1971; see also Warrington & Sanders, 1971). Making use of a questionnaire technique for assessing memory for 'public events' devised by Warrington and Silberstein (1970), these authors extended the original questionnaire to cover almost 40 years and devised a comparable technique to assess recognition of photographs of either contemporary or formerly well-known public figures. Results from 200 healthy control subjects and five amnesic patients (three cases of alcoholic Korsakoff syndrome and two of severe and chronic amnesia consequent upon carbon monoxide poisoning and temporal lobectomy respectively) are presented. On both the long-term memory questionnaire and the recognition test of 'famous faces', the findings were essentially negative. No evidence was obtained suggesting that remote memory was either spared altogether or less impaired than memory for quite recent experiences. In short, the findings gave no support for Ribot's belief that the dissolution of memory is inversely proportional to the relative recency of the events stored in long-term memory. The authors were therefore led to suggest that the scope of retrograde amnesia in Korsakoff and kindred amnesic states may well have been underestimated and that the defect was in fact operating over the whole span of the patient's adult experience. It was further proposed that the gradient often attributed to retrograde amnesia is more likely to be due not to the greater vulnerability of memories of increasing recency as to a lack of control of the difficulty of test items, i.e. questions relating to the different decades.

Although this study quite properly attracted much interest, the results of three later inquiries along similar lines have failed to endorse its conclusions. Seltzer and Benson (1974), who likewise devised a multiple choice questionnaire probing memory for public events across different decades in the lifetime of their patients (alcoholic Korsakoffs), found that the latter had a score on questions relating to the earlier years of the present century significantly superior to the score on those relating to events in more recent decades. Marslen-Wilson and Teuber (1975), in a study of particular interest, devised a face recognition test in which each item was allocated to the decade in which the individual in question had first gained fame. This test was followed by a prompting session in which all items that had not secured explicit and complete identification were re-presented and possible retrieval facilitated by a systematic cueing technique. Furthermore, the subjects included Milner and Scoville's celebrated amnesic patient H.M. as well as twelve patients diagnosed as cases of Korsakoff's disease. There were two control groups, one consisting of 34 head-injured but non-amnesic patients which was used as a control group for H.M., and the other of 12 chronic alcoholics, all without history of Wernicke's encephalopathy, to serve as control group for the Korsakoff patients.

The results of this inquiry were as follows: In the case of H.M., recognition in the absence of prompts was found to be above average for the 1920s or 1930s, to fall off slightly in the 1940s, and to drop dramatically in the next two decades. With cueing, on the other hand, H.M.'s performance was indistinguishable from that of the controls for all decades except the 1960s, when it fell below the average reached by the controls. These results are not altogether surprising when it is borne in mind that this patient underwent bi-temporal lobectomy in 1953 at the age of 24 and had exhibited a severe anterograde amnesia ever since. There had originally been a post-operative retrograde amnesia for the three years prior to the lobectomy (Scoville & Milner, 1957) which may have undergone some shrinkage in course of time (Milner, Corkin & Teuber, 1968). The slight fall-off in recognition performance for the 1940s as compared with earlier decades may be attributed to the retrograde amnesia which had been noted following operation. Nevertheless, much of this material could still be retrieved with the help of cues.

It was found that the Korsakoff patients did worse than their non-amnesic alcoholic controls for all decades until the 1960s, when the recognition rate fell off sharply. With prompting, however, the scores of the Korsakoffs and their alcoholic controls were indistinguishable for all decades. The conclusions might therefore seem to be that whereas a gradient of accessibility of remote (pre-morbid) memories appears to exist, this gradient effectively vanishes if a prompting technique is employed. This, together with the results given by H.M., provides further evidence that the deficit in retrograde amnesia is essentially one of retrieval and that a gradient consistent with Ribot's law appears only in the case of spontaneous, as opposed to cued or socially facilitated, retrieval of long-term information. This is consistent with Marslen-Wilson and Teuber's additional report that a very extensive series of biographical interviews with H.M. yielded rich recollections for the first two and a half decades of his life in contrast with both his impoverished spontaneous recollections from the year or two immediately prior to his operation and with the virtually complete absence of spontaneous recollections from the two decades subsequent to it. Although the capacity for recall in general is clearly unaffected in retrograde amnesia, there appears to be a failure voluntarily to recall more recent material acquired at a time when the brain was healthy and possibly also in states of brain dysfunction in which there is chronic memory failure for recent and current events.

The most recent study of retrograde amnesia in Korsakoff patients is that of Albert, Butters, and Levin (1979). Using a carefully designed recall questionnaire and a multiple choice recognition task and devoting particular attention to the selection of items from the standpoint of relative task difficulty, these authors find that, contrary to Warrington and Sanders' results, alcoholic Korsakoff patients possess a marked retrograde amnesia characterized by a steep temporal gradient. This gradient, they claim, does not appear to be an artefact related to the relative difficulty of the task items and it is suggested that the results obtained by Warrington and Sanders (1971) are due to a 'floor effect' and are not truly representative of the patients' retrieval capacity. (See also Butters & Albert, 1982.)

Whereas belief in Ribot's law has inevitably been shaken, it seems fair to conclude from these various studies that some relation does genuinely exist, as clinicians have long accepted, between the recency of a past event antedating the occurrence of head injury or the onset of cerebral disease and failure to recollect it spontaneously or in response to straightforward questions. At the same time, it is equally evident that retrograde amnesia is relative rather than absolute and in spite of the failure of voluntary recall, retrieval either through recognition or through appropriate cueing techniques can restore access, at all events transiently, to the ostensibly forgotten material.

Memory disorders associated with diffuse brain disease

The memory impairment characteristic of the senile and pre-senile dementias is of course the aspect of amnesia most familiar to psychogeriatricians. Some degree of memory failure is almost invariably an early – if not the earliest – manifestation of early dementia and it is often difficult, if not indeed impossible, to differentiate it with confidence from deterioration in memory inseparable from the normal ageing process. At the same time, the parallel with ageing must not be drawn too finely, in that the ageing brain commonly involves changes which are in part independent of the ageing process itself (Whitty *et al*, 1977). In particular, cerebral arteriosclerosis with consequent ischaemia and cell loss is common in elderly patients and the mental defects associated with ageing may in fact be the result of such damage rather than the effects of ageing *per se*. In this connection, it may be reported that some recent work by Huppert (personal communication, 1980) suggests that the memory capacity of some non-demented elderly persons is often surprisingly adequate and their performance on memory tasks may actually prove superior to that of much younger subjects of comparable intelligence and education. Indeed the whole issue of ageing and its effects on memory obviously stands in need of fresh inquiry.

It has been pointed out by Allison (1962) that the onset of memory failure in patients with diffuse as opposed to focal lesions is as a rule gradual and takes the form of a general forgetfulness, in particular for names and dates. The extent to which this represents a dysphasic rather than a dysmnesic syndrome is far from clear. Dysphasia is, of course, of common occurrence in Alzheimer's disease, though it is possible to minimize its effects in studying memory defect by appropriate selection of test material (Miller, 1973). As dementia progresses, amnesia for events antedating the onset of the illness becomes increasingly apparent, though a long and well-circumscribed amnesic gap, as is not uncommon in the Korsakoff syndrome, is rare. Although events of early life are on the whole retained better than those more recent, exceptions to Ribot's law are the rule rather than the exception and the patient comes increasingly to present a pattern of generalized memory impairment covering both recent and remote events (Lishman, 1978).

Under the influence of Eugen Bleuler (1924), it was at one time widely believed by psychiatrists that memory defect in the organic psychoses is without significance for the localization of memory processes. This view was undoubtedly much strengthened by the pioneer experiments of K. S. Lashley (1929, 1950) on brain mechanisms and intelligence in the rat and monkey. Lashley was led to conclude from a long series of cerebral ablation studies that the learning and retention of acquired habits and skills depends upon the extent rather than the locus of a cortical lesion and put forward a theory of cerebral mass action to account for this correlation. A critical evaluation of this theory has been presented by the present writer elsewhere (Zangwill, 1960). One may also note that a study by Chapman *et al* (1958) likewise indicates that intellectual disability in man resulting from brain damage is a function of the extent rather than the site of improperly functioning tissue within the neopallium. Although current opinion in physiological psychology is strongly critical of the mass action hypothesis and has veered increasingly towards the older localizationist position, it is still pertinent to ask whether the progressive amnesias of diffuse brain disease are attributable to general rather than to focal cerebral dysfunction.

In defence of the mass action hypothesis, it may be argued that the steadily increasing deterioration of memory with progressively advancing pathology indicates that the cerebral involvement in Alzheimer's disease is diffuse rather than focal. On the other hand, several authors have laid stress on the high incidence of pathological changes in the hippocampal region in both non-demented old people (Gellerstedt, 1933) and in cases of Alzheimer's disease (Corsellis, 1970; Tomlinson, 1979). A relatively high incidence of electroencephalographic abnormalities in the temporal region in elderly people has also been claimed, most pronounced in cases in which learning capacity is said to have been most markedly defective (Busse, 1962). These observations suggest that dementia is particularly liable to involve defect of memory in cases in which the stress of the lesion falls upon the hippocampus and related structures. This would be in keeping with the extensive evidence involving bilateral mesial temporal lobe lesions in the aetiology of circumscribed amnesic syndromes.

On the other hand, Brierley (1961, 1965, 1977), who has devoted particular attention to possible correlations between circumscribed cerebral lesions and disorders of memory, concludes that it is only rarely that a striking memory defect for recent events can be correlated with a high incidence of senile plaques and of neurofibril changes in the hippocampal formation and the mamillary bodies. Further, neither the neuronal nor the glial alterations in the ageing brain show any selective concentration in these two regions of the brain, damage to either of which is so regularly linked with amnesia. Clearly, therefore, no very clear or consistent correlations emerge between the amnesia of diffuse brain disease and selective involvement of areas of the brain, local damage to which is reliably known to produce gross memory disorder in non-demented patients.

At the same time, the possibility remains that memory disorder in pre-senile dementia is governed by a combination of focal and general symptoms. For example, Miller (1971, 1972, 1973) has adduced evidence that short-term memory capacity, while typically intact in hippocampal amnesia, is appreciably reduced in pre-senile dementia. Although dysphasic disorders do of course occur in Alzheimer's disease, Miller studied only patients without clinically evident dysphasia and the material used in his word-span tests comprised only common monosyllables likely to remain within the patients' usable vocabulary. He therefore concluded that the short-term memory defect is a consequence of the dementia rather than the expression of a lesion selectively involving the temporal lobes.

Miller further studied rote learning in pre-senile patients of lists of items exceeding the length of the memory span. For many years, 'supra-span' rote learning tests have been widely used as clinical tests of memory impairment (Zangwill, 1943) and have more recently been applied in more highly standardized form by Drachman and Arbit (1966) in their study of patients with involvement of the hippocampal complex. Using Drachman and Arbit's technique, Miller was led to conclude that, in addition to the short-term memory deficit, the demented patient has an additional defect in his ability to establish new material in long-term memory. Although cautious in his interpretation of this finding, Miller suggests that it might represent a retrieval defect comparable to that described by Warrington and Weiskrantz (1970) in their work on non-demented patients with severe organic amnesia. Such a defect might conceivably involve the mesial temporal lobes and their midbrain connections. At all events, his work suggests that further analysis of amnesia in relation to the neuropathology of Alzheimer's disease might throw interesting light upon the neuropsychology of memory.

A related issue, liable to attract increasing interest, is the demonstration of psychological impairment resulting from chronic alcoholism in patients other than cases of Korsakoff's syndrome (Ryan & Butters, 1980; Lishman *et al.*, 1980). Of particular importance is the interim report of Lishman, Ron, and Acker (1980) of the incidence in chronic alcoholics of intellectual deterioration, together with radiographic (CT scan) evidence of appreciable cortical shrinkage in young as well as in older patients. These findings were elicited after a period of total abstinence and, in spite of the lack of significant positive findings on clinical examination, the data indicate that the larger the size of the ventricles, the greater the verbal/performance discrepancy on the Wechsler Adult Intelligence Scale and the poorer the performance on certain non-verbal memory tests. Publication of the detailed findings of the study, particularly as regards the differential effects of age (if any), reversibility or otherwise of the psychological deficit, and the relationship of memory defect to intellectual loss, is eagerly awaited.

Amnesias associated with electro-convulsive therapy (ECT)

In view of the extensive use made of ECT in psychiatric treatment, mention should be made of its well-known effects on memory, which can on occasion become a matter of genuine concern both to patients and their relatives. Though it is somewhat misleading to compare these normally transient adverse side-effects of ECT with the more persistent memory impairment following temporal lobectomy, as Inglis (1970) has done, it might seem reasonable to compare the memory deficit which may follow a course of ECT with the after-effects of head-injury. As after mild head injury, a transient confusional state of brief duration is generated by a single treatment which is characterized by brief retrograde and slightly more prolonged anterograde amnesia, often with transitory disorientation (Williams, 1977). Not infrequently, the retrograde amnesia may initially be of longer duration and undergo rapid 'shrinkage' much as after mild head injury with brief loss of consciousness. The anterograde amnesia, likewise, may outlast the confusional state by some hours. A good account of the recovery of psychological capacity after ECT has been provided by Williams (1977, 1979).

Appreciable memory defect may at first be noted after the completion of a course of ECT lasting from one to four weeks. While patients themselves not infrequently complain of forgetfulness, as a rule in the small matters of everyday life and more especially in the recall of personal names, the memory deficit has been more convincingly demonstrated through the use of standardized psychometric tests (Hetherington, 1956; Cronholm & Blomquist, 1959).

Cronholm and Molander (1957) have produced convincing evidence that this deficit is essentially transient and restitution of memory was found to be complete in 28 patients who were tested on a variety of memory tests one month after the last electroshock in the series. The mean number of treatments in this series was 5.3 and treatment was given over a period of 18 days. On the other hand, the occurrence of more persistent and in some cases relatively severe memory impairment has been reported by some earlier authors in the case of patients who had undergone intensive and sometimes prolonged treatment with ECT (Brody, 1944; Stengel, 1951). Such cases are seldom reported today and may have been due, in some cases at least, to psychogenic perpetuation of a mild organic memory deficit.

Although some psychiatrists are reluctant to give ECT to elderly patients, Ottoson (1970) has produced psychometric evidence that the side-effects of ECT in older people are no more adverse than in younger subjects. It has also been claimed that the use of flurothyl is an equally effective antidepressant and gives rise to less impairment of memory than conventional ECT (Small, 1974).

While bilateral administration of ECT was for many years the standard method of treatment, the use of unilateral ECT has more recently attracted lively interest. It is claimed that ECT applied to the non-dominant (right) hemisphere gives equally good results in psychiatric treatment and produces a lesser degree of confusion with more rapid recovery of orientation. There is also evidence suggesting that ECT applied to the non-dominant hemisphere produces less memory disturbance than either bilateral ECT or ECT applied to the dominant hemisphere (Halliday et al, 1968; Strain et al, 1968; D'Elia, 1970, 1976; Dornbush et al, 1971). Of particular interest is the fact that whereas application of ECT to the dominant (left) hemisphere gives rise to learning and memory defect predominantly in the verbal sphere, its application to the non-dominant hemisphere produces a comparable disability more marked in the non-verbal or spatial sphere (Halliday et al, 1968; D'Elia, 1976). This observation is in keeping with the fact that an analogous, though far more persistent, pattern of memory deficit is regularly found after unilateral anterior temporal lobectomy (Meyer & Yates, 1955; Milner, 1968 a, b). The finding of more severe memory deficit following bilateral rather than unilateral ECT is also of course compatible with the well-established finding that bilateral temporal lobe involvement appears

to be essential to the genesis of global amnesia in man.

Paramnesia and confabulation

The term paramnesia was introduced by Kraepelin (1886) to denote errors and illusions of memory of pathological extent. He distinguished three main varieties: (1) simple memory deceptions; (2) associative memory deceptions; and (3) identifying paramnesia. Although these terms are seldom used today, the phenomena to which they refer are widely recognized.

(1) *Simple memory deceptions.* In these, events imagined, dreamed, or hallucinated are treated as being genuinely remembered. Such deceptions are of course commonly noted in delirious or confusional states as well as in paranoid or kindred schizophrenic disorders. As they commonly involve disorders of consciousness or belief (or both) rather than circumscribed memory disorders, they will not be considered further in this section.

(2) *Associative memory disorders.* These are typified by memory errors of a kind common in confusional or amnesic states. For example, a person seen for the first time is treated by the patient as having been encountered once or many times previously. Or he may say that he was previously in a hospital bearing the same name as that of the present hospital. This type of memory error has been called reduplicative paramnesia by Pick (1903) or simply *reduplication* (Weinstein & Kahn, 1951, 1955). Reduplication is often noted in the course of remission of the post-traumatic confusional state (Paterson & Zangwill, 1944; Benson, Gardner & Meadows, 1976), as well as in the alcoholic Korsakoff syndrome (Coriat, 1904; Zangwill, 1967).

(3) *Identifying paramnesia.* This refers to faulty recognition, in particular that variety commonly known as *déjà vu*. This odd sense of repetition of an entire experience which is felt to have occurred once before is common among entirely healthy individuals, particularly in youth or when fatigued. It has attracted considerable attention ever since a dramatic personal experience of the phenomenon was described by A. L. Wigan in his once well-known book on *The Duality of the Mind* (1844). This book anticipated in some degree the recent interest in cerebral disconnection syndromes (Geschwind, 1965; Sperry, Gazzaniga & Bogen, 1969). The *déjà vu* phenomenon has even found its way into literature, having been described by, among others, Shelley, Dick-

ens, Hawthorne, Tolstoy and Proust. Many of these reports have obviously been based on personal experience and one of them (Hawthorne) has been discussed by Zangwill (1945). The curious sense of intense familiarity, called by Kinnier Wilson (1928) 'hyperfamiliarity' may be limited to a single sensory modality (usually vision or hearing, though occasionally smell) but the full-blown *déjà vu* experience is typically generalized to the whole of current experience for a brief period, seldom exceeding a few seconds. In some epileptics, however, it may be much more prolonged (Pick, 1903). It is not uncommonly linked with an illusory sense of pseudo-prescience, in which the individual feels that he knows in precise detail what will happen next.

In view of the occurrence of *déjà vu* in ostensibly healthy individuals, it has commonly been regarded as psychogenic and as owing its origin to a partly forgotten experience, phantasy, or dream, the memory of which is triggered off by some feature of the current environment (MacCurdy, 1928). This line of explanation has been popular among psychoanalysts (see Zangwill, 1945) and has gained some support from demonstrations that states resembling *déjà vu* can be induced by post-hypnotic suggestion (Banister & Zangwill, 1941 a, b). On the other hand, an organic basis for *déjà vu* is strongly indicated by its frequent incidence in temporal lobe epilepsy, first clearly recognized by Hughlings Jackson (1879), in which it is frequently reported either as an ictal or inter-ictal phenomenon. It is a matter of some interest that it appears to be more frequent in cases with a right-sided than with a left-sided temporal lobe focus (Mullan & Penfield, 1959; Cole & Zangwill, 1963). Unpublished work by the present writer has failed to reveal any obvious difference between reports of *déjà vu* experienced by patients suffering from temporal lobe epilepsy and those of healthy individuals who have experienced the illusion in the course of everyday life. It may therefore be suggested that in both healthy and epileptic subjects, the illusion arises from dysrhythmic activity in some portion of the temporal lobes, the activities of which are closely related to memory. It is not, however, necessarily motivated or possessing emotional connotations.

Confabulation

Spurious memories or fabrications are of course encountered in a variety of psychiatric states but only those arising upon a primarily organic basis will be considered here. These can of course be classified as examples of Kraepelin's associative memory deceptions, and when confabulation is relatively sparse and confined largely to the covering-up of memory defects to evade social embarrassment, this term would be more or less appropriate. Some confabulators, however, give accounts of supposedly recent experience so florid and improbable as to extend far beyond simple memory deception into the domain of imaginative fabrication.

Confabulation was at one time regarded as an essential element of Korsakoff's syndrome and undoubtedly occurs frequently in the acute phase of Wernicke's encephalopathy or after severe head injury during the post-traumatic confusional state. But it is much less common in the chronic Korsakoff syndrome, at all events in its more florid manifestations (Talland, 1961, 1965; Berlyne, 1972). According to Talland, confabulation results from the more or less total disruption of chronological memory and orientation which characterizes this syndrome and its content is not uncommonly a genuine, if misplaced, memory divorced from its proper temporal context. In consequence, memories drawn from different periods in the patient's history may be condensed, confused one with another, or related to a context wholly different from that to which they actually belong. As Talland (1965) has pointed out, the confabulation is only superficially autobiographical and the Korsakoff patient when asked about his activities on the previous day often produces an answer which might well have been acceptable had the question been addressed to him several years ago. That is to say, he gives an account of habitual activities undertaken during a period for which he now presents a dense retrograde amnesia. More generally, confabulation reflects a response governed by a combination of retrograde amnesia, disorientation and defective sense of chronological sequence. It is a form of paramnesia rather than an instance of pseudologia phantastica.

At the same time, florid confabulation based wholly on phantasy does occasionally occur in amnesic states, as in a case of a post-traumatic amnesic syndrome reported in some detail by Flament (1957) and in the cases of Korsakoff syndrome following spontaneous subarachnoid haemorrhage briefly described by Walton (1953). According to Berlyne (1972), confabulation is by no means specific to Korsakoff states and may occur in a relatively high proportion of patients with dementia (37 percent in his sample of 62 cases). In only three of these, however, was the confabulation of a truly florid and phantastic type, which according to Berlyne has a wish-fulfilling character and is often associated with paranoid traits. A patient studied by the present writer developed an amnesic syndrome following excision of a frontal lobe meningioma in which she was convinced that she had been admitted to hospital to have her baby (she was childless) and confabulated accordingly. This delusion and associated fabrication persisted for several weeks. It has been alleged that the superficially sociable though basically secretive individual is particularly given to confabulation (Williams & Rupp, 1938), though no very convincing evidence has been adduced in support of this claim. Suggestibility, however, may well be a potent predisposing factor. In general, it may be said that a combination of an amnesic state with denial of illness provides the most fertile soil for confabulation to flourish.

Organic and psychogenic amnesia

In a discussion on amnesic syndromes, Sir Aubrey Lewis expressed the view that 'there is nothing in the known pathology of hysterical amnesia that has not been observed in the organic cerebral syndrome' (Lewis, 1961). In the same vein, he had written a few years earlier that 'hysteriform disorder in organic cerebral syndromes is fairly common and that there can be no question that the dynamic processes familiar in "non-organic" memory disturbances come into play in 'organic' psychoses, determining their content and to some extent their form' (Lewis, 1953). This last statement was apropos of a once much-studied patient who had for years been supposed to present a complex hysterical memory disorder but who eventually turned out to be a case of partially arrested GPI. As Lewis saw it, the problem is not so much to explain the co-presence of organic and functional disorders of memory in the same patient as to account for their relative rarity. None the less, the incidence of brain injury or dysfunction in at any rate a significant proportion of patients diagnosed as cases of psychogenic amnesia has been stressed by several authors, among them Sargant and Slater (1941) and Stengel (1966). A few exceptional cases have also been described in which the differential diagnosis between organic and psychogenic amnesia has aroused extensive controversy and has yet to be brought to a final outcome.

Among these controversial cases two call for

brief comment. The first is the famous patient of Grünthal and Störring (1930a, b) whose case was diagnosed with confidence as one of organic amnesic syndrome consequent upon carbon monoxide poisoning. This patient was studied in depth both clinically and by psychometric methods and few doubted the essentially organic nature of the memory disorder. None the less, a re-examination of the patient some twenty years later by Scheller (1950, 1956) left little doubt that, whatever its original cause, the amnesia had been perpetuated on an essentially functional basis. Indeed Gruünthal and Störring themselves, while insisting that the disorder had been purely organic in its early stages, were eventually convinced that it had later been maintained for many years as a fixed hysterical pattern of reaction. (Grünthal & Störring, 1950, 1956).

In a review of the history of this patient's illness and of the many inquiries which have been made into his case Zangwill (1967) directed attention to a number of features which even in the early stages of the illness might appear to have been inconsistent with an organic aetiology. Among these were the gross impairment of short-term memory, the lack of appreciable retrograde amnesia and the remarkable fixity of the patient's disorientation for place and time. At the same time, Zangwill pointed out that existing attempts to explain the amnesia in terms of motivational or emotional factors appeared distinctly far-fetched. In consequence, he was led to conclude that this patient's amnesic state failed to conform to any of the generally accepted patterns of memory disorder, whether on an organic or psychogenic basis. In accordance with the views expressed by Sir Aubrey Lewis, it might be said that we are in this case fast approaching the limits of utility of this particular dichotomy.

Although the best-known, the Grünthal-Störring case is certainly not unique of its kind. A case of traumatic amnesia communicated a few years later by Syz (1936, 1937) presents a number of somewhat similar features, though in this case the patient's amnesia was successfully resolved by hypnotherapy. This patient was a 45-year-old foreman who developed a severe and persistent amnesia following on what appears to have been a relatively mild closed head injury with loss of consciousness for about an hour. He was examined in hospital six weeks after the accident and found to present minor neurological signs, including a partial right hemiplegia, which appears to have been at least in part organic. In consequence of these and of his severe global amnesia, the patient was diagnosed as a case of traumatic dementia and obtained maximum compensation for total disability in a lump sum settlement. There were hence no medico-legal sequelae.

This patient was re-examined by Syz three years after the accident and it was noted that the antero-grade amnesia was still present and virtually complete. Indeed, he closely resembled the Grünthal-Störring patient in his rapid and apparently total forgetting of recent events and his prevailing state of perplexity. He was approximately oriented for place and persons though not for time. On psychometric tests, there was evidence of slight retention over short periods of time but no coherent day-to-day memory could be established. As has been said, the patient responded well to a course of hypnotherapy which led to virtually complete recovery of continuous memory and disappearance of the residual neurological signs. On the other hand, a retrograde amnesia for the entire period since the accident was now in evidence which appeared to undergo no shrinkage in response to hypnotic suggestion. Although a few features of possible psycho-dynamic significance were unveiled during the course of the hypnotic treatment, it is difficult to view these as wholly responsible for the persistent amnesic state. But as Syz points out, this case differs from typical cases of psychogenic amnesia, in which there is commonly forgetting of a circumscribed series of events in the patient's past life and which may occasionally comprise the whole of the life history, including knowledge of personal identity (Abeles & Schilder, 1935; Kanzer, 1939; Parfitt & Gall, 1944; Stengel, 1941). In these studies, the close relation of amnesic state to fugues has been discussed at length and the role of what Parfitt and Gall (1944) have called the 'refusal to remember' much emphasized, with special reference to medico-legal issues. In Syz's case, on the other hand, as equally in that of Grünthal and Störring, the compensation issue appears to have played a very minor, if indeed any, real part in perpetuating the memory disability. Nor was the pattern of amnesia at all typical of psychogenic amnesias as usually encountered in clinical practice.

There are a few earlier cases in the literature that do appear closer to the 'quasi-organic' pattern that has been described in these two cases. In his review of the Grünthal and Störring case, the present writer refers to three in which the anterograde amne-

sia was so 'pure' as to suggest a psychogenic syndrome (Rieger, 1888–9; Mabille & Pitres, 1913; Conrad, 1953) though in all three there was abundant evidence of organic pathology and one (Mabille & Pitres) came to autopsy. One should perhaps also mention an even earlier case of anterograde-retrograde amnesia, that of Charcot (1892, see Janet, 1911), in which the condition, superficially at least, was surprisingly similar to Korsakoff's syndrome but in the opinion of Pierre Janet (1911, pp. 78–90) was indisputably hysterical. To the present writer, on the other hand, it seems conceivable that it may have had a minimal organic basis (? encephalitis) but had been perpetuated as a chronic hysterical disability. At all events, one may agree with Pratt (1977, p. 225) that the clinical features displayed by patients with organic neurological disease may be expected to show little difference from those of patients with psychogenic amnesia, and with Lishman (1978, p. 47) that the somewhat rigid distinction between psychogenic and organic disorders of memory has created a distinctly artificial dichotomy.

Another group of cases of interest in the present context are cases of Korsakoff's psychosis in which temporary improvement in memory has been alleged to result from interrogation under barbiturate narcosis. Davidson (1948) has discussed eight such cases in which striking improvement is said to have occurred in five; in the remaining cases the amnesic state was unchanged. In the patients showing improvement, it was said that the prevailing euphoric mood was replaced by an aggressive and truculent reaction accompanied by a marked increase in spontaneity, partial remission of anterograde amnesia and in certain cases improved orientation. In some cases there was a striking cessation of confabulation. Davidson attempts an interpretation along conventional psycho-dynamic lines but offers no explanation of the marked individual differences in response to intravenous amytal injection. On the other hand, investigation under barbiturate sedation failed to reverse the amnesic syndrome in two cases of severe post-encephalitic amnesic syndrome reported by Rose and Symonds (1960) or in an equally severe post-meningitic amnesic syndrome briefly communicated by Zangwill (1977). More extensive study of amnesic patients under barbiturate sedation is evidently indicated.

These atypical forms of amnesia, whether organic or functional, appear to be essentially unrelated to motivation and the patients do not appear to derive any obvious advantage from the perpetuation of their illness. Moreover, they do not seem to fit easily into the conventional framework of psychogenic explanation. It may therefore prove more profitable to consider them in relation to the organization of memory itself. In this connection, the present writer has considered elsewhere the resemblance between restitution of normal memory in traumatic and psychogenic types of amnesia respectively. He has pointed out that in both types, recent memory appears to reconstitute itself in a decidedly piecemeal fashion and to reflect an endogenous process of restitution (Zangwill, 1961). In both types, too, the reversible memory deficit appears to involve a failure of associative linkage resulting in a lack of continuity in memory with failure of spontaneous or voluntary recall. In the words of Henry Head (1926, p. 494), it is '. . . a lack of mental cohesion that lies at the basis of Korsakoff's psychosis'.

4.3.
Intellectual function and its disorders

EDGAR MILLER

'Intelligence' is a word that is readily used in everyday speech but it represents a concept that has proved extremely difficult to define. One way round this problem is to follow a school of thought which simply claims that 'intelligence is what intelligence tests measure'. This definition has some appeal but it is far from satisfactory in that it has an inbuilt circularity. Tests are devised to measure intelligence and intelligence is then defined in terms of these same tests.

Scientifically, the justification for the use of the concept of intelligence arises from the well attested fact that subjects' performances on a wide range of tasks that might be considered to bear some relationship to intellectual functioning show a strong tendency to intercorrelate. Thus a subject who is better than average on, say, a test of verbal reasoning is much more likely than would be expected on the basis of chance variation alone to score highly on other kinds of intellectual task (e.g. those involving mathematical skills or making complex judgements about spatial relationships). The argument then follows that these different kinds of intellectual task must represent to different degrees some common characteristic or trait which can be identified with intelligence. Psychometric measures of intelligence (the so-called IQ tests) have been developed to measure this common characteristic. The value of these tests is further reinforced by their ability to predict things like educational attainment which presumably reflect intellectual capacity to some degree.

One issue that has caused controversy in discussions about intelligence is the extent to which intellectual ability is capable of being represented by the single variable of intelligence as opposed to a cluster of more specific abilities (e.g. verbal, numerical, or spatial abilities). This debate is reviewed by Butcher (1968) but it is probably fair to say that most authorities now accept the value of the central concept of intelligence whilst allowing that a full account of intellectual functioning will require the inclusion of some more specific abilities. This issue will come up again in a different context in a later section when the effects of focal brain lesions on intellectual functioning are considered.

Another, and better known, controversy relating to intelligence, concerns the extent to which, if at all, intellectual ability is inherited. This issue received wide public attention with the arguments arising over the work of Sir Cyril Burt who had been a leading protagonist in disputes about the heritability of intelligence (see Hearnshaw, 1979). The topic is still capable of generating great controversy and there is no scope to elaborate on the relevant evidence here. In this writer's opinion there is evidence consistent with the notion that intelligence is, to some degree at least, influenced by heredity (Vernon, 1979). This is the case even when Burt's work is discounted. There are other data on twins apart from those reported by Burt, and studies of adopted children have indicated that their IQs are more related to those of their biological parents than they are to their adoptive parents (Munsinger, 1975). Furthermore, it seems unlikely that a characteristic such as intelligence which can be affected by many variables should remain untouched at every point by heredity. It is also important to remember that to claim that hereditary influences are present does not also automatically deny that environmental factors play a significant role in determining intelligence. This would be absurd since there is also good evidence of environmental influences (e.g. Husen, 1951). The realistic questions therefore relate not to whether intelligence is determined by heredity or environment, but to how, and under what conditions, hereditary and environmental influences operate and interact.

It is not the present purpose to elaborate the concept of intelligence any further nor to discuss the technicalities relating to its measurement by intelligence tests. This has been done very competently elsewhere by Butcher (1968). Although not primarily concerned with these basic points, Jensen (1980) also provides a more detailed account of the arguments justifying the concept of intelligence and those for the use of the conventional psychometric tests of intelligence in its measurement.

The following sections are designed to look at general intellectual functioning as it relates to some of the concerns of psychiatry. Four particular topics will be raised. These are the changes in intellectual functioning that occur as a result of normal ageing, the problem of dementia, the question of intellectual decline in certain functional psychiatric disorders, and intellectual change in relation to focal brain lesions. Since space does not permit a comprehensive coverage of any one of these topics the reader must bear in mind that certain aspects will either be glossed over or not covered at all. In each case references to more extensive discussions will be provided.

Age and intellectual ability

No one is likely to dispute the assertion that intellectual ability changes markedly with age. Intellectual capacity increases throughout childhood and appears to reach a peak in early adult life. It is also generally accepted that, after a short period of relative stability, intellectual capacity starts to decline and that the rate of decline starts to increase in later life.

The development of intellectual skills in childhood is not under dispute but ideas about the nature of intellectual change throughout adult life have undergone considerable reappraisal in recent years. For this reason the effect of ageing on intellectual functioning merits closer examination. It is also a topic of relevance since it is now generally recognized that the proportion of elderly people in the population is increasing dramatically in Western countries. This is especially so in the case of the so-called 'elderly elderly' (i.e. those over the age of 75). If the number of old people is increasing and they must necessarily undergo appreciable intellectual deterioration, then this has important implications for both social and psychiatric services.

If the standardization data of a commonly used test of intelligence (in this case the Wechsler Adult Intelligence Scale) are examined and the performance of representative samples of the general population is examined at different age levels, then a graph like that shown in fig. 4.3.1 can be obtained. This shows the maximum level of intellectual performance to be in early adult life with a slowly accelerating decline thereafter. This confirms the common prejudice that older people suffer a marked loss of intellect.

Although this picture was accepted for some considerable time and is still well entrenched in the belief systems of some people, it is increasingly being realized that graphs such as that in fig. 4.3.1 are over-pessimistic. The reasons for this lie in the considerable methodological problems inherent in examining age changes over the whole of the adult life span. A complete discussion of these is not possible here but a comprehensive account has been provided by Botwinick (1977). For present purposes just a few major points will be outlined.

The kind of data on which fig. 4.3.1 is based are cross-sectional in nature. Different groups of subjects have been tested at different age levels in order to provide the information from which the graph can be drawn. In order to accept this as a valid indication of age changes it must be assumed that the only variable of consequence which separates the different groups is that of age. This assumption is likely to be false. The 70-year-olds in the sample will have been born 50 years before the 20-year-olds and at a time when standards of infant nutrition, ante- and post-natal care, and educational opportunities would have been less favourable. These factors are known to relate to intellectual performance. In consequence, it is likely that the older groups will perform less well than the younger groups for reasons other than just that of age. Cross-sectional studies will therefore exaggerate the rate of intellectual decline with age.

The alternative is to study age changes by

Fig. 4.3.1. Intelligence test performance as a function of age with the level at 25 years assumed to be 100. Data extracted from Wechsler (1955).

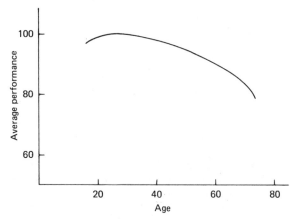

means of longitudinal studies whereby the same group of subjects is followed for significant periods of their life span. The practical problems involved in following the same group for several decades are immense. There are also methodological difficulties. In a follow-up of any group for long periods there will inevitably be some loss of subjects in the sample on account of death and other reasons. This attrition is unlikely to be random and so the results run the danger of being biased (Botwinick, 1977). As might be expected, there are no studies which have followed subjects throughout the whole of their adult life. There have been a few (e.g. Owens, 1966) that have tested middle-aged subjects and then retested them a number of years later. These indicate that up to the age of about 60 intellectual decline may be slight and is much less than is implied by fig. 4.3.1.

By far the most sophisticated investigations in this field have been carried out by Schaie and Strother (1968a & b). Their design involved both cross-sectional and longitudinal elements. They had several samples of subjects drawn in a cross-sectional manner with the ages of each group fitting every five-year interval between 20 and 70 (both ages inclusive). Subjects were tested on a particular intelligence test (the Primary Mental Abilities) which allegedly splits general intellectual functioning into a number of separate components. The subjects were then retested seven years later to give a longitudinal aspect to the investigation. When the first testings were examined on their own the results showed the typical age effect on intellectual performance illustrated by fig. 4.3.1. However, when the later retests were also taken into account they confirmed that cross-sectional studies do over-estimate the amount of intellectual decline with age. In fact Schaie and Strother's data indicate that some aspects of intellectual functioning do not deteriorate until the sixties are reached. The only major exception occurs when speed is a very significant aspect of performance. Here the pattern of decline is much more like that of fig. 4.3.1.

Another aspect of more recent discussions of changes in intellectual status with age is the phenomenon that has become known as 'terminal decline' or 'terminal drop'. A number of investigators have tested and retested older subjects and have noted that in the period just prior to death there is an especially marked deterioration in intellectual capacity. The length of this period of terminal decline varies from about six months to a few years in the different studies. As Palmore and Cleveland (1976) have pointed out, many of the reports of this phenomenon have been unsatisfactory, with large scale generalizations being derived from poorly collected data obtained from small and unrepresentative samples of subjects.

Fortunately there is more reliable information. For example, Riegel and Riegel (1972) examined and re-examined several hundred elderly people and obtained clear evidence of lowered intelligence test scores in the few years just prior to death. These authors also point out that the notion of terminal decline has implications for our general view of the effects of age on intellectual functioning. As subjects get older an increasing proportion within a group of a given age will be within the last few years of their lives and so will be exhibiting a terminal decline. This in itself would produce an apparently accelerating decline in ability with increasing age in graphs like that depicted in fig. 4.3.1. Possibly intellectual level remains more static over adult life than has hitherto been generally imagined and then shows a fairly dramatic decline as death approaches.

It is unlikely that the question of the pattern of intellectual change with age has been finally resolved. Some decline has probably started before middle age in those tasks where speed is of crucial importance. Even where the importance of speed is minimized it seems unlikely that the whole of the apparent intellectual decline with age can be explained away as a consequence of terminal decline. In looking for causal mechanisms it is important to remember that age by itself cannot produce any effect. The passage of time is important because it provides other variables with an opportunity to operate. A significant factor in explaining some intellectual deterioration in older subjects is likely to be ill-health. Cardiovascular disease, for example, is more prevalent with advancing years and results in intellectual loss (Wilkie & Eisdorfer, 1971). Neuropathological changes may also be important. Within groups of elderly demented patients there is a significant inverse relationship between intellectual status and plaque counts in the brain (Blessed *et al.*, 1968). Whether appreciable correlations could be found for normal elderly subjects is not clear.

Dementia

It cannot be seriously disputed that dementia is produced by organic changes within the brain. Nevertheless the concept of dementia is basically a psychological one in that it implies, above all else, a deterioration in intellectual capacity. As has already been indicated, the proportion of elderly people in the community is rising. This means that the problems associated with the elderly will place an increasing burden upon the health services. Dementia is prominent among these and can afflict approximately 6–10 percent of those over 65 years of age (Miller, 1977). It is therefore a problem of considerable renum. This section is largely concerned with the nature of the intellectual changes which occur in dementia of the kind commonly described as Alzheimer's disease or senile dementia, but there are other publications which consider dementia in a much wider context (Miller, 1977; Wells, 1977). In particular, the topic of arteriosclerotic or multi-infarct dementia will be left aside.

The most commonly used tests of intelligence that have been applied to clinical groups are those devised by Wechsler, of which the most recent is the Wechsler Adult Intelligence Scale (Wechsler, 1955). Besides giving an overall intelligence quotient (IQ), the Wechsler scales subdivide intellectual performance into two major subcategories. These are known as the Verbal and Performance IQs. As the name implies, the Verbal IQ is based on a series of subtests which have a strong verbal component (e.g. defining words and giving the answers to problems involving verbal reasoning). The Performance IQ is more concerned with the practical aspects of intelligence and the subtests contributing to this scale tend to have a strong visuo-spatial component (e.g. fitting coloured blocks together to make complex designs) although other things are also involved.

Miller (1977) has tabulated the results of a number of studies involving the application of one of the Wechsler intelligence tests to demented patients (these are mainly patients with senile dementia, although some data from cases of pre-senile dementia are also reported). There is a strong tendency for the mean full-scale IQs to be appreciably lower than the population mean of 100. This is hardly surprising. If it were not the case it would be necessary to challenge the concept of dementia and/or the measurement of intellectual functioning by means of intelligence tests. The interesting question lies in whether it is possible to describe the intellectual changes associated with dementia in any greater detail.

Almost universally these same studies of intelligence test performance in demented subjects show that the Performance IQ is depressed more than the Verbal IQ. It is just possible that this might be the consequence of an uninteresting technical artefact in that, as a measure, the Performance scale in the Wechsler tests might happen to be more sensitive to the deleterious effects of any change than the Verbal scale. Assuming, as seems likely, that this is not the whole explanation for the difference there are a number of ways in which the Performance scale differs from the Verbal. One is that the subtests on which the Performance scale is based all involve time limits, whereas this is the case for only one of the Verbal subtests. It could be that demented subjects show an exaggeration of the tendency found in normal elderly people for all kinds of performance to be particularly likely to suffer when speed is a crucial factor. Again, this is unlikely to be the whole story since corresponding differences can be obtained using other tests which do not involve time-limits at all (Miller, 1977).

Another difference is that between intellectual tasks involving visuo-spatial manipulations as opposed to those requiring verbal manipulations. It is possible that visuo-spatial abilities may be particularly affected by whatever processes underlie dementia. Finally, it is the case that the kind of verbal and arithmetical skills involved in the Verbal scale are frequently used and heavily overlearned in everyday life. In contrast, the Performance scale items are much less familiar and require the subject to adapt to new situations. In view of the very marked disturbances in learning that are known to occur in dementia (Miller, 1977) it seems very plausible to suppose that the Verbal-Performance discrepancy might best be explained in terms of the demented patient's inability to cope with new situations.

A basic question that can be posed about the nature of intellectual deterioration in dementia is whether it can be best described as a decline in a single intellectual variable (like overall IQ or the ability to adapt to new situations as suggested above) or as an amalgamation of a number of different abilities which have all suffered deterioration. It is difficult to obtain a satisfactory answer. The general approach to this kind of problem that is commonly used by psychologists is the application of a large number of measures to a sample of subjects and the subjection of the results to complex statistical procedures (various types of multivariate analysis) applied to the data. There are two relevant studies. One by Dixon (1965) suggested that deterioration occurs along a single dimension. That by Gustafson and Hagberg (1975) imputed several different facets to intellectual

change in dementia. From a purely impressionistic point of view the very wide range of psychological changes manifest in dementia (see Miller, 1977) implies that it represents a general disintegration of most, if not all, types of ability and that any attempt to identify a particular kind of intellectual function as being the one factor underlying the whole picture is doomed to failure.

A further point that has been raised is whether the intellectual decline that occurs in dementia is no more than an exaggeration of the changes observed in normal ageing. This is of wider interest since it relates to one of the most commonly expressed theoretical ideas about dementia; viz., that it is caused by an accelerated ageing of the nervous system. A number of investigators have examined the pattern of scores on the 10 or 11 subtests of one of the Wechsler intelligence scales to see whether those in dementia matched those found in normal ageing. The results have been completely equivocal, with every report of similarity between the pattern of subtest scores in dementia and ageing (e.g. Whitehead, 1973) being matched by one claiming the reverse (e.g. Dorken & Greenbloom, 1953). In fact, studies comparing the changes in dementia with those of normal ageing raise important methodological difficulties (Miller, 1974). These are potentially soluble but no investigation has so far used the appropriate controls and so the question remains unanswered. Nonetheless, it appears unlikely that the changes in dementia are merely those of normal ageing writ large when the evidence from all psychological functions is considered (Miller, 1974).

Intellectual functioning is adversely affected in dementia, but it is difficult to go beyond this bold assertion with any certainty. On present evidence it is unlikely that the intellectual changes in dementia will turn out to be identical with those of normal ageing, and it is similarly unlikely that the change can be characterized as lying along a single dimension. Although other factors are likely to be involved, some of the deterioration in functioning on intellectual tasks may be attributable to difficulties in adaptation to the demands imposed by new situations.

The functional psychiatric disorders

The idea that some degree of general intellectual deterioration might be involved in the functional psychiatric disorders is not new. The original term for schizophrenia was 'dementia praecox', which implies that the condition is a form of dementia.

However, it is also open to question whether the concept of 'dementia' carried quite the same connotations for writers like Kraepelin or Bleuler as it does in modern times, with the implication of a deterioration in intellectual functioning of the kind associated with conditions like senile dementia and Alzheimer's disease.

Regardless of the conceptual issues surrounding the term 'dementia', psychologists and psychiatrists have been looking for and arguing about the possibility of intellectual deterioration in those suffering from functional psychiatric disorders for some considerable time. There is now a very large literature which has been competently reviewed in detail by Payne (1973). Apart from the influence of some more recent work to be described below, the picture has changed very little since Payne's review. W. R. Miller (1975) has also provided a detailed review of all forms of psychological change, including intellectual impairment, occurring in depression. This section will be largely concerned with recent research on schizophrenia but will begin by outlining the position as revealed by Payne (1973). Before doing so it must be noted that the evidence considered comes substantially from the USA and Britain. This raises the complication that diagnostic practices differ in the two countries (Cooper *et al.*, 1972) and this introduces another variable that might have to be taken into account. Fortunately, findings from both sides of the Atlantic tend to be reasonably consistent for the matters described here.

The extensive evidence considered by Payne (1973) gives no convincing indication of intellectual change in neurotic disorders and so the real concern lies with the functional psychoses. As a general rule, studies reporting mean IQ levels in groups of subjects diagnosed as suffering from either schizophrenia or affective disorders show their average IQs to be below the population mean of 100. As Payne correctly indicates, this kind of finding is by no means proof of intellectual deterioration in such patients. It could be that psychiatrically disturbed individuals who are of lower than average intelligence are more likely to be diagnosed as psychotic. In fact, Mason (1956) found that, in general, men inducted into the US armed forces who later developed psychiatric problems did not have lower IQs than had controls. When the sample was broken down to look at specific diagnostic categories those who were later considered to have simple or hebephrenic schizophrenia did have lower average IQs when tested earlier. Those

diagnosed as manic-depressive tended to have higher IQs.

Crucial evidence relating to a decline in intellectual ability in association with psychosis can only come from investigations in which it is possible to compare IQ levels obtained pre-morbidly with those obtained during the illness. Information of this kind is difficult to obtain, but this has sometimes been possible and Payne (1973) outlines several such studies. People who have become schizophrenic during or after military service have had their IQs compared with those obtained on induction into the services. Similarly, patients in some large American hospitals have had their IQs when ill compared with those obtained when they were pupils in the local school system. Most of these investigations provide evidence of a decline in IQ in schizophrenia which may be up to about 10 IQ points (in terms of the Wechsler scales). On the other hand, a few of the reports are negative (e.g. Griffiths *et al.*, 1962), but Payne draws attention to some technical reasons that would suggest that the methodology of these negative studies was such as to make them less sensitive in detecting any change that might have occurred.

The picture is less clear with regard to affective disorders. Lowered levels of performance can be found on various kinds of intellectual task but there is not the evidence based on premorbid comparisons that exists for schizophrenia. In his detailed review of psychological changes in depression W. R. Miller (1975) argues quite strongly that there is no clear demonstration that any of the apparent changes in depression are specific to that condition. The question of intellectual decline in affective disorders will not be taken any further, and the rest of this section will concentrate on schizophrenia.

Interest has recently re-emerged quite strongly in the question of a 'dementia in dementia praecox'. One particular reason for this was a finding by Crow and Mitchell (1975) that some chronic schizophrenics appreciably underestimate their age when asked how old they are. The body of work that followed from this is summarized by Crow and colleagues (1979) but is worth describing in a little more detail here.

In this research 'age disorientation' is considered to occur in patients who apparently regard their age as being five years or more different from their real age. In the vast majority of cases with age disorientation the patient gives an age that is lower than his true age, although the occasional over-estimation does occur. This phenomenon occurs in about

25 per cent of chronic schizophrenics resident in hospital. It does not appear to be sex related, nor does it occur in other diagnostic groups (Stevens *et al.*, 1978). Despite having been resident in hospital for a mean time of almost 30 years, 11 percent of the subjects studied by Stevens and colleagues gave their age as being within 5 years of that on admission. Chronic schizophrenics with age disorientation tended to have been in hospital longer than those who did not exhibit this phenomenon. As might be expected from these findings, those subjects with age disorientation were also older but the longer hospital stays of age-disoriented subjects still emerged when the effect of this group's older average age had been partialled out. Stevens and colleagues (1978) suggest that schizophrenics who develop age disorientation may fall into a particular subgroup which has an early onset and a poor prognosis.

The meaning and significance of age disorientation obviously require further analysis. A question raised by Crow and Stevens (1978) is whether the patient's apparent belief that he is younger than he really is can be regarded as an isolated delusion or is it a manifestation of a more extensive temporal disorientation? The same subjects that had been studied by Stevens and colleagues (1978) were asked a range of questions regarding their date of birth, year of admission, length of stay in hospital, etc. When age-disoriented subjects were compared with the majority of chronic schizophrenics who provided a more realistic estimation of their true age, then the former showed a strong tendency towards an underestimation of the present year and the length of hospital stay. There were a few anomalous responses like that of the subject who seriously underestimated his own age but gave the then current year correctly. Nevertheless, the results were generally consistent with the notion that 'time stands still' for these age-disoriented subjects, at least from about the time of their hospital admission.

In a further investigation (Johnstone *et al.*, 1978) the same group carried out a much more detailed study of 18 long-stay schizophrenics selected from the same basic population as that used in the previous studies. These were compared with 10 physically handicapped people who were also long-term hospital residents and 8 normal controls. The differences between the two non-schizophrenic groups were small and insignificant and can thus be disregarded. This suggests that any differences between the schizophrenics and the other subjects are not simply the

consequence of long-term residence in an institution. (The caution should also be entered that the two non-schizophrenic groups are small, thus possibly masking real differences. Also, work on the effects of institutionalization, especially in relation to institutionally reared children, shows that the quality of care offered is of great importance in determining whether institutionalization has deleterious effects on intellectual functioning.) As compared with normal controls, the schizophrenics had larger ventricular sizes as demonstrated by the CT scan. In addition, they performed significantly less well on intellectual tests and tests of memory.

The schizophrenic groups could be subdivided in different ways. They had been deliberately selected so that half were age-disoriented and half were not. There was a consistent tendency for the age-disoriented subgroup to do less well on all the cognitive measures that were used, but the difference only achieved acceptable levels of statistical significance in 2 out of 6 instances. The schizophrenics could also be subdivided into those showing the more positive features of schizophrenia (e.g. hallucinations and delusions) and those with predominantly negative features (poverty of speech, flattening of affect, etc.). There was a marked tendency for those with the negative features to do worst on the cognitive tests and this was statistically significant in most cases.

The series of investigations just described have been performed by the same research group at Northwick Park Hospital on what appears to be essentially the same subject sample. In view of its significance it is desirable that the findings be replicated. There has as yet been no direct replication of this work, but some results broadly consistent with the reports from Northwick Park have been obtained. For example, Golden and colleagues (1980) have found evidence of increased size of brain ventricles in chronic schizophrenics and also showed that a measure of ventricular size derived from the CT scan correlated quite appreciably with depressed scores on a battery of tests related to various aspects of cognitive functioning. The report by Johnstone and colleagues (1978) that patients with negative features of schizophrenia do less well on cognitive tests is largely in line with the results of an earlier study by Lilliston (1973). Furthermore, preliminary analyses of an investigation into chronic schizophrenia conducted by a Cambridge-based group with which the present writer is associated also imply that chronic schizophrenics have impaired cognitive functioning on a number of tests, some of which match those used by the Northwick Park studies.

It therefore does appear to be the case that there is a 'dementia in dementia praecox' at least for a proportion of chronic schizophrenics. There is also an association between this cognitive deterioration and structural changes within the brain as revealed by increased ventricular size. This mirrors the association found between intellectual decline and cerebral atrophy in cases of dementia of the kind involved in Alzheimer's disease or senile dementia. This, of course, does not mean that all cases of schizophrenia show cognitive deterioration. It is likely that this type of deterioration will be most prominent in those in whom the negative symptoms of schizophrenia are predominant.

Intelligence and focal brain lesions

Since the brain is the organ most closely identified with psychological functioning it is not surprising that intellectual changes should result from damage to or disease of the brain. In a previous section the effect of generalized brain pathology (in dementia) was discussed. Focal lesions present a different but very interesting set of problems. These can be looked at in two ways. Firstly, there is the question of identifying the changes in intellectual functioning as measured by intelligence tests that are produced by lesions in different parts of the brain. Secondly, it is well recognized that focal brain lesions can produce a wide range of impairments in such functions as language, memory, and the perception of spatial relationships. These things bear some relationship to intellectual functioning. It is then possible to ask to what extent, if at all, these specific impairments are a manifestation of a loss in general intellectual ability. Of more purely psychological interest is the possibility that studying the effects of focal lesions may throw some light upon theories of intelligence, as Piercy (1969) amongst others has suggested.

A common impression is that the kind of intellectual impairment resulting from brain damage will differ in quality according to the hemisphere involved. In the terminology of the Wechsler scales, damage to the left hemisphere is associated with a decline in Verbal IQ (at least in the majority of people who are left-dominant for speech). Performance IQ is thought to be more likely to be depressed by right-sided lesions. Walsh (1978) covers much of the relevant evidence, although in a slightly different context.

That left-hemisphere lesions should produce a decline in verbal intelligence is hardly surprising in view of the association between such lesions and aphasia. However, the lowering of Verbal IQ that can occur with left-sided lesions cannot be fully explained simply on the grounds of dysphasia interfering with test performance, although this factor could be considered partially responsible in some instances. There are numerous studies that have demonstrated Verbal IQ deficits after such surgical procedures as left anterior temporal lobectomy for the removal of epileptic foci and left frontal lobectomies to excise tumours where dysphasia has not been present (e.g. Meyer, 1959; Milner, 1958; Smith, 1966).

The association between right-hemisphere lesions and deficits in Performance IQ has been less clear cut. To take studies of right temporal lobectomy as an example, some workers have reported depressed Performance IQ as a result of this procedure (e.g. Blakemore & Falconer, 1967), but others have not (e.g. Milner, 1958). While it is possible, or even likely, that the abilities tapped by the Performance IQ are not as clearly lateralized to the right hemisphere as those measured by the Verbal IQ are to the left, there are other reasons why the picture with respect to Performance IQ has become blurred. In the case reported by Milner (1958), subjects were tested both pre- and post-operatively when subjected to either left or right temporal lobectomy. The left-sided cases showed a large and statistically significant decline in Verbal IQ, while those operated upon the right side only revealed a small, but statistically insignificant, drop in Performance IQ. This led Milner to suggest that right temporal lobectomy did not affect Performance IQ. These same results were re-analysed by Miller (1972) who pointed to other evidence showing that when subjects are retested on the Performance scale there is a substantial increase in Performance IQ solely as a result of practice effects. Milner's observed slight drop in Performance IQ can then be considered as the resultant of an appreciable gain which is due to practice effects and a decline of a similar amount which is due to the removal of brain tissue. Walsh (1978) mentions other methodological problems which would also tend to explain why performance decrements would not be so easily detected after right-sided lesions.

The relationship between frontal lesions and intellectual disturbance has proved a much more contentious issue. In the past some have claimed that the frontal lobes are the seat of man's highest intelligence, whereas others have totally rejected this view.

One opportunity to study this question was provided by the numerous investigations into the effects of psychosurgical procedures carried out on the frontal lobes. In reviewing this evidence Miller (1972) found a number of studies claiming to demonstrate a decline in measured intelligence but also many that did not. A similar confusion emerges from Walsh's (1978) survey of the psychological consequences of frontal lobe pathology. One likely solution to the difficulty lies in the complex nature of intelligence tests. Performance on a given test may suffer for a variety of reasons. It is fairly well established that the frontal lobes are involved in aspects of behaviour that might relate to intelligence test performance. For example, patients with frontal lesions are less well able to switch from older and well-established methods of responding when these become inappropriate (Milner, 1964). The posterior parts of the brain are more involved in other functions, like the appreciation of visuo-spatial relationships, which might relate to intellectual activity in a different way (Walsh, 1978).

Before leaving this aspect of the relationship between intellectual functioning and focal lesions we would inject a note of caution. It is sometimes argued that because Verbal and Performance IQs appear to be differentially affected by left- and right-sided lesions then the direction of the discrepancy between Verbal and Performance IQs can be used to indicate the side of any brain pathology within the individual patient. This is not so. Many normal people do not show an even pattern of intellectual ability. A patient who, say, has always had a much higher Verbal than Performance IQ may suffer a left-sided lesion with some drop in Verbal IQ and yet still have a Verbal IQ that is slightly higher than the Performance IQ.

The problem of trying to decide whether, and to what extent, neuropsychological impairments associated with focal brain lesions (the aphasias, apraxias, etc.) can be understood as a manifestation of general intellectual impairment is more difficult to resolve. Not only are there a large number of identified neuropsychological symptoms to be considered, but questions of definition are involved. To take aphasia as an example, there is a definite tradition of defining aphasia in such a way that it must involve intellectual deterioration (see Hécaen & Albert, 1978; Zangwill, 1969). If aphasia is a disturbance of language, and language is held to be essential for thought, then intellectual loss and aphasia must be closely associated. If this view is questioned practical problems emerge. An aphasic subject's apparent failure on an intellectual task may be due not to an inability to perform the necessary operations but to a difficulty in expressing his response.

The evidence relating aphasia to intellectual performance has been recently reviewed by Hécaen and Albert (1978). The evidence is not entirely consistent, but the overwhelming impression is that there is no simple relationship between aphasia and general intellectual performance. McFie and Piercy (1952) found that a decline in intellectual functioning did occur in patients with left-hemisphere lesions but that there was no association with the presence of aphasia. Zangwill (1964) used Raven's Progressive Matrices, a test of general intelligence with a minimal overt verbal component: marked degrees of dysphasia were quite compatible with good performance on this test. On the other hand, Basso and colleagues (1973) used the Coloured Progressive Matrices and did find an association between poor performance on this test and left-sided lesions producing aphasia. It is particularly interesting that in this latter study poor scores on the matrices were not related to a measure of oral comprehension, thus suggesting that intellectual loss in aphasic subjects is not just the consequence of language disorders. Basso and colleagues suggest that there might be an area in the left hemisphere which is associated with certain aspects of intellectual performance that may be both verbal and non-verbal and that this area overlaps with the speech areas. Hécaen and Albert (1978) reach a conclusion that is not incompatible with this view by suggesting that disorders of general intelligence may be selectively associated with certain types of aphasia, particularly those exhibiting impaired auditory comprehension and semantic paraphasias.

If the relationship between intellectual functioning and aphasia is confused and difficult to disentangle, the picture appears clearer with regard to some other impairments. Although there are probably some rather subtle intellectual impairments in the amnesic syndrome, a normal range of performance on intelligence tests is usually found in patients with the alcoholic Korsakoff syndrome (Talland, 1965; Zangwill, 1977). In the study of the apraxias and related disorders, ideational apraxia does not appear to be associated with general intellectual deterioration (De Renzi et al., 1968), although loss of gestural behavior is so related (Goodglass & Kaplan, 1963).

The study of focal lesions in relation to intellectual change has certain implications for theories of intelligence. The evidence clearly does not support the notion that intellectual ability can be conceived of as a single, monolithic function. If this position is rejected two major alternatives remain. The first is to regard intellectual functioning as a collection of discrete abilities (verbal, spatial, numerical, etc.) which exist more or less independently. The second is a hierarchical model which involves an over-all general intellectual function but which subsumes a number of more specific abilities. In discussing this issue Piercy (1969) opts for the first of these two possibilities. While Piercy could prove to be correct it could be argued quite strongly that the evidence so far obtained is not clear enough to reject the second model. What does seem established is that specific abilities do have an important role within any satisfactory theory of intellectual functioning.

Conclusion

Intelligence is not a simple concept and its measurement poses considerable problems. Work on intelligence has resulted in a number of controversies. Some of these have become quite heated, such as those relating to the inheritance of intellectual ability and the use of intelligence tests in educational and occupational selection. Nevertheless, how we view and measure intelligence does have important implications for a range of social and educational issues as well as for some clinical problems.

In order to bring the present task down to a manageable size it has been assumed that the major psychometric tests of intelligence (especially the Wechsler scales) represent a reasonable attempt to measure intellectual ability. Discussion has therefore centred on work using these scales, although there has been some reference to other kinds of investigation. This does not mean that other approaches to the definition and measurement of intellectual functioning are necessarily of lesser value. A full consideration of intellectual ability and the factors that influence it would need to look far beyond work based upon the traditional psychometric tests. Since some selection of material was necessary, and the major intelligence tests are often used with psychiatric populations, it has seemed appropriate to concentrate upon this aspect here.

The preceding discussion has shown that intellectual ability is influenced by a number of factors. It develops during childhood and declines towards old age, but this decline is less marked and occurs later in life than the more pessimistic estimates of the past would allow. Brain pathology, whether generalized as in the case of dementia or the result of focal lesions, does have a deleterious effect on intellectual ability, with the particular effects being determined by the nature of the pathology. There is also evidence that a form of intellectual deterioration occurs in a proportion of people with chronic schizophrenia and is particularly prominent in those exhibiting the negative features of the condition.

Finally, it is appropriate to enter a word of caution with regard to a point that is of some clinical significance. A demonstrated decline in performance on the standard intelligence tests (like the Wechsler scales) in the absence of contaminating factors such as clouding of consciousness, can be taken as a good indication that there is some disturbance in intellectual functioning. It is important to note that the reverse is not the case. Intelligence tests are constructed in such a way as to be robust and therefore insensitive in detecting change. The fact that the measured IQ does not appear to have declined does not mean that all aspects of cognitive functioning are intact. To take one instance, IQ does decline after severe head injury but typically the drop is temporary in nature and the IQ returns to the previous level within a year. Despite this finding there is very strong evidence that those who have suffered severe head injuries suffer appreciable psychological impairments in such functions as memory and speed of information processing which are probably permanent (Miller, 1979). Intelligence test performance should never be used as evidence of a lack of intellectual deterioration.

4.4
The neuropsychology of emotion

T. W. ROBBINS

Introduction

The specification of central nervous structures which mediate emotion gained great impetus from the work earlier this century of Cannon (1927), Bard (1929) and Papez (1937). These investigators, integrating both clinical anecdote, and data from early animal experiments, implicated specific neural structures and processes within a scheme that amounted to a simple conceptual analysis of emotion. Since then, it is evident that further advance, in general, has not kept pace with developments in neuroscience or in psychology. It is not difficult to see why. 'Emotion' is riddled with dualism of all varieties; mind–body, mind–brain, brain–body, emotional experience, and emotional expression. These dissociations, rather than serving as keys to elucidation, have instead resulted in mistaken interpretation of experimental results, in pursuit of one aspect of the dichotomy to the exclusion of the other, or even in denials that the concept of emotion is of scientific validity (e.g. Duffy, 1934).

Another major obstacle has been the difficulty of measurement. Reliance upon subjective experience as scientific data is fraught with all the problems of using human language as data-language. Weiskrantz (1977) for example, has pointed out difficulties of using verbal report with amnesic or perceptually-impaired subjects. In particular, the use of 'commentary' questions (e.g. do you see this?) often provides different and sometimes conflicting information compared to questions requiring forced choice or identification (e.g. where is this?). Such discrepancies can be interpreted as illustrating a dissociation between a capacity and its acknowledgement within the same individual. There seems little doubt that analogous and probably more severe problems afflict the experimental study of emotion. Thus the relative insensitivity of human subjects to their autonomic states has been viewed as of great significance by certain theorists (e.g. Schachter & Singer, 1962; Mandler, 1975) as will later be described, but this insensitivity could be due in part simply to limitations of descriptive vocabulary rather than to lack of perceptual discrimination *per se* (c.f. Brener, 1977).

Even if we could be sure that language-data were precise, it would be difficult to escape the different philosophical interpretations of mind and body which may be irrelevant to the scientific problem at hand. However, there seems little doubt that a classification of the ways in which natural language is used to discuss emotion may serve as a basis for advances not only in communication, but also in formulating scientific hypotheses. Ryle (1949) for example provides an admirable clarification of the use of emotion-words. He distinguishes between four main uses of the term 'emotion':

(1) inclinations or motives
(2) moods
(3) agitations or commotions
(4) feelings

'Inclinations' refer to tendencies or dispositions to perform specific actions. The tendency to exhibit aggressive responses to certain stimuli in cats might fall into this category; so might the tendency to eat large meals in stressful circumstances. Ryle emphasizes that since inclinations are not events, they cannot be *causes* of behaviour. Inclinations may however be *reasons* advanced to explain observed behaviour. 'Moods' are more general, short-term propensities, such as depression or elation, which monopolize feelings and actions in diverse situations. 'Agitations' are disturbances, of which movements and autonomic activity may be signs, produced in situations involving conflicting or thwarted inclinations. Agitations may then include 'anxiety', 'irritability' and 'distractibility'. Ryle does not clearly distinguish mood from agitation, since he considers that the former can include the latter. 'Anxiety' can refer to a mood or to an agitation. Moreover, if the anxious mood is chronic, then it becomes a character trait. 'Feelings' may arise from inclinations, moods, or agitations, and come closest to what is often called 'emotional experience'. 'Feelings' are events or occurrences, such as the 'pangs' or 'thrills' that may accompany particular experiences. However, again, these events may not always have causal properties. As Ryle puts it:

> They are things for which diagnoses are required not things required for the diagnoses of behaviour (p. 114).

Thus the notion of a 'feeling' that motivates or energizes action is repudiated. What the concept of 'emotion' then implies is a cognitive evaluation of the interoceptive stimuli that are generated under particular circumstances. The next section now describes some of these circumstances.

The conditions for emotion

As Ryle's analysis shows, we should seek causes of emotion in events which occur internal or external to the organism. There have been many classifications of the stimuli eliciting emotional behaviour or feelings. The most obvious distinction is between unconditioned and conditioned stimuli. The emotion 'fear', for example, may depend upon intense, novel or incongruous stimuli such as loud noise or rapid movement. However, a previously innocuous stimulus may also come to elicit fearful behaviour, because of its association with other events in the history of the organism, and is then called a conditioned stimulus. Any theory of emotion therefore requires a contingency analysis, that is, an account of how inputs are analysed for meaning, so that the significance of an input is assessed, and a decision for action is made. Simple schemes for specifying the types of event which cause internal 'emotional states' have been proposed (e.g. Mowrer, 1960; Millenson, 1967, Gray, 1972). These schemes postulate intervening 'emotional states' produced by the presentation or omission (or termination) of types of conditioned or unconditioned reinforcing event, which may be either positive ('reward') or negative ('punishment') (see table 4.4.1).

Thus, for example, the termination of food is assumed to produce a state of 'frustration' that has particular behavioural and physiological consequences. Gray (1972) has attempted to reduce the number of basic 'emotional states' required from this type of analysis on empirical grounds, in order to facilitate the search for underlying neurophysiological mechanisms, e.g.:

There is very good evidence, both from purely behavioural experiments, and from experiments in physiological psychology, that the effects of signals of punishment, and those of signals of non-reward are functionally identical and work through the same structures in the neuroendocrine system (p. 90).

The operational cogency of this approach in generating research, as well as its parsimony, are generally upheld in this article. There are however certain criticisms of the approach which revolve around: (1) the classification of stimuli as positive ('rewarding') and negative ('punishing'). This classification depends either upon assumptions concerning the inherent properties of these stimuli or upon a *post hoc* judgement depending on the nature of the behaviour observed; (2) the implication that the positive-negative bipolarity necessarily depends upon subjective feelings; and (3) the assumption that 'positive' subjective feelings are necessarily associated with certain types of action (e.g. approach), whereas 'negative' feelings are necessarily associated with other types of action (e.g. withdrawal). These are simplifying assumptions which may, ultimately, obscure, rather than facilitate, the search for mechanisms underlying emotion.

Old notions about the inherent positive or negative qualities of stimuli are beginning to be shaken by demonstrations that a stimulus may have both positive and negative attributes. For example, Morse, Mead, and Kelleher (1967) showed that squirrel monkeys, under certain conditions, will self-administer painful electric shocks. This work has since been confirmed and extended (e.g. Morse & Kelleher, 1977) and does not appear to depend upon artefacts of conditioning. The most surprising demonstration is that the same physical stimulus, i.e. electric shock, can act as a reinforcer and as punisher for the same organism, *in different situations* (Barrett & Spealman, 1978). These results do not apply merely to aversive stimuli. Intracranial stimulation (ICS) has been regarded as a powerful reward or positive reinforcer since Olds' and Milner's initial discovery (1954) that rats would work for pulse trains delivered to particular regions of the brain. And yet Steiner, Beer, and Shaffer (1969) showed that rats would work to escape from a tape-recorded presentation of trains of ICS they had self-administered on a previous session. Analogous results have been obtained with drugs such as cocaine (Spealman, 1979) and even food

(Clark & Smith, 1977). Clearly then, a stimulus cannot be regarded as simply negative or positive. This property appears to depend upon its *context*, that is upon the past contingencies and the current situation in which the stimulus is presented. Thus, in an extreme case a squirrel monkey will work under a schedule that produces electric shock, but will not work for food if shock is superimposed upon the performance. Such results have powerful implications for the ways in which brain function is analysed. One can regard a stimulus such as shock as a complex event with both positive and negative qualities that are revealed in different conditions. How such a stimulus is represented in the central nervous system (CNS) will then presumably depend upon the ongoing pattern of neural activity engendered by the present conditions and previous experience of the organism.

Behavioural results such as these also render difficult attempts to equate 'positive' events with 'pleasant' subjective feelings and 'negative' events with 'unpleasant' feelings. The electric shock in the above example is clearly a positive reinforcer by behavioural criteria since the monkey apparently works to receive it. However, even given our ignorance of subjective experience in infra-human primates, it seems unlikely that the monkey experiences feelings of pleasure; indeed, signs of pain and discomfort are observed. On a wider scale, it is also unlikely that drug-taking in human addicts or overeating in certain types of obese subject is maintained purely by pleasant subjective experience. The suspicion in both of these cases is that the behaviour is maintained to some extent independently of the subjective states of the organism.

Finally, some of the evidence mentioned above suggests that neural mechanisms of emotional expression and experience may be dissociable, and not synonymous. This suggestion is bolstered by the study of physiological reactivity and anxiety in novice and experienced parachute jumpers by Fenz and Epstein (1967). Novice jumpers exhibited a monotonic increase until the jump, both in sympathetic activation, as measured by galvanic skin response (GSR) and heart rate, and in verbal reports of fear. Experienced jumpers however, while exhibiting broadly similar changes in sympathetic activation, reported feeling most fearful on the morning of the jump, and immediately after the jump. Hodgson and Rachman (1974) analogously report different rates of change for different aspects of fear in subjects undergoing phobic desensitization. These findings support the notion that different aspects of emotional experience and expression depend upon parallel, but distinctive, neural mechanisms. Commonly, of course, their functions are correlated, and, as one might expect of an associative relationship, activation of one mechanism may come to evoke activity in another. However, we may have to learn about the subjective consequence of stimuli and actions in the same type of way in which we manage cross-modal integration and sensori-motor co-ordination. A major task is then to define how different types of emotional expression, and emotional experience, are co-ordinated in the central nervous system, and how this co-ordination can become impaired.

Table 4.4.1. *Classification of reinforcing events (loosely based on Mowrer, 1960; Gray, 1972)*

	Unconditioned		Conditioned	
Presentation	R	P	R 'hope'	P 'anxiety'
Omission or termination	$\overline{R}$	$\overline{P}$	$\overline{R}$ 'frustration' or 'disappointment' leading to 'sorrow' or 'anger'	$\overline{P}$ 'relief'

R = reward (positive event), P = punishment (negative event).

An alternative way of considering the stimulus conditions for emotion is to emphasize the dimensions of stimulus intensity and novelty. Both of these depend upon context; a familiar stimulus in an unexpected context leads to an incongruity that may prove as disturbing as if the stimulus were totally novel. The subjective intensity of a stimulus depends upon habituation and adaptation. These processes result from the ways in which stimuli are presented in relation to the responses of the organism. Thus, stimuli predicted by the passage of time or by the organism's own behaviour may evoke rapid habituation, unless these stimuli are either themselves physically intense (e.g. electric shock) or are associated with other intense stimuli. Even the effects of intense stimuli such as electric shock may be modified by the predictability of their occurrence (see Seligman, 1975). It is these factors that may determine in part whether the events charted in table 4.4.1 are 'positive' or 'negative'. Thus, the removal of a positive reinforcer (extinction) constitutes a novel situation; so too does the presentation of an unpredictable 'negative' event. The occurrence of even a predictable 'positive' event is similarly a stimulus change, although admittedly one of minor proportions. Perhaps it is this stimulus change quality that underlies its 'positive' nature in maintaining behaviour. On the other hand, if a stimulus is sufficiently intense or novel, it may interrupt ongoing behaviour, and produce what Ryle (1949) would call an 'agitation'. Several authors, including Melzack and Casey (1970) and Berlyne (1967) have described the possible aversive effects of highly intense stimuli and Miller, Galanter, and Pribram (1960, p. 114) have also referred to the emotional consequences of interruption of planned actions. Mandler (1975) suggests that the availability of an alternative plan leads to less disruption, and consequently less emotional effect. This notion appears to be analogous to the well-known 'coping' response to stress. (Levine, Weinberg & Ursin, 1978).

Identifying the stimulus conditions or dimensions eliciting emotion is only a step towards specifying which neural structures mediate emotion. A preliminary specification will be an aim of later portions of this chapter. In brief, I shall suggest that intense stimuli have almost direct access to the action systems of the central nervous system responsible for emotional expression. The effects of these stimuli upon the action systems are modified greatly by context, and its representation by limbic and cortical parts of the brain. Intense stimuli also produce autonomic,

endocrine, and other bodily changes, the perception of which constitutes emotional experience. Context will similarly influence this perception. Meanwhile, however, I shall consider how these and related contentions have developed from the illustrious theories of the nineteenth century.

Theories of emotion
James–Lange theory

William James (1884) rejected the common-sense view that emotional expression is impelled by emotional experience. Indeed, he turned this causal sequence completely round, maintaining instead that the sensation of bodily changes 'which follow directly the perception of the exciting fact' was the emotional experience. The diversity of emotional feeling was supposed to derive from the patterning of changes in voluntary musculature and the autonomically innervated viscera. In 1885, Lange independently arrived at a somewhat similar conclusion, although his theory emphasized the role of the vasomotor changes which produced secondary effects upon muscular tension, cerebral blood supply, and so on (Lange & James, 1922).

James seems to have been initially uncertain of the mechanism by which bodily changes are converted to emotional feeling. In his 1884 article, while subscribing to the notion that the emotional feeling was produced from afferent feedback of the viscera to the brain, he also states the possibility 'of our being conscious of the outgoing nerve currents starting on their way downwards towards the parts they are to excite' (1884, p. 16). This 'psychic' mechanism contributes importantly to many current theories of emotion and was to be James's saving clause from later refutation.

Both James and Lange advanced tentative formulations of which brain structures mediate emotion. James actually proposed that no special brain centres were required:

> An object falls on a sense organ, affects a cortical part and is perceived; or else the latter, excited inwardly, gives rise to an idea of the same object. Quick as a flash, the reflex currents pass down through their pre-ordained channels, alter the condition of muscle, skin and viscus; and these alterations perceived, like the original object, in as many portions of the cortex, combine with it in consciousness and transform it from an object simply appre-

hended into an object-emotionally-felt. (James, 1890, pp. 473–4.)

Lange was adamant that emotional events produced effects upon the 'vasomotor centre', that group of nerve cells, lying between the brain and spinal cord, which regulate the innervation of the blood vessels. His emphasis upon the afferent control of the vascularization of particular organs accounts for many of the expressive signs of emotion, and, indeed, goes further, by suggesting a mechanism for what later were called psychosomatic symptoms (Ciba Symposium, 1972). Chronic exposure to emotional events may produce dysfunction in bodily organs, perhaps leading to somatic lesions. Clear evidence of the role of psychological variables in organic dysfunction is now to be found in the recent work of Weiss (1972) showing the development of gastric ulceration in rats subjected to electric shocks. The greatest amount of ulceration was found in rats exposed to inescapable, unpredictable shocks. Rats given equal amounts of shock that was both signalled and could be terminated also exhibited ulceration but to a much lesser extent than in the other group. The strength of Lange's formulation is that he makes it clear that such somatic lesions could actually be the only expression of emotion, especially since human subjects suffering organic dysfunctions might actually deny the significance of emotional events or the perception of bodily feeling. Therefore, he was understandably vague on how emotional feeling might be perceived from somatic change. However, he implies the possibility of sensory afferent feedback, but also mentions changes in cerebral blood flow which might alter mental functioning. This latter idea seems to be a forerunner of 'activation' or 'arousal' theories of emotion.

Critique and developments of James–Lange theory. Cannon's 'thalamic' theory of the emotions was born from his test and rejection of the James–Lange theory. His five major criticisms (Cannon, 1927) are famous, and bear repetition:

(1) Total separation of the viscera from the CNS does not impair emotional behaviour.
(2) The same visceral changes occur in very different emotional states and in non-emotional states.
(3) The viscera are relatively insensitive structures.
(4) Visceral changes are too slow to be a source of emotional feeling.

(5) Artificial induction of the visceral changes typical of strong emotions does not produce them.

The theoretical debates that have revolved around these five points have been legion, and yet, in many cases indecisive (see Cannon, 1927, 1931; Schachter, 1966; Mandler, 1975; Strongman, 1978). However, as is commonly the case with theoretical disputes, elements of opposing positions find their way into important new formulations. Discussion here is restricted to three crucial notions that have developed from this debate:

(a) arousal or activation
(b) the role of context in emotion
(c) 'autonomic imagery'

(a) *Arousal or activation.* Both criticisms 2 and 3 of Cannon stress that the autonomic nervous system (ANS) may be incapable of providing the differential feedback that the James–Lange theory requires for the perception of different emotional feelings. Both points are arguable. The autonomic system may not be the sensorily impoverished structure it is claimed to be (see Fehr & Stern, 1970). And some investigators have demonstrated qualitative variations in output for the ANS that may be correlated with different emotional feelings. For example, Ax (1953), in conditions designed to elicit feelings of 'fear' or 'anger' in human subjects, found different patterns of blood-pressure change, heart rate, skin conductance, and muscle potential, when he came to compare subjects' individual responses in the two conditions. Thus 'anger' was characterized by increases in diastolic blood-pressure, in frequency of GSR, and in muscle tension, with concomitant slowing of heart-rate. However, 'fear' was accompanied by increase in respiration rate, cardiac rate, muscle tension peaks, and skin conductance. Ax, and later Funkenstein (1956), related the patterns of change to those produced by systemic injections of adrenaline or noradrenaline, the adrenal hormones. Adrenaline was suggested to mediate patterns of response corresponding to 'fear', and noradrenaline those patterns corresponding to 'anger'.

These results are particularly relevant when considered together with Brady's (1967) research with rhesus monkeys in a variety of aversive conditioning procedures. He, too, found specific patterns of cardiovascular response, as well as changes in plasma levels of noradrenaline, adrenaline, and corticosteroids, as a function of well-defined environmental contingencies. These complex somatic, autonomic, and endocrine changes could clearly provide the substrate of physiological change required of James's theory. However, none of these patterns of response has yet been shown to be a *cause* of emotional feelings or, in Mandler's (1975) terms, 'the psychologically functional stimulus'.

In fact, the majority of investigators have failed to demonstrate patterning of autonomic states. Averill (1969), for example, found subtle differences in autonomic response for the feelings of 'sadness' and 'mirth', but the main feature of the results was the rather gross sympathetic discharge found for either type of feeling. Similarly, Pátkai (1971) measures adrenaline excretion in 'pleasant', 'unpleasant', and 'neutral' situations, discovering that adrenaline excretion was enhanced in both the 'pleasant' and in the 'unpleasant' situations relative to the neutral situation.

Recent emphasis, therefore, has rested upon an undifferentiated autonomic feedback function termed 'arousal' or 'activation' elicited by the types of condition outlined earlier. The concept of non-specific arousal has, of course, been central to the thinking of many behavioural theorists (Hull, 1943; Lindsley, 1951; Malmo, 1959; Duffy, 1962; Berlyne, 1967). Therefore, some care will be taken to describe the various usages of this concept, and to explicate the use employed in this article.

'Arousal' has been used as a drive which energizes behaviour (e.g. Hull, 1943), as a process linked with the ascending reticular formation in the brain which provides a suitable background of cortical activity for the efficient processing of information and co-ordination of response output (e.g. Hebb, 1955), and as a stimulus derived from ANS activity (Mandler, 1975). The usage in this chapter will concentrate on the role of arousal as a stimulus, and as a modulator of sensori-motor activity. Mandler (1975) has suggested that ANS arousal may have several consequences, a major one of which is to provide an undifferentiated stimulus which produces 'feelings' that the organism perceives and interprets according to its past history and current situation. The other consequences of ANS activity will affect attentional processes in two ways. First, the stimulus will provide a signal to the organism that 'something has happened' which will then engage attentional mechanisms such as the orienting reflex. Second, depending upon its subjective intensity, the ANS stimulus will compete with other information, and thus may restrict the attention of the organism to other (exteroceptive or interoceptive) stimuli, thereby producing

indirect effects upon selective attention. These dual actions may have emotional consequences. Thus Valins (1970) has shown that when human subjects were provided with false feedback of their heart rate when viewing slides of nudes their subsequent appreciation of these stimuli was enhanced. Even when informed of the deception, subjects retained their original preference for stimuli apparently correlated with changes in heart rate. Valins interpreted these results as an indirect effect of attention; the changing feedback was thought to induce the subject to observe the slides more closely, and thus to appreciate their positive qualities.

For Mandler, therefore, ANS feedback is the 'psychologically functional stimulus' for emotional feelings. This view does not preclude the existence of highly differentiated response patterns involving the co-ordination of both sympathetic and parasympathetic divisions of the ANS, and the neuroendocrine system, with discrete somatic output. However, because of the apparent lack of differentiation of feedback, and because of the apparently poor ability of human subjects to discriminate patterns of autonomic feedback (e.g. Mandler, Mandler & Uviller, 1958), these differentiated response patterns may play little part in emotional feeling.

The present argument will tentatively accept many of Mandler's notions, but make the following disclaimers and modifications. First, although autonomic perception is poor, it may yet be premature to deny absolutely any role for autonomic patterning in the discrimination of emotional feelings. As already noted, inability to verbalize feelings may apparently mitigate the effects of such patterning. Secondly, reverting to James, I see no reason why other interoceptive stimuli, such as proprioceptive and kinaesthetic feedback from postures and facial expression should not contribute to the general feedback function. Fenz and Epstein (1965) and Buss (1962) have collected subjective reports of muscular tension in anxious subjects, and Gellhorn (1964) has argued quite strongly that proprioception can affect mood. Thirdly, ANS arousal may contribute directly to the initiation of action patterns. Mandler has described how such arousal may produce an orienting response and hints at an 'activation' effect of the arousal upon response output (1975, p. 119). I would go slightly further and suggest that bodily feedback can directly contribute to the modulation of effects of other stimuli impinging on the organism, and thus deliver a complex signal to the appropriate action system. This modulation may occur in the short or longer term, in the latter case producing changes in 'mood'. Finally, possible neural mechanisms for these effects will be advanced to meet a criticism of Mandler's theory, namely that it fails to provide a neuropsychological account of emotion.

Before these aims are achieved, it may still be asked to what extent is 'arousal', autonomic or otherwise, a necessary or sufficient cause of emotional feeling. According to Cannon's fifth criticism, artificial induction of arousal does not generate emotional feelings. Indeed, Marañon, (1924) who had injected volunteers with adrenaline to produce an artificial sympathetic reaction, reported that his subject's introspections were devoid of real emotional response. Most of the volunteers merely reported their physiological sensations. Some felt 'as if' they were anxious or angry etc. Schachter and Singer (1962) have since managed, however, to rescue the arousal position by showing that situational *context* is an important modulator of how autonomic feedback is interpreted by human subjects.

(b) *The role of context in emotion*. Schachter and Singer (1962) repeated Marañon's experiments while manipulating two types of variable: (1) information given to the subject concerning the drug's side-effects, and (2) the social context in which the adrenaline took effect. They misled volunteers into believing that they were receiving injections of a newly discovered vitamin, 'Suproxin', and for three separate groups described the expected effects of the drug thus: (i) no expected side-effects (i.e. misinformed group), (ii) sympathetic side-effects (i.e. adrenaline-like effects; informed group), (iii) parasympathetic side-effects (i.e. misinformed group). Social context was varied by having the volunteers complete a rather insulting questionnaire in the presence of an angry 'stooge' (angry condition) or an euphoric 'stooge' (euphoric condition). Measures were taken of the behavioural and subjective responses of the volunteers, and their heart rate was also monitored both before and after the questionnaire was completed. The data, unsurprisingly, were complex, and the manner of their collection and interpretation has been both criticized (Plutchik & Ax, 1962) and defended (Mandler, 1975). However, the results and conclusions, while requiring further substantiation, have been largely supported. The main results were that subjects ignorant of the effects of the injection, from the behavioural observation and subjective reports, both exhibited and felt more emotion than informed subjects. Further-

more, the type of emotional response depended on the context; those in the angry condition felt angry, those in the euphoric condition felt euphoric. Schachter (1966) argued from these, and other results that emotion was jointly dependent upon autonomic arousal and cognitive factors. The presence of an obscure, undifferentiated autonomic feedback is postulated to demand explanation or interpretation by the subject (in a manner perhaps similar to that postulated by Gregory (1966) for ambiguous figures or other visual illusions). This interpretation will depend upon the cues the subject has available to him for explanation. In the case of Marañon's subjects, many had an adequate explanation in the form of the injection itself, which generated the emotionally neutral physiological reports. In the case of Schachter and Singer's misinformed groups, however, no such ready explanation was available. Hence they utilized social cues for explanation.

Schachter and Singer's study has important implications for the study of emotion and its neuropsychological basis. First, it provides a compromise between the extremes of James and Cannon. Secondly, it had been commonly assumed that the degree of arousal determined the quality of emotional reaction (Berlyne, 1967). Although there is perhaps some truth in this, as will be later discussed, the introduction of a cognitive element allows arousal a role in the induction of emotion, without requiring it to account for emotional differentiation as well. Thirdly, while the role of context may seem at present to provide neuroscientists with more than it seems possible to explain in terms of brain function, the evidence suggests that it should not be ignored.

There are several other facts which suggest that an intense interoceptive stimulus that produces diffuse arousal may be especially susceptible to emotional interpretation in the absence of clear contextual cues. Patients suffering from phaeochromocytoma have progressively increasing amounts of adrenaline and noradrenaline released into the circulation as a result of a benign tumor in the adrenal medulla (Winkler & Smith, 1972). This state causes increased sympathetic activity often associated with feelings of anxiety. One might well expect anxiety to be the major emotional interpretation of interoceptive stimuli for which the subject has no explanation. Similarly, some anxious subjects complain of predominantly somatic symptoms of anxiety, such as palpitations (tachycardia) and sweating, that can be treated with drugs such as propanolol, a β-adrenergic antagonist which blocks sympathetic cardiovascular effects. Tyrer (1976) has advanced the hypothesis that this 'somatic' anxiety arises because the subject cannot identify and label the environmental stimulus which elicits the autonomic activity, and which would normally elicit feelings of 'psychic' anxiety such as apprehension and tension.

The subjective effects of psychotropic drugs such as marihuana (Schachter, 1966) and amphetamine may also depend upon recognizing and labelling interoceptive feelings. It is noteworthy that whereas a major reported subjective effect of amphetamines in adults is euphoria or dysphoria, 'hyperactive' children treated with the drug frequently report 'feeling funny, not like myself' (Rapoport et al., 1980). Presumably, children have difficulties in labelling and interpreting the internal cues produced by the drug, perhaps because of lack of experience of these cues in different circumstances. Adults, on the other hand, may be sufficiently sophisticated to label their internal cues as emotional experience. These drugs have central as well as peripheral effects. Amphetamine, for example, is known to release the central catecholamines, noradrenaline and dopamine, in various regions of the CNS. Other agents, such as the electrical stimulation of the brain commonly used in the treatment of intractable pain, or temporal lobe epileptic foci, may similarly induce non-specific stimuli that are interpreted by the subject as depending upon extraneous circumstances. In the therapeutic situation one might expect reports of predominantly pleasurable feelings. For example, Sem-Jacobsen (1976) says about the reported experiences of human subjects given intracranial electrical stimulation: 'If a patient feels "something" he might wonder precisely what is the nature of this sensation? What am I feeling? Let me try it once more? Once more! Is it tickling, is it real pleasure?' (p. 511).

Reports of pleasurable feelings in subjects not being treated for intractable pain are less common (see Valenstein, 1973, pp. 104–14). Similarly, subjects given hypothalamic stimulation rarely report evocation of specific motivational states. Valenstein describes some of Heath's patients who spoke instead of 'abdominal discomfort, feelings of warmth, fulness in the head, pounding heart' in response to hypothalamic stimulation. Even when specific inclinations or memories are evoked, there is evidence of contextual control over the behaviour. Thus, feelings of anxiety or aggression may alternate in subjects

given stimulation of the amygdala (Ervin & Mark, 1969), and the specific memories elicited by cortical stimulation of Penfield and his collaborators (e.g. Penfield & Jasper, 1954) have been shown to be influenced by such factors as the personality and history of the individual and by momentary predispositions (Mahl, Rothenberg, Delgado & Hamlin, 1964).

The nature of the interoceptive stimulus produced by intracranial stimulation (ICS), by ictal seizures, or by centrally-acting drugs in these instances still remains unclear. Although ICS could be directly mimicking input of afferent visceral or somatic information, it could also be producing indirect effects by eliciting automatic or somatic responses in the periphery. Sem-Jacobsen (1976) again provides a relevant example, citing the case of a woman for whom ICS caused reflex contraction of the pelvic-musculature sufficient to elicit apparently pleasurable responses.

If ICS actually aids in eliciting certain types of movements or sensory change, the stimuli produced thereby may also add to the context of the situation and affect the subject's interpretation of the effects of stimulation. In studies of behaviour elicited by electrical stimulation of hypothalamic regions the effect of the stimulation often depends upon the nature of the goal object present. Thus, Valenstein, Cox and Kakolewski (1970) discovered that responses of eating, drinking, or gnawing in the rat could each be elicited from the same hypothalamic placement, with identical parameters of stimulation, if the appropriate goal-object were present. However, the elicited behaviour generally developed over several trials, an effect suggesting a gradual learning process, rather than the facilitation of 'hunger' or 'thirst' 'centres'. Analogously, in human Parkinsonian subjects treated with levo-dopa, Sacks (1973) has also noticed the elaboration of a motor tic or tardive mouth movements into fully organized action sequences such as an adjustment of the spectacles or voracious eating. The initially fragmented actions presumably provide feedback that is interpreted by the subjects and 'rationalized' into a coherent sequence. Similar considerations apply to the work of Flynn and his colleagues (Flynn et al., 1970) on predatory aggression elicited in the cat by stimulation of the lateral hypothalamus. This effect depends upon the facilitation of certain sensori-motor reflexes, so that the cat becomes more responsive to stimuli applied to the part of the face or mouth contralateral to the stimulation. However, the unfolding of a response sequence probably results from the sequential effects of preceding elicited motor elements. Thus elicited orienting of the head or locomotion may bring the prey into view, and so allow the facilitation of other responses (striking, biting) that result in killing of the prey. Previous experience may also contribute to the elaboration of the response. Rats cannot easily be induced to kill mice in response to similar electrical stimulation of the hypothalamus unless they have had a previous history of mouse-killing (Panksepp, 1971). The intracranial stimulation in this case seems to activate previous dispositions or inclinations of the organism.

In summary, I have argued that context is an important determinant of the perceptual and emotional interpretation of visceral sensation, but also of action sequences. These two effects of context may often occur in unison, but there is no reason to expect them to be inextricably connected and dependent upon the same neural machinery. There are many situations in which emotional expression, emotional arousal and subjective experience may be dissociated. Marañon's volunteers injected with adrenaline provided one such example since sympathetic activation produced few subjective reports of emotion. In the next section, I shall discuss a complementary type of dissociation, namely, emotional report in the absence of bodily reactions.

(c) *'Autonomic imagery'*. Cannon's fourth criticism pointed to a dissociation that seems damaging to the James–Lange position. A sluggish visceral reaction cannot antedate, for example, a phobic subject's panic as he perceives the feared event and takes evading action. Therefore, stimulation of the visceral afferents cannot be the cause of these immediate 'emotional' responses, or of the immediate subjective feelings that are often reported. The criticism is reinforced by Cannon's additional claim that emotion is unimpaired when autonomic feedback is absent, and it is convenient to meet his objection by first considering evidence relevant to this claim.

Many of Cannon's examples using transected animals with unimpaired emotional expression failed to make the vital distinction between expression and feeling. More recent studies have indicated that emotional behaviour in animals is often altered by procedures that result in functional sympathectomy, such as immunosympathectomy or destruction of catecholamine terminals in sympathetic ganglia by the neurotoxin 6-hydroxydopamine (e.g. Lord, King, & Pfister, 1976). Perhaps the most theoretically important of these experiments is that of Wynne and Solomon (1955), which achieved an almost total autonomic blockade in rats by surgical removal of the paravertebral ganglia in conjunction with pharmacological antagonism of parasympathetic outflow via the vagus. These rats showed subtle impairments of escape and avoidance learning. There was, however, little disruption in animals which had already learned to avoid footshock. These results suggest that the 'emotional' effects of autonomic feedback may be important for the acquisition of responses rather than for their maintenance. There seem to be two possible explanations for this. An obvious possibility is that the avoidance situation becomes associated with autonomic consequences of footshock, and the response is then maintained by a memory (or representation, or image) of this autonomic activity, even in the absence of actual autonomic discharge. This could be called 'autonomic imagery' (see Mandler & Kremen, 1958). An alternative possibility is that the avoidance behaviour has become an habitual response, maintained for example by the presentation of 'safety-signals', which have acquired positive properties now divorced from the original learning situation. Although either hypothesis is an adequate counter to Cannon's critique, the two hypotheses are difficult to discriminate because one cannot easily infer subjective states in animals.

Hohmann's (1966) investigation of emotional feelings in human paraplegic subjects with spinal transections at varying levels is more germane. Hohmann found that feelings of anger and rage were diminished in subjects with progressively higher transections of the cord (and therefore, with progressively reduced autonomic and bodily feedback). These subjects could apparently make emotional responses in the appropriate context, but reported feeling none of the affective colouring that normally accompanies these responses. As one subject said, 'it's a mental kind of anger'. Thus the other side of Marañon's 'as if' reaction is revealed: the cognition of emotion in the absence of emotional feeling. The ANS, and possibly proprioceptive and kinaesthetic feedback also, then play a more important role in this aspect of emotion, as James had believed.

Hohmann's data suggest that 'autonomic imagery' as such is not actually very vivid, otherwise the paraplegics would presumably have reported more feeling than they did. However, in the protracted absence of real autonomic feedback, it is possible that 'autonomic imagery' would eventually become degraded. There is actually suggestive evidence of this. McKilligott (1959) a few years earlier was apparently unable to find evidence of reduced emotional feelings in the very same population of paraplegic subjects. Now, whereas it is desirable to know of possible reasons for this failure to concur with Hohmann's results, the alternative possibility, of deteriorating autonomic imagery in the paraplegics, obviously remains.

Recent psychopharmacological research has provided rather more compelling evidence for 'autonomic imagery'. Patients complaining of predominantly 'psychic' symptoms of anxiety, such as apprehension, or specific fears, can be treated effectively with drugs of the benzodiazepine class, such as diazepam (Valium), but not with the β-adrenergic antagonist propanolol which, as mentioned above, produces an attenuation of peripheral effects, such as palpitation. Tyrer (1976) has shown how subjects with psychic anxiety believe that many of their peripheral symptoms may be reduced under diazepam, although thorough objective measurement reveals that physically some of these symptoms remain. In contrast, the same patients believe that their cardiovascular symptoms may, if anything, be exacerbated under propanolol although of course this drug reduces heart rate! These important results show clear dissociations between the imagined self and the actual self which are perhaps as dramatic as the analogous discrepancies in subjects with 'phantom limbs'. In addition to providing evidence of autonomic imagery, the results have other implications. First, Tyrer presents evidence that anxiety in normal subjects is more akin to psychic than to somatic anxiety, and so 'autonomic imagery' is not to be restricted to subjects from a morbid population. Secondly, the fact that propanolol led to reports of *enhanced* somatic effects suggests that the degree of *change* in autonomic activity is of greater importance than the direction of change in producing 'arousal'.

The dramatic effects of diazepam probably depend upon a mixture of central and peripheral effects. However, although the neuropharmacological mechanisms of action of the benzodiazepines are far from completely understood, recent evidence (Squires & Braestrup, 1977) has located specific receptors for such compounds in limbic areas and in portions of occipital and frontal cortex. These results suggest that diazepam exerts its anti-anxiety action on structures which are probably involved in mediating those effects of context and contingency

analysis that may contribute to 'psychic' feelings of anxiety.

Neural basis of emotion
Bodily afferents and emotional feeling

The interpretation of undifferentiated information from the body is held to underlie much of emotional experience, and yet no psychological theorist has suggested how this undifferentiated input is mediated in neural terms. Classically, a stimulus has two roles: a cue function, providing specific information necessary for discrimination, and an arousal function, whereby specific information about a stimulus is traded for non-specific aspects that are integrated with other forms of input to provide a 'suitable background' of activity for efficient processing of cue information by the cortex (Hebb, 1955). The problem is whether degraded bodily input from the visceral and vascular inputs is mediated by pathways subserving 'cueing', or 'arousal' functions. If hypotheses such as Mandler's are to be maintained, then the input must presumably be mediated through pathways mediating 'cueing' function, otherwise a special role for autonomic or bodily feedback will not be required. The undifferentiated nature of the bodily feedback in the emotions could then be seen as a consequence of poor sensory representation of the viscera, rather than as a contribution to non-specific arousal. The input for emotional experience would be transmitted via the classical lemniscal sensory projection pathways rather than via the reticular activating system of Lindsley (1951) and others. The non-specific aspects of the already poor input from the viscera and vascular systems may nevertheless contribute to arousal via the reticular formation and modulate sensori-motor responsiveness, possibly resulting in forms of emotional expression and autonomic imagery. This hypothesis requires, of course, precise identification of the neuroanatomical structures carrying bodily information which are, at present, poorly defined.

Although the innervation of the ANS has been comprehensively defined, evidence of autonomic afferents has been meagre. This judgement may also apply to central representations of the ANS. Nevertheless, Pick (1970) has marshalled sufficient information to conclude that afferent fibres travel with autonomic efferents and pass, without synapsing, through the autonomic ganglia to the spinal cord and the hindbrain.

Among these fibres are inputs contributory to

the medullary reflex circuits controlling respiration and blood pressure. Fibres from the tractus solitarius of this region probably supply the hypothalamus and the amygdala with information concerning blood pressure (Palkovitz, 1979). Some of the central noradrenaline-containing neurones have their cell-bodies of origin (e.g. the so-called A1 and A2 cell groups of Ungerstedt, 1971) close to this region, and as well as descending to the spinal cord (bulbo-spinal system), have ascending projections to the hypothalamus and limbic system. Functional effects of blood pressure changes on responses such as 'sham rage' in the cat have also been observed by Bacelli, Guazzi, Libretti and Zanchetti (1965), and so it is apparent that autonomic feedback may affect emotional expression.

Some of the neuroendocrine correlates of autonomic activity may also affect brain function. Dell (1957) has described how blood-borne adrenaline may activate the reticular formation. Reticular activity is probably similarly influenced by gonadal hormones and by stress hormones such as the adrenocortical steroids or adrenocorticotrophic hormone ACTH, which is secreted from the pituitary gland (e.g. McEwen, Gerlach & Micco, 1977).

However, in general, autonomic afferents are difficult to distinguish from somatosensory afferents, and it seems likely that bodily feelings depend upon interaction between these and other sensory modalities. Amassian (1951), for example, found that afferent impulses are conducted in an A beta group of splanchnic fibres with origins in the viscera, and represented in somato-sensory areas of cortex in rabbit, cat, dog, and monkey. There is also evidence of considerable interaction of autonomic and somatosensory inputs in the production of visceral pain (Melzack & Casey, 1970).

In fact, a detailed consideration of the afferent mediation of painful experience encapsulates many of the problems of the perception of bodily feelings in general. Melzack and Casey (1970) have emphasized that pain has at least three interacting dimensions; sensory–discriminative, motivational–affective, and cognitive. Thus, as well as considering its spatial, temporal, and intensity attributes, the effects of painful experience in producing withdrawal or aversion reactions and the effects of previous experience and current circumstance in determining the response to pain must be taken into account. Superimposed upon this complexity is the time-course of pain. Acute pain, usually caused by an obvious stimulus, has a rapid onset (phasic component) followed by a tonic component which persists until the injured tissue has healed. Pain persisting after this healing is called chronic pain, and is the most commonly encountered form in clinical practice (Sternbach, 1978).

It is hardly surprising that pain sensation is not found to be the result of stimulation or damage to a fixed sensory pathway to a central pain 'centre'. This conclusion is reinforced by failures to eliminate chronic pain syndromes such as low back pain or neuralgias by neurosurgical intervention along pain pathways (Melzack & Dennis, 1978). Among the more dramatic refutations of the hypothesis that painful experience necessarily results from input along sensory pathways comes from studies of paraplegic subjects with 'phantom body' pain. These patients continue to suffer severe pain from abdomen, groin, or legs despite a generally heightened pain threshold and a complete removal of the appropriate sensory information by cordectomy and sympathetic blockade (Melzack & Dennis, 1978). Evidently, some sensory experience results from central processes, in a manner perhaps akin to sensory imagery, and hence recalling the inferred 'autonomic imagery' of Hohmann's paraplegic subjects described above. Phenomena such as these have encouraged the concept of pain resulting from a 'pattern generating mechanism' produced by pools of neurones at several levels of the spinal cord and brain. The activity of this mechanism is hypothetically modulated by multiple inputs, including not only tonic and phasic sensory inputs, but also autonomic and visceral input, and descending influences from the brain. Pain results from imbalances in activity of the patterning mechanism, and can be modulated by cognitive and motivational biases emanating from other neural levels (Melzack & Dennis, 1978). This model, of course, fits well with the type of contextual control over emotional feelings postulated earlier, and can also account for the analgesic effects of 'hyperstimulation' (e.g. acupuncture), hypnotic suggestion (e.g. Hilgard, 1978), and placebo.

The essential afferent components of the pain-patterning mechanism involve several major somatosensory tracts which may have distinct, but interactive, roles in mediating different aspects of pain sensation. Some of these pathways, such as the dorsomedial columns, the spinocervical tract, and the neospinothalamic tract are more rapidly-conducting than others. These pathways carry predominantly temporal, spatial, and intensity information to the thalamus and somatosensory cortex. The dorsomedial tract has been suggested to function as a 'feedforward' projection enabling rapid cognitive processing and subsequent efferent control of input via descending pathways (Melzack & Casey, 1970). A more recent speculation by Melzack and Dennis (1978) is that the same noxious stimulus could evoke activity in one or other of these pathways, depending on the state or current behaviour of the organism, and thus result in different responses depending upon the situation. This consideration may also be relevant to determining whether a stimulus has positive or negative affective qualities. Other somatosensory pathways from the spinal cord such as the spinoreticular tract and the paleospinal tract are slow-conducting and probably contribute to chronic and affective components of pain. These projections are portions of a 'paramedial ascending system' which consists of short, densely-branched neurones capable of both temporal and spatial summation, and which innervate the reticular formation and thence project to limbic system, mid-line thalamic nuclei, and frontal cortex. Many of these areas are involved in aversive reactions; for example, electrical stimulation of midline thalamic structures may evoke unpleasant experiences in man (Ervin & Mark, 1969), or signs of discomfort in animals (Melzack & Casey, 1970). However, somatic input can also elicit approach reactions with similar neural substrates, and the mechanisms determining approach or withdrawal to a particular stimulus remain to be defined. Melzack and Casey (1970) suggest that this tendency is determined in part by the intensity of input, since the 'paramedial' cells apparently transform spatio-temporal information into intensity information. Whereas relatively low levels of input may produce approach tendencies, and possibly pleasant effects, high levels of input may produce withdrawal and aversive effects. The critical values of stimulation producing approach or withdrawal are presumably subject to other factors such as experience, hypnotic suggestion, and so on. This model forms a basis for considering the neural mediation of approach and withdrawal in later sections of the chapter.

The neospinothalamic and dorsomedial tracts eventually constitute portions of the medial lemniscus, through which it is possible that some autonomic and bodily information is conveyed to the thalamus and cortex. Sensory representation of bodily feelings within the cortex, however, seems poor.

Penfield and Rasmussen (1950) described how it was possible to elicit intra-abdominal sensations by electrical stimulation of that 'buried plot' of insular cortex, the island of Reil, just above the Sylvian fissure on the precentral gyrus. Penfield & Jasper (1954) later concluded on the basis of many cases that abdominal and thoracic aura preceding epileptic seizures are produced by discharge in insular cortex or in neighbouring grey matter. These sites are quite close to the sites in the temporal cortex that may elicit associated emotional feelings such as fear or sadness (Williams, 1956).

Flanigin, Nashold, Wilson, and Nebes, (1976), also found subjective reports of anxiety, fear, and 'a non-specific rushing sensation', coupled with autonomic phenomena following stimulation of the amygdala. Hippocampal stimulation induced myriad effects, including 'chest and abdominal sensations'. Reports of cardio-vascular feelings, by contrast, are rare, although palpitations were reported by one subject of Penfield and Rasmussen following stimulation of the supplementary motor region. The difficulty in these cases is in knowing whether the stimulation was producing the sensations indirectly from the feedback of effector mechanisms.

The problem of bodily feelings interested both Papez (1937) and MacLean (1958). Papez' original idea was that the cortex of the cingulate gyrus was 'the receptive region for the experiencing of emotion as the result of impulses coming from the hypothalamic region.' The source of input to the hypothalamus was postulated to be primitive sensory areas in the subthalamus which were believed to receive afferents from a variety of sensory channels, including the spinothalamic tract and the medial lemniscus. Additional afferent impulses were thought to reach the cortex via the internal capsule, and via the dorsomedial thalamus. 'Imagination', and other 'psychic' afferents were assumed to arise from the cortex and hippocampus areas and to travel via fornix, mammillary body, and the anterior thalamic nucleus again to the cingulate cortex. This constituted the 'Papez circuit'.

MacLean (1958), in contrast, laid less emphasis upon the cingulate cortex in favour of the hippocampal and amygdaloid components of a 'limbic system' formation. He thought that the dentate and hippocampal gyri had primary sensory functions analogous to the somatosensory cortex. Detailed evidence for sensory projections of the types postulated by Papez and by MacLean is lacking. For example, the subthalamic input proposed by Papez probably receives itself only a limited sensory input. However, the hypothalamus almost certainly does receive a rich supply of bodily information (Pick, 1970) and hypothalamo-cortical projections may potentially provide cortical representations of bodily 'feeling'. Le Gros-Clark and Meyer (1950) pointed out that 'viscero-somatic' impulses could probably reach frontal cortex via the massive projection through the dorsomedial thalamus (see also Ingram, 1960). There are a few relevant experimental data provided by both old and recent work. Bailey and Bremer (1938) reported that stimulation of the vagus in the cat evoked synchronized activity in the orbital gyrus. MacLean (1975), though finding few electrophysiological units responding to interoceptive stimuli in the hippocampus, reported that 20 per cent of units sampled in cingulate and supracingulate cortex of squirrel monkey were responsive to vagal volleys. Furthermore, these units are unresponsive to exteroceptive stimuli, such as somatosensory input. MacLean (1975) suggests that these impulses reach cingulate cortex from a pathway including the tractus solitarius, Gudden's dorsal tegmental nucleus, the mammillary bodies, and the anteroventral thalamic nucleus, possibly involving noradrenergic fibres.

Despite the paucity of information on sensory representation of the ANS, there is considerable evidence of cardiovascular and visceral responses following stimulation of anterior cingulate cortex, posterior orbital frontal lobe, motor and pre-motor regions, and the temporal lobe, both in man and animals (Wall & Davis, 1950; reviews by Ingram, 1960; Kaada, 1960). Thus, another possible source of the bodily 'afferents' could be their perception as efferent impulses to effector organs, as James himself speculated. Perhaps he also considered the possibility that the 'autonomic imagery' that this theory requires is a corollary of this efferent discharge.

The reticular formation: activation, arousal, and mood. The reticular formation (Lindsley, 1951) is the traditional substrate for arousal, although the neuroanatomical definition of this structure has never been precise. Briefly, the term 'reticular formation' refers to a diffuse collection of ascending and descending pathways from the level of the brain stem to the diencephalon. Nauta and Kuypers (1957) have defined two major ascending projections; (1) several pathways corresponding to a 'limbic-midbrain' circuit, including ascending components of the medial fore-

brain bundle and the dorsal longitudinal fasciculus, and (2) a component of Forel's tractus fasciculorum, comprising fibres originating in portions of the medullary and pontine reticular formation, and projecting to the 'non-specific' thalamic nuclei and the subthalamic region. Specific neurotransmitter pathways course through these regions, as revealed by recent mapping studies. In particular, discrete projections containing noradrenaline, dopamine, serotonin, or acetylcholine have been identified along the medial forebrain bundle (Ungerstedt, 1971, Lindvall & Björklund, 1978; Azmitia, 1978; Lewis & Shute, 1978). All of these substances have been connected with emotional behaviour and mood states such as manic-depression as well as with the action of certain psychotropic drugs, including the antidepressants and lithium salts (Schildkraut & Kety, 1967; van Praag, 1978; Robbins & Sahakian, 1980).

The reticular formation certainly receives inputs from what Melzack and Casey (1970) called the paramedial ascending system, which carries information mainly about the total intensity of undifferentiated input. As suggested earlier, the main role of this input is to modulate sensori-motor responsiveness, which may occur via diverse mechanisms, at several levels in the CNS.

Processing of sensory input, including bodily feedback, depends upon cortical arousal, as reflected in desynchrony of the EEG. The subcortical structures producing cortical arousal include the non-specific thalamic nuclei (Lindsley, 1951) and probably include some of the ascending neuro-transmitter pathways of the medial forebrain bundle. Destruction of the dorsal noradrenergic projection from the locus coeruleus in the rostral hindbrain for example, produces cortical synchrony, and lesioning of ascending serotonergic projections appears to have opposite effects (Jouvet, 1978). Cortical arousal may also depend on an ascending reticular cholinergic projection to the midline thalamic nuclei (Lewis & Shute, 1978).

Another role of non-specific stimulation is to facilitate response output. This effect upon motor disposition can be called activation rather than arousal, particularly in view of evidence that cortical arousal and behavioural activation are dissociable phenomena (Feldman & Waller, 1962). Activation may provide a tonic excitatory influence that is necessary for motor output, although the precise form of the output depends upon phasic and discriminative aspects of input, and upon the context of the situation. Thus high levels of activation may be associated with both anxiety and elation. Very high degrees of activation have been hypothesized to lead to behavioural competition and disorganization of motor sequences (e.g. Lyon & Robbins, 1975). Interruption of behavioural sequences or plans of this kind may well produce autonomic arousal and aversive emotional experience (Mandler, 1975).

Activation and cortical arousal depend upon ascending pathways of the medial forebrain bundle. Animals with electrolytic bilateral lesions of this structure at the level of the lateral hypothalamus exhibit impairments in regulatory behaviour, such as eating and drinking, but also in performance of shock-avoidance tasks and conspecific fighting. These changes in behaviour are initially accompanied by cortical EEG synchronization and a cataleptic hypokinesis which appears to contribute to the behavioural deficit observed. The disabilities of animals with hypothalamic lesions resemble in part those of human Parkinsonian subjects, and there is a neurochemical connection between the two conditions since both are accompanied by depletion in brain dopamine content, particularly in the nigro-striatal pathways (Marshall & Teitelbaum, 1977). Brain dopamine – and its interactions with other neurotransmitters, including noradrenaline, serotonin, and acetylcholine, in several forebrain terminal areas, including the caudate/putamen, the nucleus accumbens septi, the central nucleus of the amygdala, the lateral septum, and the frontal cortex – is a major neurochemical substrate of activation (Antelman & Caggiula, 1977; Marshall & Teitelbaum, 1977).

Environmental stimuli of many kinds have been found to change the turnover of neurotransmitters that modulate activation and arousal. For example, stimuli as diverse as inescapable electric footshock, handling, cold temperature, restraint, electroconvulsive shock, omission of food, 'rewarding' brain stimulation and pinching the tail have been shown to increase noradrenaline turnover in rats (Stein & Wise, 1969; Sparber & Tilson, 1972, Anisman, 1975; Antelman, Szechtman, Chin & Fisher, 1975). Prolonged exposure to inescapable shock may actually increase turnover to the point where depletion of central noradrenaline occurs (Weiss, Glazer, Pohorecky, Brick & Miller, 1975). Rats exposed to stress in this way are deficient in learning to escape from shock, and they have been proposed as a cognitive animal model of human depression (Seligman, 1975). According to this model, organisms become 'depressed' or deficient in

acting upon new environmental contingencies because of the previous experience of lack of control over environmental events. The most dramatic examples are provided by dogs previously subjected to inescapable shocks, who subsequently are apparently unable to learn a simple avoidance response. 'Helplessness' has also been produced in human subjects by exposure to inescapable loud noise or insoluble problems (see Seligman, 1975). Although it is tempting to ascribe these behavioural deficits to cognitive changes, an alternative view considers the deficiency to result from reduction in arousal or activation produced by depletion of noradrenaline (Anisman, 1975, Weiss et al., 1975). It is possible that deficits in activation may also lead to cognitive change. McEntee and Mair (1978) have recently shown that patients with a Korsakoff syndrome exhibit depletion in brain noradrenaline.

In the shorter term, the increased noradrenaline turnover produced in rats by shock may be involved in the increased running ('flight') or aggression directed towards another animal following electric shock (Stolk, Conner, Levine & Barchas, 1974; Anisman, 1975), with obvious affective consequences.

Further evidence that activation may have affective consequences is provided by the discovery of Olds and Milner (1954) that rats would self-administer ICS to certain areas of the brain. Many of the effective sites were along the trajectory of the medial forebrain bundle, and in limbic sites (see Olds, 1976, for details). The suggestion that the structures involved in activation and in the reinforcing effect of ICS are largely identical is supported by important recent studies which link brain dopamine to the self-stimulation phenomenon. Phillips, Carter and Fibiger (1976) obtained self-stimulation with electrodes implanted in the caudate/putamen, and administered the neurotoxin 6-OHDA either to the ipsilateral or to contralateral substantia nigra. Ipsilateral lesions, which reduced striatal dopamine levels to about 4 per cent of normal, produced permanent reductions in responding. Thus the reinforcing effect of the stimulation was presumably mediated unilaterally by release of striatal dopamine. Koob, Fray, and Iversen (1978) have extended these results to show that self-stimulation at other sites such as the locus coeruleus is also mediated by the ipsilateral release of dopamine, which presumably alters the activational disposition of mid-brain or thalamo-cortical motor mechanisms. In the experiment by Koob and colleagues, it is apparent that ICS must affect dopamine only indirectly since the stimulating electrode is located relatively far from dopamine cell bodies, but close to noradrenergic neurones. The result illustrates how changes in noradrenaline functioning caused by environmental stimuli, as well as by ICS, can be converted into an activational influence via a dopaminergic mechanism. Changes in noradrenaline turnover induced by environmental stimuli such as foot-shock might similarly be converted to an activational influence via a dopaminergic mechanism.

Human subjects with impaired dopaminergic neurotransmission often suffer from definite changes in emotional experience that are sufficiently general and persistent to be called mood changes. Major tranquillizers like haloperidol, which act as dopamine antagonists, induce dysphoric effects (see Randrup *et al.*, 1975), and depletion of brain dopamine in Parkinsonian patients induces impairment of emotional expression and experience greater than could be attributed to the illness *per se*. Dramatic examples are provided by some of Sacks' (1973) remarkable case studies. For example, in describing the state of Magda B. following a severe form of encephalitis lethargica, Sacks relates how this subject showed few signs of anger or frustration in circumstances which warranted such reactions, such as intolerable abuse by other patients.

> Mrs B. seems amiable and appreciative of help, but docile, *bland* and perhaps incapable of emotional reaction. (Sacks, 1973, p. 55; his italics.)

In contrast, the partial reversal of motor incapacities by the precursor of dopamine (and of noradrenaline), levo-dopa, led to almost catastrophic swings in mood in some cases. Hester Y. frequently became excited emotionally as well as overactive following the administration of levo-dopa.

> Mrs. Y's favourite and most typical excitement is a hilarious excitement ("*titillatio et hilaritas*') and she loves to be told jokes, to be tickled . . . anguish, rage and tears are alternatives to hilarity but are shown much less often. (Sacks, 1973, p. 90).

These observations provide support for Gellhorn's (1964) hypothesis of the intimate relationship between mood and movement or posture and also show that high levels of activation can result in negative as well as positive affect.

Behavioural irritability is often attributed to an apparent removal of cortical or limbic inhibition

(Cannon, 1929; Bard, 1939). Animals with transections above the hypothalamus exhibit rage in response to only a gentle touching of the forepaw. In the absence of specific lemniscal input, it is likely that this effect depends upon non-specific reticular pathways (Zanchetti, 1967).

Lesions of the ventromedial hypothalamus in animals also produce an exaggerated response to peripheral stimuli which may contribute to their hyperphagia and aggression (Grossman, 1966; Marshall, 1975). Comparable behaviour in a woman with bilateral ventromedial lesions has been described by Reeves and Plum (1969). Hyperphagia was accompanied by wide fluctuation in affect, and episodes of rage, and inappropriate laughter and crying. Poeck (1969) also describes several cases where the mere appearance of a person in the visual field, innocuous gestures, touch, or noise could elicit outbursts of rage with unrestrained acts including screaming, biting, and utterance of obscene remarks. In other examples, similar mild stimuli could elicit uncontrollable laughing and crying. The relationship of many of these phenomena to emotional experience is problematical. The existence of syndromes of sham rage and uncontrollable laughter in man again raises the question of dissociable emotional experience and emotional expression. Neither of these pathological responses appears to be accompanied by appropriate affect. Many of the subjects remain indifferent to the elicited movements, although they would probably wish to escape from them if at all possible. In animal studies, brain regions from which it is possible to elicit signs of pain such as 'flight' and 'defensive' aggression, sometimes produce 'aversive' effects. Rats will turn off ICS administered to the ventromedial hypothalamus, the central grey of the midbrain, the periventricular region and the dorsal tegmentum, suggesting the existence of a 'punishment system' parallel to the earlier-mentioned 'reward' system (Olds & Olds, 1965).

However, though useful as heuristic models, concepts of pre-programmed, and differentiated 'reward' and 'punishment' systems may be premature. Thus rats will turn off ICS of even 'reward centres' of the brain, if the current exceeds a critical level, (Valenstein & Valenstein, 1964), and Steiner and colleagues (1969) demonstrated that control over the onset of ICS appeared to be an important determinant of its reinforcing value at a region normally considered to be a reward site. There is only slight evidence that animals will learn to *avoid* as well as *escape* from ICS, suggesting that the onset of stimulation, even in a 'punishment' region, may not be aversive (see also Valenstein, 1973). Ball (1972) has even observed reliable self-stimulation of the ventromedial hypothalamus in rats, an area considered to be a portion of the 'punishment' system. Perhaps it is safest to conclude at this stage that withdrawal-type responses have predominantly negative effects and 'approach' responses have predominantly positive effects, depending however upon the degree of activation of each response and upon the context in which it is elicited.

Neural mechanisms of emotional expression

Midbrain and hypothalamic influences. Darwin's monumental work on emotional expression (Darwin, 1872) perhaps laid the foundation for the later quasi-ethological exploration of underlying brain mechanisms by Bard (1928), Hess (1954) and others. By providing detailed descriptions of different action patterns, Darwin revealed the complexity of the co-ordinated autonomic and motor organization contributing to emotional responses. For example, 'defensive' rage or aggression in cats involves a hunched posture, ear retraction, growling, hissing, piloerection, pupillary dilation, and other signs of autonomic discharge. By contrast, 'predatory' aggression in the same species involves 'quiet' stalking, and a biting attack upon contacting the prey. These different patterns may have differentiated neural mechanisms. Thus, 'defensive' rage tends to be elicited by electrical stimulation of medial hypothalamic regions, whereas similar stimulation elicits predatory attack at lateral placements within the hypothalamus in cat, opossum, and rat. (Wasman & Flynn, 1962; Roberts, 1970; Panksepp, 1971).

The motor and autonomic elements of these patterns of aggression are present in the mid-brain. Bard (1928) showed that 'automatic', uncoordinated, and ill-directed elements of sham rage could be elicited in cats with transection of the mid-pontine region. More recently, lesions of portions of the mid-brain, such as central grey, have been found to abolish elements of rage (such as hissing or growling) elicited in cats by natural stimuli or by ICS (de Molina & Hunsperger, 1962). Evidence reviewed by Hunsperger (1968) suggests that different elements of the rage and flight patterns are controlled by different projections of hypothalamus to midbrain, probably along descending components of the dorsal longitudinal bundle of Schütz (the periventricular region).

Chi and Flynn (1971), using a combination of lesion and stimulation techniques, have also traced degenerating pathways subserving defensive aggression to the central grey of the midbrain, with pathways subserving predatory aggression being located more ventrolaterally. It is of interest that the medial–lateral relationship between the two forms of aggression at the hypothalamic level is preserved in the midbrain.

The midbrain and hindbrain are also important in executing expressive forms of emotion in man, although we are as yet ignorant of precise projection pathways. For example, spontaneous moaning and crying may occur in human subjects with hemicephalic malformations, in which only the medulla oblongata and (perhaps) the caudal pons are present. Laughter or smiling, however, are rarely if ever observed (Poeck, 1969).

Areas at the level of the hypothalamus in the forebrain probably contribute to the co-ordination of these brain-stem response elements. Bard's work with decorticated cats revealed that although the threshold for rage was lowered, the response was co-ordinated and directed towards external stimuli. Similarly, stimulation of hypothalamus evokes well-coordinated aggression (Hess, 1954; Wasman & Flynn, 1962). This co-ordination may depend upon the sequential effects of specific sensory input provided by lemniscal influences, in combination with the tonic activation of mid-brain mechanisms, as earlier described (Sprague, Chambers & Stellar, 1961; Flynn *et al.*, 1970).

Poeck (1969), in a detailed survey, has also linked pathological laughing and crying in many clinical cases with damage involving such structures as the cerebral peduncles and caudal hypothalamus and with nearby structures, including the substantia nigra, and the caudate/putamen and claustrum. Not surprisingly, these phenomena are present in other syndromes involving extrapyramidal damage, including Parkinsonism, chorea, athetosis, hypokinesis and hyperkinesis. The movements differ from case to case in their fatigability and ease of elicitation. They can be part of a spastic motor weakness, or other forms of 'motor release' phenomena.

Limbic–cortical influences. Elicitation of emotional behaviour and autonomic effects is not confined to hypothalamic and brain stem structures. Patterns of somatic, endocrine, and autonomic response can be elicited from cortical and limbic structures, although these patterns may differ in subtle ways from those at lower levels. For example, Ursin and Kaada (1960) found a dissociation between 'flight' and 'defensive' aggression with electrical stimulation of different portions of the amygdala in the cat. Flight responses were lateral, whereas aggressive responses tended to be more medial. Electrical stimulation of the amygdala may elicit rage and fear in man (Ervin & Mark, 1969), and uncontrollable laughing, crying or rage are exhibited as seizure manifestations or interictal phenomena in psychomotor epilepsy of the temporal lobe (Poeck, 1969). The aggressive behaviour in both cases appears to be in reaction to hallucinations or delusions as distinct from the sham rage elicited by midbrain or hypothalamic damage. Analogously, King (cited in Isaacson, 1974, p. 112) finds the aggression elicited from the amygdala in the cat to be less 'time-locked' to the stimulation than that elicited from the hypothalamus.

Autonomic responses, including changes in heart-rate and respiration, can be elicited from widespread limbic structures, including the amygdala, septum, cingulate cortex, and orbitofrontal cortex. No conclusions are possible about the direction of these changes, which depend on many factors, including precise site of placement and temporal parameters. If a generalization can be made it is that hippocampal stimulation is rather ineffective in eliciting autonomic or, indeed, somatic changes, a fact rather surprising in view of this structure's connections with the hypothalamus (see Kaada, 1960; Isaacson, 1974).

Probably the most effective metaphor for integrating data on limbic/cortical and brainstem influences in the control of emotion is the familiar concept of 'levels of control' introduced by Hughlings Jackson (Taylor 1958), which suggests that a function may be organized at several interactive levels in the brain, with progressive sophistication of control at higher levels. The excessiveness of the rage displayed by thalamic preparations originally suggested to Cannon (1929) and to Bard (1939) that it might result from a release of descending inhibition of cortical origin. Other more recent lines of evidence also indicate higher spheres of control emanating from limbic, as well as neocortical structures. Egger and Flynn (1963) found that the 'defensive' aggression elicited by electrical stimulation of the hypothalamus can be inhibited or facilitated by concurrent stimulation of different amygdaloid nuclei. The amygdaloid stimulation had no effect on aggression by itself, so it appears that the amygdala can 'modulate' the form of response induced by hypothalamic stimulation through descending pathways such as the ventral amygdalofugal projection. Septal lesions in the rat (although not apparently in all species) can result in a transient aggression in response to handling and a hyperreactivity to intense stimuli such as foot-shock or bright lights that may similarly depend upon inhibitory interactions with the ventro-medial hypothalamus (see Grossman, 1978, for a review). The relevance of the 'septal rage' syndrome to clinical observations is unclear, but Zeman and King (1959) found that patients with tumours of anterior midline structures such as the septum, fornix, anterior thalamus, and subcallosal bundle exhibited heightened startle and emotional lability. The frontal lobe, in particular the orbitofrontal cortex, also exerts descending control upon hypothalamic structures through well-defined projections (Nauta, 1971). In conclusion, the existence of modulating influences, including both inhibition and facilitation, from limbic and cortical structures provides a neural substrate, however poorly defined, for contextual control over behaviour.

Context, comparison and the limbic system. Books and symposia on the limbic system proliferate (e.g. Isaacson, 1974; Ciba Foundation Symposium, 1978), and this review concentrates on the theme that the limbic system is involved in the mediation of context, and in formulating plans involving present circumstances with previous experience. The definition of the limbic system has been clearly discussed by Nauta (1973). To the structures earlier described by Papez (1937) can be added Yakovlev's (1948) 'basolateral limbic circuit', including the orbito-frontal, insular, and anterior temporal cortex together with their connections with the amygdala and the dorsomedial nucleus of the thalamus. It is evident that assigning functions to heterogeneous structures with such ramifying connections is a perilous enterprise, and the functions of the limbic system cannot be considered in isolation from those of brainstem and neocortical structures.

Temporal pole and amygdala. Almost coincident with Papez' original speculation, Kluver and Bucy (1937) rediscovered the bizarre behavioural effects of bilateral temporal lobe ablation in rhesus monkeys that had already been noted by Brown and Schäfer (1888). Other investigators have confirmed the presence of the following behavioural patterns listed in the order of their frequency of occurrence; increased tameness, visual agnosia ('psychic blindness'), compulsive oral behaviour, increased attention to or handling of objects ('hypermetamorphosis'), dietary changes, and hypersexuality (see Gloor, 1960). Incomplete forms of the syndrome arise clinically from rapid degenerative diseases of the brain (e.g. Pick's disease and Alzheimer's disease) with bilateral involvement of mediobasal portions of the temporal lobes, from bilateral vascular accidents, from surgical intervention, and from epileptic foci (Poeck, 1969). Marlowe, Mancall and Thomas (1975) have described a patient with a full-blown Kluver–Bucy syndrome resulting from extensive, but relatively selective, destruction of the temporal lobes and associated limbic structures associated with a necrotizing viral encephalitis of presumed herpetic origin. Studies with monkeys have implicated bilateral damage of the amygdala in the production of the syndrome (Pribram & Bagshaw, 1953), with the exception of the visual agnosia, which has been attributed to damage of the temporal lobe (Mishkin & Pribram, 1954). The importance of the connections between these structures is supported by the discovery of an incomplete Kluver-Bucy syndrome in monkeys following damage of neocortical areas (Akert, Gruesen, Woolsey & Meyer, 1961). A less clear picture emerges from clinical studies. Poeck (1969) considers the bilateral involvement of the medial temporal lobe, including Ammon's Horn to be essential, but bilateral amygdalectomy, as used in psychiatric surgery does not always produce the Kluver-Bucy symptomatology (Narabayashi & Shima, 1973).

Whereas many of the behavioural changes of the Kluver–Bucy syndrome may depend on different mechanisms, certain theorists have preferred to stress their common elements. Thus, Weiskrantz (1956) suggested that the lesion of the amygdala produces a dissociation of the sensory and affective qualities of stimuli. The tameness, hyperorality, and hypersexuality could all be counted as failures of stimuli to become associated with bodily change. In a later study, Weiskrantz (1960) found that bilateral lesions of the medial temporal lobe in the monkey enhanced the intake of high concentrations of saccharine, while leaving the taste threshold for this substance unchanged. This finding is congruent with the notion that the temporal lobe/amygdala lesion does not produce a primary sensory loss, but rather changes the affective properties of stimuli. Jones and Mishkin (1972) found that lesions of the amygdala/temporal pole in rhesus monkeys – in contrast to other lesions,

of hippocampal areas or of orbitofrontal cortex – produced apparent deficits in acquiring or reversing place or object discriminations that seemed to depend upon deficits in acquisition, rather than upon hindrance from perseveration or other behavioural impediment. These impairments of acquisition could arise from a failure to produce differentiated autonomic reactions, from a failure to perceive such reactions, or from a failure to associate the reactions with appropriate stimuli. The possibilities are difficult to separate, especially in view of the capacity of these portions of the brain to produce autonomic effects. There is limited evidence, however, to suggest that the failure of amygdalectomized monkeys to habituate to repeated presentations of a tone, is correlated with reduction in autonomic measures such as the GSR, respiratory rate, and heart rate (Bagshaw & Benzies, 1968). Such changes were not observed in animals with hippocampal damage (Bagshaw, Kimble & Pribram, 1965). A probable interpretation of such a result would be that the lesion of the amygdala selectively disrupts the autonomic components of emotional responses. However, the autonomic response mechanisms are apparently intact after amygdala lesions. GSR changes occurred readily in response to electric shocks with no apparent change in threshold, although the amplitude of the GSR responses lacked the normal correlation with increasing shock intensity (Bagshaw & Pribram, 1968). In a more detailed review of the GSR results Pribram and McGuinness (1975) suggest that 'registration' processes are impaired following amygdala lesions, which may be another way of saying that a stimulus fails to become encoded appropriately because of the lack of differential reinforcement it receives through bodily feedback. This hypothesis may explain the lack of habituation to novel stimuli, the impairment in acquisition and the indiscriminate affective reactions of amygdalectomized animals to changes in size of food reward (Schwartzbaum, 1960), to saccharine concentrations (Weiskrantz, 1960), and, possibly, to electric shock intensity (Bagshaw & Pribram, 1968). The apparent lack of affective differentiation may lead to both increases and decreases in appetitive behaviour. Thus, the Kluver–Bucy syndrome is characterized by a suppression of normally aversive reactions to foods, and Weiskrantz (1960) found enhanced intake of high and normally aversive concentrations of saccharine. On the other hand, impairment of appetitive acquisition may also result from amygdalectomy. The amygdala, therefore, may be involved in encoding reinforcement from bodily reaction, regardless of hedonic polarity.

As the opposite side of the coin, Bear (1979) has suggested that the paranoid or grandiose responses of patients with seizures of the temporal lobe and amygdala may conversely result from the enhanced associability of normally innocuous events produced by exaggerated activity of these areas. It is important to emphasize that Bear is referring mainly to interictal phenomena rather than to experiences elicited by the seizures themselves. Therefore, it is not necessarily a paradox that other writers have denied that the emotional effects directly resulting from temporal lobe seizures result in such permanent and marked changes in cognition as the bizarre associations posited by Bear. For example, Williams (1956), after a detailed analysis of one hundred cases, writes:

> if cognition is related to ictal emotions, it is of a rudimentary kind and is secondary to them. No convincing example of primary and isolated 'compulsive thought' as an ictal event has been found in the series (p. 64).

Williams emphasized the absence of elaborate emotional reactions, dividing the feelings experienced by his subjects into fear (61 per cent), depression (21 per cent), pleasant (9 per cent) and unpleasant (9 per cent), although in some cases feelings from more than one category could occur together, including 'pleasant' and 'unpleasant' ones. These simple categories of feeling, which could occur with wide-ranging degrees of intensity, were commonly associated with visceral sensations (e.g. in the abdomen), but there were no specific patterns of visceral sensation associated with the different categories. Williams speculated that he was dealing with simple 'units' of emotional feeling in the absence of an integrative structure (in our terms, context) because of the limited nature of the emotional experiences. Indeed, in some instances (e.g. case 17, J.Q.) some visceral sensations produced a reaction 'as if I had been frightened, but I am not' (p. 46), recalling some of Marañon's observations of subjects injected with adrenaline to which reference has been made. On the other hand, fear-like viscerosomatic responses could be evoked, and although aggressive activity was observed in eighteen subjects, accompanying feelings of anger were reported in only one (psychopathic) case. Most subjects exhibiting or reporting fear had focal activity in the anterior temporal lobe, but isolated seizures in this structure evidently do not generally lead to integrated emotional experience.

Links between temporal lobe epilepsy and schizophrenic psychosis have been proposed on the basis of ictal and inter-ictal phenomena, but these comparisons may be simplified by the use of psychiatric diagnostic criteria rather than by detailed behavioural comparisons. Nevertheless, there are interesting clinical implications of the hypothesis that the amygdala and other parts of the temporal lobe are involved in the registration of reaction to environmental stimuli, and hence in associative processes. Gruzelier (1978), for example, has likened the impaired GSR reaction of a subpopulation of human schizophrenics to possible amygdaloid dysfunction. The flattened affect of Parkinsonian subjects described earlier may result from depletion of dopamine from limbic structures, including the amygdala, as well as from the nigrostriatal projection.

Finally, although many of the studies reviewed suggest that it may be dangerous to infer emotional feelings from overt behaviour in animals, it is still possible to use results from animal experiments for critical assessment of neurosurgical procedures in man. Thus, the use of amygdalectomy for treating otherwise uncontrollable aggression (e.g. Narabayashi, Nagao, Saito, Yoshida & Nagahata, 1963) should perhaps be tempered with the knowledge of wide-ranging disruptive effects upon animal behaviour of amygdaloid damage, not only in artificial situations, but also with regard to the complexities of social behaviour in a natural setting (Kling, Lancaster & Benitone, 1970).

Septo-hippocampal influences. The classical theories of Papez (1937) and MacLean (1958) both emphasized the role of the hippocampus in mediating emotion, although in different ways. For Papez, the hippocampus was an important relay station for the conduction of 'psychic' emotional influences of cortical origin via the fornix to the mammillary body, and thence through the anterior thalamic nucleus to the cingulate cortex. In almost complete contrast, MacLean considered the hippocampus to be a reception area for visceral impulses.

Direct evidence for these points of view, as discussed above, has not been strong, and subsequent interest has focused on the possible role of the hippocampus in memory processes, and in human amnesia (e.g. Weiskrantz, 1978). Electrical stimulation of hippocampal areas in man produces complex effects which include anterograde amnesia (if the stimulation is bilateral), déjà vu phenomena, and hallucinations (Ervin & Mark, 1969). Occasionally evoked memories will have an emotional quality, such as embarrassment (Flanigin *et al.*, 1976). Accounts of the human amnesic syndrome (e.g. Zangwill, 1977) do not emphasize gross emotional changes, although there are suggestions that patients with Korsakoff's syndrome are unduly apathetic, and lack motivation (see Glanzer & Clark, 1979, p. 474). The relationship between amnesia and motivational state is unclear; memory and motivation are interdependent to some extent. It is possible that the recent finding (McEntee & Mair, 1978) of central noradrenaline depletion in Korsakoff's patients is a central correlate of their apathy.

Notwithstanding these observations, there remains support for some role of the hippocampus in emotion. Considering the septo-hippocampal region as a functional unit on the basis of certain shared neuroanatomical and neurophysiological relationships, Gray, Feldon, Rawlins, Owen and McNaughton (1978) have proposed that 'anxiety' and 'frustration' as well as the effects of 'anti-anxiety' drugs, are controlled in part by these structures. The evidence favouring this position is controversial as well as complex, but depends mainly upon the behaviour of operated animals in situations assumed to reflect those emotional states (see also table 4.4.1), viz:

(1) Hippocampal or septal animals generally take longer to extinguish a previously learned response when this response is no longer rewarded.

(2) The so-called 'frustrative' effects of non-reward upon response persistence in extinction are generally attenuated.

(3) Suppression of appetitive-behaviour by presentation of electric shocks or other punishers is generally reduced in hippocampal animals.

(For details see Isaacson, 1974; O'Keefe & Nadel, 1978; Gray *et al.*, 1978; Gray, Rawlins & Feldon, 1979).

A full critical analysis is beyond the scope of this review, but a prevailing impression would be that these 'specific' impairments may result from more global deficits in the ability to detect, or act upon, novel contingencies. Thus, Gaffan (1972, 1974) found that rats and monkeys with fornical transections are impaired in the discrimination of familiarity, a deficit that might also be expected to result in the observed impairments in exploratory behaviour (O'Keefe & Nadel, 1978). There is in fact neurophysiological evidence that the hippocampus can potentially act as a

'comparator' or 'match–mismatch' device in the sense used by Sokolov (1960), and Douglas and Pribram (1966). Vinogradova and Brazhnik (1978) have shown that the normal habituation of hippocampal units depends upon an interaction between septal and cortical inputs. The idea is that a triggering input from reticular structures (possibly non-specific activation, or visceral impulses) reaches the hippocampus via the septum, disturbing its spontaneous activity. The cortical signal to the hippocampus is thought to develop more gradually and eventually to antagonize in some way the reticular influence. Thus, in the normal case, mismatch between the context (or 'expected' input) and the obtained input (which may depend upon the cortical and septal inputs respectively), will generate interruption of ongoing behaviour, with accompanying autonomic and emotional effects. In organisms with hippocampal damage, however, there will be fewer signals of interruption, and consequently fewer emotional effects. This formulation therefore assigns to the hippocampus a role in response selection, that is in directing attention to salient inputs and acting according to changed circumstance. Consideration of the role of the hippocampus in encoding and retrieval processes in memory is not relevant to the present argument. That contextual information gains access to the hippocampus is, however, necessary for its postulated match–mismatch function. There is supporting evidence that single units in the hippocampus begin to fire to conditioned stimuli as learning proceeds (e.g. Olds, 1970; Sideroff & Bindra, 1976; Berger & Thompson, 1977), although the hippocampal inputs responsible for this firing remain largely unspecified.

In general, it is clear that the theoretical naivety represented here will eventually benefit from knowledge of the nature of sensory input reaching the hippocampus, and of the mechanisms by which the hippocampus affects response output. There is a good deal of relevant neuroanatomical data on afferent and efferent projections of the septo-hippocampal system which may eventually contribute to such knowledge. For example, Swanson (1978) emphasizes the polysensory input derived from the sensory and association cortex which reaches the hippocampus via the entorhinal area, as well as inputs from the amygdala to the septal region. There are, in addition, catecholaminergic and serotonergic projections to the septal area and hippocampus from the brain stem. (Lindvall & Björklund, 1978; Azmitia, 1978). On the efferent side, direct and indirect projections of the septo-hippocampal system to cingulate cortex and to the habenula provide routes for hippocampal output to reach striato-thalamo-motor systems. The functions of some of these inputs and outputs are only just beginning to be explored. For example, Mason and Iversen (1975) found that destruction of the dorsal noradrenergic tegmental projection, which innervates mainly the hippocampus and the neocortex, produced increased resistance to extinction in rats. In parallel with this work, Tye, Everitt and Iversen (1977) showed that the destruction of ascending serotonergic projections, which also innervate the hippocampus among other areas, produced in rats a 'resistance to punishment' similar to that produced by anti-anxiety drugs such as chlordiazepoxide. Although both of these effects of monoaminergic depletion mimic effects of hippocampal lesions, further interpretation of this work within the rubric of emotional behaviour and the hippocampus awaits a more precise specification of the neural relationships and behavioural processes involved.

Cingulate and orbitofrontal cortex. Of all the neocortical structures the frontal lobes have the greatest variety of limbic connections, and so it is not surprising that frontal areas are commonly implicated in emotion. Lewin (1973), for example, arguing for the use of selective leucotomy in human subjects, has suggested that bilateral cingulectomy can be efficacious in reducing uncontrollable aggression and obsessive-compulsive behaviour, whereas orbital leucotomy is preferable for treating anxiety and depression. If one can accept the evidence of sometimes poorly-controlled behavioural observations, often based upon rating scales, within a framework of loose diagnostic criteria, this type of conclusion may be valid. There is certainly a good deal of evidence that cingulectomy, for example, reduces obsessive-compulsive symptoms (Meyer, Mcelhaney, Martin & McGraw, 1973), but given the lack of understanding of the psychological aetiology of obsessionality, one might question to what extent the ameliorative action depends upon the elimination of emotional antecedents. Specific roles for the frontal lobes are also thrown into doubt by the use, for example, of subcortical psychosurgery of midline thalamic structures and the internal capsule in treating obsessive-compulsive neurosis, or posterior hypothalamotomy (Bingley, Leksell, Meyerson & Rylander, 1973; Hassler & Dieckman, 1973) and the use of temporal lobectomy or amygdalectomy in treating aggression (e.g. Nád-

vornik, Pogády & Sramka, 1973; Narabayashi & Shima, 1973).

Valenstein (1973) has provided a popular, but critical, account of psychosurgery, and points out the inconsistent changes in personality coupled with subtle intellectual deficits that can occur in frontal patients. Some of the patients display emotional 'blunting' of affect; others with similar brain damage show by contrast a vacuous euphoria, or emotional instability, reminiscent of manic-depressive behaviour. In short, this vast corpus of clinical information adds very little to our understanding of the neuropsychology of emotion.

Much of the rationale for psychosurgery depends upon a few experiments on monkeys or chimpanzees with frontal lesions. For example, Pribram and Fulton (1954) found that the disruptive effects of omission of reward in chimpanzees were less enduring after lesions of anterior cingulate cortex, an effect attributed by Pribram (1971) to a deficiency of short-term memory. The effect is also somewhat reminiscent of a hippocampal deficit, and neuroanatomical evidence confirms that two major projections of the frontal lobe – from its dorsal convexity and from the orbitofrontal region – innervate the hippocampus (Nauta, 1973).

A phenomenon possibly related to the emotional 'blunting' described above is the curious indifference to chronic pain exhibited by some frontal patients that may render unnecessary the use of narcotic analgesics (Sweet, 1959). This indifference contrasts markedly with the 'pain asymboly' connected with damage to the insular cortex and supramarginal gyrus (Rubins & Friedman, 1948). Pain asymboly refers to the lack of withdrawal reactions to painful stimuli, but in the absence of discriminative sensory loss. Pain asymboly, then, appears to be a 'disconnection' syndrome (Geschwind, 1965) in which the sensory and affective attributes of stimuli are dissociated, possibly because of a lack of communication between the somato-sensory cortex and the limbic system. The analgesia due to cingulectomy, however, does not appear to have this property. The patients respond normally to brief or novel painful stimuli, but they appear oblivious, at least temporarily, of chronic pain. Ortiz (1973) postulates that the lesion somehow disrupts the particular neural patterning which may contribute to chronic pain. The two syndromes may then result from the dissociation or disruption respectively of different aspects of complex sensory input. In general, the rationale underlying surgery for psychiatric disorders appears to rest upon the simple premise that patterns of neural activity controlling response output can be altered by leucotomy and related procedures (e.g. Freeman, 1949). Modern developments in neurochemistry may provide a more rational basis for understanding these examples of central analgesia. Cannon, Liebeskind & Frank (1978) have reviewed evidence that analgesia produced by manipulation of brain stem structures in animals may depend upon the release of the newly-discovered enkephalins. It is possible that one or both of the syndromes discussed results from release of similar substances in the cortex.

Despite the rather confused state of knowledge concerning the frontal lobes and emotion, the discovery of several neuroanatomical projections has permitted speculation that may guide future research. Nauta (1971, 1973) has pointed to several rather special features of these projections. First, the frontal areas receive polysensory input from all the sensory association areas, a property shared by few other cortical regions. Secondly, visceral information may reach the frontal cortex through extensive inputs to the dorsomedial thalamus from the septo-hypo-thalamic-midbrain continuum. In theory, this input would provide the potential for the considerable cross-modal matching and integration of several sensory modalities that are required for the utilization of contextual information and the formulation or retrieval of appropriate response strategies. Pribram (1971) has noted examples of socially inept behaviour in frontal subjects which are consistent with this type of view. Thirdly, the frontal lobes, probably in conjunction with the hippocampus and the striatum as well as by direct projection of the orbitofrontal cortex to the septum and hypothalamus, can presumably modulate both somatic and autonomic output. Evidence viewed by Kaada (1960) is certainly consistent with a role in autonomic output, and the theory that the frontal cortex aids in some way the sequential ordering of motor behaviour (Nauta, 1971) is also in agreement. Some of the occasional irritability of frontal patients may arise primarily because of the interruption of plans, rather than because of a specific effect on 'emotion'. The sometimes 'catastrophic' emotional effects, including anxiety and irritability, in patients with Broca's aphasia (Gainotti, 1972) may arise in a similar way. Fulton (1949) has suggested a possible function for the frontal lobe in 'co-ordinating' the several aspects of response output. This type of function may be required, given the evidence of

Hodgson and Rachman (1974) described earlier of 'emotional desynchrony' of responding. There is, indeed, limited evidence that brain-damaged subjects exhibit different patterning of somatic and autonomic output in reaction-time type tasks (Holloway & Parsons, 1972), but there is little indication that this is primarily a disturbance of frontal lobes. Our further speculation on the matter, though, is not encouraged by Denny-Brown's (1951) condemnation of Fulton's particular suggestion as being 'physiologically preposterous'.

Cerebral asymmetry, emotion and language. I suggested earlier that a further analysis of human emotion may depend upon clarifying the different functions of language in emotional behaviour. In this chapter, I have emphasized a 'commentary' function (see Weiskrantz, 1977) which results from an idiosyncratic interpretation of internal stimuli ('feelings') according to external circumstance ('context'). According to this view, language provides a sometimes inaccurate commentary about bodily feelings which includes an interpretation or rationalization of moods or actions that may have no obvious antecedents for the subject. Lang (1978) has discussed an analogous 'perceptual' function as well as two others he denotes as 'expressive' and 'control' functions. The 'expressive' function is simply the repertoire of verbal expression used by a subject for describing particular situations (e.g. 'it's horrible') and appears to correlate quite well with autonomic measures of emotion. The 'control' function refers to the verbal instructional context provided to a subject which may influence his perception of internal or external events. This function interacts with the 'perceptual' one to produce rather poor correlations of actual autonomic events and reported experience. Consideration of these functions of language may contribute to neuropsychological analysis of emotion. There is evidence, both from subjects with hemispheric damage and from 'split-brain' subjects who have undergone transection of the corpus callosum to prevent the spread of epileptic seizures (Sperry & Gazzaniga, 1967), that affective response may be dissociated from verbal commentary.

For instance, Gardner, Ling, Flamm & Silverman (1975) have reported anomalous responses to humorous cartoons in subjects with damage to the right hemisphere. Largely in contrast to aphasic subjects with left hemisphere damage, the subjects with right hemisphere damage exhibited diverse emotional responses. They tended either to exhibit a lack of emotional response even when the point of the cartoon was grasped or, more rarely, in the absence of intellectual comprehension, would exhibit inappropriate hilarity. Gainotti (1972) also reported a greater proportion of 'indifference' reactions, including anosognosia, in subjects with right hemisphere damage. Whether these findings lend support to these authors' notion of hemispheric specialization of affective experience (see also Schwartz, Davidson & Maer, 1975) would seem to require a good deal more research. However, such results provide evidence for a degree of independence between the induction of an emotional state and the verbal commentary upon it.

Further evidence, although largely in anecdotal vein, is provided by 'split-brain' subjects. One such subject (P.S.) has undergone callosal section with sparing of the anterior commissure (Ledoux, Wilson & Gazzaniga, 1979). This subject can exhibit an interhemispheric transfer of emotional experience, possibly through the intact subcortical or commissural connections between the two halves of the brain. For example, when an emotive command ('laugh') was presented to the left visual field (right hemisphere), P.S. indeed laughed, but his left hemisphere attributed this act not to the command but to an imaginary antecedent ('You guys are really something'). If the command 'kiss' was made to the right hemisphere, the verbal response of the left was of indignation, although it could not verbally identify the command presented. Ledoux and colleagues interpret these data as meaning that emotional words are encoded in a manner which includes an emotional assessment even prior to their recognition as words. They suggest that this is in conflict with Schachter's (1966) concept that nonspecific emotional arousal is given emotional valence only after cognitive appraisal. This interpretation would seem to go beyond the data, since it essentially identifies cognitive appraisal with the verbal output from consciousness of the left hemisphere, and underestimates the cognitive faculties of the right hemisphere. However, as Ledoux and colleagues indicate, the results do provide evidence of the non-verbal attribution of emotional valence, and suggest that there may be separate mechanisms processing different attributes of stimuli that could result in differential emotional assessment. As argued earlier, this could begin to explain why stimuli can have both positive and negative attributes and why a motor 'approach'

tendency might be to some extent independent of positive attribution. Part of the task of a verbal commentary system may then be

> to make sense out of the emotional and other mental systems and in so doing allow man, with his mental complexity, the illusion of a unified self (Ledoux *et al.*, 1979, p. 553).

Acknowledgements

I should like to thank Drs P. J. Fray and B. J. Sahakian and Messrs S. B. Dunnett and R. Bush for their comments on the manuscript, and Ms E. Carl for her prodigious typing.

4.5
Disorders of language

MARIA A. WYKE

Introduction

The assessment of language function forms an integral part of the examination of the psychiatric patient. It relates to every stage of the psychiatric evaluation, from the taking of a patient's clinical history in a free interview situation to the more subtle analysis of his mental state. The ability of a patient to understand spoken language, to relate information, to express his ideas and to convey his emotional state is of fundamental importance to the interpretation of his case.

The psychiatrist is frequently faced with the problem of analysing 'specific incapacity' (see Slater & Roth, 1972) associated with known or suspected disorders caused by brain damage. For this reason it is essential to be aware of the presence of dysphasia (*i.e.* the loss or distortion of language that may result from cerebral lesions) and to be able to distinguish between dysphasic and other, non-dysphasic, language disorders.

In the following pages an attempt is made to draw together relevant information, derived from experimental and clinical studies, which may provide some basis for a better understanding of the neuropsychological mechanisms involved in language behaviour. To this end attention is drawn first to the analyses of language disorders occurring during the initial stages of verbal development, and then to the description of the breakdown in adulthood, when the pattern of language function is already firmly established.

Disorders of language in children

(1) *Language development and hemispheric specialization*

The traditional view with regard to specialization of hemispheric function has been to consider the two halves of the brain as equipotential at birth. That is to say, both left and right hemispheres have an equal capacity to develop language function. This evidence has been derived from three main sources: studies of the effects of localized brain damage sustained in early childhood (McFie, 1961; Basser, 1962; Wilson, 1970) which result in no significant retardation of language development; the transient and mild nature of dysphasic symptoms (Guttmann, 1942); and the fact that dysphasia in children is likely to appear with damage in either hemisphere (Basser, 1962). The age at which lateralization of language function occurs has frequently been questioned. It has been claimed (see Hécaen, 1976) that there is no specialization before a child reaches two years of age, although some authors consider (Krashen, 1973) that transfer of language representation may still be possible up to the age of five and probably not fully completed until adolescence. Although the age at which specialization actually occurs is still under debate, most investigators until now (Hécaen, 1976) seem to have accepted the concept proposed by Lenneberg (1967), that is, the existence of a critical period for the acquisition of language, which corresponds to the development of cerebral dominance.

More recently, however, the issues of age and acquisition of hemispheric specialization have been questioned on different grounds. For instance, it has been suggested (Kinsbourne, 1975) that the transfer of language function from one hemisphere to the other is not necessarily indicative of the equipotentiality of the two hemispheres in subserving language function. It is argued that the presence of damage to the dominant hemisphere may result in a dynamic compensation by the unaffected side of the brain, and that the extent of such compensation would be determined by the age of the individual at the time the damage occurs. Such an interpretation necessarily implies that cerebral dominance is not developed but that it is present, most probably, before birth.

The possibility of some form of left hemisphere specialization present before the appearance of language has gained support from recent studies. The observations of Woods and Teuber (1973), for instance, have shown that subjects with early left-sided lesions were consistently inferior in their performance of verbal tasks to those with right-sided lesions. There are also the findings obtained in a study of the laterality of childhood hemiplegia and the growth of speech and intelligence (Annett, 1973) which showed that there were more instances of speech defects in children with righthemiplegia than in those with lefthemiplegia. These observations indicate that in many cases hemispheric specialization for speech cannot be fully subserved by the right hemisphere in the event of an early left-sided lesion. Moreover, recent work on the linguistic analysis of children who have had early hemidecortication (Dennis & Whitaker, 1976) has shown deficits in the organizational, analytical, and hierarchical aspects of language function when the removal was carried out in the left hemisphere, whereas such deficits were not present in the cases of right-sided hemidecortication. These findings clearly argue against the established concept of an equipotentiality of the two halves of the brain.

Recent anatomical and physiological observations also appear to favour the concept of some form of cerebral asymmetry present in embryonic life. An anatomical examination of the structural asymmetry of the two hemispheres in a small group of foetal, premature and infant brains (Teszner *et al.*, 1972; Wittelson & Pallis, 1973) has shown the region of the planum temporale (the cortical area lying between Heschl's gyrus and the posterior margin of the Sylvian fissure) to be predominantly larger in the left than in the right hemisphere. These findings have been confirmed in another recent study (Wada *et al.*, 1975), which demonstrated that similar discrepancies existed in 90 per cent of a large sample of infant brains. The examination of averaged evoked potentials has provided neurophysiological evidence of hemispheric specialization in infants. Molfese (1977), for example, reports that, in response to verbal stimuli (syllable sounds and spoken words), averaged evoked potentials were greater from the infants' left hemisphere. Similarly, electroencephalographic tests have been used to demonstrate this hemispheric specialization of the infant brain. Gardiner and Walter (1977), in a study of four normal infants aged 6 months, found a difference between the hemispheres which closely resembled that of adults, *i.e.* a decrease in the proportion of alpha band activity in the left hemisphere during the presentation of verbal stimuli.

The increased interest in establishing anatomical and physiological asymmetries has been accompanied by a significant number of studies which deal with the inheritance of lateralization in the nervous system (see Harnard *et al.*, 1977; Diamond & Blizard, 1977). Particular emphasis has been placed on the problem of inheritance of handedness. The basic familial characteristic of handedness is not in question, and several interpretations of the ways in which it may be transmitted have been suggested, although no one theory has gained general acceptance. Levy and Nagylaki (1972), for instance, proposed a model involving two genes with four alleles. One gene determines which hemisphere will be dominant for language, the allele for the right hemisphere being recessive, and a second gene determines whether hand control will be contralateral or ipsilateral to the hemisphere subserving language – ipsilateral control being recessive. Annett (1972, 1979) has suggested that though there may be a gene for the transmisson of right-handedness, there is not one for the transmission of left-handedness; Morgan (1977), on the contrary, argues that handedness cannot be genetically determined because genes are 'left–right agnostic', *i.e.* able to produce asymmetries but unable to code the direction of the asymmetries; while Collins (1977) concludes that the inheritance of human handedness does not appear to be compatible with patterns one would anticipate according to Mendelian principles, although it does appear to be compatible with simple, non-Mendelian patterns of inheritance, that is, they represent a form of cultural inheritance.

Unfortunately, this increased interest in analysing anatomical differences and the ways in which they may be transmitted has not been matched by a parallel interest in defining the relationship between anatomy and function (see Galaburda *et al.*, 1978), and until this has been established the precise meaning of anatomical and functional relationships will necessarily remain unclear. There still remains, for instance, the unanswered, though important, question of why the hand areas (left and right sensorimotor cortical areas) do not display the same striking asymmetries in size as seen on the planum temporale.

(2) *Childhood aphasia*

Language disorders in children are being considered here under two main headings: acquired aphasia which refers to those disturbances of language occurring after language acquisition, and developmental dysphasia which refers to the limited and defective development of language function in children of normal, or above normal, intelligence whose hearing ability would permit the perception of speech sounds and who show no evidence of neurological or psychiatric disabilities.

Acquired aphasia. The clinical picture of this type of childhood aphasia has been reviewed by Critchley (1970) and more recently by Hécaen (1979).

The pattern of impairment is characterized by the following features: Deficits of verbal comprehension are said to be rare. Guttmann (1942) reported difficulties in this area in only two of the 16 cases he examined. Other authors (Alajouanine & Lhermitte, 1965; Collignon *et al.*, 1968) have claimed that the proportion is higher, with at least one in three of the children showing deficits in the comprehension of both oral and written language. In only a few cases, however, was the defect severe. Deficits of language expression are marked by the poverty of spontaneous speech, loss of ability to communicate, and, not infrequently, total mutism (Hécaen, 1976). There is also a poverty of gestural activity (Alajouanine & Lhermitte, 1965). Articulatory disorders are very common, although the pattern of dysarthria (Critchley, 1970) differs from that seen in adult patients, with the child showing a more marked dyslalia, representing an attempt to avoid difficult sounds and replace them by easier ones. It is important, here, to note that certain of the features which are often displayed by adult dysphasics are seldom seen in children. These include logorrhea, phonemic and semantic paraphasias, and perseveration. In particular, jargon has never been reported in children (Geschwind, 1964), although instances of jargon aphasia have been observed in written material (Alajouanine & Lhermitte, 1965).

Several factors have been shown to determine the pattern of impairment. Among these the most important seems to be the age at which injury occurs. In children under 10 years the disorders of verbal expression and also of reading are usually severe, and articulatory disorders are always present. On the other hand, when the injury is sustained between the ages of 10 and 15 the disorders of articulation are less frequent (Alajouanine & Lhermitte, 1965).

It is important at this stage to draw attention to the growing body of evidence of the existence of a syndrome of acquired aphasia associated with seizure disorders. This was first described by Landau and Kleffner (1957) and more recently by Gascon *et al.* (1973), Rapin *et al.* (1977) and Koepp and Lagenstein (1978). This acquired seizure disorder is characterized by short absences or staring attacks, and is associated with bilateral temporal EEG discharges and the development of severe receptive and expressive aphasia – although up to this point language development has been normal. The deficits are not always reversible but can sometimes be compensated for by learning the sign language of the deaf. These children may also develop reading and writing skills if taught by appropriate methods. The impairment appears to be similar to the pure word deafness seen in adult aphasics. The failure to speak has been interpreted as secondary to the receptive deficits, and similar to that seen in children who suddenly lose hearing.

Developmental dysphasia. The study of children with developmental dysphasia poses numerous theoretical and practical problems, and a great deal of research into the subject has been carried out by neurologists, psychologists, linguists, speech therapists, and remedial teachers. A comprehensive account of this topic, including reports and critical evaluation of current research, has been provided in a recent publication (Wyke, 1978). The debate focuses on three main issues: (1) the essential nature of the disability; (2) the cognitive deficits associated with the failure to develop language; and (3) the problems associated with the differential diagnosis of developmental dysphasia and other, non-aphasic disorders of language, for instance those seen in cases of autism, mental retardation, and deafness.

(1) In attempting to explain the nature of the disability some authors have sought a unitary cause (e.g. Tallal & Piercy, 1978; Cromer, 1978), others argue that developmental dysphasia is not the product of a unitary deficit but results from multiple causes. Similarly, debate has surrounded the relative emphasis to be placed on neurophysiological mechanisms or on its behavioural aspects. Rapin and Wilson (1978) argue that, except in rare cases of severe environmental deprivation, the failure to develop language should be seen as a consequence of a dysfunction affecting those neural pathways responsible for the comprhrehension and expression of language. Although few will question the organic basis of the disability there are, at this stage, undoubted limitations to a purely neurophysiological explanation. In fact the behavioural analysis – that is, the description and classification of the language deficits observed in these children – has been more profitable in attempting to understand the possible mechanisms which underlie the failure to develop language. In this con-

text, several possible explanations have been advanced for the presence of developmental dysphasia (see Cromer, 1978, for a detailed review). Among such possible explanations are: auditory imperception, and in particular the inability to interpret sounds in a phonetic context (McReynolds, 1966; Eisenson, 1968); impairment of short-term auditory memory (Rosenthal & Eisenson, 1970); impairment of rhythmic ability (Griffiths, 1972); deficits of temporal sequencing (Monsees, 1961; Tallal & Piercy, 1978); and deficits which are specific to the linguistic system, i.e. a defect not of sensory perception but rather of language itself (Cromer, 1978). These theoretical interpretations, and the extensive research from which they have been derived, have made considerable advances towards an understanding of developmental dysphasia. But, as yet, these differences remain unsolved and the question of the essential nature of the disability is still far from being answered.

(2) The specific cognitive deficits found in children with developmental dysphasia have been reviewed by Benton (1978). The problem has been approached in two ways. Some authors have analysed those cognitive functions which they regard as the prerequisites for the normal development of speech; others have studied defective aspects of cognition which are thought to result from the linguistic disability.

The first approach – the identification and analysis of pre-existent deficits which might preclude the development of language – has been the main source for the various theories of the essential nature of developmental dysphasia. The problem which has attracted particular attention has been the analysis of defects of sequential perception. This originates from Lashley's (1951) views on the problem of serial order in behaviour. He considered that both language comprehension (auditory perception) and language expression (organization of movements) require an orderly temporal integration of the elements of speech. Following this, a great deal of research has been carried out in children with developmental dysphasia, using tasks requiring spatial and temporal ordering. Defects in sequential perception in the auditory modality were first reported by Monsees (1961) who considered them to be central to the language disability. More recently, Tallal and Piercy (1978) have drawn attention to the importance of specific variables which affect this deficit, for example the duration of the stimuli and the intervals

between their presentation. Similar disorders have been shown to exist in other, non-auditory tasks. Monsees (1961) commented on the presence, although to a lesser extent, of sequential deficits in the visual modality amongst dysphasic children. Similarly, Furth (1964) has demonstrated that dysphasic children have specific difficulties with the Picture Arrangement test of the WISC – a test which requires the temporo-spatial ordering of information. So far, it has been consistently found that children with developmental dysphasia perform poorly in all sequential tasks, although the majority of studies do suggest that the auditory defect is more severe than that found in other modalities (Stark, 1967; Poppen *et al.*, 1969).

The second approach – how defective language development might impinge on other, non-language, cognitive functions – has been poorly investigated. Attention has been drawn recently, however, (Wyke & Asso, 1979) to the growing number of reports of memory defects in children with developmental dysphasia. These deficits are demonstrable with both linguistic and non-linguistic material (Griffiths, 1972), and have been shown to be present by means of tests which require the use of either the auditory or the visual modality (Doehring, 1960; Withrow, 1964; Poppen *et al.*, 1969; Wyke & Asso, 1979). Furthermore, memory deficits in aphasic children have also been found in the performance of motor tasks (Levy & Menyuk, 1975). Most of the above-mentioned observations have been made using tests which require the recall of sequences, and consequently many authors have concluded that it is a sequencing deficit which is the primary cause of these language disorders. Wyke and Asso (1979) have argued that as the complexity of the sequencing task has been found to be of critical importance, and since an increase in complexity necessarily involves a time factor, it is possible that the basic defect in these cases might be one of memory rather than one of sequencing.

(3) The problem of differential diagnosis is the most important one in clinical practice, since the physician is usually the first to encounter a child suspected of language retardation.

In diagnosing developmental dysphasia it is essential to distinguish between an 'aphasic' disorder and a language disability resulting from mental retardation, deafness, or autism. A subnormal child frequently displays articulatory disorders (Benton, 1964), inadequate vocabulary (O'Connor & Hermelin, 1971), and a slowness in the acquisition of syntactical and phonological rules (Lenneberg, 1967). Consequently, it is not unusual to misdiagnose a child with developmental dysphasia as being mentally retarded. This danger is increased when psychometric evaluation has been made from tests which have an emphasis on language items (the Terman-Merrill, for example). For this reason the use of non-verbal tests, for example the Hiskey-Nebraska test (1955) and the Raven Coloured Progressive Matrices (1962) should be strongly recommended.

It is also important to draw attention to the distinction between the severe deficits of verbal communication which characterize autism and developmental dysphasia. Autistic children tend to be more mute and echolalic (Rutter, 1971) and often the language deficits reflect a severe impairment of symbolic behaviour. However, it is interesting to note that, in common with dysphasic children, they find difficulty in tasks which require a series of items to be thought of in an orderly sequence (O'Connor & Hermelin, 1971). The differential diagnosis, however, is made much easier by the striking behavioural differences that exist between autistic and aphasic children. For example, the autistic child shows marked difficulty in forming human relationships; he gives the impression of detachment and does not engage in co-operative play. The dysphasic child, on the other hand, will usually show adequate patterns of socialization (Cantwell *et al.*, 1979).

The most difficult differential diagnosis to make is between hearing impairment and developmental dysphasia. This topic has recently been reviewed by Rapin and Wilson (1978) who stress the importance of a comprehensive screening for hearing loss, using both behavioural and physiological tests. The advantage of the behavioural tests (*i.e.* those which are based upon the ability of the child to respond to certain sounds with specific gestures) is that they test the 'whole system', that is to say the whole acoustic pathway from peripheral receptor to the programming of a motor output. Unfortunately, behavioural tests are not always possible or reliable and for this reason physiological tests, which do not require the full co-operation of the child, are encouraged. Amongst these, the most frequently used are the recording of the stapedius reflex in response to loud noise, cochleography and auditory evoked responses. The screening for high frequency losses is particularly important as, in severe cases, the children are totally incapable of discriminating between consonant sounds and are therefore apt to be misdi-

agnosed as cases of developmental dysphasia. A proven adequacy of the hearing of verbal sounds is fundamental to the diagnosis of developmental dysphasia, and for this reason the above-mentioned tests should be an essential part of the examination.

Disorders of language in adults
(1) *Hemispheric specialization*

Contemporary lines of enquiry into language and hemispheric specialization have followed rather divergent paths. Increasing attention has been paid to the demonstration of anatomical asymmetries of the human brain in an effort to provide a basis for the explanation of a left hemisphere dominance for language function. On the other hand, neurological and psychological studies have been gathering proof for the presence of language function in the minor hemisphere.

A large number of papers has been published on the subject of anatomical asymmetries of the human cerebral cortex, and reviews of this literature have been provided by Rubens (1977) and Galaburda and colleagues (1978).

Morphological differences (visible to the naked eye) have been shown to exist between the left and right planum temporale (see Wada *et al.*, 1975). The increased size on the left has been put forward as anatomical evidence of the importance of this region in language functions. The planum temporale lies posteriorly to the Heschl's gyrus, which is known to be the primary acoustic cortex and therefore of critical importance for the auditory processing of speech sounds.

Morphological differences have also been described in the courses of the left and right lateral (sylvian) fissures. These studies have been carried out using carotid arteriography (Le May & Culebras, 1972; Hochberg & Le May, 1975), and simple measures of length on superimposed photographic slide projections (Rubens *et al.*, 1976; Rubens, 1977). Both methods of analysis demonstrate that after pursuing similar courses the right lateral fissure angulates sharply upwards into the inferior parietal area, while the left continues posteriorly – the sharp angulation in the right resulting in a smaller parietal operculum in this hemisphere.

Pneumoencephalography has also been used to demonstrate asymmetries in the human brain. McRae and colleagues (1968) have shown, in a group of unselected neurological patients, that in over 50 per cent of cases the occipital horn of the lateral ventricle was longer in the left than in the right, and in the case of right-handed patients the percentage was higher.

The morphological differences seen in the left and right hemispheres that consistently favour the size of the left temporal auditory region support the notion of an anatomical superiority of the left – dominant – hemisphere. But, as pointed out previously, the actual relationship between size and superiority of function has not been unravelled. It has been suggested (Szentagothai, 1974) that gross morphological asymmetries might not be sufficient to interpret microscopic differences, and that connectivity rather than size may be a more important factor.

The second topic of investigation related to hemispheric specialization has been the definition of the role of the non-dominant hemisphere in subserving language functions.

The term 'dominant', 'major' or 'leading' hemisphere – usually the left – refers to the cerebral hemisphere in which disease or damage may produce dysphasia. For many years these terms were used in their literal sense, implying that the anatomical bases of language were vested exclusively in only one cerebral hemisphere. Nowadays these terms have lost their strict meaning, since evidence has come to light indicating that the 'minor' hemisphere – usually the right – has some capacity to subserve language functions.

Evidence that the non-dominant hemisphere is concerned with language has been derived from different sources. The first of these comprises investigations of patients who have undergone surgical removal of the dominant hemisphere in adult life (Hillier, 1954; Smith, 1966, 1972). This operation – hemispherectomy – was developed to treat patients with otherwise incurable malignant tumours. After surgery the patients are found to be profoundly aphasic, but a little later recover comprehension of spoken language, as shown by their ability to follow simple commands. They can also produce isolated words (mostly expletives and stock words) and short phrases. They are, however, unable to communicate an idea in terms of the spoken word. With the passage of time, speech comprehension and expression improve slightly and some patients have recovered the rudimentary ability to read and write.

The second source of evidence derives from electrical stimulation of the exposed cerebral cortex of conscious patients (Penfield & Roberts, 1959): It has been shown that when applied to the appro-

priate regions of the right cerebral hemisphere this produces vocalization (usually consisting of the utterance of a sustained vowel sound) as well as arrest of speech, an inability to vocalize spontaneously, and a distortion of words and vowels. Thirdly, evidence that the right hemisphere serves some aspects of speech has come from injecting sodium amylobarbitone (WADA test) into each carotid circulation (see Milner *et al.*, 1964), for these studies have shown that when the injection has been made into the dominant hemisphere the patients become speechless but nevertheless can still follow verbal commands.

Finally, the most detailed information regarding the role of the non-dominant cerebral hemisphere in speech has emerged from studies of patients in whom the interhemispheric connections have been divided surgically for the relief of epilepsy (Sperry, 1974). These patients offer a unique opportunity to examine left and right cerebral functions independently in the same patient, for after the operation the interhemispheric transfer of complex information is abolished, so that each cerebral hemisphere is restricted to using information gained through its primary pathways. For instance, if the patient's eyes are closed, an object which is actively explored by the left hand cannot be recognized by the right, and vice versa. Similarly, if these patients are shown printed words for a short time in the left visual halffield (thereby restricting the visual input to the nondominant hemisphere) they can identify, by touching with their left hand, objects corresponding to the words presented, although they cannot as a rule describe them in speech or writing (Gazzaniga & Sperry, 1967; Sperry & Gazzaniga, 1967). These reports have indicated that the disconnected right hemisphere is concerned with verbal comprehension but not with verbal expression.

The possibility that the non-dominant hemisphere may nevertheless possess some latent ability for verbal expression has been explored by Gazzaniga and Hillyard (1971), who claim that some limited language capacity exists in the right cerebral hemisphere in right-handed adults, though there is little or no capacity for syntax. They conclude from their studies that there is no clear evidence that the right hemisphere subserves spoken language. Others, however, have suggested that the minor hemisphere may serve rudimentary spoken and written language, assuming that the restriction of verbal expression stems from the predominance of the left – dominant – hemisphere in the control of the neuromuscular mechanisms involved in speech (Butler & Norrsell, 1968; Levy *et al.*, 1971). Such inhibition is thought to be mediated, in patients whose brain has been bisected, by midbrain pathways. Release of the inhibition of speech mechanisms by the left hemisphere has also been demonstrated in the case of some aphasic patients. Thus, Kinsbourne (1971) studied three right-handed patients who had suffered left hemisphere strokes which caused aphasia, all three subjects having some residual speech functions. Although injection of sodium amylobarbitone into the right carotid circulation caused a complete arrest of speech, this was not the case when the injection was given on the left side. The observations were interpreted to imply that these patients' remaining capacity for speech was subserved by the right and not by the left hemisphere.

Until recently the scope of investigations carried out in patients with commisurotomies has been restricted by the method of testing, which requires brief tachistoscopic presentations of the stimuli and tactual identification of the named object. Zaidel (1975) has introduced a novel technique which permits long exposures and allows free ocular scanning, manipulation of the stimuli, and self-monitoring of the subject's hand movements. With this method virtually any type of standardized test may be used, making possible quantitative comparisons between the two hemispheres on the same patient.

Taken together, Zaidel's results have largely confirmed the functional asymmetries of the left and right hemispheres and also the findings which indicate that the right hemisphere does exhibit some degree of linguistic capacity. In a recent study Zaidel (1976) has shown that the vocabulary of the right hemisphere corresponds approximately to that of a child aged eleven years and seven months, and similar findings were obtained in another study (Zaidel, 1977) dealing with the performance of these patients in a verbal comprehension task (Token test).

(2) *Classification and localization of aphasic syndromes*

(i) *Cortical lesions.* The classification and localization of aphasic disorders has encountered many problems since the early description of Broca and Wernicke in the mid-nineteenth century. The difficulties have arisen (see Wyke, 1971) from inadequate classifications of language which in many instances do not comply with the complexity and extent of language function, and also from the techniques used in

localizing the cerebral lesions, which until recently have been technically poor and inaccurate.

At present the most widely used classification of aphasias is that proposed by Geschwind (Geschwind, 1972; Butler & Benson, 1974; Benson, 1979). He divides language disorders into two main groups: those resulting from lesions anterior to the lateral fissure and those related to lesions posterior to the lateral fissure. These two groups are then subdivided into the following: *anterior aphasias,* which comprise aphemia, Broca's aphasia, and transcortical motor aphasia; *posterior aphasias,* which are subdivided into Wernicke's aphasia, pure word deafness, transcortical sensory aphasia, conduction aphasia, and nominal aphasia. In addition, the term global dysphasia is used when there is a severe impairment of all aspects of language function.

Aphemia. This is considered a rare type of dysphasia; it presents in the form of mutism or cortical dysarthria. The patients show no defect in grammar or in other aspects of language, including reading and writing. On the whole it is difficult to distinguish aphemia from a pure Broca's dysphasia, but it has been thought that aphemia results from an undercutting of Broca's area rather than from the destruction of Broca's area itself (Brown, 1972).

Broca's aphasia. This is the most common type of language disorder resulting from cerebral lesions. The typical features are loss of verbal fluency, cortical dysarthria, and agrammatism. The speech has a telegraphic quality, and connecting words such as articles, prepositions, and conjunctions are missing. The patients' verbal comprehension is adequate, although frequently they have difficulty in following double commands. The site of the lesion is most frequently at the foot of the third frontal convolution. Recent studies, however, have shown that this type of language disorder is associated with considerably larger lesions which include Broca's area, the insula, and adjacent areas situated within the territory supplied by the upper division of the left middle cerebral artery (Mohr *et al.*, 1978).

Transcortical motor aphasia. This is also a rare condition which resembles Broca's aphasia in that it is a non-fluent type of disorder with no severe deficits of verbal comprehension. It differs from Broca's aphasia, however, in that verbal repetition is significantly less impaired. Geschwind (1965) has advanced the theory that this deficit results from the isolation of Broca's area from the remainder of the frontal lobe, the lesions being usually located anterior and/or posterior to Broca's area.

Wernicke's aphasia. This is characterized by a profound loss of comprehension. The patient's speech is fluent and is normal from the point of view of grammar and intonation. There is, however, a marked logorrhea or press of speech, paraphasia (i.e. substitution of the correct words by others related semantically or phonetically), and not infrequently there are overt neologisms. Reading and writing are impaired but to a level proportional to the comphrehension deficit. The lesion associated with Wernicke's aphasia is usually found in the posterior aspects of the superior temporal gyrus of the dominant hemisphere.

Pure word deafness. In this condition, although there are no primary auditory deficits, there is a selective inability to understand spoken language. It is usually associated with a loss of music appreciation (Denes & Semenza, 1975) and acalculia. The patients can, however, understand written material and are themselves able to write. The lesions may be unilateral or bilateral (Gazzaniga *et al.*, 1973), and most frequently affect the regions of the primary acoustic area.

Transcortical sensory aphasia. In this type of disorder, unlike transcortical motor aphasia, there is a significant comphrehensive disturbance which extends to both spoken and written language. The patient can, however, repeat isolated words and sentences without difficulty. The speech is usually fluent, and frequently the patients show marked echolalia. They are unable to name objects when shown them, and cannot write spontaneously or to dictation. The lesions are usually situated on the posterior portion of the temporo-parietal regions.

Conduction aphasia. This is characterized by a striking difficulty in repeating words and phrases. Speech is usually fluent, although marked by frequent paraphasias. There is intact or near intact verbal comprehension. The patient's difficulty in reading aloud has been said to be related to paraphasic contaminations (Benson *et al.*, 1973), and comprehension of written material was thought to be unaffected. In a recent study, however, it has been shown that these patients have subtle difficulties in processing the phonological and semantic aspects of written material (Coltheart & Wyke, to be published). The existence of conduction aphasia as an independent clinical entity has been questioned in the past. At present, however, there is ample evidence (Dubois *et al.*, 1964; Green & Howes, 1977) supporting the view that conduction aphasia is in fact a well-circumscribed clinical syndrome. The repetition defect has attracted a great deal of interest, but the

nature of the disability remains controversial. Some authors (see Kinsbourne, 1972) consider the repetition defect to be secondary to the linguistic deficit; some (Warrington & Shallice, 1969; Shallice & Warrington, 1970; Warrington *et al.*, 1971) have interpreted it as a specific defect of short-term memory for auditory verbal material, and others (Tzortzis & Albert, 1974) suggest that the impairment is one of memory for sequences and not exclusively related to the auditory modality. In a more recent paper Strub and Gardner (1974) warned that caution should be used in interpreting the defect as one of selective memory, because they have demonstrated that repetition performance improves dramatically when the stimuli are presented slowly. Furthermore, the repetition errors are primarily paraphasic and sequential. In their opinion the repetition defect should be viewed as a linguistic deficit which is specifically associated with the processing, synthesis, and ordering of phonemes. The lesions associated with conduction aphasia usually involve the perisylvian region, above and/or below the sylvian fissure (Benson *et al.*, 1973).

Nominal dysphasia, amnesic or anomic aphasia are the different names given to the type of disorder of which the primary symptom is the inability to find the correct names of objects, colours, letters, and numbers. The naming errors (see Wyke, 1962; Goodglass & Kaplan, 1972) are of three main types: circumlocutions (e.g. 'use in door' instead of 'key'), phonetic approximations (e.g. 'sieve' instead of 'thief') and semantic errors (e.g. 'pen' instead of 'pencil'). Spontaneous speech is fluent although circumlocutory; there are no comphrehension deficits, but usually the patients show other defects such as reading and writing difficulties, right-left disorientation, and finger agnosia. The naming difficulties are related to the frequency of usage (Newcombe *et al.*, 1965), with low-frequency words being more difficult to elicit than those in common usage. There is, however, no clear relation between the naming deficit and the modality in which the objects are presented (Goodglass *et al.*, 1968; Oxbury *et al.*, 1969). That is to say, the patients find an equal degree of difficulty in naming objects presented visually, tactually, or auditorily.

Most often the site of the lesion giving rise to nominal aphasia is seen in the region of the angular gyrus, although anomic defects are said to arise also from lesions in the temporal lobes (Benson & Geschwind, 1971). Using the electrical stimulation method (Penfield & Roberts, 1959) two recent studies have shown rather disparate results. Fedio and Van Buren (1974) demonstrated object-naming defects when stimulating the left posterior temporo-parietal cortex, while Whitaker and Ojemann (1977) elicited naming errors from a larger extent of the lateral cortex, for instance the parietal operculum, the mid-frontal and mid-parietal regions. This latter work has also shown that, from one person to the next, there is a marked degree of variability of response to stimulations.

The validity of the above-mentioned classification, based on a clinico-anatomical correlation, has gained ground from a recent study which correlated the type of aphasia and the localization of the lesion derived from the findings on the cranial computed tomography (CT) (Naeser & Hayward, 1978). In this study nineteen patients were assessed and classified into five different aphasic syndromes. Broca, Wernicke, conduction, transcortical motor, and global aphasia. The results showed that there was a good correlation between the type of aphasia and the localization of the lesions. A more recent study, also using the CT scan (Kertesz, 1979), has likewise shown a close association between the site of the lesion and the type of aphasia, as well as size of lesion and severity and persistence of aphasic symptoms. It is, however, necessary to regard with extreme caution a theory which proposes a strict anatomical localization of the aphasic syndromes, as many contradictions appear frequently in the literature. For instance, it has been shown (Zangwill, 1975; Mohr *et al.*, 1978) that a lesion in Broca's area is neither a necessary nor a sufficient condition for the occurrence of aphasia.

(ii) *Sub-cortical lesions.* Studies of disorders of language resulting from brain lesions have, in the past, focused their attention on the neocortical structures, despite the fact that for some time several investigators have claimed that subcortical regions also participate in the organization of language function. One of the first workers to propose such a view was Penfield (Penfield & Roberts, 1959) who considered that the thalamus played a major role in the organization of language as part of his postulated 'centrecephalic system'. At present there is a great deal of evidence indicating the participation of the thalamus in language mechanisms. This has been derived primarily from the analysis of patients who have suffered thalamic haemorrhages, from the observations of speech disturbances following stereotaxic surgery carried out for the treatment of movement disorders, and also from studies of electrical stimulation on various regions of the thalamus.

The interest in delineating more precisely the function of the thalamus in language mechanisms has clearly been reflected in the large number of papers which have recently appeared in the literature: one complete issue of the *Journal of Brain and Language* has dealt with this subject (edited by Ojemann, 1975a), and there are comprehensive reviews on language and subcortical mechanisms (van Buren, 1975; Ojemann, 1975b; Brown, 1979).

The pattern of impairment seen in patients with thalamic haemorrhages varies considerably, in respect of both the type of aphasic disorder reported and the severity and persistence of the aphasic symptoms. For instance, Ciemins (1970) reported on two patients who had suffered thalamic haemorrhage; one showed only a slight expressive aphasia, while the other showed a decrease of spontaneous speech, difficulty in carrying out commands, difficulty in writing and also defects in reporting material read. Fazio and colleagues (1973) investigated a similar patient (with a left thalamic haemorrhage confirmed at post-mortem examination), and described the language deficits as a reduction of spontaneous speech with syntactic and paraphasic errors and also stereotypies. This patient also showed difficulty in tests of comprehension. By contrast, Mohr *et al.* (1975) reported that in some instances patients with thalamic haemorrhages when fully awakened showed normal language function, although they quickly lapsed into logorrheic and paraphasic speech which resembled the language disorders seen in cases of delirium.

Another somewhat different picture has been reported recently by Cappa and Vignolo (1979). They investigated 14 patients with thalamic haemorrhages documented by the CT scan. Aphasia was present in 7 out of 8 patients with left-sided lesions and absent in 6 patients with right-sided lesions. In three cases the aphasia was characterized by a reduction of spontaneous speech with paraphasias; there was difficulty in verbal comprehension but repetition was intact. These authors concluded that the pattern of impairment resembled that seen in transcortical aphasia.

The fluctuation of the aphasic symptoms in thalamic haemorrhage is also evident when analysing the persistence of the disability. Thus, of the four cases reported by Reynolds and colleagues (1978), two patients had recovered language functions completely after one year, while the other two remained severely aphasic. These fluctuations of the aphasic symptomatology have been ascribed (van Buren, 1975) to the lack of anatomical control of the area of thalamic destruction. They are also likely to be related to the wide variations in the level of consciousness and the associated confusion seen in many of these patients. Destruction of thalamic regions, as well as electrical stimulation, carried out in the course of operations for the relief of Parkinsonism and other motor disorders have been shown to produce language deficits. These are characterized by alterations of fluency, general hesitation, and blocking of language, and also deficits in naming objects (Riklan *et al.*, 1969; Ojemann & Ward, 1971; Guiot *et al.*, 1961; Darley *et al.*, 1975; Ojemann, 1975c). There is, in addition, a clear-cut laterality effect. Thus, receptive as well as expressive verbal deficits are present after left, but not after right, thalamotomy, and similar results have been obtained with electrical stimulation of the thalamic regions (Ojemann & Ward, 1971; Vilkki & Laitinen, 1974). The deficits, however, are consistently reported when the operation, or stimulation, has been carried out on the ventrolateral nucleus of the thalamus (Ojemann & Ward, 1971; Vilkki & Laitinen, 1974; Riklan & Cooper, 1975). On the other hand, destruction of the pulvinar – the posterior and largest of the thalamic nuclei – has given conflicting results. For instance Cooper and colleagues (1973) found no evidence of speech or language deficits after destruction of the pulvinar complex in either unilateral or bilateral lesions. By contrast, Ojemann *et al.* (1968) and also Fedio & van Buren (1975) have reported naming deficits resulting from stimulation of the left pulvinar in right-handed subjects. Similarly, psychometric studies of verbal function (Riklan & Cooper, 1975) suggest that this nucleus plays a role in verbal function, most specifically that involving fluency. The persistence of speech deficits following thalamotomy is also controversial. Some authors (Riklan & Cooper, 1975) state that language function returned to pre-operative levels within several weeks after surgery, while others (Vilkki & Laitinen, 1974) report that the changes persisted for 16 to 18 months after operation.

The role of the thalamus in language mechanisms has been seen in the past as disrupting cerebral psychological processes in general, and consequently the functions of language. Recent developments, however, point to a more active role of thalamic regions beyond one attributable to a generalized intellectual loss.

It is important at this stage to mention observations on the role of other subcortical structures in the organization of language function. Darley and colleagues (1975) reported evidence of basal ganglia involvement derived from a study of language changes after surgery for Parkinsonism. More recently, Kornhuber and colleagues (1979) have shown that patients who had had infarcts in the territory of the left medial cerebral artery and were classified as having a global type of aphasia all showed evidence of massive basal ganglia involvement. The writers go further, claiming that a basal ganglia lesion is a necessary factor in the pathogenesis of the complete syndrome of global aphasia. On the other hand, a lesion restricted to the basal ganglia causes only a transient Broca type of aphasia (see also Mohr *et al.*, 1978).

(3) *Aphasic and non-aphasic disorders of language*

It is pertinent to describe here, albeit only briefly, speech disorders that occur in association with neurological pathology, but that can also occur as manifestations of psychiatric illness: for instance, mutism, palilalia, echolalia, and jargon.

Mutism can occur as a result of surgical procedures involving the supplementary motor area (Penfield & Roberts, 1959). This, however, is always transient, lasting only for a few weeks. As part of an aphasic syndrome it is rare, and even in the most severe cases of aphasia the patients usually retain a few utterances. Furthermore, the aphasic patient nearly always attempts to communicate in other ways, e.g. using gestures or grunts (Critchley, 1970). Mutism can be associated with other neurological conditions, as in advanced cases of dementia. In this instance, however, the loss of language does not represent a focal symptom but is part of a more generalized intellectual loss (Geschwind, 1964).

Palilalia is a disorder characterized by involuntary repetition of words and phrases. It can appear as a symptom of various neurological disorders. It is frequently reported in patients with basal ganglia pathology (Brain, 1961; Kornhuber *et al.*, 1979), and is regarded as a specific feature of the speech of the general paretic, although in these patients the repetition disorder appears mostly confined to syllables (Geschwind, 1964). It has also been reported in cases of encephalitis lethargica (Benson, 1979), and as a transient phenomenon it is not infrequent in patients with seizure disorders involving the supplementary motor area (Alajouanine *et al.*, 1959).

Echolalia is a disorder characterized by a tendency to repeat what has just been said by the examiner. This is a common feature of patients with transcortical aphasia, who tend to incorporate the examiner's words and phrases into their speech although they are unable to understand the meaning. It is noteworthy that the repetitions are not always a passive echo, as the aphasic patient often repeats only part of the statement and frequently makes appropriate pronoun changes (e.g. 'I' for 'you'). It is also typical for the patient only to echo the language which is directed to him (Benson, 1975). As echo responses are frequently seen in patients with schizophrenia, a patient with transcortical aphasia is not uncommonly diagnosed as psychotic (Benson, 1979).

Jargon speech or word salad is characterized by a rapid verbal output, press of speech, and logorrhea. The speech contains numerous paraphasias, substitutions, and frank neologisms, and is often incomprehensible. Jargon aphasia is frequently asso-

ciated with Wernicke's aphasia. It has also been considered a feature of schizophrenia, and several linguistic studies have been carried out in order to distinguish this from the jargon speech of the aphasic. A review of this subject is beyond the scope of the present chapter (see Gerson *et al.*, 1977; Critchley, 1970; DiSimoni *et al.* 1977), but the main clinical features of distinction rest on the following points: first, the episodic nature of the jargon speech of the schizophrenic patient; secondly, the fact that the speech of the patient with jargon aphasia suggests confusion of phonemes, especially when they have similar sounds, while this defect is not present in the schizophrenic; finally, the aphasic patient has difficulty in writing and shows great reluctance to do so, while writing may be profuse in the schizophrenic. The distinction between jargon aphasia and schizophrenic word salad remains at present obscure, owing mainly to the lack of a systematic tabulation of these patients' language output (see Rochester and Martin, 1979).

5

Socio-cultural variations in symptomatology, incidence and course of illness

H. B. M. MURPHY

The relationship of socio-cultural variables to psychiatric disorder defies easy classification, and often even understanding. It is not something which one needs to grasp in order to practise basic psychiatry, and a clinician who goes to work in a society markedly different from that in which he was trained can immediately apply that training without a knowledge of local social conditions. However, even in his own society, he will remain only a mediocre practitioner if he does not take social variables into account, and no amount of attention to the psychopathology of individual patients can make up for an ignorance of the social forces at play around them. Some authorities believe that it should eventually be possible to distinguish the nature of mental diseases from the forms in which social forces cast them, i.e. from the pathoplastic aspects, and then to attack the 'true causes' while ignoring such social variations. However, this is to ignore how much the mind is a product of its environment, particularly that in early childhood, and how far the 'true cause' might in itself be social. Moreover, even when it becomes possible to agree on the divisions between 'primary' and 'secondary' symptoms, we will still be faced with the fact that the secondary pathology, once started, is sometimes more difficult to eradicate than the primary one, as can be seen in some forms of depression. For these reasons, socio-cultural variations in mental disorder need to be studied in their own right, rather than simply as complications, and the goals of treatment should be to encompass these variations rather than circumvent them.

In this chapter the emphasis will be on empirical observations, since it is only after the facts have been properly established that one can seriously attempt to understand them. Although not entirely appropriate to the task, grouping of the material will be according to broad diagnostic category and only at the end will there be an attempt to summarize certain theories of social influence in the light of the foregoing observations. However, before the variations can be described, a few words need to be said about some non-psychiatric terms to be employed. Many social descriptors are ambiguous, either because popular usage chooses to blur logical distinctions, or because alternative meanings have not yet been disentangled. For instance, when we refer to sex differences, we are still often uncertain whether we are referring to the biological or to the social. Among these terms are role, culture, and community.

A *role* is a pattern of behaviour which has been learnt from social sources and which is thus different from patterns that are biologically determined, as well as from behaviour which is in response to a particular situation and not repeated. The sick-role is something different from the state of being sick, and not every sick person assumes the sick-role. The standard sick-role in one society (i.e. the way in which a sick person is expected to behave) may be very different from that in another; and it is not necessary to have male gender to play male roles. Borrowed from the theatre, the term implies an actor, a script, an audience and usually fellow actors. 'Role conflict', which has considerable relevance in family psychiatry, can imply either that the actor is trying to play two disparate roles at the same time, or that there is disagreement between the actor and the others regarding how a role should be played (Spiegel, 1957).

Culture is often used synonymously with *ethnic group*, but the two should be kept separate. As indicated by their derivations, the first refers to the cultivation of the mind and hence to characteristics induced by the social environment, while the second refers to racial or political labelling. In the anthropological sense, culture refers to the body of shared attitudes, values, and habits which is conveyed by a society to its members, and 'a culture' refers to a social group in which such shared transmission takes place (Kluckhohn, 1952). Not all members of an ethnic group need share the same culture, and not all members of a culture need be of the same ethnic group. It is customary to refer to ethnic group when reporting observations but to culture when trying to explain these observations, and erroneous conclusions can be drawn if the distinction is not remembered.

Community is a term which gets used in many ways, not just in psychiatry but in the social sciences, sometimes being synonymous with and sometimes antithetical to *society*. In this chapter it will be used in the latter way, carrying approximately the same sense as the German *Gemeinschaft* has been given in the classic sociology of Ferdinand Tonnies (1957). In a community (*Gemeinschaft*), most typically a traditional European village, each individual is known as a whole person rather than as an assemblage of roles; in the looser society (*Gesellschaft*), most typically a large city, each individual is usually known to other specific persons only in particular roles. In theory, therefore, someone in need of care will be more likely to have all his wants appreciated in a community than in a looser society, but will also have all his defects more widely known in the former than in the latter. The community psychiatry movement seeks to exploit the former fact but tends to forget the latter.

Socio-economic status (SES) is often used synonymously with *social class*, and may appear to be only a clumsier paraphrase of the latter; but there is an important difference. Where true social classes exist, as in nineteenth-century Britain, individuals tend to compare themselves only with others of the same class; where they are absent, as is broadly true in twentieth-century America, they tend to compare themselves with the whole range of society, something which improves the self-image of those higher up the ladder, but is more harmful to that of those lower down, although changing from one class to another tends to be more traumatic than changing socio-economic status. In this chapter, reference will be made principally to SES, since the existence of distinct classes is usually difficult to ascertain today.

For each of the major mental disorders sociocultural variations will be examined first as respects symptoms and other clinical features; then in terms of incidence; and then in terms of course, prognosis, and factors affecting treatment.

Schizophrenia

Symptomatology. In psychiatry, as compared with most other branches of medicine, diagnoses are unusually dependent on symptoms. In consequence, it is convention rather than knowledge or logic which leads us to stop applying a diagnostic label when certain symptoms are absent, and if the term schizophrenia, for instance, were in the future to be applied only to disorders in which a certain neurochemical defect was present, then the degree to which symptoms vary with social conditions might prove to be much greater than that which we currently recognize. It has been shown that the use of the term 'schizophrenia' is much broader in New York than in the UK (Cooper *et al.*, 1972), but it cannot be said which usage is the more correct; nor do we know whether schizophrenia should be regarded as a single entity or as multiple entities, as Eugen Bleuler (1950) suggested in the subtitle to his famous book. In this chapter it will be treated as a single entity possessing most of the symptoms categorized as 'concordant' in the International Pilot Study of Schizophrenia (IPSS) (WHO, 1973).

Delusional content is the feature of schizophrenia which varies most with social background, as for instance the displacement of religious by scientific or technical content when the poorly educated rural populations of South America move to the cities and abandon traditional beliefs for more modern ones. Though this tells us little more than that such content comes from acquired knowledge rather than pure fantasy, familiarity proves not to be the only factor. For instance, delusions of being watched by the secret police are said to decline rather than increase in societies where political change has made such an improbable idea much more possible, perhaps because what is projected then becomes either too threatening or too mundane.

The complexity of the delusional system is another feature which varies with education and setting, paranoid schizophrenia being usually commoner in urban than in rural populations while simple schizophrenia is proportionately commoner in illiterate rural peoples (Murphy *et al.*, 1963). In part that difference may be an artefact, deriving from the greater ease with which city patients communicate with the city-trained doctor, but in rural settings unpredictable and inexplicable events are more common than in purely man-made environments, and the lower-educated patient does not expect to be able to explain as much as a person with a higher education. Hence when the disease generates hallucinatory or other purely subjective stimuli, both education and environment can be expected to affect the degree to which the patient constructs explanatory delusions.

An exception to this rule occurs in illiterate peoples who believe in witchcraft, since their cultures usually demand that all misfortunes be given an explanation, and the patient complies with that demand.

Thought disorder and lack of insight do not show any consistent variation with social background, but this could be merely because psychiatrists tend not to diagnose schizophrenia if these symptoms are judged absent. Affective flatness and social indifference, which Bleuler treated as 'fundamental' symptoms, do vary in this fashion. Thus, when standardized and extensive rating schedules were used, it was found in the IPSS that only 10 per cent of schizophrenics in Washington and London showed flatness, although the frequencies were 50 per cent and 32 per cent in Moscow and Denmark (WHO, 1979). When carefully matched samples of young male schizophrenics were studied by similar means in Montreal, it was found that those of French-Canadian origin showed much less social indifference than those of British-Canadian origin. Probably, therefore, these are defensive reactions somewhat comparable to the once-common catatonic states, rather than states which the schizophrenic patient absolutely cannot avoid, the choice of defence arising partly from the cultural background and partly from the way in which the patient finds himself treated after the first signs of his illness appear. Hallucinations also vary considerably across societies, depending partly on the culture's encouragement or discouragement of suggestibility.

Incidence. The most striking – and probably the most neglected – demographic feature of schizophrenia is its low incidence before the late teens, the average onset being still later in women than in men. Although the hormonal changes of puberty would seem to be the most likely factor here, it is difficult to explain on this basis why the average onset is not then earlier, or why it is later in females than males. An alternative explanation could be that the onset is linked to the expected assumption of adult responsibilities and abandonment of childhood dependency, a link which is unproven but which acquires added probability from the fact that when decisions are communally shared and little individual initiative is expected or needed, as in some South Pacific communities, the rates of schizophrenia seem to be low. The second most obvious demographic feature in schizophrenic incidence (particularly in comparison with the depressive psychoses) is the high percentage of unmarried persons, something which is definitely social rather than biological in origin, but where the relation between cause and effect is unclear. The schizophrenia-prone individual often lacks both the social skills to attract a marriage partner and the desire to enter into an intimate and demanding relationship. Hence the demographic feature can be secondary to the psychiatric. However, if such a person does marry, and the partner is sufficiently supportive and undemanding, this may prevent the development of the disease and the psychiatric feature is then secondary to the social.

Further evidence that social support is important in protecting the schizophrenia-prone is to be found in the rates for ethnic or linguistic minorities living in the same society. Other things being equal, one finds an inverse correlation between the size of the minority group and its schizophrenia rate, something which is most easily explained by the fact that members of small minorities must deal more with 'strangers' than members of large minorities need to. From this it seems reasonable to expect that the schizophrenia-prone will do better in a community (*Gemeinschaft*) than in a looser society. In fact, this does not necessarily follow. Communities which provide much support to their members often also impose many demands, and quite high rates of schizophrenia in village communities are found if the demands are such that persons with certain types of mental defect find difficulty in making adequate response. Thus, although there is a tendency for schizophrenics to drift into certain 'anonymous' districts of cities and frontier regions, the schizophrenia rate in some rural districts of Eire is much higher than in Dublin, and the latter still higher than in Irish communities overseas. In Canada, similarly, rates have been found to be higher in cohesive than in less cohesive rural communities of the same culture.

The third prominent demographic feature of schizophrenia is its inverse relationship to social class and status, the association being strongest in long-established industrial societies, less strong in immigrant populations and least strong in rural ones with castes. Neither theories based on social selection nor those dependent on social stress appear adequate to account for the variations observed, since there are populations under great economic stress which have relatively low schizophrenia rates, and if social selection were the sole factor one might have expected the disease to have disappeared by now. When groups of similarly low SES are compared, evidence from the USA suggests that the actual social pressures and deprivations are less important than the disparity between what people aspire to and what they actually possess (Parker & Kleiner, 1966). With regard to selection, it has been hypothesized that schizophrenia-bearing families may have other, positive traits which enable them to re-ascend the social ladder, something for which there is slight support from Icelandic historical data.

Course of illness. One of the major findings regarding schizophrenia in recent years is that it runs a less chronic course in some tropical, developing countries than in temperate, developed ones (WHO, 1979). There are exceptions to this rule, with quite chronic schizophrenia occurring in preliterate tribes, but the finding appears genuine, and although the reason for it is unknown the most likely explanation seems to relate to social demands. Studies in Britain and elsewhere have shown that schizophrenics are more likely to relapse when the family imposes many expectations (usually hostile) on them than when it imposes few, and although it cannot be said that mutual hostility within families is any milder in developing countries than in developed ones, it is possible that the role-demands (both intra-and extra-familial) in the former are lighter than in the latter. A second possible explanation is that the patient's explanations for having been ill are more easily accepted in the former; and a third is that the more elaborate services of the more developed countries may be tempting patients to remain in the sick-role, or trapping them there.

In developed countries, social status used to be a powerful prognostic factor (Hollingshead & Redlich, 1958), the patients with fewest material resources outside the hospital being the most likely to remain long in the hospital. However, where forced evacuation of mental hospitals has taken place, and community boarding care has replaced the old chronic ward, as in California and Saskatchewan, that disadvantage seems to have been reduced. Prognosis is still poorer for the community-placed schizophrenic without private financial resources than for the one with some, since being a customer at local stores is one partial route to social reintegration; but the odds are less heavy against those without private means, particularly when the patient can be protected from excessive social demands (Segal & Aviram, 1978). If that protection is given, then even when the condition is chronic, passive symptoms tend to predominate, whereas active symptoms are more likely if the pressure of demands continues, regardless of SES.

The affective psychoses

Symptomatology. The most marked social variation in the symptomatology of the affective psychoses concerns depressive guilt feelings and self-accusations. In much of Africa and Asia these are still very rare among non-Westernized patients, whereas paranoid symptoms, i.e. complaints against others, are common. In Europe they were similarly rare until about the mid-seventeenth century, but then became so familiar that psycho-analysts were able to build whole theories of depression on this feature, although in recent years they seem to be becoming rarer again. In some respects these variations appear to be related to differences in religious belief, but an alternative theory, fitting the data better, concerns the degree of internalization induced by different styles of child-rearing (Murphy, 1978). As well as the paranoid symptoms, depression in Africa and Asia tends to show a relative abundance of somatic complaints (hypochondria), something which can be variously attributed to a concreteness of expression, to the body being more involved in the image of the self than is true among higher-educated Europeans, and to somatic symptoms being more likely to receive attention. In Europe such somatic symptoms, which dominated the picture before the seventeenth century, have remained important in patients of lower SES, and today are said to be regaining favour with higher SES patients as well, as the self-accusations decline.

Variations in the symptomatology of mania are less easy to assess, due to the unreliability of that diagnosis in the past and the overlap with reactive psychoses and schizophrenia. However, grandiose ideation seems particularly common in lowly-educated rural patients who move to a city or overseas, the reason for this being easy to infer. In Russia a form of mania with pseudoparesis has been reported, an unexpected combination.

Incidence. Lack of agreement on diagnostic boundaries both within the affective psychoses and where their overlap with the schizo-affective psychoses makes interpretation of the data difficult here, particularly as regards sex ratio. However, there is no doubt that these psychoses are precipitated or induced by inadequately anticipated drops in the amount of emotional (social) support received, and that they are infrequent in true community (*gemeinschaftlich*) settings. Thus, rates are frequently above average in widows, refugees, military conscripts, inadequately prepared immigrants, mothers whose children have left home, and residents of districts where social interaction is weak, but low in villages (e.g. India, Israel) and religious communities, and during social movements such as the student protests of the late 1960s. Rates tend to be higher in cultures, such as the French-Canadian, which emphasize social interaction, than in those which emphasize individualism, but if that individualist teaching is combined with ideas of guilt and duty to God, affective psychoses may be frequent in the absence of emotional loss. Thus, in the Hutterite colonies in the North American prairies, where affective disorders should have been infrequent because of the combination of communal living with an emphasis on individual responsibility before God, a form of psychotic depression called *Anfechtung*, with rich delusions, was relatively common (Eaton & Weil, 1955). The age distribution can vary considerably from one society to another, if one counts depression in children (anaclitic), adolescents, and the aged, and the same applies to social status; but the reason can usually be linked fairly easily to the emotional support factor already mentioned.

The incidence of mania and ratio of mania to depressive episodes in the cyclic psychoses vary greatly with culture. Thus, the rate of mania in Czechoslovakia is stated to be less than a fifth of that in Denmark, while that for male West Indian immigrants to Britain is over five times as high as for British-born males, neither difference being explainable in terms of unequal criteria. In some developing countries, for instance New Guinea, mania with grandiose delusions is the major type of affective psychosis coming to official notice, and may result in whole revolutionary social movements (e.g. cargo cults) as other people become caught up in the patient's delusions.

Course of illness. Before the introduction of imipramine, textbooks customarily made a clear distinction between manic-depressive psychosis and involutional depression, the latter being considerably more chronic and less episodic. Although both forms respond to the same drugs today, and although an organic basis for the difference is not impossible, the most likely explanation relates to impending loss of roles or status. Chronic involutional depression was rarely found in societies where status increased with age and was not dependent on physical or sexual powers. Another European observation in the pre-chemotherapy era was that depression was more chronic when excessive guilt feelings and self-accusations were present than when they were absent, something which harmonizes with the fact that in India, where these symptoms were absent in even severe affective psychoses, recovery could be very rapid if the patient received news that some recent social loss had been reversed.

Other functional psychoses and 'borderline states'

The majority of conditions falling into this group are reactive. Their character thus depends to a considerable extent on the trauma or threat reacted to, and on the teachings of the local society regarding the threat. In consequence, the clinical pictures to which some diagnostic terms refer vary from one national school of psychiatry to another; the same syndrome can carry different labels, and a single label may cover several syndromes.

Paranoid states are most commonly encountered by the average psychiatrist among immigrants with little education who do not know the local language adequately, and who have insufficient contact with others sharing the same cultural background (Kino, 1951). Ideas of reference predominate in these cases and it is easy to see why they should, since such a person has the narcissistic trauma of feeling incapable, and his ignorance of what local people are meaning by their words and gestures leaves an empty page on to which his unconscious can project feelings of hostility and resentment. For obvious reasons, the condition tends to occur fairly early after migration, but a less clear-cut form can occur at a later stage, particularly among refugees, when the time comes for the person to choose between his old and his new societies. At this stage it is not just the local but also the originating society that is seen as persecuting, and the ideas of reference derive less from hostility than from ambivalence. In Africa a similar state develops among migrants to the towns, since success there carries the disadvantage of separating the person still further from his community. However, cultural background has a strong influence here, some cultures encouraging suspiciousness and projection and others not. In Britain, such paranoid ideation has been particularly described among Polish immigrants.

Confusional states can arise under similar conditions, when immigrants are inadequately prepared for what to expect but are not trained to be so suspicious or projecting. However, the key factor here is education rather than change of setting. Such conditions, and the type midway between paranoid and confusional states, which the French call *bouffée délirante* (Ey, 1950), are very rare in Europeans with higher education, but comprise up to 30 per cent of admissions to some psychiatric services in West Africa. The frequency with which such states occur is probably related to the degree to which groups share vague anxieties, but within any such group the more dependent members are likely to be the more susceptible, so that in Cuba, for instance, the rate is higher among persons still living in the parental home than among those who have left that home, allowing for age. Organic factors can also play a part, and it is frequently impossible with such patients to assess whether an intercurrent infection, chronic malnutrition, the use of a drug such as marihuana, or a recent social trauma has been the major precipitating factor. The duration of a confusional psychosis is usually short, but it may merge with a more chronic state of depersonalization or derealization in more educated subjects, and with severe reactive depression in less educated people if the trauma which precipitated the psychosis is perceived as continuing and as threatening existence ('Voodoo death').

Paranoia, in the narrow sense of a nuclear delusion in the presence of otherwise good reality contact and the absence of deterioration, tends by contrast to be found most frequently in persons of higher education, perhaps because it needs considerable mental agility to maintain reality testing in other spheres while permitting the delusion to continue. The content is highly determined by the culture, so that in India one can meet relatively many delusions of marital jealousy, in France (in the past?) delusions of high descent, in the USA delusions of being a defrauded inventor, and messianic delusions among the Bantu; whereas these varieties are met much less frequently in most other societies. Paranoia is usually reported more frequently in males than in females, but it is unclear whether this difference would persist if one included all cases of *de Clérambault's syndrome* and similar erotomanias, which in European societies are predominantly found in women. It is also unclear whether the linking of paranoia to homosexual desires suggested by Freud and Ferenzi is culturally based or not. Kretschmer's *sensitive Beziehungswahn* (1927), a milder but persistent form of paranoia, was in its original form probably linked to the culture of that time and place, and now seems much less frequently described in Europe than formerly. However, a very similar condition has been reported among males in North Africa, where affectionate relations between older and younger men can engender intrapsychic conflict. In the latter setting it seems to be more susceptible to psychotherapy than the original German version.

Infantile autism is another condition which appears to occur predominantly among the higher social classes, or at least the higher educated. Cases are less frequently reported in continental Europe than in Britain and the USA, and in the latter country they seem to occur disproportionately among Jews; but this could be due to differences in the diagnostic criteria being used by different clinics.

The *puerperal psychoses* are no longer recognized as a diagnostic entity, but they invite consideration here because of the marked social variations that can occur in respect of the incidence and form of psychoses developing in the puerperium. In some societies, notably European, they used to comprise less than 3 per cent of female mental hospital admissions; in Israel over 10 per cent; and in some places in Africa they are alleged to comprise one case in three, differences which are only partly accounted for by frequency of pregnancies. Where rates are highest, the psychoses are predominantly of a confusional type occurring in primipara within the first week after delivery, the condition often being precipitated by inadequate physical care and by the culture shock which admission to an overcrowded maternity service can induce in women who have never been to hospital before. However, even when that aspect is discounted, there remain many variations. In Bristol, schizophrenia developing in the puerperium had a very poor prognosis, whereas in Dublin it had a good one. In West Africa the majority of patients seem to be in their late teens, whereas in Tunisia the majority are in their thirties although age at marriage is not so different, the stress in the one instance being apparently the entry into the maternal role and in the other instance the burden of continuous child-bearing. As goes almost without saying, the incidence is lower in stable marriages than in other family settings, being considerably more frequent in unmarried mothers. In the USA it is twice as frequent in the black as in the white population.

Hysterical psychosis (Hirsch & Hollender, 1969) is also a term which has disappeared from official classification but which it seems useful to mention here, since socio-cultural variations are marked.

When used loosely as an umbrella term for the reactive psychoses, transient psychoses, and possession states in general, it is misleading. However, when confined to cases where psychotic behaviour is being appropriated for manipulative purposes and where socially endorsed possession or suggestion states have escaped control, it seems helpful, permitting the assembly under one rubric of a variety of conditions which otherwise are hard to classify. Among the latter are the 'Puerto Rican syndrome'; the 'wild man' syndrome in New Guinea; *pibloqtok* of the Eskimos; hysterical pseudodementia in Indian troops; most cases of the Ganser syndrome; and the transitory erotomanias which are found in societies which still believe in love potions. As the list suggests, the condition is mainly found in non-Western societies with limited education and is very rare in the higher educated strata of Western societies. In comparison with other types of transitory psychosis, it tends to occur in societies where (a) suggestibility and auto-suggestibility are common; (b) certain types of feeling (hostility towards superiors, sexuality in women, etc.) are not permitted sufficiently direct expression; and (c) limited expression through states of possession is not sufficiently institutionalized or controlled.

Amok has some of the social characteristics of a hysterical psychosis also, but in its most typical form differs from these in being suicidal (Murphy, 1973). Relatively common in Malaysian peoples during the nineteenth century, it made a surprising reappearance in Laos during the 1960s and 1970s, when the weapon used to attack others was the explosive grenade and not the sword or kris. It occurs almost exclusively in men, and is distinguished from other forms of homicidal insanity in that, typically, the people whom the amoker attacks bear no particular relationship to him: they are not, for instance, those supposedly persecuting him. Instead, there seems to be a blurring of ego boundaries, with suicide directed against a non-specific 'we' rather than against the 'I'. Another culture-linked psychosis in which homicide and suicide used sometimes to be involved was the *windigo* of some northerly Amerindian tribes, in which the victim believed himself possessed by a cannibal spirit; but here the suicide took place to avoid attacking people, not as part of the attack.

The organic psychoses

The *infectious, toxic, or traumatic psychoses* are considerably commoner in people who are exposed to multiple environmental insults than in those whose general health and social welfare are good. The form is most commonly that of a confusional state, but local social factors can superimpose other pictures. Thus, in Malaya during the nineteenth century somatic illnesses were often the precipitators of amok attacks, and there is a description of a physician struggling throughout one night to prevent a local ruler from running amok during a febrile, malarial delirium, there being no other apparent cause for this threatened amok behaviour. Where the psychosis assumes a schizophreniform or manic-depressive character, prognosis is usually better if there has been a somatic precipitant than if there has not been, but that association is not constant and in East Indians the prognosis is considerably poorer when such a somatic illness is present than when it is absent. Where brain tissue has been destroyed as the result of an abscess or wound, any resultant psychosis, and in particular any 'catastrophic reaction', (Goldstein, 1959) is likely to be a consequence of the person's efforts to respond to the demands made on his brain by himself and by others rather than the direct product of the injury. In consequence, the degree of disturbance in such cases is likely to be related to the degree to which individuals have been taught by their culture to undertake certain types of thinking, notably abstract thinking, and the degree to which the milieu also imposes such demands. There are pictures from developing countries of patients with large parts of the brain exposed or damaged, but who continue to function as long as the demands made on them are limited. In more developed societies such patients would usually show more disturbance, because they would be accustomed to demanding more of themselves.

The *chronic, progressive organic psychoses*, as typified by the senile and arteriosclerotic group, are of much more practical concern to the average psychiatrist, and socio-cultural variations are more reliably documented. In the first place, there has been a marked change in the rates of mental hospital admission for these conditions in most developed countries during the present century. For instance, in New York State, the age-specific rates increased 200–300 per cent between 1910 and 1950 and dropped again quite sharply in the 1960s, whereas admissions for other psychoses increased during the earlier period by less than 20 per cent. Secondly, rates appear to be much higher in developed countries in general than in developing countries, this proving true not only with regard to hospital admissions but also to cases discovered through community surveys. Thirdly, there is a well-established association between such

psychoses and social isolation, old persons who live alone being considerably more liable to develop such psychoses than those who live with relatives. Immigrants tend to need hospitalization more frequently for these disorders than non-immigrants, possibly because they have fewer social supports but perhaps too because they are more liable to cerebrovascular arteriosclerosis. Persons who have to move residence in old age are more liable to such psychoses than persons who do not, and if a residential move takes place after the disorder has developed, they also tend to die sooner.

Some of these associations might disappear if we were able to distinguish more consistently between organic disease and depression and between senile deterioration and dementia in the elderly. Many associations can be expected to remain, however, the key being the degree to which the demands made on the old person harmonize with his remaining abilities. Where too little is demanded, abilities decline with unnecessary rapidity. Where too much is demanded, as when respect can only be retained by retaining the role of wage-earner, there is liable to be confusion or an attempt to deny the mental deterioration that is taking place, for instance with fictive memories. However, even when the attitudes of the surrounding society are uniform, earlier cultural indoctrination may play a role, and an acceptance of declining abilities can be much easier for persons from one culture than for those from another. The Hindu doctrine of *vanaprastha* (disengagement) can be particularly beneficial in this matter, provided circumstances permit the disengagement to take place; by contrast, British-Canadian cultural emphasis on independence is probably a disadvantage, leading their elderly members to be less accepting of family and community support and hence probably contributing to the fact that this subculture has higher rates of senile psychoses than have most other Canadian subcultures.

Where a chronic neurological disease produces mental disorder before old age, as with *general paresis* (GPI), Parkinsonism-dementia, or kuru, then the major social variables are naturally those affecting the persons' risk of acquiring that disease, and these are not of direct socio-psychiatric concern. However, even among persons who have acquired the basic disease there can be social factors affecting the subsequent risk of mental disturbance. At the beginning of this century, Krafft-Ebing's aphorism that GPI was 'a product of Syphilisation and Civilisation' was widely accepted, since the mental disorder was then more frequent among the higher than among the lower educated in Western society, whereas syphilis itself had probably the reverse distribution, something which was repeated in urban India. Another association is with migration, the ratio of GPI to tabes being considerably higher in the migrant populations of Asia than in the non-migrants. Since the discovery of penicillin treatment for syphilis, the picture has tended to be reversed, since the better-educated are now the more likely to have their primary lesion properly treated; and there has been a change in symptomatology as well. Formerly, grandiose delusions were a common feature of GPI; today they are quite rare, most probably because it was mainly the more educated patients who were exhibiting them (Dewhurst, 1969).

Drug psychoses and drug abuse

The psychoses due to drugs could have been included with the organic group above, but they may be placed more appropriately with the other pathological effects of the non-medical use of drugs.

Of the drugs so used, *alcohol* undoubtedly induces most pathology, although the nature of that pathology and the question of whether we should think in terms of a single disorder, 'alcoholism', or of several disorders remains unclear. The most constant feature of the epidemiology of alcohol abuse, regardless of its type, is the sex difference in consumption levels, and although it has been argued that this occurs because women are allowed freer expression of emotion than men, the universality of the finding suggests a biological basis. Probably the second most constant feature of alcohol abuse is its increase in populations or sections of populations which experience and resent a loss of power over their own lives, something which was observed in Britain during the Industrial Revolution (as illustrated in Hogarth's cartoons) and can still be seen in many native peoples who have been overrun by colonial powers and have not yet learnt either to exploit the intrusive culture or to re-establish a value system which can compete with it. This fact, among others, had led to the theory of excessive alcohol consumption being related to power needs (McClelland *et al.*, 1972); but this can be only a partial explanation since the Jews seem never to have resorted to alcohol when oppressed, and the notorious Irish alcoholism persists after better opportunities for self-determination have been reached overseas. In consequence, an alternative

theory has been proposed relating alcohol need to dependency conflicts, but this does not account for all the facts any more satisfactorily.

In some types of alcoholism, notably the Delta type (Jellinek, 1960), where the psychological effect is mainly a dependency and a dulling of faculties, incidence is quite closely related to mean level of consumption in the surrounding society and is also related to age. The pathology depends on a high daily consumption over a long period and that consumption tends to be related to, although higher than, the local norm. With the forms of alcoholism which are more often brought to the psychiatrist's attention, however, there need be no relationship with either the mean per capita consumption or age. Some types of alcohol abuse occur particularly in youths, and some types of alcohol abuser disregard completely the local drinking norms. It is here that one is most liable to find alcohol being used to mask some deeper disturbance, perhaps social as much as psychological. Thus, for instance, low status individuals may act out blatantly after only a few glasses and show no real signs of toxic damage when tested the next day, while a company director may prove on testing to be suffering from quite severe neurological damage from his heavy drinking and yet to have been showing very little behavioural abnormality. For this reason, the developmental sequence of alcoholic symptoms which Jellinek described should only be considered as an average picture, more applicable to middle than to lower SES groups and to Anglo-Saxons rather than to, say, Finns or Celts.

The incidence of *alcoholic psychoses* is linked to style of drinking, being commoner in subjects who deliberately drink to unconsciousness or have periods of abstinence after heavy drinking than in the regular, heavy drinkers who do not seek unconsciousness. These styles of drinking vary greatly with ethnic group but so, apparently, does susceptibility to certain types of alcoholic psychosis, independently of the drinking style. Thus until recently (the picture is changing) Japanese men used to indulge in episodes of very heavy drinking scattered among longer periods of virtual abstinence, but the incidence of psychosis from this behaviour was apparently much lower than it would have been in a Western society. Conversely, the Melanesians of New Caledonia are unusually susceptible to epileptiform fits after heavy drinking. It is not known how far such differences are biologically and how far culturally determined, and even the fact that Oriental peoples suffer from more skin-flushing with alcohol than Occidentals is not unquestionably of genetic rather than cultural origin.

Cannabis use results in two main types of mental disturbance: a semi-panic reaction in naive users and a chronic state approaching dementia in heavy, long-term users. The first is observed particularly among young Western smokers who are insufficiently prepared for what they will experience and who may project into the experience quite disturbing expectations and unconscious feelings, the same being true with hallucinogens such as *LSD* and *peyote*. The second has been reported mainly from North Africa, where the traditional form of hashish may have a different chemical composition from the forms used elsewhere. Dependency, as with alcohol, relates in part to duration of use and in part to the psychological characteristics of the user.

Factors which distinguish preferences for cannabis, alcohol, and opium when all these are available have been described by Carstairs (1954). Regarding *opium* and *heroin*, the most vulnerable section of a population is undoubtedly that which has a chronic, painful burden to bear, and which out of a sense of duty to self, family, or society is not prepared to rebel against that burden. Thus it was that the drug could get such a grip on the South Chinese labourer earlier in the century, and on the US soldier in Vietnam, a similar situation existing with respect to coca use in the Andes. Severing dependency on these drugs was once thought very difficult, but experience with returned soldiers from Vietnam (Robins, 1974) indicates a better prognosis, provided the burden is lifted and the basic personality not too weak. Stimulants such as *amphetamines* and *cocaine* (the latter functioning in contrary fashion to the coca from which it is derived) appeal not to the overburdened but to those who seek to achieve or at least experience more than the average, notably students, and the psychoses which can result from their use have a similar social focus. *Barbiturates,* which are often forgotten when drug abuse is discussed, sometimes appear to be the female's substitute for alcohol in developed societies, their use being much greater in women than in men and often high where alcoholism is rife. However, that substitution is inconstant and in Australia, where the prevalence of alcoholism is high, it has been analgesic powders to which women mainly turned in the past. There are a number of other drugs which are employed widely in particular cultures – betel, kava, khat, etc. – and which can produce either a psychosis or some degree of brain damage; but few psychiatrists encounter them.

The psychoneuroses

The true social distribution of the psychoneuroses is very difficult to assess. The phenomena of many neuroses are often purely subjective and unrevealed by behavioural abnormalities; many cases never come into care; and although it is easy to obtain self-reports of symptoms in community surveys (see below), there is no agreement on how far these reported symptoms should be thought of as indicating neuroses or not. Moreover, the same type of stress can produce quite different forms of neurosis in the same society, if certain conditions change. Thus, battle conditions during the American Civil War resulted in relatively numerous cases of a nostalgic depression; the same types of condition during the 1914–18 war, however, yielded hardly any with this character, since the condition would then have been thought close to 'malingering', and most neuroses assumed a somatic form, the commonest conditions being 'shell shock' and 'disordered action of the heart.' Anxiety neuroses replaced the latter during the second world war, thanks to a better understanding and a better orientation of officers and medical personnel. Their incidence at that time was high, whereas it was quite low in the American war in Vietnam even though the fighting was no less fierce. That drop was caused partly by assuring each soldier that he had only to sit out the situation for a limited time before he could return home, but also by the wide availability of illicit drugs to allay anxiety, widespread drug addiction functioning as a substitute for neurosis. Even when the data seem consistent and reliable, therefore, it may be difficult to generalise from them.

The most consistently observed association between the psychoneuroses and any social variable relates to education and/or SES. At the higher levels, the obsessive-compulsive, phobic, and neurasthenic neuroses are relatively common while at the lower levels it is the hysterias and mixed states which predominate, this being as true today, allowing for the improvement in public education, as it was when Freud visited Charcot, and as true in India as in Europe. In part these associations may arise from the types of care available, the poor finding it easiest to obtain attention when they present somatic or dramatic features; but they may also be related to the forms of internalization and ego defence which different levels of education promote. Probably the second most consistent social association of the neuroses, particularly the depressive neuroses, is to the female sex, whose rates are nearly always higher than those of males. Much has been made of this fact as indicating the disadvantaged status of women in human society, but the argument neglects the psychosomatic stress disorders and alcoholism, both of which show the opposite bias, and it is possible that what is represented here is a difference in choice of ego defence rather than a difference in the pathogenic stresses experienced.

Whether there is a stable relationship between neurosis and social class or status, other than that mentioned above in relation to education, is much debated, because of the conflicting results obtained by different methods. It is my impression that there is no essential relationship here, but that the commonest picture is a U-shaped curve, frequency being least in the skilled blue-collar group. Other social factors which have been scrutinized with respect to incidence of neurosis are residential density and location, e.g. suburban, city tenement, new town; but here also the findings are mixed, and the most probable general conclusion is that these factors are also not directly relevant to the neuroses, even though enforced crowding or enforced isolation, as in a prison, may produce the latter. Undoubtedly, a subjective sense of isolation is frequently associated with the neuroses, particularly of the anxiety or depressive type, but objective measures of relative isolation have yielded mixed results. Thus, immigrants who are pursuing a chosen plan tend not to show any such pathology even though they may have relatively few social contacts, whereas those who have migrated without any clear plan (including quite often the wives of the former group) may show excess pathology. 'Tropical neurasthenia' was at one time a remarkably frequent disorder among Europeans and North Americans who had gone to tropical countries to take up high-status positions and who had not foreseen the problems of adjusting to the majority population there; by contrast, the condition was virtually unknown in Queensland, Australia, with a comparable climate, since there was no aboriginal majority and most immigrants did not expect to receive a high social status.

Social crises, as at the start of a war, often result in a drop in the number of reported neuroses, with the lower rate continuing as long as the public is given clear and simple priorities, such as defeating the enemy or keeping alive. However, if leadership is lacking or if a crisis brings with it a conflict of goals or loyalties, as when people who consider themselves loyal citizens are treated as potential traitors by their own government, then the incidence of reported neurosis may rise significantly, just as it tends to do when such a crisis is over and people have to readapt to the complex relationships of an everyday life which has changed in the meantime. Returned prisoners-of-war often have poor mental health for this reason, as do survivors of some civilian disasters, and one of the results may be an increased mortality, as happened after the 1968 Bristol floods. Chronic occupational stress, with or without the threat to life, increases the risk of neurosis, but so does work requiring a skill inappropriate to the worker's intelligence, or providing too little scope for initiative, or being too monotonous, as has been repeatedly reaffirmed since Russell Fraser's (1947) classic work on this subject.

Culture, as one might expect, has a strong influence on the symptomatology of the neuroses, and it might be said that every culture stamps its own imprint on the clinical picture, whether we assign shared or separate labels to what results. Between neighbouring mainstream European populations speaking the same language, such as the Bavarians and the German-Swiss, differences in the average clinical pictures can be found once psychiatrists start looking for them, and even so-called 'culture-bound' neuroses may be found there, as in the case of *Putzwut* (cleaning madness) described among the German-Swiss. However, for an easy example of cultural variation it is better to go further afield, for instance to Japan, whose psychiatrists have paid special attention to the ways in which the local neuroses differ from what is described in Western textbooks.

The most specifically Japanese neurosis is that called *shinkeishitsu*. Although assuming a number of forms – obsessional, hypochondriac, neurasthenic – its basic characteristics are an egocentric oversensitivity towards one's mental and somatic processes, and a sensitivity also respecting the image which one achieves in the eyes of others. Other neuroses which are considerably commoner among the Japanese than among other peoples are a range of phobias – fear of blushing, of smelling offensively, of coming in contact with sickness and, most importantly, fear of looking another person in the eyes – which are usually grouped under the term anthropophobia. It has been suggested that the specifically Japanese features in the patients with these disorders stem from a disturbance in a type of dependency relationship which Western styles of child-rearing do not encourage but which Japanese do, this type of relationship conducing to pathological feelings of shame rather than to pathological feelings of guilt so that the symptomatology of depression in Japan also differs from that in the West, even when self-accusations are present (Lebra & Lebra, 1974).

Shinkeishitsu and the Japanese anthropophobias can be chronic, but the majority of other culture-linked neuroses are typically of brief duration, often acute attacks of anxiety or hysteria which disappear within hours or days but which occasionally deteriorate rapidly, threatening death. Thus, Eskimos have acute anxiety attacks while at sea in their small kayaks, whence the name *'kayak Angst'*, even though the water be calm and the shore within sight; but recovery occurs within a day or less and the individual is unlikely to have another attack for a long time. The Chinese and some other Asian groups get acute attacks of fear lest the penis (very occasionally the clitoris) shrink into the abdomen and death result, the condition usually going by the name *koro* or *shook yong*, but these episodes likewise last only hours or days. However, if the anxiety arises from the belief that one has been bewitched or cursed, and if traditional countermeasures either fail or are unavailable, then 'malignant anxiety' (Lambo, 1962) may develop and may even lead to death ('Voodoo death') without adequate somatic cause. The latter has been described from many parts of the world, with the patient having sometimes predicted the day of his death. In some alleged instances there is good reason to think that the psychological aspect was irrelevant, but tropical physicians and anthropologists have reported too many others in which fear and despair were the major or the only detectable factors.

'Psychosomatic' illness

It is a familiar observation that mental and somatic illnesses, particularly cardiovascular, tend to cluster in the same individuals and that the gravity of any somatic illness tends to increase when a mental disturbance, particularly depression, is also present. Moreover, even where a socio-cultural variation in the distribution of an illness has a clearly physical basis, there is often a psychosocial factor affecting exposure to that physical element, as for instance in lung cancer, where tobacco smoke is the key organic factor but where the use of tobacco by some individ-

uals and not others is psychosocial. Here, attention will only be given to those conditions with which the psychiatrist is most likely to be implicated, but the wider picture must not be forgotten.

Hypertension is probably the condition in which socio-cultural variation has been most frequently reported, but there are many apparent contradictions in the results (Scotch & Geiger, 1962). Thus, urban blood-pressure levels are higher than rural ones in South African Blacks, but the reverse is true among Germans; reports from Russia and Czechoslovakia indicate considerably higher rates in administrators than in labourers, whereas in the USA it is those with the lowest SES who have the highest levels. Also, where theory would lead one to expect a difference there may be none, as between the Fijians and the Indians of Fiji, the former being apparently much more relaxed than the latter. Viewing such results, some physicians have argued that psychosocial factors in the disease must be unimportant; but this is to take too simple a theoretical position. In one society, rural life may be more strenuous or anxiety-provoking than urban, and in another the reverse may be true. In one ethnic group there may be much more obesity than in another, something which is relevant to the Fijian situation, and the psychosocial variation may only become apparent after comparison with groups of similar body weight. It seems broadly true that populations which feel themselves frustrated have more hypertension than those that do not, but this concept needs to be refined and allowance has also to be made for different styles of reacting to such frustration.

Coronary heart disease (CHD) is another disorder in which organic factors – diet, smoking, exercise – have been shown to play an important role and in which, consequently, it has been argued that the psychosocial elements are unimportant. However, it can also be argued that the former do not sufficiently account for the reported variance. Thus, the extreme concentration of angina pectoris in (mainly upper class) males during the nineteenth century in Britain seems linked to smoking, but the rise in female cases to reach 40 percent by 1950 is not adequately explained by such a linkage. The relative immunity of Japanese males to CHD was initially attributed to genetic or dietary factors, but extensive studies among Japanese-Americans suggest that these and other organic factors do not account for the variance, psychocultural factors thus remaining implicated (Marmot & Syme, 1976). What the psychiatrist needs before he can use socio-cultural variations to guide his interventions in this disorder are more studies such as that just cited; but he should not abandon his right to be involved in CHD prevention, both at the individual and at the mass level, even if the theories at his disposal here are incomplete.

Peptic ulcer is a condition in which sex differences have been marked but changeable, and where ethnic differences are also great. Gastric ulcer was relatively common in women but uncommon in men in the nineteenth century, while duodenal ulcer became much more frequent in men than in women during the first half of the present century (Wastrell, 1972). Gastric ulcer tends to increase inversely with SES whereas duodenal ulcer shows the opposite trend and is virtually unknown in many rural populations. Japanese and Chinese have relatively high rates of peptic, notably duodenal, ulcer, whereas Malaysians have strikingly low ones, and although genetic factors have obviously to be considered here, the two former groups do develop among their males the traits which resemble those hypothesized by Alexander and other psycho-analysts as belonging to the 'peptic ulcer personality', whereas the Malaysian modal personality is very different.

Anorexia nervosa was formerly almost always confined to the upper SES, but since World War II it is apparently both increasing in frequency in Western societies and becoming more widely distributed. In the nineteenth century, some of its features could be found in the more frequently diagnosed 'chlorosis'. Subsaharan Africa and many other underdeveloped regions of the world scarcely know it, but it is recognized in Japan. One is tempted to say that it does not occur where the symbolic meanings of food and eating are greatly overshadowed by their primary meaning. The age and sex distribution of this disease are too well-known to need comment. *Ulcerative colitis* is another condition which has been alleged to occur mainly in persons of high SES, but in this case the data are much less unanimous, and there is also doubt regarding the consistency of the sex and age distributions. The one feature which does stand out, at least in US studies, is the disproportionate presence of persons of the Jewish religion. *Asthma* also affects Jews disproportionately, at least in the Western Hemisphere, but there are so many forms of this condition that the data can appear contradictory unless one distinguishes between them. Thus, in Singapore, asthma in children occurs disproportionately among the Malays, perhaps because they are disproportionately exposed to plant aller-

gens but more probably because they experience a greater (unwelcome) change from home to school than indigenous children of the other ethnic groups. In adult life, however, it is not the Malays who show the excess of asthma, but the local Indians, the women having a hospitalization rate for this condition which is over ten times that of the other ethnic groups, a finding which may be linked to the fact that they tend to feel more (repressed) anger and resentment against their assigned roles than the women of the other ethnic groups. The 1960s saw a sharp rise in the mortality from asthma in several Western countries, but it was probably due to organic causes.

Sociopathic and other borderline conditions

Analogous to the 'psychosomatic' diseases are certain psychosocial disturbances, not primarily psychiatric in character, and hence not to be routinely taken into psychiatric charge, but benefiting from judicious psychiatric intervention. *Delinquency*, both juvenile and adult, is the most obvious of these. In homogeneous societies it derives mainly from families of low SES and unstable structure, in which a parent has had a criminal record (Rutter & Madge, 1976). However, low SES alone may not be a consistent correlate if the society is made up of many subcultures, and a parent's criminal record may also not be prognostically useful if there exists a cultural minority which does not accept the majority's laws. An obvious, underlying factor in this matter is the extent to which persons outside the nuclear family assist in the upbringing and informal education of the offspring; another less obvious factor is the degree to which the paternal role facilitates or exacerbates the resolution of Oedipal conflicts. Jewish and Chinese minorities have in the past been examples of groups where the nuclear family was supervised and assisted; family traditions in the Singapore Indian, urban US Negro and rural Polish societies are among those in which Oedipal conflicts seem to be exacerbated. Adverse prognostic indicators in low SES subjects tend to be different from those in higher SES groups, an 'affectionless character', laziness, and drinking being important for the latter.

Psychopathy, theoretically something quite distinct from delinquency and hence probably having a different social distribution, is unfortunately not as easy to distinguish in practice, so that most statements about its social distribution are based on delinquency statistics and hence are untrustworthy. However, if one's theory concerning this mental state links it to the extreme forms of *narcissism*, then there may be some relevance in the findings of those anthropological studies which link this phenomenon to situations where cultural traditions interfere most radically with the husband-wife bond (Slater & Slater, 1965) and hence produce maternal ambivalence. Such interference occurred most blatantly during the slave-owning period in the Western Hemisphere, but it could be said to persist for US Blacks today, thanks to the giving of more generous welfare support to mothers having no admitted male partners than to mothers who admit to having one. The same mechanism has been attributed in lesser degree to ancient Greece and modern India.

A wholly different condition with psychiatric implications is religious *possession*. The mental mechanism operating in possession is a dissociation comparable to that which occurs in cases of multiple personality, and which psychiatrists are accustomed to regard as pathological. However, under socially controlled conditions, which are found in very many societies (Bourguignon, 1973), it is a form of ego defence or support, no more and no less pathological than the distortion of mental states by alcohol or other drugs. By its means, repressed feelings are allowed time-limited expression, and since all socially-approved possession states take place before an audience, usually under the guidance of an experienced person, they serve as a means of communication, giving warning of otherwise hidden tensions and making ego control at other times easier. In Western Europe, where rationalism both within and outside of religion has almost entirely abolished the social settings in which such controlled dissociation can take place, persons exhibiting a possession syndrome should usually be treated as patients; elsewhere, however, the psychiatrist may be of less assistance in such cases than religious leaders and traditional healers. Sometimes, in religions which encourage such dissociation, the leaders (shamans) may be preferentially appointed from among persons who have gone through a type of transient psychosis, perhaps drug-induced; but that does not necessarily prevent their influence from being beneficial and it can demand delicate judgement from the psychiatrist to decide to intervene or not.

Societies in which possession states are commonest are usually those which encourage auto-suggestion or hetero-suggestion. In a small number of such societies there occur states which deserve to be regarded as pathological but are not usually seri-

ous and do not fit comfortably within our category of the neuroses. These are the *latah-type disorders*, whose main symptoms are an excessive susceptibility to being startled, the involuntary expression of socially-disapproved acts or words while in the startle state, with perhaps some echolalia and echopraxia; the resulting clinical picture can therefore be quite similar to that of Gilles de la Tourette's syndrome, although no organic features are present (Murphy, 1976). Today they occur mainly in middle-aged women, but usually no treatment is sought and their interest is mainly theoretical.

General mental health ratings

Social conditions which are associated with a high morbidity for one mental disorder may both in theory and practice be associated with low rates for some others. However, it is both more simple and more satisfying if one can conceive of social conditions which are associated with unduly high or unduly low rates of mental disturbance in general, and there have been many attempts to identify and study these. Such attempts encounter great difficulties of method and interpretation e.g. deciding whether a transient neurosis should receive the same quantitative weight as a chronic schizophrenia. In the first half of this century such studies tended to focus on cases needing hospitalization, ignoring the lesser disorders, while in the third quarter it is the major disorders which tended to be forgotten, symptoms reported by persons living in normal households being then emphasized and diagnosis being by-passed. Despite their weaknesses, however, surveys yield interesting and instructive information.

A first generalisation is that extreme physical deprivation seriously harms mental health in time, a point which might seem obvious but which needs to be made, since lesser degrees of deprivation can apparently improve mental health, through suppressing all but the most basic needs. The key work here is that of John Cawte (1972) among Australian aborigines, but the same impression is given by anthropological studies of marginally surviving tribes elsewhere.

A second generalisation concerns the adverse effect of city as opposed to country life on the mental health of *children*, this being most systematically recorded in Britain (Rutter *et al.*, 1975) but also noted more impressionistically in Africa and elsewhere. A third point concerns social organization, the total amount of mental disturbance being higher in a community which is disorganized than in one which is more organized, and the level of mental health improving as social organization improves. As noted earlier in respect of schizophrenia, this is not a uniform relationship, and some types of mental disturbance can increase with increased social organization (few societies are more fully organized than that of a prison). In general, however, the finding has been supported.

In community surveys employing symptom-check-lists, women nearly always report more symptoms than men, and the lower SES's more than the upper ones, exceptions being among persons on welfare relief, where males can score as highly as females, and in some rural populations where the less educated may be uncommunicative. It goes almost wihout saying that persons who have grown up in broken homes have, on average, poorer mental health ratings than those who have not, and that those whose adult social history has shown instability through multiple work changes, divorces, etc. do the same. People who remember their parents as being either strongly religious or non-religious generally receive poorer ratings than those reporting their parents to be moderately religious, and those on whom major social changes have been imposed – for instance by the closing of a town's only factory, or the flooding of tribal land for a dam – show poorer average mental health than neighbouring people whose lives have not been so disturbed.

Theories of social influence

No one theory can account for all the variations to which this chapter has referred or even, probably, for the variations affecting a single disorder. Guides on sources of excessive rates and abnormal features are still desirable, however, and even if our theories are inadequate they still deserve attention.

Social selection and social disadvantage were the two main competing theories used to explain socio-cultural variation in the nineteenth century. The excess vulnerability of the poor, of immigrants, and of the unmarried was explained on the one hand by their mental weaknesses having led them into these situations (some migrations were thought 'of poor human stock') and on the other hand by these situations having been loaded with too great difficulties and by those affected being given too little support. Both ideas carry some truth but there are large bodies of data which neither can alone explain. Psychoanalysis, drawing its patients from the more privileged strata, could not easily blame either disadvantagement or genetic weakness and turned instead to the mistakes made by parents as an explanation, this idea being extended even to schizophrenia through the 'double-bind' and related theories; but only a little of the social variance has ever been explained on this basis. Hans Selye's theory of adaptation strains and most recently the concept of 'learned helplessness' deriving from conditioning theory have each claimed to account for a certain amount of psychopathology, but that amount seems very small.

To imagine how these different, hypothesized, influences can combine in particular patients or populations one may remember that, like all organs or systems, the mind is most likely to become disordered when it is given work beyond its capacity. The capacity is determined in part by genetic inheritance and in part by training, including the damage done by faulty training, as in the case of an athlete's muscles. The work to be tackled is determined in part by the external material on which it must operate, but still more by what it is desired to extract from that material, i.e. by what are considered as needs. Some of these needs are innate, but in larger degree for most people they are learnt, and as primary needs are satisfied it is customary for people to create new and more complex ones for themselves. This is basically what was meant by another nineteenth century theory to the effect that mental disorder is part of the price which we have to pay for the benefits of civilization. In assessing any social setting or group, the psychiatrist would do well to ask himself first: what do these people want of themselves; and then ask how far their mental capacities are liable to be overstrained in trying to satisfy these wants, given the realities around them. Relief may be achieved by changing circumstances, but it may also be effected by simplifying needs.

6
Medico-legal aspects

T. C. N. GIBBENS

The criminal law of most English-speaking nations, in so far as it incorporates the 'common law', is largely based on ancient custom refined by successive judicial decisions. It incorporates the principle of *mens rea* which establishes that to be guilty of crime a person must not only have done the act prohibited (*actus reus*) but have the mental accompaniment of knowing that it is illegal. It tends to secure much more sensitive justice, and the principle is continually upheld and even extended. There are, however, offences of 'strict liability', often referring to new offences, which do not require *mens rea* but only that the act should be voluntary. If a person drives at night without lights he is responsible, even if he did not know that they had fused or were broken. Even if a person falls asleep, he is responsible; he should have stopped at the first sign of drowsiness.

The same emphasis upon *mens rea* occurs in the McNaughton rules which still remain the test of legal insanity or irresponsibility as a result of mental disorder in England. This provides that the offender, through defect of reason due to disease of the mind, did not know what he was doing or that what he was doing was wrong. It was only quite recently that Lord Goddard ruled that 'wrong' meant merely illegal (and not sometimes morally wrong). The new version of the test of responsibility to replace the McNaughton rules suggested by the Butler Committee (1975) is still that the patient did not 'know . . . and also suffered from mental illness or severe subnormality' (but not psychopathic disorder or subnormality). Any consideration of psychopathology in relation to criminal law calls for discussion of the controversy which surrounds the problem of consciousness.

Amnesia

Amnesia for a crime raises the question of consciousness of wrongdoing. The processes of memory used to be divided into perception, registration, retention, and recall or recognition, but Whitty (1978) maintains that 'to assign memory loss to one part of it is often difficult' and he prefers merely to say that it is due to inability to recall past experiences and record recent experiences for recall. 'What emerges from experimental and clinical studies is the complexity of memory mechanisms and their defects. Not only must some loss of memory be regarded as normal, but some distortion or alteration of all memories must be accepted. Psychologically, the effect of emotion in distorting, repressing, or even maintaining memories in a selective fashion is pervasive.' Recently it has been shown that one of the legitimate uses of hypnosis or brief narcosis is to demonstrate that a great many more memories are recorded than are ordinarily available, e.g. that witnesses of a crime carried out publicly can be persuaded to remember details and give identifiable descriptions of other people in the street at the time that have enabled the police to trace them. In relation to offenders, therefore, the traditional decisions about whether an amnesia is organic, or due to hysteria, or to lying or malingering, are much less important or clear cut than they used to be. They rarely affect the issue before the court concerning whether 'he knew what he was doing at the time'.

The scepticism and caution with which claims of amnesia for the crime by offenders are regarded need not disguise the fact that in most cases the amnesia 'protects' the offender's mental health or balance just as genuinely as it does that of honest and truthful non-offenders. Amnesia frequently protects individuals from unbearable memories, especially in war-time when, for example, it may shield a professional soldier from an intolerable memory of running away in battle (and if recovered under hypnosis may drive him into a state of acute depression). Conversion symptoms, e.g. blindness, paralysis, are also fairly frequent.

In offenders, logically planned behaviour before and after the crime, variable accounts of the duration of amnesia, and absence of any organic or other pathological signs usually make the situation clear. O'Connell (1960) has reviewed the extent of amnesia in 50 murderers. Forty per cent had either no memory or the haziest recollection of the crime. Those affected tended to have low intelligence, immature or histrionic personalities, and there were precipitating factors in the crime which would cloud or restrict attention, such as alcoholic intoxication, extreme sexual excitement, or rage. Sadistic impulses are normally so heavily repressed that it seems doubtful whether the recollection of sadistic emotion is tolerable except in a very few cases.

Nevertheless, genuine amnesia may be concealed by false recollections as a result of hearing frequent accounts of events, and amnesia from an organic noxa like a head injury may be prolonged by psychogenic factors. Podola was arrested for an armed robbery, but managed to escape after fatally shooting the arresting policeman. Four days later he was arrested in a violent struggle with the police in which he was knocked out. On coming round he claimed to remember nothing either of recent events or the whole of his past life. The defence claimed that he was unfit to plead because he did not have access to any information which would help his defence; but the Appeal Court concluded that since it was quite legal for an offender to be convicted, although he is unable to trace the witness who could allegedly exonerate him, Podola could stand trial although he had lost the witness of his own recollection.

Automatism

The use of the word probably derives from post-epileptic automatism, but refers in Lord Goddard's words to 'someone performing acts in a state of unconsciousness'. It has assumed considerable legal importance.

Automatism can affect responsibility in normal circumstances e.g. the motorcyclist who, losing control when a bee gets inside his helmet, consequently runs over somebody. It can, however, arise in such conditions as epileptic (especially temporal lobe) states, in hypoglycaemic attacks, sleepwalking, and arteriosclerotic states of confusion.

It is rare for post-ictal automatism to be the cause of serious crime – though Gunn (1978b) has reported a recent case – and in the past it was too easily accepted as justifying a verdict of guilty but insane. However, hypoglycaemic attacks are well attested. A diabetic clergyman, for example, took his usual dose of insulin but forgot to have breakfast before taking early Communion; in the vestry he became confused and seriously assaulted his verger without any motive. There have been several reported cases of causing death in a nightmare, and of committing an assault while sleepwalking and, especially, on being awakened suddenly.

A further type of disability was described in an early and dramatic case of matricide by Hill, Sargant, and Heppenstall (1943). A young man, after drinking a few pints of beer, had a verbal argument with his mother and killed her for most inadequate reasons. It was shown that his EEG was normal except at fasting blood sugar levels, but when he was given equivalent quantities of beer and made to overbreathe, as he would have done in an argument, the EEG became pathologically abnormal and he was seen to become mentally confused. This was in the days of the death penalty, and the offender was found not guilty by reason of insanity. The condition relates to the hyperventilation syndrome of Pincus (1978) in which marked psychosomatic and mental symptoms with confusion occur when anxiety induces overbreathing.

The legal issue, which has undergone considerable evolution, is that if a person acts involuntarily he cannot be guilty of crime and is entitled to be acquitted and set free. If, however, his act is due to a pathological condition affecting his mind, then the proper verdict is not guilty by reason of insanity, entailing indefinite detention. Under what circumstances should one be entitled to be acquitted and set free? In Charlson (1955), an arteriosclerotic man in a state of confusion had attacked his small son, to whom he was devoted, with a mallet and pushed him out of the window into the river. He was acquitted. In Kemp (1956) however, where an elderly arteriosclerotic irrationally attacked his wife with a hammer during the night, the judge ruled (1) that disease of the mind in the McNaughton Rules includes clinical disorder of the brain and not only any form of psychosis; and (2) that in arranging his defence Counsel had raised the issue of a verdict of not guilty but insane, which would result in detention. As Lord Denning observed later: 'any mental disorder which has manifested itself in violence and is prone to recur, is a disease of the mind'.

The issue appeared to be settled by the case of Bratty (1961) who killed a girl he had taken for a ride in his car. He said that an attack of blackness came over him and he did not know what he was doing.

He claimed to have had previous attacks of a similar nature. He was dull, suffered from headaches, entertained religious preoccupations, and showed odd behaviour. The possibility of psychomotor epilepsy was raised on very inadequate evidence. The jury was invited to bring in a verdict of automatism, or manslaughter, or guilty but insane. The judge withdrew the verdict of automatism from the jury and the accused was found guilty of murder. The appeal reached the House of Lords which ruled that there were two types of automatism, sane and insane. The verdict of automatism could be left to the jury only if the judge ruled that, in his opinion, there was positive evidence to support it; otherwise the verdict must be either not guilty or guilty but insane.

This procedure was subsequently used in the case of a sleepwalker called Harvey. He had been out of work for some time and learnt one night that his family was to be evicted the next day for non-payment of rent. He went to bed in great anxiety as to how he was going to break the news to his wife, with whom he was on good terms. He woke in the early hours to the sound of screaming, and found himself at his wife's bedside; on putting on the light he found that he had blood on his hands and a hammer in his hand, with which he had beaten his wife in the face. His statement that he could remember nothing never varied, and his wife never doubted that he was sleepwalking. The medical evidence was to the effect that there was no indication of epilepsy or suggestion of malingering and that what had occurred was sleepwalking, which was unlikely to recur. The judge instructed the jury that they could acquit the accused if they shared that opinion; this they did.

The procedure seemed settled until the case of Quick (1973), a mental nurse who claimed that when he assaulted a patient in hospital he was suffering from diabetic hypoglycaemia. The judge ruled that the proper course of action was to invite the jury to bring in a verdict of insanity, whereupon Quick pleaded guilty to one of the two charges. On appeal, Lord Justice Lawton reviewed the history of automatism and considered that difficult borderline cases should be resolved by asking whether the mental condition could fairly be called a disease of the mind. In Quick's case the mental malfunctioning was deemed to be due to an external cause, the using of the insulin prescribed by his doctor, and not to a bodily disorder constituting a disease. The jury, it was concluded, should have been allowed to consider automatism; in doing so, however, they would have needed to consider a number of other factors, such as Quick's consumption of alcohol, his neglect of the doctor's instructions about regular meals, and whether he had had advance warning of the onset of hypoglycaemia. The judge's comment on the particular circumstances raised the question of whether a defence of automatism might be called into question if the accused had in some respects contributed to it himself.

In a post-concussive or post-epileptic state of automatism an individual may behave for some time as usual: a concussed footballer may get up and play on vigorously before recovering consciousness some moments later, the epileptic may button or unbutton his clothes or tie his shoelaces. Some neurologists maintain that the only real evidence of consciousness is a person's capacity to remember. The question arises whether habitual criminal behaviour can be included in such habitual automatic behaviour. For example, a man aged 30 with 13 previous convictions for housebreaking had a head injury at 9 years and at 15 developed jerkings of the arm and cramps in the right leg which occasionally spread to become fully-developed epileptic fits. He claimed that the jerking of his arm was so embarrassing that he took to going out only at night and came to live by burglary. On his last offence he had no recollection of the evening until awakened 'by a policeman, sitting on the steps of the house he had just burgled'. He knew 'something was wrong' because, he claimed, apart from the amnesia, he had burgled the house before (this was very unusual), he was in his best clothes, and had no gloves or housebreaking equipment; none the less, he pleaded guilty 'to save time'. In prison he mentioned his perplexity to the medical officer and was referred for a psychiatric opinion. Neurosurgery was recommended, and at operation a scar was excised from the superior margin of the left cerebral hemisphere. The fits ceased apart from a single convulsion five years later, which was associated with excessive drinking. Even more remarkably, his criminal behaviour also ceased. Ten years later his criminal record revealed only one offence, that of deserting ship in Australia after he had become a cook in the Merchant Service.

Alcohol and other drugs

Here there are many problems in common with automatism and amnesia, and some which seem less satisfactorily resolved at present. At times alcoholism is a mitigating factor and at other times, in persistently aggressive individuals, an aggravating one

which greatly increases the offender's potential dangerousness. When severe, as in delirium tremens, alcoholism may lead to a psychotic state within the framework of the McNaughton Rules. It is only a defence against a criminal charge if it is of such a degree as to render the accused incapable of forming the intent required by law. The ordinary person is assumed to know what effect alcohol is likely to have, and the man taking insulin should know the consequences of not following regular eating habits. Between these two extremes, however, there are conditions in which alcohol, either by causing liver damage or leading to dietary deficiency, upsets carbohydrate metabolism and causes neurological disability affecting behaviour.

By way of an example, an Irish labourer of law-abiding character lived largely on whisky, with only occasional ham rolls as food. He lived in a rooming-house with an elderly landlady who took a maternal interest in him, washing his clothes and cutting his hair. One evening he returned home drunk, bringing a half-bottle of whisky, with which he drank himself to sleep in the chair. He awoke next morning to find that the landlady had been brutally battered to death. No one could have entered the house, and forensic evidence showed that he was responsible. He wandered the streets for some hours with no memory of the night's events, but gradually concluded that he would be blamed and gave himself up to the police. Investigations showed that his resting blood-sugar level was so low that it would have produced faintness and disturbance of consciousness in a normal man; these he had not experienced. The blood-sugar curve rose normally to low normal levels and then sank to abnormally low levels. He was found guilty of manslaughter and sentenced to seven years' imprisonment.

Similar situations arise in the case of drugs. Many people are familiar with the effects of hallucinating drugs from personal experience and by parallel reasoning can be held responsible for the consequences of taking them. The effects of new drugs, however, are uncertain. Lipman (1969), an American who came to England largely because he could obtain LSD more easily, was given a large tablet of an 'extra strong' hallucinogen which might have been STP or one of the various derivatives. He gave half to himself and half to his girl friend and after drinking a certain amount they retired to bed. He had hallucinations of flying to the stratosphere and then plunging to the centre of the earth, where he wrestled with snakes. Next morning he awoke to find the girl dead, he having fractured her skull with a heavy tumbler and asphyxiated her by stuffing the counterpane down her throat. He was charged with murder but convicted (on a majority verdict) of manslaughter, sentenced to seven years' imprisonment, and ordered to be deported. This was upheld on appeal on the grounds that there is no reason in law to distinguish between the effects of drugs voluntarily taken and drunkenness voluntarily induced. The crime of manslaughter does not require the formation of an intention to kill or do grievous bodily harm; it includes any unlawful behaviour which a sober or responsible person would recognize as involving a risk of death.

In the case of driving offences, where the same issue is often raised, magistrates have sometimes dismissed cases where a driver has been affected by drugs whose effects he could not anticipate but were prescribed by a doctor, on the basis that the driver was 'not driving'. Unconsciousness coming on insidiously as a result of carbon monoxide poisoning has been accepted as a defence. In *Watmore* v. *Jenkins* (1962) a driver, who had given himself a higher dosage of insulin than usual because of the effects of infective hepatitis, drove erratically for some time and collided with a stationary car. He was found in a dazed condition and claimed that he had no memory for the last five miles or so. The magistrates acquitted him of dangerous driving and of driving under the influence of drugs; on appeal against this decision, however, a plea of automatism was accepted only as a defence to a charge of being under the influence of drugs, and not as a defence to the charge of dangerous driving and driving without due care and attention. The court held that the evidence that the accused had driven some miles and shown some degree of control was incompatible with automatism.

In practice, many difficulties arise in assessing the effects of alcohol in combination with other drugs. When mandrax and alcohol were taken together, the combination was particularly liable to produce explosive violence; and several murders and crimes of violence occurred before mandrax was taken off the market.

Violence

Violence is a feature of a large number of psychopathological conditions, from functional psychosis (affective and schizophrenic) and organic psychosis to non-psychotic conditions connected with head injury and other forms of brain damage or deterioration.

Homicide

Homicide (murder, manslaughter, and infanticide) is the most important form of violence and receives much publicity. It tends to set the pace of public opinion concerning the nature of all forms of violence, though its relationship with mental abnormality is probably exceptional.

The frequency of homicide in different societies varies very widely according to social tradition and culture, and tends to vary inversely with the frequency of suicide. To a surprising extent it varies also with climatic temperature, the homicide rate rising sharply as one nears the equator. The rate in the northern European countries, including England and especially Scandinavia, is exceptionally low and the suicide rate high. The exceptions to the tendency – USA, Finland, and to some extent Scotland – are partly due to social habits of carrying weapons which are predominantly guns in the USA and knives elsewhere. Homicide in New York is 16 times higher than in London.

In many parts of the world homicide is considered laudable and necessary in certain circumstances, much as the Western world accepts homicide in war. For example, in some Moslem countries an adulterous wife or a girl who loses her virginity before marriage must be killed traditionally.

When homicide is rare but suicide frequent, as in England, it tends to involve extreme mental states, including psychosis. In England the special Mental Health Law, passed during the days of the death penalty as a result of the Royal Commission on Capital Punishment, (1953) represents an attempt to resolve the protest about the ineffectiveness of the McNaughton Rules in exempting mentally disordered murderers. Under the Homicide Act of 1957, a person accused of murder can be convicted of manslaughter with diminished responsibility if he suffers from a 'mental abnormality which substantially diminished his mental responsibility'. Although this leaves many doubts about what the terms 'mental responsibility' or 'substantial' mean, these were much easier questions for doctors to answer than McNaughton's questions. 'Diminished responsibility' has rapidly replaced the McNaughton Rules which are now used in only a handful of cases a year, and these not always in relation to homicide. If responsibility is diminished, the offender is found guilty of manslaughter, which allows the judge to pass any sentence from probation to life imprisonment. As already stated, manslaughter does not have the specific intent of murder, which is with malice aforethought to kill or do grievous bodily harm. If convicted of murder, an offender is compulsorily sentenced to life imprisonment. The issue of whether the accused had diminished responsibility under the Act is left to the jury; the judge's function is not to direct the jury, but to explain the law. Legally it has always been the case that the jury can reach a decision and under the McNaughton Rules, with or without medical evidence.

In 1967 the death penalty was abolished in England and much of the justification for the Homicide Act disappeared. The Butler Committee on the law in relation to mental abnormality (1975) even suggested that there would be no objection to replacing the distinction between murder and manslaughter by one offence, that of homicide, the sentence for which would rest with the judge after he had heard any medical evidence as to whether a hospital order, with or without restriction of discharge, was appropriate. At the same time the Committee realized that murder and manslaughter were hallowed words in popular imagination, carrying a different sort of stigma, especially for the relatively minor forms of manslaughter.

In 1978 in England and Wales though 500 cases of suspected homicide were recorded by the police (10 per million of population), many turned out to be accidents, suicides, lesser offences, or unsolved events. A large proportion of the unsolved cases refer to children under the age of one year. Infanticide in England, unlike the USA, is a separate offence in which the mother's responsibility for causing death in the first year of life is diminished if the balance of the mind was disturbed as a result of not having recovered from the effects of childbirth. The age criterion has always been the dominating one, the great majority of such cases occurring in the first three months of the child's life. Most infanticidal mothers show no psychiatric evidence of abnormality, except for a disinclination to bear the child, for whom none of the ordinary preparations are made; sometimes even an awareness of pregnancy is repressed. Mothers who later batter or kill their children often have very underweight babies; it is as if rejection occurs from conception and leads to suppression of the psychophysical maternalization processes, below the level of detectable psychopathology. By contrast, child homicide that is due to a clear-cut puerperal psychosis is uncommon but usually occurs after the first three months of the child's life; as a consequence of maternal depression it may occur any time until the child is capable of taking evasive action.

Infanticide as a charge is nowadays virtually obsolete in England since the crime is fully covered by the Homicide Act. Only about 8 cases a year are convicted and all are put on probation or enter a hospital under a condition of probation or a hospital order.

The psychopathology of child killing is exceptionally complex. Intelligent and educated couples with much marital disharmony may become reconciled by what appears to be a process of making the child a scapegoat for their problems, and often deny responsibility for murder in the most convincing way (Gibbens, 1972). Thus, a middle-aged woman, cheerful and apparently unconcerned about her situation but certainly not psychotic, admitted to pushing her baby out of a window on to a concrete pavement many feet below. Two other children had died, one when a baby by accidentally falling into a bath of boiling water prepared for the washing; and the second, some years old, by falling in an outhouse so that the stick of a toy propeller had driven down its throat and it had allegedly been found dead. She admitted to being only 'occasionally bad-tempered'. In some developing countries, it may be recalled, maternal rejection appears to be almost unknown but an imperfect child is traditionally left at birth to die of exposure in some recognized place.

In England in 1978 355 persons were convicted and sentenced for homicide 44 per cent being convicted of ordinary manslaughter. Of the remaining 188 the conviction and sentence were for murder in 59 per cent, but in 41 per cent were for murder reduced to manslaughter with diminished responsibility. However, if the 30 persons not brought to court because they committed suicide immediately after the homicide are included, 55 per cent were mentally abnormal. Among those persons whose charges were reduced to manslaughter the majority were sentenced to shorter forms of imprisonment, and only 11 per cent were sent to hospital under a hospital order with or without restriction. Many murderers convicted of manslaughter are therefore not psychotic, but suffer from such conditions as morbid depression, serious subnormality, or senility. The judge retains the option of imposing a life sentence, as he would for murder. Among the cases of diminished manslaughter, however, over half had no previous convictions and a quarter had previous convictions including offences of violence. Among convicted murderers, on the other hand, less than a quarter had no previous convictions, and 40 per cent had previous convictions which included violent offences. Organic defects frequently play an important part in homicide and lesser crimes of violence, such as those committed by the persistently aggressive individual whose control gradually lessens as a result of repeated head injuries in public house brawls. Even so, substantial reduction in responsibility usually applies only to persons with psychoses secondary to organic causes, post-encephalitic children or persons with temporal lobe epilepsy.

The frequency of serious mental disorder in those charged with murder, along with the publicity it receives, naturally create the unfortunate impression that psychotics are especially likely to be dangerous. Böker and Häfner (1973) studied the 410 males and 126 females medically detained in West Germany between 1953 and 1964 for homicide, limiting themselves strictly to functional and organic psychoses and to severe degrees of subnormality. Though finding that homicidal behaviour, especially directed towards strangers, was distinctly higher among schizophrenics, they calculated that only 0.05 per cent of known schizophrenics commit homicide (i.e. 5 in 10 000) compared with 0.005 per cent in depressive psychoses and 0.006 per cent in subnormals. However, a suicide rate of between 6 per cent and 10 per cent is recorded in schizophrenics, who are a hundred times more dangerous to themselves than to others; the corresponding figure for depressive psychotics is between 1000 and 10 000 times.

The period of illness at which homicide took place is of much interest, not least because of the prospects for prophylaxis. Böker and Häfner found that homicide occurred within a month of the onset of psychosis in only 3 per cent of cases. A great deal of psychiatric literature has been devoted to this group, giving the impression that it is much more common. Eighty-four per cent of their schizophrenics had been ill for over a year and 55 per cent for over 5 years. Among depressed psychotics, however, a third had only been ill for up to 6 months, in one-third of these for the first time: but those who killed their young children in an extended suicide would not be recorded. For all varieties of psychosis the greatest risk was to the nearest members of the family (wife, children) and members of the household.

This is especially true of depressive illnesses, most markedly among women. Strangers or the general public were victims of a minority of schizophrenic homicides, mostly when paranoid delusions suggested that a neighbour or stranger was responsible for persecution.

In this study, therefore, homicide was a feature of schizophrenics who had sometimes not been diagnosed or treated, but was more often a feature of those who had lost contact with the hospital, having received no after-care or follow-up treatment. Most, however, had been discharged with the doctor's approval because they were sufficiently well-preserved to press for discharge if they had families to care for them. Homicide occurred most often within six months of discharge from care. In view of the frequency of threatening paranoid delusions, homicide may be accounted a relatively rare event. One of the disadvantages attached to the maintenance of outpatient care was the reliance placed on the patient's statements, insufficient attention being paid to the reports of wives or relatives. Many homicidal patients had given prodromal evidence of impulsive physical violence, and it was suggested that the patient and his spouse should be under separate psychiatric supervision so that information from both sources could be monitored and the situation explained to the wife.

Böker and Häfner emphasize that in two-thirds of cases there was no evidence of recurrence or exacerbation of symptoms; the patient had simply not had the mental capacity to cope reasonably with a sudden critical or worrying situation which most would have been able to surmount. All this accords with English clinical experience. It is an artefact of the criminal law that once a person is legally declared to be mentally disordered no further explanation is required about how or why the offence came to be committed. In the majority of schizophrenic homicides, the motivations are clear and similar to those encountered among normal offenders who act violently – understandable anger, resentment, jealousy, or fear. The pathological element resides in the response, not the motivation. Few patients entertain such delusional motives as divine inspiration, or the duty of exterminating an enemy or class of enemies, for the good of mankind. There are, nevertheless, certain dangerous syndromes, especially those relating to ideas of marital infidelity (Shepherd, 1961), where there is an almost continuous gradation from the unusual but still normal degree of jealousy, through clearly excessive jealousy, to morbid jealousy of psychotic intensity in which trivial phenomena are interpreted as evidence of infidelity. If acutely psychotic, such individuals must be regarded as dangerous to their wives. By contrast, patients with 'litigious paranoia' are seen more frequently by judges than by psychiatrists. Here there is a persistent and possibly satisfying continuous litigation about imaginary injustice or persecution, with little risk of an irrationally violent outcome.

Provocation

Physical aggression is so common in society, and so widely accepted in at least a large section of society as a normal means of dealing with interpersonal conflict, that the criminal law has to take this into account. Neither side in many disputes would regard the involvement of the police as appropriate even if blood were shed and weapons were used. English criminal law recognizes a detailed hierarchy of offences, ranging from common assault (which is not an indictable offence and is not included in a criminal record) to assault occasioning actual bodily harm, grievous bodily harm, or manslaughter, mainly based upon the consequences rather than the intention, which is clearly very difficult to decide reliably.

The situation is further complicated by the need to introduce the idea of provocation. For some years provocation was admissible only if the victim or complainant of a physical assault had struck the first blow, which was taken to excuse, totally or in part, a violent response. This can at least be proved by reliable evidence. Quite recently it has been allowed that verbal taunts, without blows being struck, can constitute provocation.

Provocation in law, however, is strictly limited to the immediate, hot-blooded situation. A man cannot claim provocation if he gets the worst of a fight, goes away and broods on revenge, and collects a few friends to waylay the assailant on his way home a few hours later. His response to violence must also be limited to the minimum force necessary for self-defence; it would not apply to a man who responded to minor violence by producing a gun and shooting his assailant. In other countries much greater latitude is permitted. In France, for example, a husband may be exonerated if he kills a man whom he finds in bed with his unfaithful wife – the *crime passionel;* and a farmer would be exonerated for firing a rifle after a chicken thief who is running away.

The peculiarity of the defence of provocation, which psychiatrists often find baffling and contrary to reason, is that it is limited to the response of the 'average' or 'reasonable' man, with whom the jury can readily empathize. It cannot apply, as is clearly the case so often in real life, to special sensibilities. A homosexual cannot claim provocation by a lover who taunts him or permit himself to be provoked by finding his lover in bed with another man, though in such a case the provocation may actually be more severe than that of the ordinary man. The reasons for this restriction are that provocation constitutes an extremely easy defence to concoct or exaggerate and that reliable evidence is very difficult to obtain. The judge may well take such factors into account in sentence, if it does not involve murder, but they cannot be considered in relation to conviction. Thus homosexuality itself cannot be represented as a mental abnormality which substantially reduces responsibility if a person is charged with murder. The Criminal Law Revision Committee (1980) has recently suggested ways to resolve this dilemma.

Psychopathic personality

The psychopathology of this condition, and especially its relevance to the criminal law, presents a number of problems which for the moment remain unsolved. We will assume here that the terms psychopathic personality, psychopathy, personality disorder, and pathological personality (as used in the International Classification of Diseases) are synonymous, though the text of the glossary is somewhat ambiguous on this point.

In relation to the English criminal law the situation is complicated by the fact that psychopathic disorder is a legal term in the 1959 Mental Health Act. Legal draftsmen usually maintain that it is a mistake to include any technical term in the criminal law, since scientific progress may alter the meaning of such terms suddenly and thus frustrate the purpose of an Act until this is changed. From this point of view it is perhaps fortunate that 'psychopathic disorder' has not hitherto shown any likelihood of becoming a technical term with an agreed meaning.

The International Classification of Diseases (ICD) is rightly taken as the touchstone of the consensus of opinion among psychiatrists concerning the meaning of psychiatric terminology. In the World Health Organization international conference on the personality disorders section of the ICD held in 1970 the participants were presented with sample case histories complete with all relevant pathological

investigations, accompanied by videotaped interviews with the patients. Their collective views were
then examined to reveal the dimensions of agreement or disagreement among experts. The results
displayed the extent to which culture affects both the
perception and definition of behavioural and mental
deviance. In the report of the conclusions of the conference (Shepherd & Sartorius, 1974) it was stated that
'despite diagnostic imprecision and terminological
confusion, the concept of personality disorder
remains indispensable to clinical psychiatric practice'.

The Glossary of Mental Disorders prepared by
the Registrar-General's Advisory Council on Medical
Nomenclature (General Register Office, 1968) in the
past had defined personality disorders as 'a group of
more or less well-defined anomalies or deviations of
personality which are not the result of psychosis or
any other illness. The differentiation of these personalities is to some extent arbitrary and reference to a
given group will depend initially on the relative preponderance of one or other group of character traits'.
The glossary prepared by the World Health Organization (1971) states that personality disorder includes
'deeply engrained maladaptive patterns of behaviour
generally recognisable by the time of adolescence or
earlier and continuing throughout most of adult life,
although often becoming less obvious in middle or
old age. The personality is abnormal either in the
balance of its components, their quality and expression, or in its total aspect. Because of this deviation
or psychopathy the patient suffers or others have to
suffer, and there is an adverse effect upon the individual or a society'. The definition goes on to point
out that any variety which is related to malfunctioning of the brain, or is directly related to any neurosis
or psychosis, should be classified under the relevant
disorder.

Shepherd and Sartorious emphasize that the
present classification of personality disorders is particularly inadequate in three respects. First, the subcategories (there are seven varieties of pathological
personality, and four types of immature personality)
are not comprehensive and do not make clear how
far personality 'traits' are included in the various definitions; secondly, it is unclear how far the deviations are related to mental disorder on the one hand
or to an ill-defined notion of normality on the other;
and, thirdly, that there is no indication of the degree
of severity necessary for the diagnosis of a personality disorder. The last problem, one may suggest, is

largely the cause of the first two, unless one emphasizes differences in quality as opposed to differences
in degree. The WHO report emphasizes that the only
solution to inadequate knowledge is not to ignore this
amorphous group as falling outside the scope of psychiatry, but to initiate research which at least achieves
the identification of groups which are more fully
understood and classifiable under firm diagnostic
sections.

Even so, much information is lost if, for example, deterioration of personality after pre-frontal
lobotomy is classified as an organic disorder exclusively. There have been over a hundred murders after
lobotomy in the USA, and chronic inadequate criminality in a man with an XYY syndrome hardly constitutes a congenital disorder. It was suggested that
personality disorder might be best described by some
modification of the tripartite system, such as Rutter
and colleagues (1969) had suggested for child psychiatric disorders, with symptoms, family or social situations, intelligence or personality factors comprising the three axes.

Some varieties of personality disorders – schizoid, paranoid, cyclothymic – are clearly intelligible
when viewed as being allied to psychoses, requiring
careful differentiation but constituting a serious burden upon health in themselves. The most vague and
unsatisfactory category, however, and the one most
relevant to the criminal law is 'antisocial personality'. In the English glossary this was said to 'include'
the characteristics of psychopathic disorder as defined
in the Mental Health Act – a mental abnormality
leading to seriously irresponsible or abnormally
aggressive behaviour, and requiring or being susceptible to medical treatment. Sexual deviancy, alcoholism, and drug addiction in themselves are
excluded from the definition, although their pathological consequences or accompaniments can, of
course, be included in their own right.

Walker and McCabe (1973) have pointed out
that in clinical terms a diagnostic label can have one
or more of four functions: explanatory, prognostic,
therapeutic, or descriptive. They examine each in
relation to psychopathy and conclude: 'as a description the diagnosis tells one nothing . . . prognostically it exaggerates the difference between psychopaths and ordinary recidivists on the one hand, and
on the other schizophrenics and subnormals . . . it
cannot be an explanatory label; and . . . as a method
of indicating suitable forms of treatment it tells us
that none has been found very profitable. What can-

not be argued away is the fact that psychiatrists seem to feel the need to use it'.

The Butler Committee recommended that it should be accepted that some criminal psychopaths should be recognized as suitable only for imprisonment, but attempted to define those who were 'treatable' by suggesting that detention in hospital should not be made 'in the case of an offender suffering from psychopathic disorder with dangerous antisocial tendencies unless the court is satisfied (a) that a previous mental or organic illness, or an identifiable psychological or physical defect, relevant to the disorder is known or suspected; and (b) there is expectation of therapeutic benefit from hospital admission'. The Review of the Mental Health Act (1978), which sets out the Government's decision as to the form of the new Mental Health Act, found that adopting the term 'personality disorder' had little backing from the profession. It recommended that the category of psychopathic disorder should be retained and that there was nothing to be gained in practice from including the suggested attempt to define 'treatability'. It proposed to delete the clause 'and requires or is susceptible to medical treatment', and substitute only a 'likelihood of benefit from treatment'.

In practice, the inference of the Mental Health Act is such that no use is made of the ICD in the psychiatric service in general, but only in research institutes. The general category of psychopathic personality alone is deemed to be sufficient without subcategorization. Advantage was taken of the systematic use of the ICD as part of the thorough postgraduate training in psychiatry at the Institute of Psychiatry, however, to study the differences between criminal and non-criminal psychopathics and neurotics admitted to hospital in the 10 years 1952 to 1962 (Gibbens *et al.*, 1968). This procedure enabled matched controls to be selected by age and subcategory e.g. a schizoid non-offender with a schizoid offender. The overwhelmingly important difference, as expected, was that the offenders had been subjected much more often to traumatic and depriving experiences in the first five years of life which had tended to continue. By contrast, among non-offenders this finding was absent or was possibly more concealed and susceptible of compensation later in life; more non-offenders were middle-class in origin and tended to be protected by the concern of their families. One of the subsidiary points of some interest to emerge from a comparison between psychopaths and

neurotics, offending or otherwise, was that insomnia and other sleep disturbances were largely confined to those individuals diagnosed as neurotic. The fact that an aggressive psychopath may have an untroubled night's sleep immediately after committing a murder emerges as a striking characteristic.

Lee Robins (1966) has approached the problem of psychopathy by attempting to construct social measures of severity. Her category of 'sociopath' is arrived at by adding up several aspects of social deviation – unemployment, receipt of public relief, sexual promiscuity, marital maladjustment, mental symptoms, alcoholism, and crime – to permit some cumulative estimate of severity. In the USA the term sociopath has tended to supplant that of psychopath. On this basis, any persistent form of criminality proves to be a serious form of deviance, often involving all the others; sexual disorders or alcoholism, unless extreme, are by contrast often partial and compatible with a valuable pro-social existence, reminiscent of Henderson's group of 'creative psychopaths'.

Gunn (1976, 1978a) has traced the particular problems of research into the effectiveness of treatment at Grendon Psychiatric Prison. Non-psychotic prisoners of average intelligence or above were selected by judges and medical officers as 'treatable' psychopaths, and it was asked how they differed from a control group of prisoners of similar age, criminal record, and other social factors. With two observers rating the subjects for reliability of assessment, Gunn intercorrelated a number of personality factors, including many resembling those of Robins, and also the responses to the General Health Questionnaire (Goldberg, 1972) with regard to neurotic and anxiety symptoms. He concluded that in this population of psychopaths only 5 scales form a significant relationship to one another: this was in the area of anxiety and depressive symptoms in relation to conflicts in interpersonal, family, and group relations. He concluded that 'the majority of so-called psychopaths could be happily accommodated under the diagnostic category of neurotic. The diagnosis 'neurotic (antisocial behaviour)' would decide whether or not a patient qualified for this ill-defined and heterogeneous label of psychopath'. This conclusion would free the psychiatrist to concentrate the treatment of the neurotic element in the disorder.

The marked difference in both the extent and characteristics of female and male crime and psychopathy is a fruitful area for research. Guze (1976) has noted that the problem of hysteria was exceptionally high in women offenders – more than 20 times greater than in the general population. Even when the additional diagnoses of psychopathy, alcoholism, and drug addiction were excluded, hysteria alone (15 per cent) was increased more than fourfold by comparison with the rest of the population. There appeared to be a significant association between sociopathy and hysteria (sociopathy alone 39 per cent, hysteria alone 15 per cent, and both together 26 per cent), leading to the suggestion 'that at least some cases of hysteria and sociopathy share a common etiology or pathogenesis. Since hysteria is predominantly a disorder of women while sociopathy is predominantly a disorder of men, it was suggested that, depending on the sex of the individual, the same etiological and pathogenetic factors may lead to different, though sometimes overlapping, clinical pictures'. (Cloninger & Guze, 1970). Put less tentatively, the idea that hysterical psychopathy in women is often equivalent to aggressive sociopathy in men may account for the psychiatrist's perception that women offenders are much more seriously 'disturbed' than male offenders. Whether or how much this depends upon biological or constitutional factors in women or on an early inculcation of gender–role differences in a particular society is of course uncertain.

Sexual disorders

Like aggressive behaviour, acceptable sexual behaviour varies so widely throughout the world that the real nature of sexual deviance is still a matter of doubt. Paedophilia is accepted as normal in wide areas of the Middle East and extensive bisexuality is a matter of no concern. Yet sexual orientation is not infinitely variable, and the many minor perversions, e.g. exhibitionism, frottage, fetishism, are strictly limited. Most societies seem to have some exclusive homosexuals; even in Central Africa, where homosexuality is rare, there is a class of men who are allowed to live as women in women's clothes, and who suffer no discrimination once the choice is made.

In England and most European countries it has been widely accepted that there are great difficulties in applying the criminal law to sexual behaviour with any uniformity because of the wide range of attitudes adopted, and that it is wise to limit it to three aspects of behaviour which interfere with the rights of others and are universally condemned: namely, (1) the use of force, (2) the exploitation of the young, weak or handicapped, and (3) behaviour which affronts public decency. Several offences were redefined in the nineteenth century which again emphasized moral repugnance in addition to the protective function of law. In the last 10 years there has been further criticism that the law interferes unnecessarily with human rights.

According to Halsey (1978), one of the most dramatic social changes in the last hundred years has concerned the status of children. This has progressed from the view of minors as simple possessions of their parents with no rights until adolescence, to according them many individual rights, almost from conception, against both state and their parents or parent substitutes. One of the most controversial legal issues to have emerged is the age at which the child or young person is accorded the right to determine its own sexual behaviour.

The age of consent for independent sexual choice varies widely in different countries. In England a girl is considered incapable of giving consent to sexual intercourse until 16, though there are many suggestions that with the steady decrease in the average age of puberty it should be lowered to 14 or even 12. Meanwhile many civil rights depending upon the age of adult responsibility – of voting, making an independent will, joining the Army – have been lowered to 18, and it would be anomalous for adult status in respect of sexual activities not to follow suit.

Although a girl may not consent to sexual intercourse until 16, it is unusual for anyone to be prosecuted for consensual intercourse with a girl aged 15, and in some cases aged 14. It has been a judicial rule for some time that a young man under 21 who has intercourse with a girl of 15 believing her to be over 16 is entitled to acquittal on the first occasion. In practice, a youth who systematically seduces girls of 14 with their consent is warned that he will be charged if this conduct continues. One difficulty associated with the use of such discretion is that different police areas have been shown to differ widely in its exercise. The second difficulty is that it also gives considerable discretion to parents, who may angrily demand prosecution. Professor Antilla, for some years Minister of Justice in Finland, has suggested that one consequence of the autonomy of young girls and the frequency of conflict with their parents, should be their right to decide whether their lover should be prosecuted. Pressure by strict parents may induce a frightened girl to give false evidence of having been raped rather than admit that she fully consented to intercourse. Even if the power of criminal prosecution is held in reserve, it is felt by many schoolteachers to be useful in warning girls of 15 that they are breaking the law and so preventing them from exercising pressure, by public ridicule as peculiar exceptions, upon other sixth-form girls who wish to remain virgins. Research, admittedly carried out some years ago, showed that girls who do not have sexual intercourse until 16 or 17 form a much larger proportion of young people than reports in the media would lead one to suppose (Schofield, 1965). By contrast, unlawful sexual intercourse with girls under 13 (USI) is regarded as a very serious crime, carrying the maximum sentence of life imprisonment. Since the 1956 Sexual Offences Act in England the tendency has been towards prosecution of some cases of USI under 13 on a charge of rape. The statistics of rape and USI, which include separate estimates of these offences, show that a surprising number of victims of rape or USI or attempts at these offences are directed at children aged less than eight years (Gibbens *et al.*, 1980).

It is still a serious offence for anyone to have sexual intercourse with a severely subnormal girl or woman. The new Mental Health Act proposes to define 'severely mentally handicapped' (or retarded) more widely than the 'severe subnormality' of the 1959 Act, stressing social competence rather than estimated IQ. With the growing policy of substituting hostel or foster-homes in the community for institutional care there will be wider opportunities for social and sexual contact between the sexes and it is becoming increasingly difficult and inappropriate to prevent such conduct. On the whole, the medical profession dealing with the handicapped takes the view that it is an excessive interference with human rights to deprive any class of person completely of the right to a sexual life, or even of marrying if at all possible, and it seems probable that in this respect the law will be changed (Policy Advisory Committee, 1979).

Paedophilia

The age of consent for sexual behaviour presses hard upon the paedophiliac. In England the Paedophilia Information Exchange (PIE) takes the view that the age of consent should be abolished, that children are as capable of accepting or rejecting sexual advances as adults if the relationship is affectionate. Few will accept that this could be regarded as 'informed consent' but it remains true that many of these offences are relatively trivial (touching, peep-

ing, masturbation, etc.), consensual, and only marginally traumatic. Others, however, are extremely serious, consisting in virtual rape by usually drunken assailants who perpetrate physical damage on the child. PIE is punitive towards this group and maintains that those who 'molest, pester and use violence' to children should receive long sentences of imprisonment. Most members of the public, not only parents, have a deeply shocked and punitive attitude towards all such offences, and the courts have somewhat limited ability to differentiate between the consensual and violent varieties by varying the sentence.

In terms of their psychopathology paedophiliacs are a complex group. Some are exclusive homosexuals, interested only in young boys; others do not differentiate much between the sex of the children. About 40 per cent, moreover, are elderly men who have been married and are either widowed or divorced, leading very solitary lives, and being unable to make ordinary friends. Some of these people are possibly products of the destruction of human relationships caused by repeated imprisonments. In some young paedophiliacs under 25 it has been suggested that the cause is the development of a phobia of pubic hair produced by some childhood experience, since some of them are also attracted by old women (gerontophilia) and have mutually satisfying sexual relations with women of 70 or 80 whose pubic hair is equally sparse.

Incest

Incest, which carries a maximum sentence of life imprisonment, is also very varied in respect of psychopathology and severity. In England it only became a criminal offence in the 1908 Punishment of Incest Act, after two Bills had failed in the previous eight years on the ground that to make it illegal would merely advertise a rare anomaly which could perfectly well be dealt with as an indecent assault. In 1908 the Act was passed after the Archbishop of Canterbury had maintained that in deteriorated sections of cities the new service of moral welfare workers had reported their inability to persuade fathers to desist when they came upon a case.

Incest tends to occur in large and overcrowded families where it causes, in my own experience, remarkably little trauma to adolescent girls if the father is steady and affectionate at other times. Often the mothers are dull, invalid, or nagging and the father is touched by the apparently artless affection of his adolescent children; in many such cases the mother tends to connive at or ignore the offence. A second group, emphasized by Virkkunen (1974), is much more serious, consisting of heavily alcoholic fathers, often with previous aggressive convictions, whose wives reject sexual intercourse because of drunkenness. These men then brutally rape or bugger their very young children, sometimes causing physical damage. Incest between mother and son is relatively rare.

About a quarter of cases of incest occur between brother and sister. Most of these cases are in overcrowded delinquent families, the boys having many previous (and subsequent) offences against property. They are mostly detected because the boy is on probation or under social supervision. The offenders are much more lightly punished. Among them are an adult group which barely meets the criteria of incestuous behaviour: a half-brother and half-sister who have not been brought up in one family and meet late in life. The genetic risks are here the same as for father – daughter incest, but it seems likely that this group may be de-criminalized, if both are over 18 or 21.

Homosexuality

Homosexuality is the most controversial form of deviance. Its causes are still quite obscure in the exclusive forms of early origin, but in those arising in later life various forms of inhibition of heterosexual development appear to be demonstrable, and bisexuality is widespread in psychopaths. The incidence rates – approximately 10 per cent of the general population and 30 per cent with some transitory homosexual feeling or behaviour in adolescence – are probably equal in the two sexes, though in women it often does not reach physical expression and is more often compatible with marriage.

An amendment to the law, which would permit homosexual behaviour in private between those over 21 was recommended by the Wolfenden Committee in 1954 (1957) but became law only 13 years later, in 1967. Since the age of majority in England has become 18, the age of 21 has become an anomalous criterion. There is, however, a widespread view that the age of consent should be lowered to that of 16 (or even 14), not only on the general grounds of sexual equality but also because it is widely believed that the direction of the young adolescent's orientation is relatively fixed by the age of 16 and is unlikely to be affected by homosexual seduction or social pressures. At present very few young men of 18 or over are arrested for co-operative homosexuality and the numbers of those aged between 16 and 18 is very small. None the less, the effects of lowering the age to 16 might cause great problems for parents or schoolteachers, and such a move would almost certainly be bitterly opposed by public opinion. In the armed forces and merchant navy the law still preserves the age of 21 and seems unlikely to change.

Pornography

Pornography has long caused great legal difficulties, partly because of the difficulty of distinguishing between artistically erotic creations and pornographic material concerned exclusively with sexual titillation, and partly because of such technological developments as videotapes. The old criterion of pornography that 'it tends to corrupt' was notably inadequate and always difficult to determine. Though some psychiatrists have been ready to give clear-cut evidence on whether a particular example was or was not liable to corrupt, it has never been clear why psychiatrists should be regarded as better equipped to judge these matters than any other members of the community. Physicians, however, were also often called by the defence to give evidence on whether pornography could be therapeutic to some, if only a very small proportion, of society.

The remarkable experience in Denmark of abolishing all censorship of pornography, carefully studied by Kutchinsky (1974), has shown that the effect was a very temporary increase in the sales of pornographic material, rapidly followed by a fall to a steady, very low level of local sales; there was, however, a marked increase in production for sale to nearby countries, especially Germany. More importantly, arrests and prosecutions for almost all minor perverse sexual offences – exhibitionism, indecent assaults on children and adults, but less so for rape – have all fallen to much less than half their former figure. It has been suggested that the increasing liberalization of sexual attitudes might have led to this result because the public simply failed to report such offences. This explanation, however, could hardly apply to those offences involving violence to children. Kutchinsky has examined the findings carefully and has observed that samples of the female population report that they are definitely not the victims of sexual exposure to the same extent as hitherto.

From the standpoint of psychopathology, there appears to be a group of very handicapped or inhibited males who cannot masturbate to orgasm without the help of pornographic pictures. This has long been a problem with mentally handicapped patients and plays a part in the build-up of tension and impulsive behaviour. Attempts are now being made by male nurses to teach the mentally handicapped how to masturbate to satisfaction, a procedure which causes some anxiety as to whether they are breaking the law relating to the sexual conduct of hospital staff in the Mental Health Act. Such issues, however, refer to a small proportion of the community and a recent committee on obscenity (Williams Committee, 1980) has wisely recommended that the accent of any law should be firmly placed on the concept that insults to the public by unwelcome advertisements and displays should be the main focus of prohibition. The practice of pornography in private, on the other hand, need not be restricted.

Juvenile delinquency

Child psychiatrists are much more often involved in the assessment and treatment of juvenile delinquents than are other psychiatrists in respect of adult offenders. Except in certain hospitals whose catchment area includes very busy central urban courts, the average consultant psychiatrist in England does not have to deal with an offender on remand or under a Mental Health Act more often than three or four times a year.

If the juvenile delinquent is subject to the care and control of his parents, his status before a court is modified. Moreover, it has been a steadily developing policy in successive Children's and Young Person's Acts to remove any specifically criminal connotation from a delinquent act; delinquency is regarded as no more than one of several other indications of being in need of social care. The current Act leaves little scope to juvenile magistrates to do more than dismiss, fine, place under supervision, or commit the delinquent to the care of the local authority. This authority has the power to take any action regarded as necessary, including sending the delinquent home again. Research (e.g. Weeks, 1958) has suggested that the congregation of delinquents in special institutions creates a self-image in the young adolescent of belonging to a special criminal class, as well as exposing him to an education in more sophisticated delinquency. In general, the new policy of 'decriminalization' or destigmatization of minor offenders has worked well, though it has gradually emerged that there is a small proportion, perhaps 3–5 per cent, who are uncontrollable because no facilities for control exist.

West & Farrington (1977), in a study of 400 children in a poor urban area, showed that those who became recognized delinquents tended to come from poor homes, with criminal fathers or siblings, to belong to large families, to have parents considered unsatisfactory in their child-rearing methods, and to be of below average intelligence. In self-reporting studies by the boys themselves, those who admitted to much undetected delinquent activities tended to be similar, and the same group had been picked out beforehand by their teachers and contemporaries as difficult and undisciplined in school. In various studies, including West's, between 15 per cent and 28 per cent of boys in these areas become recognized delinquents by the age of 18. It is thus inherently improbable that many of them can suffer from serious mental disorders.

The relative significance of the factors listed above was open to various interpretations, but the concentration of delinquency in multiproblem families was impressive. A minority of 45 (11.4 per cent) of such families accounted for nearly half of all registered convictions. The high rate of family crime was not explained merely by the size of such families.

The psychopathology of delinquency is thus very complex. A specific child psychiatric disorder is found rather rarely, in only 1 to 5 per cent of cases. Such influences as prematurity, birth trauma, later brain damage, encephalitis, the hyperkinetic syndrome, physical handicaps, and genetic influences or psychoses can be implicated in particular groups, but the nature of their relationship to delinquent conduct is uncertain. Twin studies, which once seemed to furnish strong evidence of genetic factors in aetiology, have since been largely discounted by more systematic research (Dalgard & Kringlen, 1976).

Despite the difficulties, however, some sort of classification is necessary for the purposes of scientific enquiry. Classification, according to Scott (1965), can be based on varieties of specific behaviour, those based upon personal qualities including motivation, and those based upon his interaction with others. In fact any classification which is to have more than academic interest must involve all three elements. Scott's own classification was based upon 'personal qualities' primarily, but also took account of some aspects of learning theory. It consisted of four broad groups: (1) The 'ill-trained', brought up with the necessary minimum of care and affection but provided with no consistent lessons, and liable to be easily influenced by stronger characters in their delinquent locality. (2) The 'pseudo-trained', who have either been brought up in criminal families to have deviant conceptions of honesty, usually regarded by observers as likeable rogues with many emotionally normal responses but including more subtle variants who have been unconsciously trained to fulfil their parents' wishes, e.g. in families with quarrelling parents who use the child as a means of antagonizing their spouses. (3) The 'reparative', by analogy with the learning theorists' conditioned avoidance reaction. Here a lesson in the avoidance of anxiety and conflict is learnt so thoroughly that the boy never learns to abandon it. Such a group contains echoes of Freudian 'reaction formation' and of inappropriate sublimation, as well as of 'neurotic' reactions. (4) The 'maladaptive', who appear to have suffered such great anxiety from fluctuating and contradictory experiences that they adopt pointlessly repetitive and unconstructive self-damaging behaviour.

Several classifications have been employed in the study of delinquency. Of those specifically designed as a basis for differential treatment the most influential and thought-provoking has been the classification of Grant and Warren, of 'levels of maturity in interpersonal relations', used in the California Community Treatment Project (Warren, 1969; Palmer, 1974). Those individuals committed to the care of the Youth Authority were (with some exceptions) submitted to a programme of intensive personal care by probation officers and other selected care officers in the community as an alternative to expensive institutionalisation. Each officer was allocated only 8 cases. The hypothesis was that 'low maturity' developments would fail to respond since they needed some form of social structure; it was expected, on the other hand, that high maturity types, including neurotic delinquents, would respond better than in institutions. The project was continued for 10 years and though at first highly successful, it tended in time to show that the early successes were often reversed by institutionalization two or three years later for relapses at a time when those initially institutionalized were doing rather well on supervision after release. When Lee Robins interviewed her disordered children as adults 30 years later, those who had long ceased to break the law could attribute their response to only two factors: first, to 'getting older and wiser' and, secondly, to getting married, achieving new satisfactions in life, and being motivated not to risk destroying them.

The criminal law continues to define the different offences committed by children in exactly the same way as with adults, but the offenders are managed with much greater flexibility since the Children's Acts require magistrates to 'consider the welfare of the child', a requirement that does not exist in the adult criminal law. Adult law applies in the same way to one offence, that of murder by children. On a conviction of murder, the High Court can order a child to be detained in custody for a limited or unlimited time. Many murders by children are not associated with gross psychopathology, and the offender can be integrated into the general system of child care after two or three years. A few, however, with very disordered personalities can present serious problems of assessment for long periods of time.

Criminal responsibility

Hitherto certain aspects of responsibility have been briefly considered. The issues are considered in rather more detail below.

The concept of criminal responsibility is very old. The Hammurabi Code of ancient Babylon (about 2000 B.C.) describes a sophisticated system of law, distinguishing between accidental, negligent, and intentional crime, and preserving graded punishments or exoneration for each. The criminal law must rest upon a moral concept of justice if it is to command respect; history has demonstrated the terrible consequences of employing social efficiency as the criterion of justice. At the same time an absolute decision as to whether an offender may be deemed responsible for his crime is unrealistic when there are so many intermediate grades between full moral responsibility and total irresponsibility.

There are two main ways in which a person is declared criminally irresponsible by English law.

Disability

An offender may be found 'insane on arraignment' or 'unfit to plead'. Under the Criminal Law Amendment Act of 1967 this was changed to 'under disability' in defending himself. The Act, however, did not change the criteria which have long been established: that the accused is so mentally confused or disordered that he is unable to understand the court proceedings, to distinguish between a plea of guilty or not guilty, to challenge jurors, or to instruct Counsel in his defence. The issue can be raised by the judge, the prosecution, or the defence. The special risk is that if found 'under disability' the accused is ordered to be detained indefinitely 'during Her Majesty's pleasure' without proof in a court that he ever committed the act. Under the present Act, the issue can be postponed until the prosecution has outlined the case against him.

It is important in practice that the plea of disability should be used only in cases where there is no doubt whatever. If an accused psychotic, calm, and seemingly capable of rational argument, insists on his innocence he should not be denied a trial. By way of an example, a highly intelligent African lady, the last descendant of a royal family, had qualified as a barrister but ultimately developed a chronic paranoid schizophrenic psychosis of some 10 years' duration though she was fully able to live in the community. A middle-aged homosexual lived in the room across the corridor in her rooming-house, and she frequently complained about his noisy parties. On the day in question the man had slammed the door in her face, whereupon she had broken down a door panel and threatened him with a large carving knife. Having dismissed a succession of counsels as incompetent to defend her, she was eventually reported to be fit to plead and conduct her own defence. She cross-examined her accuser with such vigour that he became faint in the witness box, and when the judge intervened she rebuked him for interfering with her conduct of the defence. Medical evidence was given that she suffered from a paranoid psychosis. The jury acquitted her of any offence and she was set free.

In cases where a psychotic offender is so acutely ill, especially when suicidal, that he requires urgent treatment and cannot be observed in prison as well as he would be in hospital, he can be removed to a special hospital without trial until sufficiently well to face trial. This procedure is used also in only about a dozen cases a year.

The second main procedure for determining criminal responsibility is by the McNaughton Rules, which have been described earlier (p. 172). This is essentially a defence of 'not guilty by reason of insanity', to which the accused must agree, although in practice he is usually persuaded by counsel to have it advanced. If the offender refuses, then he must be found either unfit to plead or face trial, at which counsel may find it impossible to accept his psychotic instructions. Again, the McNaughton defence is nowadays used very rarely. In these two procedures the jury makes the decision with, or if necessary without, medical evidence. It is open to the defence counsel to put forward the plea, even if the medical evidence maintains that the accused is sane in law.

It has been pointed out that an individual accused of murder may be found guilty of manslaughter with diminshed responsibility if two doctors give evidence that he suffered from a mental abnormality which substantially reduced his mental responsibility. This question has proved so much easier for doctors to answer, and a jury to decide in the light of conflicting evidence provided by psychiatrists for the prosecution and the defence, that it has tended to supplant the McNaughton Rules even when these could be clearly applied.

There are a number of technical issues with regard to the burden of proof in these procedures. The defence is only required to prove its case on the 'balance of probabilities', even with a defence of automatism. Once the issue is raised, however, the prosecution must establish its case that the accused is sane or responsible 'beyond reasonable doubt'.

In England about 98 per cent of all crime is dealt with by the magistrates' courts, including most of those crimes by offenders who are committed to a mental hospital under Section 60 of the Mental Health Act (Hospital Order). In retrospect, it is apparent that the Act made a great advance by making no reference to criminal responsibility in such cases; it merely requires two doctors to agree that the prisoner is disordered in a defined way and requires treatment. In this manner the issue of criminal responsibility has been virtually eliminated in practice, though no doubt it remains a moral concept in the minds of the magistrate, the judge, and the jury. There have been several instances in which an offender has appealed against a hospital order on the grounds that, although psychotic or mentally disordered under the Act, his condition had nothing to do with the offence, which was normally motivated. Often this plea was intended as a means of avoiding detention for up to 12 months, whereas a sane man would be sentenced to a fine, probation, or a much shorter period in prison. The Appeal Courts have rejected this procedure on the grounds that the Act makes no reference to any connection between the illness and the crime, merely stating that the most appropriate way of disposing of the case is by medical treatment. Conversely, if a magistrate refuses to accept a firm recommendation from several doctors that the offender needs hospital treatment, the Appeal Court has usually upheld the doctors against the magistrate or judge.

PART III

Taxonomy, diagnosis and treatment

7
The principles of classification in relation to mental disease

R. E. KENDELL

The classification of its subject matter is one of the most fundamental activities of any science or any branch of learning. It is fundamental in two senses: because it is a necessary preliminary to almost any useful communication; and because all classifications involve assumptions about the relationships between the different components of the system which largely determine the questions that are, or can be, asked. If these assumptions are correct, as they were in the classification of plants developed by Linnaeus and the classification of chemical elements proposed by Mendeléef, the subsequent development of knowledge is greatly facilitated. But if they are incorrect it is seriously, perhaps fatally, retarded. Our understanding of many diseases, for example, was hindered for a long time by their classification as deficiencies or excesses of one of the four Galenical humours, and understanding of the life cycle and evolutionary origins of whales was hardly possible until it was realized that they should be classified not as fish but as mammals. It follows from these two considerations – the necessity for some kind of classification even in the early developmental stages of a subject, and the pervasive influence for good or ill of the assumptions involved – first that classification is too important a matter to be treated lightly, and second that all classifications must be provisional. However long they have been in use and however appropriate they may seem they must never be allowed to ossify.

Menninger (1963) listed many of the diverse classifications of mental disorders of the past 2500 years as an appendix to his book *The Vital Balance*. This fascinating collection, starting with Hippocrates, Plato, and Celsus and including most of the influential classifications of the seventeenth, eighteenth, and nineteenth centuries, clearly illustrates how faithfully all classifications reflect the theoretical ideas of their time. Indeed, these now abandoned classifications constitute the framework of the history of man's changing assumptions about the nature of mental disorders.

The inevitability of classification

From time to time in the history of psychiatry it has been suggested that the attempt to classify mental illnesses was pointless and should be abandoned. It is doubtful, however, whether those who made the suggestion – Prichard and Neumann in the nineteenth century and Carl Rogers and Karl Menninger a generation ago – realized the full implications of their proposals. In the first place some form of classification is virtually unavoidable. Even our language involves classification; every noun – apple, ape, neutron, or fairy – embodies the recognition of a class of objects. Moreover, any decision to recognize only one form of mental illness would involve two assumptions as crucial as any to be found in more elaborate schemata: namely that mental illness is different and distinguishable from mental health, and that all mental illness is basically the same.

It helps to clarify the issues involved if one reflects that every psychiatric patient has attributes of three kinds:

(A) Those he shares with all other psychiatric patients
(B) Those he shares with some other patients, but not all
(C) Those that are unique to him

The potential value of classifying patients depends on the relative size and importance of these three, or more precisely on the size of B relative to A and C. If all patients were the same there would be no need to distinguish between one type of patient and another, or indeed any means of doing so. If this were the case, however, or if we decided for other reasons to disregard the differences between them, it would be impossible for us to develop rational criteria for using different treatments for different patients. Either every patient would have to be given the same standard treatment, or the application of

treatments to patients would have to be haphazard, determined by whim or the throw of dice. Alternatively, if every patient were unique, or if we chose to concentrate our attention on their unique features, we would find it impossible to acquire any useful knowledge. In the course of treating an individual patient we might well learn important things about him and become better able to help him as a result, but that knowledge and skill would be irrelevant when we came to treat other patients, because they would be quite different. Indeed, if our patients really differed from one another in all their most important characteristics it would be impossible to learn anything useful from teachers, colleagues, textbooks or even our own previous experience. In short, insistence on a unitary concept of mental illness condemns us to giving the same panacea to everyone, and insistence on the uniqueness of every individual prevents all learning and all useful communication about disease. Those who have argued in the past that classification should be abandoned may well have been correct in maintaining that where mental illness was concerned category B above was small in comparison with A and C, but our attention still has to be focused on B if we are ever to acquire any useful understanding and pass that understanding on to others. In fact, of course, as soon as one begins to recognize features that are common to some patients but not to all, and to distinguish between those which are important and those, like eye colour, which are not, one is classifying them whether one recognizes it or not. The only points at issue are whether that classification is overt or covert, public or private, stable or unstable.

The different classificatory criteria available

Although we talk loosely of classifying mental illnesses it is not illnesses as such that are classified, it is people suffering from illnesses. The object to be classified is a sick human being, or in biological terms a malfunctioning organism, and the decision that has to be made is whether that person is suffering from schizophrenia or alcoholism, or possibly both, not whether a disembodied illness is schizophrenia or alcoholism. In principle any characteristic of an organism that is capable of being observed and described can be used to classify it. However, the observable characteristics of human beings are almost infinite and most of these lack any obvious relevance to the issues of sickness and health. It is often assumed that classifications of mental illness should be based on one or other of the following attributes of illness:

(1) *Symptomatology* – the patient's complaints, his descriptions of abnormal subjective experiences and the observable abnormalities of his behaviour.

(2) *Prognosis* – the temporal course or response to treatment of these symptoms and the disabilities associated with them.

(3) *Aetiology* – the fundamental abnormalities of structure or function known, or believed, to underlie and antedate the overt symptoms of the illness.

It is generally agreed that an aetiological classification is the most desirable because aetiological distinctions are more fundamental, and therefore useful in a wider range of situations. A classification of infections based on the identity of the causal organism, for example, is more useful than one based on the characteristics of the fever and other symptoms observable at the bedside. However, where mental illnesses are concerned we understand so little of the aetiology of most of them at present that an aetiological classification can be little more than an aspiration.

At first sight, classification on the basis of prognosis is an attractive option, and one with respectable historical precedents. Kraepelin's classification of the functional psychoses was based on the different prognoses of dementia praecox and manic-depressive insanity, was it not? The issue is not so straightforward as it looks, however. One of the most important functions of a diagnosis is to determine the choice of treatment and to predict outcome. In order to influence that choice, however, the diagnosis must be based on information that is available before treatment starts. To define mania as a psychosis which responds to lithium carbonate would not help one to decide whether or not to give lithium to a man running around the ward declaring that he was the Prince of Wales. If diagnoses were based on prognosis they could only be made in retrospect, in the extreme case only after death, and so could never be used either to determine treatment or to predict outcome. In fact, strictly speaking, Kraepelin did not define either dementia praecox or manic-depressive insanity in terms of their prognosis. He defined them in terms of their symptomatology, but delineated the two syndromes in such a way as to maximize the difference in outcome between them. Outcome was thus a *validating criterion*, rather than a *defining characteristic*. and if a patient with the typical symptoms of dementia praecox recovered completely this did not justify changing the diagnosis.

Symptom-based classifications

Because an aetiological classification is not yet feasible and a prognostic classification inappropriate, most classifications of mental illness have generally been based primarily on symptomatology, sometimes augmented with demographic and other data. In Scadding's terminology (Scadding, 1967) the *defining characteristic* of most psychiatric disorders has usually been their *clinical syndrome.*

A syndrome consists of a cluster of symptoms which tend to occur together and which often have a more or less characteristic time course. The relationship between the constituent symptoms of the syndrome and the corresponding diagnosis is usually 'polythetic' rather than 'nomothetic'; that is, the diagnosis is established by the presence of several of the constituent symptoms of the syndrome, without any single one being essential. (This is characteristic of biological classifications in general. Mammals, for example, are distinguished from other vertebrates by being warm-blooded, covered in hair, delivering their young alive, and suckling them with specialized mammary glands, but none of these four characteristics is possessed by all mammals.) As a result, unless it is carefully stipulated which combinations of the various symptoms constituting the syndrome are adequate to establish the diagnosis and which are not by means of an *operational definition** different clinicians will tend to use different criteria, and diagnostic assignments will consequently be very unreliable.

This reliance on symptomatology has often been criticized. In the 1950s clinical psychologists fre-

---

* An operational or semantic definition is one which provides clear cut *rules of application* for the diagnosis in question. Let us assume that diagnosis X is commonly based on the presence of some combination of symptoms, a, b, c, d, e, and f. A traditional textbook or glossary description might say that in condition X a and b were 'characteristic', c 'a valuable diagnostic clue' and d, e, and f 'commonly present'. This is useful information but it does not spell out which of the many possible combinations of a, b, c, d, e, and f are adequate to establish the diagnosis. As a result, one clinician may diagnose X whenever a, b, or c is present, another may insist on the presence of a, and a third be prepared to make the diagnosis if he can elicit any two of the six. An operational definition eliminates this ambiguity by stipulating precisely which combinations of these characteristics are and are not adequate to establish the diagnosis. It might state, for example, that 'to establish diagnosis X either a or b must be present, together with at least two of c, d, e, and f'.

quently suggested that symptoms should be replaced by scores on cognitive or other psychological tests, or by rating of interpersonal behaviour or social role functioning, while psycho-analysts repeatedly advocated a classification based on pyscho-dynamic defence mechanisms. More recently a new generation of clinical psychologists has advocated a classification based on a comprehensive analysis of behaviour in a wide range of different situations. Indeed, it is hardly an exaggeration to say that at some time or another every group professionally concerned with the care of the mentally ill has advocated a classification based on whichever mechanisms or responses were of most interest to them personally. None of these suggestions has come to fruition, however, largely because the advocates of change have never persevered with the task of testing and refining successive versions of their novel classification to the stage where it provided a viable alternative. There is, however, no reason in principle why characteristics other than symptoms should not be used. At the same time, it is important not to be too apologetic about our continuing reliance on symptoms. They are, after all, what the patient complains of, which is in itself sufficient reason for treating them seriously. They are also readily observed or elicited, they can be recorded with adequate reliability if suitable definitions are provided, and the psychiatric literature contains a great wealth of information about them.

Defining characteristics change as knowledge increases

In the long run symptoms are almost certain to be displaced by other more fundamental abnormalities described in physiological, psychological, or biochemical terms. It is characteristic of classifications of disease for the defining characteristic of an illness to start as its clinical syndrome and then, as understanding of its pathogenesis develops, to change to a structural, physiological, or biochemical anomaly, and there is no reason to expect that mental disorders will be exempt from this general trend. Identification of the syndrome is an essential preliminary to this process because attention cannot be focused on the condition, or its antecedents and pathology studied, until the syndrome has been recognized and defined. Once useful research is made possible in this way, sooner or later some crucial abnormality is detected which antedates and accounts for the overt symptoms, and when that occurs the defining characteristic changes from the clinical syndrome to that abnormality. The discovery of an additional chro-

mosome in children with Down's syndrome or of a deficiency of thyroxine in patients with myxoedema are typical examples of this process. Often when this transition occurs the disease changes its name; Down's syndrome became trisomy 21 and myxoedema became hypothyroidism in recognition of this change in their defining characteristics. This is not invariable though; GPI and tabes dorsalis retained their names even after the discovery of their syphilitic origins. The population of patients embraced by the new concept may also be rather different from the old one, as it was when myxoedema gave way to hypothyroidism, but again this is not invariable. Sooner or later, therefore, we can expect that the neurophysiological defect we presume to underlie the syndrome we call schizophrenia will be identified, though when this happens it is anyone's guess whether the term schizophrenia will survive and whether the new physiological concept will embrace quite the same population of patients as the present clinical one.

Classifications of mental illness, including the present International Classification (World Health Organization, 1978), are sometimes criticized for using aetiological criteria in some areas and syndromal criteria in others. It is quite true that mixing aetiological concepts like puerperal psychosis and psychogenic psychosis with syndromal concepts like delirium and mania often causes confusion, but in practice inconsistency of this kind is almost inevitable. The only way to be consistent would be to use syndromal criteria throughout; but once having discovered, for example, that Alzheimer's disease had a specific morbid anatomy it would be folly not to make use of the greater precision and understanding that information afforded. The best answer to the problem is to utilize both types of information, syndromal and aetiological, but to keep them separate as is done in multi-axial classifications (see pp. 197–8).

Categories v. dimensions

Most classifications in everyday use are typologies. That is, they consist of a mutually exclusive set of categories with every individual assigned to one, and only one, of these categories. The majority of large typologies, like those of animal and plant species, are arranged in tiers, but this is not invariable. Most classifications of mental illness are tiered typologies of this kind with a primary division into functional and organic disorders, a further division of the former into psychoses and neuroses, and then one or two further tiers consisting of illnesses like schizophrenia and hysteria and subtypes of these. One unusual feature of classifications of disease is that it is often legitimate to make more than one diagnosis at a time, glandular fever and psoriasis for example, or schizophrenia and mental subnormality. This is because, as has been stressed already, we are dealing with a classification not of diseases or of people but of diseases *in* people.

Typologies are not the only classificatory format available, however. The relationships between the members of a heterogeneous population can also be expressed by assigning them to loci on one or more axes or dimensions. When we measure people's height in inches or centimetres, or express their intelligence as an IQ, we are in fact classifying their height or intellectual abilities in dimensional terms, in preference to describing them in categorical terms as tall or short, clever or stupid. Dimensional representation has a number of important advantages over categorization. In the first place it is more flexible and capable of providing more information. Compare, for example, the information provided about the intelligence of a population by a set of IQ scores and by the information that x members of that population were clever, y unremarkable and z stupid. Two individuals with IQs of 120 and 160 would both, presumably, be allocated to the 'clever' category, although this would obscure an important difference between them. Two individuals with IQs of 114 and 116, on the other hand, might find themselves in different categories although in fact the difference between them was trivial. Moreover, a distribution of IQ scores can always be converted into any number of categories as occasion demands and the boundaries of these moved up or down the scale at will. But the reverse cannot be done. Categories cannot be converted to dimensions, or the number of categories changed except by amalgamating existing ones. Dimensions have two further advantages that are particularly important where mental illness is concerned. They eliminate the use of labels like schizophrenic and hysteric which have acquired harmful pejorative connotations; and they do not distract attention from, or distort perception of, individuals lying near the boundary between two adjacent categories, as typologies habitually do. Consider, for example, the many patients with both affective and schizophrenic symptoms. The distinction drawn in categorical classifications between schizophrenic and affective psychoses generally results in one component of the symptomatology of these patients being glossed over or ignored, and for research purposes they are commonly discarded. In a dimensional classification on the other hand their intermediate status is accurately represented by an intermediate score on the appropriate dimension.

There are, however, several disadvantages to dimensional systems. A system involving more than one dimension can only be handled algebraically or geometrically, and if there are more than three only the former is possible. This is not necessarily a defect but it does mean that those using the system must have a greater familiarity with mathematics than is possessed by most psychiatrists. A more fundamental problem is that dimensional systems usually have to be converted to categories before the information they contain can usefully be applied to individuals. For example, although it may be of considerable theoretical interest to know that the correlation between response to ECT and a particular dimension of depressive symptomatology is 0.71, the important practical question is whether patients with scores between x and y on that dimension are more likely to respond to ECT than to a tricyclic drug. Partly for this reason, and partly because no one has yet produced a viable dimensional system covering mental illness as a whole, dimensional classifications have only been used up to now in a few limited areas, to express the relationship between different types of functional psychosis, for example, or the relationship between psychotic and neurotic depressions.

Although dimensional and categorical classifications can both be used in a wide variety of situations, and the choice between them may legitimately depend on the use to which the classification is to be put, dimensions are more obviously relevant in areas where variation is, or appears to be, continuous, and categories more obviously relevant where variation is, or is likely to be, discontinuous. For this reason the attractions of a dimensional classification are much greater where personality disorders are concerned than for the functional psychoses, though it is perhaps worth noting *en passant* that our traditional assumption that the various forms of psychotic illness we recognize are distinct conditions each with its own separate aetiology has remarkably little firm evidence to sustain it.

The International Classification

We have already seen that classification is essential for almost all useful communication. However, two psychiatrists or two nations can only communicate successfully with one another if both are using the same classification and until quite recently psychiatry was badly hampered by the lack of any common classification, or even any agreed nomenclature.* Most countries or administrations had their own nomenclatures; indeed so did many university departments, and even within their own territories many of these were widely ignored. In the last twenty years, however, the World Health Organization has made strenuous and on the whole successful efforts to persuade governments and national societies to agree to use a common international classification. Although the 6th revision of the International Classification (ICD–6) in 1948 was officially adopted by only five countries, and used half-heartedly even by them, the 8th revision in 1968 was formally adopted by almost every country with organized psychiatric services and its code numbers were widely used in the international literature.

The present revision, the 9th, was introduced in 1979 (World Health Organization, 1978) and, like its immediate predecessors, will remain in use for a decade. The differences between the 8th and 9th revisions, like those between the 6th and the 8th, are fairly modest but reflect none the less a steady expansion of psychiatry's sphere of interest and an increasing awareness of the importance of defining the meaning of the terms employed. Perhaps the most important single innovation in ICD–9 is the inclusion of a reasonably comprehensive classification of the disorders of childhood and adolescence. In place of the single omnibus category of ICD–8 there are now separate categories for childhood psychoses, conduct disorders, the hyperkinetic syndrome, specific developmental delays, and emotional disorders. Another important innovation is the incorporation of a comprehensive glossary as an integral part of the classification. Every diagnostic term, both major 3-digit categories like schizophrenia and personality disorder and the 4-digit categories that represent their various subdivisions, is followed by a brief description of the salient clinical features of that condition and sometimes by criteria for distinguishing it from related conditions as well. This built-in glossary is unique to the mental disorders section (chapter V) of the International Classification and has been provided in recognition of the great difficulties created for psychiatry by the lack of laboratory criteria, and the chaotic situation created in the past by diagnostic

---

* A nomenclature is simply an approved list of categories or titles. In order to constitute a classification its categories must be mutually exclusive and jointly exhaustive, and may have other formal relationships with one another as well, being arranged either in tiers or in a hierarchy.

terms being used in different ways in different countries.

The International Classification is necessarily rather conservative both in its format and its detailed content. Because it would be of little use unless most of the individuals and nations who contribute to the psychiatric literature were prepared to use it, all changes and innovations must have the consent of a large international committee. Like a convoy, its speed is determined by that of its slowest members. Radical changes, like the introduction of operational definitions and multiple axes, are particularly difficult to effect; and conditions like depressive illnesses, which tend to be classified in different ways in different countries and arouse strong feelings as well, cause almost insuperable problems. National representatives make it clear that their compatriots will be unable or unwilling to use the classification unless it contains their favourite diagnostic categories and the end result is the inclusion of several incompatible concepts simultaneously. This is why, although ICD–6 contained only three varieties of depressive illness, ICD–9 contains no less than 10 three-digit categories and 19 four-digit categories where patients with depressive symptoms can be coded. The participation of most governments and national associations has been assured and life has been made easier for record clerks, but in the process all coherence and unity have been lost. For all its shortcomings, however, the International Classification is an invaluable means of communication. In most respects ICD–9 is a great improvement on ICD–6 and we must all recognize our obligation to use it. We may, if we wish, use other classifications as well, but the advantages of being able to communicate freely and reasonably accurately with other workers throughout the world are so great that it is worth tolerating a classification that falls short of our personal aspirations.

The hierarchy of diagnoses

Like most other classifications of mental illness, the International Classification starts with the organic psychoses (categories 290–294). Next comes schizophrenia (295), followed by affective and other functional psychoses (296–299), neurotic disorders (300) and personality disorders (301). The order is not accidental. It is a reflection of the fact that these disorders form a hierarchy with five tiers in which each tier is allowed to exhibit the characteristic features of all lower tiers, but not of any higher level. Organic psychoses constitute the highest tier and if a patient has clear evidence of brain disease, like epilepsy or a positive CSF WR, that establishes that he has an organic psychosis regardless of which particular psychotic or neurotic symptoms he possesses. Schizophrenia comes next in the hierarchy and if a patient exhibits the characteristic symptoms of schizophrenia that is usually sufficient to establish the diagnosis, regardless of whether or not he is also depressed or paranoid, or has delusions of guilt or obsessional symptoms. Schneider's dictum that his 'symptoms of the first rank' are pathognomonic of schizophrenia 'except in the presence of coarse brain disease' is an explicit recognition of schizophrenia's status in this hierarchy, as is the convention that 'schizo-affective' patients are classified as a type of schizophrenia rather than as a type of affective psychosis (see also vol. 3, chap. 4). The same considerations apply to the lower tiers. Neurotic illness, the fourth tier, can only be diagnosed in the absence of all psychotic symptoms, though there is no objection to the presence of the characteristic features of the fifth tier – lifelong personality disorder.

It is likely that this hierarchy is man-made, though it seems to have developed unwittingly and not by design. It is one of the fundamental principles of medicine to try whenever possible to account for the patient's symptoms by a single diagnosis. In psychiatry, however, nearly every symptom of psychopathological significance is capable of appearing in the presence of nearly every other symptom, and in such a situation the arrangement of symptoms in an arbitrary hierarchy, with the least common at the top and the most widespread at the bottom, provides almost the only way of making single diagnoses. It has been claimed, however, that patients with disorders at the top of the hierarchy not only may but do possess the symptoms of all the disorders below it; that schizophrenics, for example, not only can but in practice characteristically do have paranoid, grandiose or guilty delusions, neurotic symptoms, and mood disturbances, as well as their schizophrenic symptoms. If this is so, and it is not yet clear that it is, there are obviously important implications for our theories of aetiology.

Multi-axial classifications

Reference has already been made to the fact that in most commonly used classifications, including the International Classification, although most disorders are defined in syndromal terms some, like alcoholic and psychogenic psychoses, are defined in aetiological terms. Other diagnoses, like schizophrenia, are sometimes interpreted as incorporating aetiological assumptions and sometimes simply as statements about symptomatology. The result is much unnecessary confusion. Psychiatrists who do not accept the aetiological implications of terms like psychogenic psychosis refuse to use them, although they may have no difficulty in recognizing the syndrome in question; and disagreements develop about whether, for example, a patient is schizophrenic or not because one clinician is recognizing the characteristic symptoms of the condition and the other refusing to accept that the illness is 'endogenous'. The answer to such problems, as the Swedish psychiatrist Essen-Möller (1971) has often pointed out, is to separate symptomatology and aetiology by having separate classifications for each. This prevents convictions about aetiology from contaminating judgements about symptomatology, and has other advantages for the designation of illnesses whose aetiology is known, or presumed to be known. For example, in a classification of traditional type a manic illness developing in the puerperium might be classified either as a puerperal psychosis or as mania. In practice, regardless of what instructions are given in the relevant glossary, some such illnesses are classified one way and some the other, and either way important information is lost. A dual classification, however, enables all puerperal illnesses to be designated as such regardless of their aetiology. Similar considerations apply to schizophrenic illnesses secondary to temporal lobe epilepsy or precipitated by amphetamine abuse.

The argument for recording aetiology and symptomatology separately is therefore quite strong. However, once the principle of a single comprehensive diagnosis is abandoned good arguments can also be found for providing separate classifications for several other aspects of the patient's problem as well. For this reason multi-axial classifications usually contain three or four axes and not just two. In 1969 an international working party (Rutter, *et al.*, 1969) recommended that WHO should adopt a tri-axial classification for the psychiatric disorders of childhood with separate axes for the clinical syndrome, the child's intellectual level, and 'aetiological and associated factors', and a subsequent suggestion that physical and psychosocial factors should be handled separately increased these three axes to four. Ottosson and Perris (1973) in Sweden use a classification of adult disorders with four axes (symptomatology, severity, aetiology, and course) for routine clinical assessments as well as for research purposes and the official classification of the American Psychiatric

Association (DSM–III) (1979) incorporates five separate axes (*vide infra*).

Although classifications of this type are usually referred to as 'multi-axial' or 'multidimensional' these terms are rather misleading because they have nothing in common with the dimensional classifications discussed on pages 194–5. Patients do not have scores on linear dimensions, nor do the axes have any geometric or algebraic relationship to one another. The multiple 'axes' are simply a number of important but arbitrarily chosen aspects of mental disorder, each of which is accorded a separate (usually categorical) classification of its own. It remains to be seen whether multi-axial classifications of this kind will come into widespread use in the future. Undoubtedly, they provide more information than unitary diagnoses and prevent disagreements about aetiology from contaminating other areas of discourse, but in doing so they make the process of classification considerably more complicated. To some extent they are a cross between a diagnosis and a formulation, and can be seen as an attempt to provide some of the wealth of information provided by a formulation in a form suitable for group comparisons and scientific analysis.

The American Psychiatric Association's Classification (DSM–III)

The American Psychiatric Association was the first body to produce a glossary describing the meaning of the various terms recognized in its official nomenclature and the relationship of these terms to one another. The first edition of this Diagnostic and Statistical Manual (DSM–I), published in 1952, was strongly influenced by the psycho-analytic and Meyerian schools which dominated American psychiatry at that time. The second edition, though, was based on the nomenclature and format of the 8th revision of the International Classification (ICD–8), domestic preferences being sacrificed on this occasion for the sake of international agreement. The authors of the third edition, however, were not prepared to postpone the major changes they wished to introduce and abandoned the format and terminology of the International Classification, though ICD code numbers were retained to enable either nomenclature to be translated into the other. The content and format of DSM–III are radically different from those both of its own predecessors and of the International Classification and reflect the sudden resurgence of interest in psychiatric nosology of contemporary American psychiatry.

In the first place DSM–III is a multi-axial classification with five separate axes, the first dealing with the syndromes of mental disorder and the second with personality disorders in adults and specific developmental disorders (e.g. enuresis and specific reading disorders) in children. The third axis is for associated non-psychiatric conditions which either are of aetiological significance (e.g. head injury) or influence management (e.g. diabetes). The fourth axis is a linear grading of the severity of psychosocial stressors and the fifth a similar grading of the highest level of social and occupational functioning achieved in the past year.

An even more important innovation is the systematic provision of operational diagnostic criteria. Instead of the thumbnail sketches provided in most other glossaries, unambiguous criteria are provided for every category in the manual, stipulating precisely which combinations of symptoms and other characteristics are and are not adequate to establish that diagnosis. The need for criteria of this kind has been apparent for more than a decade but extensive clinical trials, field studies, and consultations are needed before sufficiently wide agreement can be obtained on the detailed criteria for each condition to make their incorporation into a national glossary a practical proposition. Properly used – and it remains to be seen whether they will be properly used – these operational criteria should greatly increase the reliability of diagnostic assignments, not just in research but in routine clinical work as well, and in the long run this increased reliability should strengthen the therapeutic and prognostic inferences derived from these diagnoses.

The third important innovation is one of terminology. Many hallowed names like manic-depressive psychosis and hysteria have been discarded and replaced by deliberately unpretentious terms like episodic affective disorder and dissociative disorder. Doubtless many will lament the change, but it has long been apparent that antique terms like neurosis and hysteria are encrusted with so many layers of meaning and trail so many false assumptions in their wake that we are really better off without them. Much will depend on how successful DSM–III proves to be in practice. If the majority of American psychiatrists accept its many innovations and find them helpful then it is likely that the next revision of the International Classification will also incorporate them, but if they are widely misunderstood or ignored the more cautious policy of WHO will be vindicated.

8
Diagnosis and the diagnostic process

J. E. COOPER

Introduction

This chapter starts with a discussion of the concept 'diagnosis' and then examines the sequence of activities that constitute the diagnostic process, keeping clinical practice in mind. The reliability of psychiatric diagnosis is then examined, and this is followed by a brief discussion of the importance of 'operational criteria' and the use of computers in diagnosis.

The diagnostic process is more than the choosing of a diagnostic term from a classification of disorders and diseases. Before the final act of classification is possible, the clinician must work through a complicated series of activities and processes, whose importance is often underestimated. The diagnosis itself also should be seen in perspective as only one part of the wider process of clinical formulation. The interdependence of diagnostic process, classification, and formulation is a theme which is intentionally emphasized in this chapter, and it is also evident in the preceding chapter on classification. In a general sense classification and diagnosis can hardly be separated, but the specific topic of classification of disease concepts in psychiatry is sufficiently important in its own right to merit discussion separately (pp. 191–8).

What is a diagnosis?

Every society possesses healers who are consulted by those who feel unwell and who do not know how to get themselves better. The healer's task is to discover the underlying cause of the unpleasant experience – that is, he should be able to see through the presenting symptoms and signs and diagnose another and different kind of process (*dia* = one apart from another; *gnōsis* = recognition, knowledge, perception). The healer's expert knowledge and skills then enable him to alleviate the symptoms and signs by treatment of the underlying cause. In modern medical terms, the underlying cause or process is called the disease and when it has been identified the person consulting is called ill. Treatment then follows, determined by current ideas of aetiology and the technical remedies available. There are also usually important social consequences of being 'ill' and having 'treatment' from a doctor, in terms of lessened responsibility and overtly expressed sympathy and support from relatives and friends. The 'illness behaviour' of the patient as a result of these social and cultural influences (Parsons, 1951; Mechanic, 1961, 1978) needs to be separated from the effects of the symptoms of any physical disease processes that are present.

Diagnoses are made in whatever terms seem familiar and useful to the doctor, derived from current ideas of causation of illness and leading to the treatment based upon the same set of ideas. Doctors of previous generations made diagnoses couched in the medical ideas of their times which now seem strange, and doctors of the future will make useful diagnoses that we cannot now even imagine. Medical practice can also encourage illness behaviour under the guise of treatment (for instance, in the form of changing fashions for the length of stay in bed following childbirth or coronary thrombosis).

Modern medical knowledge and technology have refined our knowledge of the aetiology and pathology of many disorders to a remarkable degree in only a few generations, and doctors in most medical disciplines have come to regard an aetiological statement (with physiological or anatomical implications) as the only correct meaning of 'diagnosis'. Similarly, 'the diagnostic process' is now often seen only as the use of medical technology in the search for a tangible aetiology. It is unfortunately easy to forget that a large number of patients in many medical disciplines are never given a definite and satisfying aetiological diagnosis. The doctor often has to be content with a provisional or intermediate statement, reflecting all that he can conclude about likely causes for the presenting symptoms. But even though it is incomplete or simply descriptive, such a state-

ment is still a diagnosis in the above general sense, so long as it is the most useful and illuminating statement available according to current medical knowledge. It may well be that we need some new terms to convey different degrees of knowledge and inference about underlying processes or lesions, particularly within psychiatry. Until other acceptable terms are proposed, we must continue to make do with 'diagnosis', but preferably qualifying it by adjectives such as 'descriptive' 'psycho-dynamic' 'aetiological' or 'anatomical', depending upon which framework of ideas is being used.

Qualified diagnostic statements such as these are particularly important in psychiatry, where patients with widely differing types of disorders are encountered. For instance, for purposes of making a diagnosis in the way just described, on current knowledge psychiatric conditions can be put into three main groups:

(1) Disorders with a known cerebral lesion or physiological malfunction – traditionally called the organic psychoses whether the known cause is anatomical or physiological. In patients with these disorders, the diagnosis will be an aetiological statement and will indicate treatment.

(2) Disorders whose only measurable characteristics are behavioural and emotional, but about which knowledge is now accumulating that makes it reasonable to assume that there is a very important neurophysiological component. These are the manic-depressive and the schizophrenic illnesses, traditionally called the functional psychoses. Patients with disorders in this group cannot be said to have aetiological diagnoses, but yet current concepts of what underlies schizophrenia and manic-depressive illness have developed a long way from simple listing of symptoms. Evidence is accumulating which suggests the presence of disorders of mechanisms of arousal and perception, and in addition abnormalities of neuro-transmitters and other highly active cerebral amines may be concerned. Explanatory hypotheses are still fragmentary and provisional, but a diagnosis of this kind represents a level of meaning somewhere between the established aetiology of the organic group and the purely behavioural syndromes of the next group.

(3) Disorders whose manifestations cannot (and perhaps will not) be explained in terms other than the acquiring and persistence of maladaptive behaviour. The neuroses and the personality disorders come into this group, as do sexual and antisocial behav-

iour disorders and the large majority of psychiatric disorders of childhood and adolescence. The problems of these patients are caused by excesses of behaviour and emotions that are in themselves common and familiar to all. Most of these patients are usually viewed as having learned the unwanted behaviour, and few psychiatrists or psychologists see any need for postulating any underlying disorders of structure or of biochemical mechanisms. Instead it seems more reasonable to think of the abnormality being primarily in the nature, frequency and intensity of the learning experiences to which the individual has been subject.

Even these brief comments are enough to show that quite different types of concept are involved in searching for a diagnosis in different patients. Viewed in this way the diagnosis is an essential part of a medical assessment and is not tied to any particular model of aetiology or degree of understanding: as knowledge increases, the diagnosis will be expressed at increasingly useful levels of meaning. So long as a qualifying adjective is attached to the word 'diagnosis' it should be clear what level of knowledge is being implied. Suggestions that diagnostic terms in psychiatry are useless or even harmful (Menninger, 1963) are based largely upon a restriction of the concept of diagnosis to knowledge of organic aetiology, together with misunderstandings about the need for varying emphasis upon different sections of the overall clinical formulation in different types of psychiatric patients.

Relationships between diagnosis, classification, and clinical formulation

Classification is a central part of the diagnostic process. As a diagnostic interview proceeds, the clinician selects some of the information about the patient and uses it to fit him into a particular system of classification of psychiatric disorders – that is, he gives the patient a diagnosis. As we have seen, the way in which the diagnosis is expressed will depend upon current knowledge of underlying processes, and also upon the state of development of techniques of classification (see chapter 7).

The diagnostic process itself is only a part of the wider process of clinical formulation. In clinical work no patient has been properly assessed until a formulation has been put together which contains many things in addition to a discussion of the diagnosis. The formulation should indicate the extent to which the patient's upbringing and life experience have influenced his development, and whether these are related to his present state and current problems. In some psychiatric patients there will be a diagnosis expressed in terms of organic disease processes which will be by far the most important part of the formulation. Even in these cases, the formulation will often emphasize the interplay between the organic disease and psycho-dynamic and social influences.

In others, the diagnostic term itself will be a much less precise term, such as some variety of personality disorder, which indicates only a tendency towards certain unwanted behaviour patterns or emotional reactions. For these patients, it is likely that comparatively large sections of the formulation will be taken up by listing problems to do with personal relationships and social maladjustment; a discussion of these will determine what is to be done and the diagnostic label itself is only a general indicator of the type of problem to be expected. The importance of the formulation is that it ensures that a number of possible ways of looking at the patient have been explored, so that the most relevant issues are given precedence whatever their nature.

The components of the diagnostic process

If we consider the usual clinical situation of a psychiatrist interviewing a patient, the following components of the diagnostic process can be distinguished:

(1) The interviewing technique of the psychiatrist.
(2) His perception of the patient's speech and behaviour, whether they be spontaneous, or in response to the psychiatrist.
(3) A complicated series of processes during which the psychiatrist sorts out the information in order to make a variety of inferences and decisions. It is convenient to examine this in two stages:

(i) A first stage in which the psychiatrist sifts through all he perceives, deciding how to use the information and what to ask next. This includes separating the information out into categories such as symptoms, personality traits, social and personal problems and social disabilities.

(ii) A second stage of summarization and classification of the potentially diagnostic information selected by the first stage. Symptoms, syndromes, disease concepts, or behaviour patterns can begin to emerge, according to the type of patient and the set of ideas the psychiatrist is using.

(4) A final stage of classification, in which the psychiatrist chooses one or more terms from a stated classification of psychiatric disorders, so that the diagnosis of the patient can be recorded and communicated to others in a way they will understand.

The importance of those steps in the diagnostic process that precede the final classification is usually underestimated, probably because in ordinary clinical work they are rapid and the clinician is often unaware or only half aware of them.

Although the whole diagnostic process is a sequence of activity, these elements are too interdependent to be regarded as separate steps in the sequence. Each step is necessary for the next one to take place, but the results of each step begin at once to influence its predecessor. For instance, the interviewing technique and the content of the question will have been predetermined to some extent by the diagnostic system that the psychiatrist is using. In addition, since perception is partly a learned process, the psychiatrist's perception of the patient will be influenced by his psychiatric training and by previous interviewing experience. Each decision he makes about the meaning of the patient's behaviour and responses will influence what he is likely to ask next, within the context of his interviewing technique. All these processes go on in the psychiatrist's mind as the interview proceeds, and determine the questions that are asked; these in their turn result in more information to be processed in the same way.

Because of the complexity of these processes and the speed at which they occur, it is easy to see how differences can arise between psychiatrists when presented with the same patient. With such variation in mind, the individual elements in the diagnostic process noted above will now be examined.

(1) Interviewing technique

An interview can be regarded as a conversation with a purpose. Conversation implies that both parties will contribute, and most conscious attempts to develop particular techniques of interviewing have this mutuality in mind. The purpose of a diagnostic interview will be to obtain information in a form and sequence that will help the clinician in his search first for diagnostic clues and then for confirmation and amplification of his possible diagnostic choices.

The clinician's knowledge of possible diseases, syndromes, and symptoms and of how to detect psychopathological and psychological processes and mechanisms will determine to a large extent his efficiency in eliciting information. His own experience and personal attributes such as verbal fluency and self-confidence will also play a major part. 'Empathy' and 'rapport' are often emphasized as desirable qualities to be cultivated which will allow the search for information to be conducted while an optimal relationship is established with the patient. Neither of these is an exact term, although both are often discussed and confused. Rapport is probably best viewed as a very general term implying mutual understanding and willingness to co-operate because of the establishment of feelings of mutual respect and trust. Empathy has been studied more specifically (Truax, 1966) and can be regarded as the ability to be sensitive to another person's feelings plus the ability to communicate this understanding to the other; it is a large part of the concept of 'warmth'. Neither rapport nor empathy should be equated with the attempts to be informal and to agree indiscriminately with the patient which often occur as a result of inexperience or over-enthusiasm.

Training in diagnostic and other types of clinical interviewing is naturally a major topic in most psychiatric establishments, but surprisingly little systematic knowledge is available about the effect of such attempts to change or develop interviewing behaviour; those studies which have been reported are almost all concerned with training for special methods of rating and interviewing in research work. From the comparatively few studies done in a clinical setting, three rather chastening points are worth remembering. First, consistent differences can be demonstrated in the tendency of raters to respond in a stereotyped way irrespective of what is being observed (Grosz & Grossman, 1968). Second, clinical experience may well interfere with the ability to make unprejudiced ratings (Lehmann, Ban & Donald, 1965). Finally, the length of clinical experience may be more powerful than the type of experience or theoretical framework being used. Fiedler (1950) studied the interviewing styles of three supposedly different types of therapist (psycho-analytic, non-directive Rogerian, and Adlerian), and found that experienced experts of all three schools resembled each other more closely than they resembled non-experts of their own school.

For clinical purposes, a compromise has to be reached between the needs for structure and systematic coverage, and the need for the flexibility that allows the interviewer to participate naturally in the personal and interactive aspects of the interview. In practice, most of these points can be accommodated by following the same simple and logical set of principles that are often taught as the basis of interviewing in all medical disciplines:

(1) First ensure that the patient has ample opportunity to describe his problems, complaints, and symptoms in his own way.

(2) Ask general or open-ended questions to introduce topics that seem important, and follow up the first hints or clues with general probing questions (about time, frequency, intensity, so as to obtain specific examples of symptoms and events).

(3) Use detailed confirmatory or leading questions about specific symptoms, behaviour, and feelings after these general questions and not before.

(4) Confirm any conclusions reached about the key symptoms and behaviour by putting them to the patient in terms he will understand, to see if he agrees.

In addition to its importance as a guide to efficient and sympathetic interviewing in clinical work, this same sequence has formed the basis of a number of systematic and comprehensive standardized interview procedures used widely in research where high levels of reliability are required. This aspect of interviewing and diagnosis is discussed later.

Detailed guidance on the content and sequence of clinical interviewing can be found in convenient publications such as Leff and Isaacs (1968) and in pocket-sized note-books prepared by teaching institutions (Institute of Psychiatry, 1973). Field workers in disciplines outside medicine often take a more professional and technical look at interviewing procedures than does the medical profession, and most psychiatrists will learn a good deal by examining some of the more general publications on the subject (such as Matarazzo and Wiens, 1972; Marquis, Cannell & Laurent, 1972).

(2) Perception

It is easy for the busy clinician to forget the complexity of the processes by which we perceive and make judgements about the emotions and personality traits of other persons. These processes are also subject to the same influences as are judgements about less complicated stimuli such as colour, shape,

and movement. Some general points about perception are worth noting, since they immediately highlight a variety of possible sources of bias in judging other persons.

Perception is necessarily a selective process in which some of the information available is omitted, since all possible stimuli cannot be registered simultaneously. In addition, what is perceived is often supplemented in order to make the perceived material fit better into the observer's frame of reference. These points have been well known for many years, but are rarely discussed during psychiatric training. For striking examples there is no need for experiments using sophisticated technology; Bartlett's work (1932) on the remembering of stories and pictures contains many instances of both omission and supplementation. This whole process, by which incoming stimuli are sorted out and given meaning, was well summarized by Newcomb (1950) as 'structuring . . . a process of omitting some features, supplying others, highlighting one or a few and subordinating the rest in the interests of making sense out of the environment'.

Another way of summarizing this process is to say that the expectations of the observer will influence the conclusions he arrives at from a given set of information. In the clinical setting, an important example of this is seen in the effect that knowledge of a patient's previous state or diagnosis can have upon judgements of the present state. Bias of this sort can be demonstrated easily as a training exercise by obtaining the judgements of groups of clinicians about selected extracts of audio-tapes or video-tapes of patients, some with and some without additional information about the patient. An additional type of bias of diagnostic importance is the influence upon perception of symptoms that comes from expectations acquired during the interviewer's psychiatric training. Abnormalities whose presence is anticipated are sought more diligently and detected more readily than others, whereas any that are unexpected are liable to be glossed over, or not recognized at all (Grinker, *et al.*, 1961; Kendell, 1968).

In addition to specifically psychiatric expectations of the sort just noted, there are more general influences on interpersonal perception that have been extensively studied by social psychologists. The best known are probably the 'halo effect' and 'logical error'. Thorndike (1920) coined the term 'halo effect' to summarize a consistent error found in ratings of personality traits due to 'suffusing ratings of special features with a halo belonging to the individual as a whole'. For instance, if an observer is making a number of ratings of the traits of another person, it can be shown that he makes first of all an overall decision that the person is good or bad in general; he then makes more specific trait ratings so as to fit in with the overall goodness or badness to a much greater extent than is justified by the detailed evidence available about the specific traits. This same effect of increasing intercorrelation between judgements can also result from the 'logical error' described by Newcomb (1931) and Guildford (1954). This is the tendency of observers to give a person similar ratings on characteristics which are logically related in the opinion of the observer; for instance, a man judged to be industrious on good evidence may also be described as dependable, intelligent and a good leader on very little evidence, simply because in the opinion of the person making the judgements these traits usually go together.

These influences upon the diagnostician can be expected to be particularly strong when dealing with the comparatively subtle and minor degrees of abnormality that are common when dealing with those in whom there is doubt about the presence of a definite disorder, or when attempts are being made to identify new or unfamiliar conditions. The perceptual processes and personalities of those making the judgements can certainly have a considerable influence upon supposedly rational ratings of normal individuals, as was very obviously the case in a large study by Raines and Rohrer (1954) based upon experienced psychiatrists rating candidates for officer selection.

Judgements can never be free from bias, but unwanted effects can be minimized if the interviewing clinician is aware of the main varieties and sources of bias in general, and if he has tried to identify his own particular tendencies.

(3) (i) *Inferences, decisions, and the first stage of sorting into different types of information.*

The psychiatrist is much more aware of making decisions about the points to be examined in this next section, in contrast to most of the processes of perceiving discussed above. He needs to allocate the information about the patient into a few major types of information, each with a quite different significance. Even if the patient can give an organized chronological account of his troubles, what emerges during the interview is usually a mixture of information about symptoms, personality traits, personal

relationship problems, and social or work problems, together with accounts of any resulting social disability. The psychiatrist cannot get a balanced picture of events upon which to base his formulation until the relative importance of these different types of information for the individual patient has been determined. It is particularly important not to confuse the usually intrusive behaviour of the present illness with that of the pre-morbid personality, which is often difficult to establish in chronic or mild disorders. Another common error is to assume that symptoms are a reliable guide to social disability. Although these are both at a peak in acute conditions, they can vary almost independently in chronic disorders; a patient with an obsessional illness, for instance, may be able to conceal distressing symptoms and be almost normal outwardly, in contrast to a chronic schizophrenic patient who is socially withdrawn and incapacitated but has only a few of the 'negative' symptoms and no complaints.

As soon as the psychiatrist begins to form initial impressions about likely causes for the patient's symptoms and other complaints, he needs to decide what to ask about next. The systematic study of decision-making in clinical situations has not proved popular amongst psychiatrists, perhaps because of the uncomfortably obvious differences between individuals when faced with similar tasks. The extensive literature on decision theory, problem-solving, and the theory of games does not provide much guidance because laboratory experiments from which models and theories have been derived are usually games or tasks with very simple rules and a carefully restricted number of choices – obviously a far cry from a clinical interview. Bayes' theorem in particular (Edwards, Lindman, & Savage, 1963) cannot be used as a statistical model 'for the revision of opinions in the light of new information' unless the prevalence of what is being studied is known in the total population from which the patients are selected; this is a grave drawback in the case of psychiatric disorders.

A limited degree of understanding of clinical decisions about diagnosis has come from the writing of computer programs which mimic clinical diagnostic procedures: these are discussed in a later section. In their present forms these programs are linked to fairly cumbersome standardized techniques for obtaining clinical information suitable for research projects, but simplified forms could become widely used as an aid to ordinary clinical work if advantage is taken of the desk-top micro-processors now becoming available. So long as computer aids are used to supplement rather than to supplant common-sense and clinical experience, they can be a useful reminder of the unsystematic nature of many clinical decision processes.

The few studies of decision-making in psychiatric clinical work which do exist highlight two surprising features, first, the rapidity with which confident diagnostic decisions are made, and second, a lack of awareness on the part of the psychiatrist as to which items of information are the crucial ones. In a study of filmed interviews, Gauron and Dickinson (1966) noted that their psychiatrists often formed quite definite diagnostic impressions within the first minute of an interview. Similarly, Sandifer, Hordern, and Green (1970) found that after three minutes of film-viewing the psychiatrists they were studying had arrived at a diagnosis which was the same in three-quarters of the cases as their final diagnosis, made on average about twenty-five minutes later. These findings were confirmed by Kendell (1973) using diagnostic statements obtained from psychiatrists after two minutes and five minutes of viewing video-tapes of a variety of psychiatric patients. These studies by Gauron and Dickinson and by Kendell also showed that the psychiatrists were often unaware of which items of information they were using for diagnostic decisions, and that some items they thought to be crucial, such as behaviour and projective test results, in fact carried little diagnostic weight.

Closely allied to the timing and basis of decisions is the style of thinking and questioning adopted by the individual psychiatrists. Gauron and Dickinson (1969) made some preliminary suggestions, dividing their psychiatrists along two dimensions – one of inductive–logical versus intuitive–logical thinking, and one of structured versus unstructured method. A few studies of these issues have been reported from medical and surgical disciplines (Elstein *et al.*, 1972; Leaper *et al.*, 1973) but generalization of their findings to psychiatric problems must be tentative in view of the less clear-cut nature of many psychiatric conditions. The strengths and weaknesses of conventional diagnostic interviews in psychiatry are obviously in need of further exploration.

(3) (ii) *Summarization and classification of potentially diagnostic information*

What goes on in the clinician's mind during this stage will be largely determined by the type of classification chosen by him as most applicable to the patient. Classifications based upon symptoms and

upon disease concepts, and the use of categories and dimensions (or both) are discussed in the preceding chapter on Classification (chap. 7). For the purpose of this present review of the whole diagnostic process, only one point of major importance in clinical work will be noted.

Clinical decisions can be fruitfully discussed if the procedures and ideas upon which they are based are systematic and consistent and can be communicated to others. A few moments spent at almost any psychiatric case-discussion or clinical conference, however, will usually provide examples of clinicians making diagnostic decisions but yet finding it difficult to explain the reasons or thought processes behind the decisions. In the present state of psychiatric knowledge, different viewpoints and clinical styles are to be encouraged, but the simple opposition of different conclusions about the same problem or patient is not likely to be constructive. The development by discussion of some knowledge of one's own decision processes and prejudices should form part of clinical training and continued education, for without it there is presumably an inevitable tendency to develop idiosyncratic and inexplicable clinical habits.

(4) *The final choice of a diagnostic label*

Every clinician necessarily develops a system of classification for his personal use, and it is likely that it will bear some resemblance to one or other of the national or international systems. He will also have some beliefs and clinical impressions of his own, but so long as the more idiosyncratic ideas are subject to debate and testing, they can be a desirable and potentially constructive stimulus.

For administrative and statistical purposes, a common framework of ideas is necessary, and systems of classification such as the International Classification of Diseases (currently in its Ninth Revision) (WHO 1978) and the DSM–III (Diagnostic and Statistical Manual of the American Psychiatric Association, third edition, 1980) are the result of this need. Several other systems exist, but there has been a welcome tendency over the last few decades for most countries to show an increasing willingness to use one of the major systems as a reference point for both internal and international communication. Clinicians and teachers are often unnecessarily suspicious of 'official' classifications, apparently feeling that their use might inhibit individuality or innovation in diagnostic thinking. The opposite should be the case, particularly for DSM–III and ICD–9, since a detailed glossary of terms is an integral part of both of these. The educational potential of such officially recognized systems is considerable, and is specifically noted by the World Health Organization in the case of ICD–9: 'Apart from its primary purpose of fostering communication, Chapter V of ICD–9 with its glossary can also serve as an educational stimulus, since it was compiled by psychiatrists representing many different countries and points of view. It is hoped that discussion of these difficult and controversial points will serve to highlight the problems underlying all systems of medical and psychiatric classification, and will emphasize the need to acknowledge and try to understand the opinions of others' (WHO, 1978).

Finally, the clinician should always know what use will be made of the diagnosis he is recording for a patient, particularly when completing official documents. He should be clear in his own mind whether he is classifying only the main illness of the patient by choosing just one term out of a classification of psychiatric conditions, or whether he is making a more complicated statement in order to classify a patient who may have several conditions at the same time, of differing degrees of importance and permanence. Clinical work usually requires the second of these, and a few simple rules are needed which allow a classification of conditions (such as the ICD) to be used for classifying persons. A simple and useful example of this is to record Main, Subsidiary, and Alternative Diagnoses when using the ICD. The minimum to be recorded in the case-notes should be a Main Diagnosis, plus one or more Subsidiary Diagnoses if needed. These should be followed by an Alternative Diagnosis when reasonably probable alternatives exist, and there may be alternatives to either or both of the Main and Subsidiary diagnoses. The Main and Subsidiary Diagnoses do not conflict with or exclude each other, but are complementary since both conditions are being declared present at the same time (for instance, Main Diagnosis: Paranoid Schizophrenia; Subsidiary Diagnosis: Obsessional Personality Disorder). The Alternative Diagnoses provide another way of interpreting the diagnostic information when there is reasonable doubt about the degree of confidence with which the Main and Subsidiary Diagnoses are held. For example, a reasonable alternative to the example just given might be Main Diagnosis: Obsessional Neurosis; Subsidiary Diagnosis: Paranoid Personality Disorder. To record alternatives such as these in the case-

notes, plus explanatory comments, indicates the degree of confidence in the diagnostic assessment of the patient; this may have important implications both currently and in any future illnesses.

The reliability of psychiatric diagnoses

The reliability of diagnostic judgements between psychiatrists presented with the same information varies a great deal, depending upon the type of patient in question and upon the setting in which it is studied. When symptoms are obvious and the underlying disease process is easily conceptualized, as in organic conditions, quite high reliability between clinicians can be demonstrated. When symptoms are less well-defined and underlying processes more speculative, as in many of the neuroses and personality disorders, disagreements abound and reliability can become alarmingly low. Kreitman's study (1961) contained good instances of this variation; he found overall figures of 75 per cent agreement for organic diagnoses and 61 per cent for functional psychoses, but only 28 per cent agreement for neurotic disorders. Beck (1962) and Zubin (1967) similarly arrived at a generally gloomy view of diagnostic reliability, but these reviews (and almost all previous work) dealt with studies in which few or inadequate precautions were taken to ensure that the diagnosticians were using either common data or agreed criteria. Unfortunately these are the conditions which still usually prevail in everyday clinical work, perhaps because there is little interest shown in the study of diagnostic reliability in either general medical education or in psychiatric postgraduate training programmes.

In both clinical work and research, the procedures necessary for the establishment of a reliable diagnosis fall in practice into two stages. The first stage encompasses components one, two, and three of the foregoing analysis of the diagnostic process, and provides the psychiatrist with information about symptoms and behaviour. The second stage is the choice of a diagnostic term from a classification (component four), and for this to be reliable the diagnostic terms need to be described unambiguously and in some detail. The reliability of these two stages will now be discussed in turn, using information derived mainly from research procedures involving the use of various structured and standardized interviewing and rating methods.

The reliability of rating symptoms and behaviour

The first generation of widely used procedures attempted to bring under control only the items to be rated, and left the length and style of the interview up to the discretion of the clinician. Some procedures are confined to one particular type of symptom, such as Hamilton's rating scale for depression (Hamilton, 1960). Others, such as Overall's Brief Psychiatric Rating Scale (Overall & Gorham, 1962), and Lorr's Inpatient Multi-dimensional Psychiatric Rating Scale (Lorr & Klett, 1967) attempt a comprehensive coverage of symptoms. Self description by the patient has also been systematized, and Beck's Self-reporting Inventory for Depression (Beck *et al.*, 1961) is probably the most widely used example of this approach.

Partly controlled procedures such as these still have some uses but as research standards and needs have developed, more precise descriptions of greater reliability have been required. The most recently developed structured and standardized instruments bring both interviewing technique and definition of constituent items under control. Examples of some of these more elaborate procedures are the Present State Examination (Wing, Cooper & Sartorius, 1974) and a slightly less structured interview developed in the General Practice Research Unit (Goldberg *et al.*, 1970). At about the same time, a set of instruments was produced by Spitzer and his colleagues in New York (Spitzer, Endicott & Fleiss, 1967), and more recently this same group has devised schedules aimed particularly at describing affective disorders and schizophrenia (Endicott, J. & Spitzer, R., 1978). Procedures of this generation can be called instruments quite legitimately, and their correct use necessitates a good deal of training and assessment of inter-rater reliability. They are primarily intended for research but clinical workers are likely to benefit from being familiar with their contents, since these instruments are basically a systematic and detailed representation of conventionally accepted psychiatric symptoms and behaviour. The degree of inter-rater reliability that can be achieved by means of these instruments depends upon the amount of practice and training, and where research teams have a similar background and thorough practice together, very satisfactory levels of agreement can be reached (Wing, Cooper & Sartorius, 1974; Kendell *et al.*, 1968).

When planning a research project, it is now usually possible to choose an established set of procedures to match the degree of detail and reliability required, and it is already evident that these instruments have more similarities than differences. Before long, the major need will be to bring existing instruments together rather than to produce more.

Choosing a diagnostic term

A classification cannot be used sensibly unless its constituent terms are described in some detail, and preferably defined. Description of the terms and concepts found in widely used psychiatric classifications has gradually been accepted over the last decade or so as a necessary although at times uncomfortable development. One of the first signs of this was the provision of a glossary of terms for the Eighth Revision of the International Classification of Diseases (ICD–8) by the Office of the Registrar General of the United Kingdom (now the DHSS) in 1968 (HMSO, 1968). The American Psychiatric Association also produced their own Diagnostic and Statistical Manual to ICD–8, or 'DSM–II' (APA 1968). The World Health Organization followed by publishing an international glossary to ICD–8 in 1974 (WHO, 1974) and has recently produced an improved and extended version tailored to the current ninth revision of the ICD (WHO, 1978).

These glossaries all rely upon thumbnail sketches or brief stereotyped descriptions of their constituent conditions, which give considerable latitude to the user in deciding what to include in a category; numbers, relative severity, and duration of symptoms are not specified.

This is the traditional method of describing diagnostic concepts that has been used in textbooks for many years, and although some studies have shown that a classification of this type can be used with high reliability between trained raters working closely together (e.g. Wing *et al.*, 1967), this approach has failed over the years as a means of communication between psychiatrists. For instance, during the 1960s, studies in both the United States of America and in the United Kingdom showed the remarkable extent to which diagnostic concepts in the two countries had diverged, in spite of a common language and a shared European psychiatric heritage. Striking differences in routinely collected hospital admission statistics remarked upon by Slater (1935), Lewis (1946) and Kramer (1961) were shown to be almost entirely due to differences in the concepts used by the psychiatrists rather than to differences between the patients (Sandifer *et al.*, 1968; Katz, Cole & Lowery, 1969; Cooper *et al.*, 1972). The last of these three studies confirmed that most American psychiatrists were using a very broad concept of schizophrenia and a very narrow concept of manic-depressive illness, when compared to British psychiatrists. Some of the differences in diagnostic concepts that have been demonstrated are so great that publication about patients identified only by a diagnosis are likely to lead to grave misunderstandings when read by a psychiatrist from another country. Details of history and mental state are required before the research results of other workers can be interpreted with any confidence.

Practical recognition of this major problem in communication has become evident only recently, in the form of published lists of specified and detailed clinical criteria for psychiatric diagnoses, often referred to as 'operational criteria'. The St. Louis group have been prominent in this development, and have produced a detailed set of criteria recommended by them for use in research (Feighner *et al.*, 1972; Spitzer, R. L., Endicott, J. & Robins, E., 1978). The compilers of 'DSM–III' (the third edition of the Diagnostic and Statistical Manual of the American Psychiatric Association) have been heavily influenced by this example, and a detailed and comprehensive set of operational criteria will be an integral part of this new classification.

To use the detailed criteria of others is often an uncomfortable procedure, but it has no substitute if high standards of reliability and comparability are required. Disagreements and differences of emphasis become immediately identifiable, instead of being hidden or tacitly ignored. Nevertheless, the virtues of operational criteria for comparative research must not be allowed to elevate them beyond their arbitrary and completely practical nature. They must be distinguished sharply from attempts to describe disease concepts or underlying processes, and they must not be confused with characteristics of symptoms or illnesses that are used as indications for treatment or management. For instance, the operational definition of schizophrenia used by the St. Louis group contains an unusually long time-criterion. This diagnosis cannot be made on their system unless signs of the illness have been present continuously for at least six months, and briefer illnesses, however severe or typical the symptoms, are given other labels. For the purposes of a specified research study, criteria such as this are quite legitimate even though they are debatable. Many psychiatrists would be uncomfortable at the exclusion of

patients with illnesses of four or five months' duration, but at least they know what to do if they wish to replicate the study or compare it with their own data. The point at issue here is that the use of such a criterion in research does not imply a recommendation to clinical workers that the diagnosis of schizophrenia or the instigation of treatment should be withheld for at least six months. Only indirectly, by being a valuable aid to research, may operational criteria influence the eventual development of new diagnostic ideas or treatment procedures.

In summary, it can be said that so long as some control is exercised over the components of the diagnostic process, the reliability of choice of diagnostic terms can reach acceptable levels. The use and further development of operational criteria should result in a significant increase in the meaning of diagnostic statements in research, and should also increase the awareness and interest of clinicians in the use of clear and agreed diagnostic criteria.

Computers and diagnosis

Computer programs have been written that mimic ways of arriving at diagnostic decisions, and by their use the normally unavoidable human processes of variable bias and forgetting are avoided. By their nature, programs are completely reliable, since any given set of symptom ratings or other clinical information will necessarily generate the same diagnosis every time. Such programs have an important place in research, particularly where comparisons are needed between large groups of patients about whom there is abundant diagnostic information.

Before such a program can be written it is necessary to stipulate quite precisely the steps in the decision process, and the criteria upon which each step is based. This is in itself an educative process and existing programs have clarified some aspects of the nature and variety of possible diagnostic styles. Three different decision styles form the basis of existing programs, namely, a logical decision tree, probability theory, and multiple discriminant function. The decision tree is the simplest, consisting of a series of questions each of which has to be answered by yes or no; the answer eliminates some possibilities and also determines the next question to be asked. This step-by-step process goes on until every diagnosis except one has been eliminated. The two most widely used structured and standardized interviewing and rating procedures already mentioned have computer programs of this type attached to them, and they have both been used in large-scale comparative studies of diagnosis (Spitzer & Endicott, 1969; Wing *et al.*, 1974). Catego, the program developed for use with the Present State Examination by Wing and his colleagues, depends also upon a series of condensations of symptoms into syndromes and categories, and is more complicated than a simple decision tree.

Diagnostic programs based upon probability theory (Bayes' theorem) and upon discriminant function procedures depend upon more involved statistical techniques, and have been used much less widely than those based upon a logical decision tree. Further details and discussion of their comparative merits can be found in reports by Fleiss and colleagues (1972), by Kendell (1975), and in the report from the World Health Organization International Pilot Study of Schizophrenia (WHO, 1973).

The merits and uses of computer programs in diagnostic research are considerable and are likely to increase, but it is worth repeating the truism that computer programs can only do what they are told to do. They cannot improve the reliability or meaning of inadequate data.

Diagnosis in an interdisciplinary perspective

The emphasis in the preceding sections upon the psychiatrist's task being to search for a diagnosis should not be taken to suggest that he is interested in nothing else. As a doctor with medical, legal, and ethical responsibilities for the patient, a psychiatrist may often seem to his colleagues from nursing, social, and psychological disciplines to be initially preoccupied with signs and symptoms. This is a necessary safeguard for the patient, who will be subject to avoidable hazards if symptoms which can be alleviated only by the use of physically based treatments are allowed to remain obscured by social and interpersonal problems. But having checked this possibility, the psychiatrist will realize that for many patients models of disease processes or disordered neurophysiology will be helpful in understanding only a small part or even none of the patient's symptoms. Even in those patients with clear-cut organic diagnoses it is usually found that there is an important interaction between the manifestations of the disease process and a variety of social and interpersonal influences. In other words, successful diagnosis, treatment, and management for most patients will include the assessment and manipulation of unwanted behaviour patterns or attempts to alleviate problems originating in social and interpersonal relationships.

The psychiatrist has to learn to acknowledge the extent to which he depends upon colleagues from other disciplines, since their professional skills allow them to provide not only large sections of the information necessary to make the diagnosis and formulation, but also to carry out much of the treatment and management. In return, the non-medical members of the team should acknowledge that a competent psychiatrist shares with them some knowledge of topics of joint medical and social interest, such as 'illness behaviour', the importance of family networks, and the effects of institutions.

Diagnosis and the diagnostic process can therefore be seen as central features of the clinical work of the whole therapeutic team, in that the type of diagnosis and the concepts underlying it will indicate the relative roles of the professional workers from different disciplines. But this prominence in the early stages of assessment and decision should not be allowed to hinder the subsequent development and use of social and psychological ideas and procedures. In conceptualizing and managing the patient's problems in relation to his social network and environment, these other non-diagnostic activities may need much thought and effort from all members of the team and may become just as important as the diagnosis itself.

9

The clinical assessment of mental disorders

FELIX POST

Introduction

Comprehensive and correct clinical assessment is not possible without some understanding of both descriptive and dynamic psychopathology. Mastery of the techniques for eliciting psychopathological phenomena is equally necessary. Finally, a patient's clinical assessment is only the first, but perhaps the most important step in his treatment, and therapeutic success can easily be jeopardized by a psychiatric interview in which the diagnostic enquiry has smacked of interrogation.

While a volume devoted to psychopathology needs to carry a chapter headed 'Clinical Assessment', it will be assumed that the postgraduate reader will have acquired his own technique of examining psychiatric patients from the relevant sections of numerous textbooks. More advanced techniques of case-taking have been described in recent publications specifically for postgraduate students, and they run to far greater lengths than there is space available in the present volume. There are, for example, the (London) Institute of Psychiatry's *Notes on Eliciting and Recording Clinical Information* (1973), Leff and Isaacs' (1978) *Psychiatric Examination in Clinical Practice,* and the 9000–10 000 word section in Lishman's (1978), *Organic Psychiatry,* devoted to the clinical examination, to which is added a full discussion of relevant psychological tests and their indications. With these recent publications available, the intention here is not to offer an authoritative, still less an authoritarian chapter on clinical assessment, but to submit personal observations which might prove useful in complementing the reader's own techniques.

I shall begin by drawing attention to the fact that by the use of scientifically validated questionnaires and inventories a modicum of quantitative and qualitative order can be imposed on the seemingly inchoate mass of psychopathology. The usefulness of these instruments for therapeutic trials and diagnostic labelling cannot be over-estimated, but it will be shown that investigations using some of these instruments have highlighted the limitations of psychiatric diagnosis in the present state of our knowledge. For purposes of everyday practice, clinical assessment by means of history-taking and mental state exploration will remain the chief approach to the patient, and the bulk of this essay will consist of thoughts concerning both these procedures.

Some standardized clinical assessments

During the last twenty years, numerous scorable devices for psychiatric assessment have been introduced mainly in the form of self-rating questionnaires using check lists of items. They have been largely employed to assess the severity of various forms of disorder in a comprehensive and repeatable form during therapeutic trials. The reader may like to be reminded of some of these measures with dates of first publication and (where applicable) with references to further important reports concerning the various scales. There are first of all various depression scales: Hamilton's Rating Scale for Depression, (1960, 1976; Knesevich *et al.*, 1977), Beck's Depression Inventory (Beck *et al.*, 1961; Bailey & Coppen, 1976), and Zung's Self-Rating Depression Scale (1965; Biggs *et al.*, 1978). In the area of anxiety, there is Taylor's (1953) Personality Scale of Manifest Anxiety. Particularly useful in patients exhibiting both anxiety and depression, and hovering on the borders between neurosis and psychosis, have been found Shapiro's (1969; Shapiro *et al.*, 1973) Personal Questionnaires. They are somewhat time-consuming to construct, but frequent administration of these tailor-made measures, which use the patient's verbatim description of symptoms, have been shown to be valuable correctives of the clinician's assessment in difficult individual cases (Shapiro & Post, 1974). In addition, there are countless occasions on which charts registering numerous malfunctions of patients under treatment are constructed. In patients with schizophrenic conditions some successes have been

demonstrated in scoring disorders of thinking (formal schizophrenic thought disorder), but though the administration of the procedures developed from the Kelly grid (Kelly, 1963) can of course be learnt by the clinician, they are usually in the hands of the clinical psychologist (Bannister & Fransella, 1966; Bannister, 1970). Similarly, workers experimenting with behavioural techniques in the treatment of phobic and obsessional states have worked out their own techniques for measuring severity and response to treatment (Marks, 1978a, b.). Finally, the assessment of senile deterioration, and attempts to manage it, have led to measures like the Dementia Scales of Blessed and colleagues (1968), the Stockton Geriatric Rating Scale (Meer & Baker, 1966, Gilleard & Pattie, 1977) and the Clifton Assessment Schedule (Pattie & Gilleard, 1975, 1978), to name only a few.

Self-rating questionnaires using check lists of signs and symptoms have also been introduced not just to measure the severity of clinical pictures, but rather to arrive at their diagnosis. Among the better known ones have been Wittenborn's (1955) Psychiatric Rating Scales, a Brief Psychiatric Rating Scale by Overall and Gorham (1962), and Lorr's (Lorr *et al.*, 1963) In-patient Multi-dimensional Psychiatric Scale. Wing and his colleagues (1974) summarized criticisms of these measures, and described the origin and development of a more closely standardized psychiatric interview introducing set interviewing techniques and agreed sets of descriptions and definitions of clinical phenomena of the kind which lead to diagnostic statements. They claim (Wing *et al.*, 1974 – p. 6) that 'these methods indicate that it is possible to rate the presence or absence of a wide range of psychiatric symptoms reliably through the use of special techniques and [that] this fact suggests that part, at least, of the variability in making psychiatric diagnoses can also be reduced'. The book by Wing and his colleagues (1974) also contains full details of the measures which they have developed, the PSE (Present State Examination), and, in computerized form, the Catego Programme. The PSE has been adapted for the diagnostic assessment of aged psychiatric patients by Copeland and his group (Copeland *et al.*, 1976; Copeland, 1978). All these measures can be used by non-medical workers, but psychiatrists also need training in their use, though some of the constituent scales can be employed in therapeutic trials without expertise in the whole procedure.

The PSE and its derivatives have proved their worth in a number of international epidemiological studies (summarized by Leff, 1977). Employing them in multicentre international comparisons has demonstrated that differences between locally reported prevalences of conditions like mania, schizophrenia, depression, or dementia were due to differences in the theoretical background and training of psychiatrists, and that when these were eliminated the prevalences of the major psychoses, at any rate, were not culture-dependent. However, an interim report of follow-up findings of one of these international studies (WHO, 1973) has also confirmed long-standing doubts about the value of psychiatric diagnosis in the present state of ignorance: while diagnostic categorization of patients is necessary for the choice of initial management and for comparisons of psychiatric patients in different settings during epidemiological research, at the present time initial diagnosis often tells us little about the deeper origins of a patient's psychopathology. A considerable proportion of schizophrenics identified during the WHO (1973) study, and who made remissions, were reclassified during a further attack as manic-depressives by trained workers using the same instrument as that employed initially (Sheldrick *et al.*, 1977). The occurrence of patients presenting with both schizophrenic and manic-depressive clinical pictures at the same time or on successive occasions, who may therefore be labelled schizo-affective, has been discussed for a long time (summarized by Procci, 1976) and opinions as to the significance of schizo-affective illnesses differ (Perris, 1974; Post, 1971, 1980). What seems clear, however, is that the way a patient presents clinically at first contact is by no means a safe guide towards the 'final diagnosis' in a considerable proportion of cases.

Another area in which the limitations of diagnostic exercises have been obvious for some time is that of affective illness. The question as to whether neurotic and psychotic depressions were separate illnesses or represented the more extreme portions of a spectrum disorder has not so far been clearly answered. Having seen again and again in many patients, during the same attack but even more often during consecutive attacks, the picture change from apparently insightful and non-deluded to clearly psychotic and melancholic, I would be inclined to look upon every mental illness (and not only every depression), as a highly individual affair in that in the same person different clinical pictures may appear at different times on account of changing constitutional factors (e.g. through ageing, or through hav-

ing experienced earlier psychological breakdowns) as well as on account of changing external factors (e.g. social circumstances, physical illness, bereavement). Unless the provisional nature of our diagnoses in a research setting as well as in relation to our clinical work is fully recognized, and thorough reassessments are made at regular intervals, there is a grave danger that we may not notice changes in the patient's psychopathological pattern, and that in consequence we perseverate with theories and treatments which are no longer appropriate. There is a very real danger that we may fail to change our therapeutic approach because of some preconceived notion (for details, see Post, 1972).

Standardized and scorable interviews are indispensable techniques in epidemiological research and in drug trials. They are, however, too lengthy to administer in the situations in which most patients are seen: the public or private out-patient clinic or consultations in the patient's home. Opinions differ as to whether even relatively open and semi-structured scored interviews may not be therapeutically unhelpful, but they may certainly be regarded as too rigid for clinical practice. Most important, there do not seem to be any standardized and scorable history-taking schemes (Leff, 1978), and quite often the development and setting of a disorder may be more important than the mental status presented at first contact. Most patients, with the exception perhaps of a few psychotics coming from 'primitive' backgrounds (Anglo-Saxon or European, not only Third World) have some highly differentiated personal symptoms all of which cannot possibly figure in any standardized present state schedule, and subsequent changes in these clinical features may be most important in gauging progress. For all these reasons informal, free-wheeling clinical assessment remains the royal road to the patient.

The general setting of the clinical assessment

In ordinary psychiatric practice, assessment is aimed solely at planning optimal management of the patient's and his family's and friends' problems. Casting a preliminary diagnosis and estimation of the severity of any disorder will obviously be of considerable, often life-saving import. In addition, the way in which the first interviews with patients and their 'significant others' are carried out may influence therapeutic outcome profoundly: if they are badly done, the patient is unlikely to keep further appointments, and his friends will not press him to do so. If he is obliged to remain in the 'treatment situation' on account of compulsory admission or a court order for out-patient treatment, he will fail to develop the abilities towards therapeutically useful communication which are dormant in the most severely disordered persons. Compliance even with the most simple form of psychiatric treatment, the taking of tablets, is almost certainly dependent on a good relationship with the prescribing doctor. The even more central role of this relationship in the treatment of neuroses and personality disorders will find detailed consideration in the chapter on assessment in volume 4 (chap. 2).

Regardless of whether the patient is severely ill, or is a well ordered person with some specific problems asking for help, or is a child, an adolescent, a mature adult, or in his dotage, there is a conflict when carrying out any clinical assessment. The psychiatrist wishes to comprehend the patient and his disorder in terms of his own conceptual framework, whereas the patient and his friends have no theoretical interests in the matter, but solely want help, and may pour out much that seems irrelevant. Moreover, the patient himself, and even more often his friends, tend to hold definite views on the causes of his problems. This tendency to wish to 'sell' their opinions to the psychiatrist is by no means limited to the uneducated, and the views of well-spoken persons with some knowledge of psychiatric, psychological, or psycho-analytic matters might prove seductive to the psychiatrist. More often, he will tend to be irritated. Obviously, the art is not to stifle the flow of information coming from patients and informants, but at the same time to fill in all the pieces of one's own hypothetical framework. Karl Jaspers (1959, p. 825) has expressed this very well: 'We have to submit to the patients' individuality and allow them to give verbal expression to it. On the other hand we have to investigate the situation from a number of definite points in view with certain guiding aims in mind. If we neglect the latter we get a chaos of detail. If we neglect the former we simply pigeonhole the particulars into a few rigid categories which we already have; we see nothing fresh and are likely to do violence to our material'.

In trying to make fruitful his first contact with a patient, both to promote his own understanding and to establish the patient's trust, the psychiatrist will have to decide beforehand whether to see him on his own or with his companions, or whether to see the patient on his own before or after the informant. Obviously many patients will come for consultation unaccompanied, or are brought in by people who do not know them; some patients may, at least initially, refuse access to any informants. However, where it arises, the decision whom to see first is more important than is often realized, and it may have to be made in settings of considerable turbulence on in circumstances where time is limited.

Any disorder of communication on the patient's part will make it desirable for the doctor to see an informant first, and preferably on his own. Among such disorders of communication, there are most obviously deafness, speech, and language disorders, as well as disturbances of awareness and memory; but there are also slowness, mutism, and speech abnormalities in patients without gross cerebral pathology but related to one of the more severe functional conditions. The family doctor's introduction or any other information obtained before the consultation will give some idea whether serious communication difficulties are likely to be encountered. Obviously, it would be highly injudicious to see as the first person the relative, spouse, or friend of a patient referred for advice on some minor or intimate psychological malfunctioning, even though the garrulousness of some neurotics and their irrelevance or suppression of important facts would make a preliminary account by an outsider time-saving. When it is decided to try to see an accompanying informant before the patient, either on account of previously received information, or because the patient's appearance and behaviour in the waiting room suggest the presence of a communication disorder, the best tactic has been in my experience, to shake hands with both, and then to say to the patient: 'Would you mind if I saw your . . . first? It will save you from having to answer all sorts of tedious questions.' Where one is not certain about the patient's ability to give information, or about his attitude to being seen only after the external informant, it has been my practice to invite the patient first on his own, and after a few minutes of desultory exchanges to suggest a break in the interview, while the friend is seen. Most patients visited in their own homes tend to be rather ill, and therefore handicapped as historians. In the setting of the domiciliary consultation an initial interview with a relative can sometimes be arranged before the visit, as at home the patient is likely to wander in and interrupt any tête-à-tête. Finally, under what circumstances should the patient not be seen on his own, but with one or more of his friends in the room? Leaving out the obvious case of the dangerously aggressive patient, there is the patient who is too frightened, or who claims that he (usually she) is too frightened, to be left alone with the strange doctor. On the other hand, there are clinical circumstances in which the psychiatrist may find it useful to see the patient together with one or several of his friends even on the first occasion. This matter is more fully discussed in volume 4, chapter 2. Finally, where well-integrated paranoid persons are brought for consultation by one of their 'significant others', or where the psychiatrist has been called in for a domiciliary visit, it frequently occurs that the patient blandly denies all reported paranoid talk and behaviour when seen on his own, but immediately launches forth into all his over-valued ideas or delusions with the informant in the room. Once the patient's dissimulation has been by-passed, he is likely to confide his thought-content with all its ramifications in interviews with the psychiatrist alone.

In which order to record

Many case-taking schemes will be familiar to the reader. I should like to recommend the following order for the recording of information obtained during the assessment:

Obtain data both from patient and, if at all possible, from an informant. Record separately from both sources the following items of history:

    Reasons for referral ('complaints')
    Heredo-genetic family data and personalities of
      key relatives
    Family atmosphere
    Childhood development
    Schooling; higher education, if any
    Work history; date of when last at work
    Sexual and marital data, mental health of chil-
      dren
    Personality before first appearance of symp-
      toms
    Previous physical and psychiatric health
    Account of development of present symptoms

Obtain from patient:

    Physical state
    Behaviour
    Form of talk and, where relevant, of written
      material
    Mood
    Thought content: preoccupations, phobic,
      obsessive, hysterical symptoms, over-valued
      ideas, delusions and perceptual disorders

    Level of awareness, general mental ability,
      orientation, memory, and where cerebral
      pathology needs to be excluded fronto-
      temporo-parietal defects
    Self-assessment of problems

A schedule of this sort, which deviates in some parts from traditional ones, has the merit of ensuring that information in all areas has been gathered. If the information has been recorded in the suggested sequence, reading it over should allow one to build up a picture of the way in which the patient's illness fits into his family and personal background, as well as how it has developed out of his life experience. This historical account, together with the cross-sectional view of the patient's mental functioning, will yield a preliminary diagnostic formulation and permit the drafting of a plan of treatment.

It may be helpful to point out a number of tricks of the trade by going through the items of the case-taking schedule one by one. But before doing so, and at the risk of stating the obvious, it should be pointed out that while the case notes should be recorded in the logical sequence suggested here, it would be a grave mistake to impose this order on the history-taking process itself with the relative, and even more so on the exploration of the patient. With both, the interview should be divided into two parts. During the first period of the interaction, the psychiatrist should be passive and make minimal verbal contributions after inviting the informant and the patient to state what they see as the main problem, the reason for consultation, and especially in the case of longstanding difficulties the reason for seeking help now and not earlier. Contributions from the doctor should at this stage only serve to stimulate the flow of talk. There is in the great majority of instances no need to be anxious about wasting precious time by allowing the speakers to ramble on. Most people are so unaccustomed to being permitted to talk without interruption that they will soon fall silent. By then it will have become clear to the doctor whether, through lack of general or verbal abilities, the informant has begun to go round in circles during his account, or whether perhaps hints and omissions invite further enquiry during the second period of the interview. Just as in the case of the relative, the patient's first words, whether in terms of a complaint or a statement, often indicate the diagnosis, and such spontaneous, often almost pathognomonic, statements might not be obtainable if the psychiatric interview amounted to anything resembling an interrogation. This holds especially for less ill patients, who may betray depression underlying their neurotic symptom only on this single occasion ('I have changed, I've lost all interest, life has become empty, etc.') In the case of psychotic patients the *form* of their talk is best observed at the beginning of the interview, when the patient is not interrupted and the psychiatrist should suppress his inclination towards exploring even the most bizarre statements for *content*.

With both informants and patients there comes the point when their spontaneous contribution is no longer producing any clear or possibly relevant information, and one then enters upon the second period of the interaction. The psychiatrist will first of all follow up any obvious cues by supplementary questioning. Then, with the relative, I find it useful to ask his permission to go over the patient's background, life history, and illness in an orderly fashion 'to facilitate my own note-taking and comprehension'. Starting with family history, childhood, and schooling, the informant is again encouraged to hold forth on each subject, but elucidating and guiding questions will almost always be indicated. Initially, the patient will also be encouraged to tell the story of his life, and will be allowed to wander away to his preoccupations, but now the opportunity will be taken to elucidate his mental content with questions. Again, the exploration of the patient will not be along predetermined lines to fit one's case taking scheme, but will be permitted to develop by association. Finally, it will almost always be necessary to fill in any gaps of the assessment by direct questions. Also, at the end of the interview, or more often of a series of interviews, a searching enquiry into the patient's cognitive functioning will have to be mounted. Employing a psychologically sophisticated approach to the mental state examination usually ensures good co-operation for orientation, memory, specific cerebral function, and intelligence testing, except in the most seriously disordered patients.

Finally, both the patient and his friends must be told something. How and what to tell cannot be taught. In my own experience, the closer to the truth the better – avoiding any positive rebuff of their opinions (especially in the case of the 'deluded' patient) or criticism, but also avoiding the impression of an easy acceptance or optimism, except in the rare cases where this is not out of place.

Some aspects of history-taking

We may begin by pointing out that the differences between 'history' and 'mental state', i.e. between the informant's objective and the patient's subjective information are not as clear and fundamental as these words suggest. Even documentary evidence in a patient's history (just as in General History) such as school reports or accounts from employers are products of another person's mind and thus far from objective. These sources of distortion are obviously much more in evidence in the case of informants with emotional involvement of varying quality and intensity with the patient. The patient's own account of his past life, his personality and the development of his psychological disability is, of course, very much coloured by that disability. Where there is no external informant, the only information available, i.e. that given by the patient, will therefore have to be taken with a large grain of salt, though some psychiatrists may query this suggestion. We are, after all, interested in the 'true' story of the patient's life only in as far as we attempt to be scientists, but from a therapist's point of view it may be far more important to understand how the patient sees his life and illness, than to obtain the real facts. To give a rather gross example, perhaps the patient's parents had in reality led a most exemplary and happy married life, but if the patient recalls nothing but rows and perhaps also sexual approaches by her father, that is all that really matters in terms of her psychopathology. It is suggested here, however, that the psychiatrist should be both a scientist and an artist (e.g. therapist) and seek knowledge of both the objective and the imaginary truths. In general, it may be said that the more a patient is mentally disabled, the more his own accounts of his family, his life and his illness will be part of his 'mental state'. On the other hand in the case of neurotic disorders, e.g. of certain obsessional and phobic conditions, but also in the case of some slowly developing psychoses, the patient may have soldiered on without his condition becoming apparent to others, and in that case he may be the only true informant concerning his illness.

Turning to some particular issues, the conflicting claims between an allegedly coldly scientific and a warmly humane therapeutic approach are sometimes highlighted by sloppy recording of family histories. Provided that this is not done at the beginning of the interview (see previous section), neither relatives nor the patients themselves will mind being asked about mental or personality disorders having occurred in other members of the family. Many will be worried about hereditary matters in relation to the patient's illness, and glad to ventilate this side of things. A chart containing all first degree relatives is easily jotted down, and on it any psychiatric involvement may be entered. Quite separately from this, and not necessarily at the same time, information is gathered about the characteristics and the lives of members of the family who had made an impact on the patient especially during his childhood. To preserve clarity, heredo-genetic data should be recorded separately from emotional forces which almost certainly had influenced the patient's childhood development.

Information under the heading of Family History is thus seen to merge with that relevant to the heading of Childhood, and this again merges with School History. The main point is that an attempt should be made to bring to life the patient's earlier years with all relevant aspects, including early signs of pathological developments. The Occupational History gives the outer framework of a patient's life, and in a basically affluent modern society the Work History is very largely a product not only of intelligence, but also of strengths and weaknesses of personality structure. To an even greater extent Marital and Sexual History is nothing but an account of an important emotional aspect of personality.

However, an attempt to obtain a picture of the level of the patient's functioning in all aspects of his existence is made under the heading of Personality. Having dealt with his sexual adjustment, it will be natural to enquire into the nature and extent of his relationships to others in general, then into his belief systems, and habitual mood as seen by the outsider. Finally an approach will be made to potentially pathological aspects of personality: alcohol, tobacco, drugs, conspicuous food-fads, as well as evidence of earlier obsessional, phobic, histrionic-hysterical, etc. trends. From here the enquiry leads to previous circumscribed episodes of psychiatric disorder, as well as of physical illhealth. It probably does not require stressing that any diagnoses concerning past disorders volunteered by the informant should be countered by an enquiry into the nature of past symptoms and their treatment.

Though best seen in the light of the patient's background, his life story, and his earlier psychological problems, the present illness will of course, have been the first topic of the patient and of his friends, and may be briefly recorded under the first heading of 'reasons for referral and complaint'. Especially with the informant, it is often useful to go once again and in more detail into the development of the present illness. It is important to enquire more specifically into the approximate date of onset of the very first symptoms or changes in the patient, as well as into

the speed and variations of the progress of the disorder. Sudden onset or rapid recent worsening obviously point to a potentially dangerous development and situation. A more detailed investigation of the history of the present illness with an outside informant, and especially where the patient is relatively inaccessible, may be valuable in yielding information about the patient's thought content at a time when he had still been able to communicate with his friends. However, in the majority of cases, patients will themselves describe their symptoms, and it will be more important to try and find out from the informant the ways in which the patient's condition had become noticeable to others through changes in personality and appearance (including weight) through problems at night, through unusual day-time behaviour, betraying either abnormal mental content or decline in mental abilities.

As a final comment it should be observed once more how thoroughly worthwhile it is to get into the habit of recording the history of the patient and his disorder in the suggested logical order, which is designed to throw light on the development of his personality, his pre-illness adjustment, and the way in which his disorder first impinged upon his life, as well as on the course it has pursued (including treatments, the response obtained, readmissions, etc.). The importance of bearing in mind this kind of sequence is stressed by me perhaps rather *ad nauseam* because once a habit of building up a logically coherent picture has been developed, it becomes easy to obtain quickly essential information, which can be supplemented with details later. Most psychiatrists work under considerable pressure, and not too much time should be employed for initial history-taking. Much of the information will be biased, and even more likely are omissions that are due to lapses of memory or suppression. Before a general assessment of the situation has been completed, the doctor will not always know where to probe: the true story of the patient's life and illness will emerge only at a later stage and after longer exploration, in most instances.

There will, however, be a few important matters which should be clarified at first contact. I mentioned earlier that the rate of progress should be assessed, as a rapid and recently worsening course is unlikely to be affected by even the most adroit psychotherapy or social management; psychotropic drugs also usually take some time to act. Steep recent increase of disturbance or disability usually indicates the need for emergency action; powerful medication or admission according to the clinical and social circumstances. In a similar vein, even where there is ample evidence for some degree of lifelong maladjustment any recent worsening should indicate that an urgent enquiry is needed. To mention just one other point, a family history of suicide or attempted suicide, as well as previous attempts on the patient's part, should also ring an alarm bell.

Some comments on the Present State Examination

By contrast to the recommended sketchy approach to initial history taking, no time should be spared during the exploration of the present mental state. We are dealing on a unique occasion with the assessment and recording of the patient's condition at first presentation and before the picture has been modified by contact, discussion, medication, or perhaps the ceasing of some particular stress. This importance of obtaining and recording fully all pathological findings immediately is especially applicable to patients who are about to be admitted to hospital. Admission often brings about a considerable calming (usually only temporary) improvement, and it is essential to know what the patient actually did and said when first seen. Did he really report so-called first rank symptoms, was he really deluded, with guilt ideas, what precisely was the evidence for saying that he was hallucinated, disorientated, or confused? History of illness is secondhand evidence and soft currency in terms of clinical economy, while the immediacy of the mental state gives it the status of a hard currency!

The continuity which exists clinically between history-taking and mental state assessment is well exemplified by the first heading under which the mental status of a patient should be recorded: Behaviour.

In the majority of patients who consult psychiatrists there are no gross behaviour abnormalities, even though their life behaviour may have been seriously affected by their condition. The patients' problems are in most instances communicated by the patient to others in the form of verbal complaints, and obvious abnormalities of behaviour manifest themselves only when illnesses become more serious and acute, and when verbal communication tends to become increasingly disrupted. In such severely disturbed patients, behaviour during the psychiatric interview may, however, be quite unrepresentative, and an account of abnormal behaviour will have to

be obtained from informants under the heading of History of Present Illness. Where a patient has had to be admitted, a detailed description of his ward behaviour by members of the trained staff will be even more productive of pointers towards the nature of the underlying psychopathology, and should be fully recorded.

The first item to be noted during the interview itself is the patient's appearance, whether dress and hairstyle are inconspicuous or noticeably dishevelled, fashionable, elegant, unconventional, or even provocative. It is of special importance to note discrepancies between dress and hairstyle on the one side, and chronological age as well as psychomotor conduct, on the other. As an example might be given the youthfully dressed middle-aged woman, wearing a provocative blouse and make-up, but exhibiting marked emotional inhibition. Not infrequently such external discrepancies will draw attention at first contact to basic personality conflicts (Kind, 1973, p. 7), or if of recent origin to personality disruptions.

With regard to psychomotor behaviour one or two points may be highlighted from a recent comprehensive and critical assessment of non-verbal behaviour in mental illness (Hill, 1974). Just like ordinary people, psychiatrists tend to believe that they can read peoples' characters in their facial mobility, and over and above this psychiatrists used to believe that different mental illnesses had their distinct facies. However, in contrast to old textbooks of psychiatry, more recent publications no longer contain photographs of psychotic patients (as reproduced in Hill's paper). No doubt ethical considerations may have had an inhibiting effect on publishing pictures of this kind, but probably there has also been a growing realization of the lack of evidence concerning the reliability of these impressions. Measurements made from confidentially prepared and held videotapes might perhaps in future be used to test the diagnostic significance of physiognomy for different personalities and illnesses, as facial expressions continue to be regarded as valuable diagnostics by some psychiatrists. Investigations of this kind might also be used to refine some generally held notions of psychomotor behaviour in different kinds of psychoses and severe neuroses.

The patient's talk should also be evaluated in the first instance only as a psychomotor performance, and the temptation to become immediately concerned with its content should be resisted. Especially, where one has some information about the patient's earlier speech habits as well as his education and profession, minor degrees of slowing or of diffuseness may be picked up as significant. Written or tape recordings of several minutes of the patient's uninterrupted talk may reveal the presence of flight of ideas, which may otherwise be difficult to discover when one is dealing with the slow variety of this disorder of talking. A recording might facilitate the differentiation between pressure of talk and flight of ideas (usually but not always manic), incoherence (usually but not always schizophrenic), and circumstantiality (usually but not always psycho-organic). Changes in the speed and form of speech mirror shifts in disturbances of thinking, and are thus very sensitive indicators of clinical change. To assess later progress any formal disorder of talk present should be carefully documented before any treatment is given.

Both psychomotor behaviour and talk, as well as the content of a patient's talk give indications of his prevailing or changing affective state. The way in which psychiatrists evaluate whether the patient's mood is infectious, adequate, flat, or incongruous is yet another aspect of the mental status examination which might be investigated by modern methods. At the present time, all one can say is that the beginner in psychiatry is often not yet able to sense the finer shades of a patient's mood and how this may evoke a similar feeling in himself. Beginners also tend to see flatness or incongruity, where there is merely inhibition during the interview, or in severely depressed patients a subjective loss of feeling, which is reflected in their facial and other emotional expressions. For these reasons alone, a full subjective description by the patient of his mood must always be obtained, and his responses to further enquiries made in order to confirm or refute the doctor's impressions should be carefully recorded. Again, in the course of treatment it will be helpful to compare statements made by the patient initially with those voiced in later interviews.

It will have been noticed that in following the suggested sequence of observations, we have approached the patient from the periphery: first what others told us about him, then what we observed, and what disorders of communications he showed. When exploring his emotional state, we had begun to approach the patient's inner self. Regardless of the nature of the patient's thought content, communicating it to his doctor may prove to him a helpful experience, provided this part of the mental state examination is carried out sensitively. We, as it were, ask the patient to allow us to enter into his inner world, by encouraging him to tell us about his preoccupations and anxieties, and how they arose. This may in effect amount to the patient's 'History of the Present Illness'. It is most important to give him plenty of time and to stimulate the flow of talk in various well described ways (see vol. 4, chap. 2). Finally, some pertinent enquiries by the psychiatrist will always be necessary in the patient's interest. Their content will depend on the general nature of the disorder, which should have become fairly clear by the time this point in the exploration has been reached. For example, a very small minority of patients only have delusions or hallucinations, and it is a mistake to enquire into these phenomena routinely. There are certain symptoms which patients may not reveal spontaneously, and which should be enquired into by using leading questions. Where there is any hint of depression (even in the presence of obvious anxiety alone), the patient's ideas about suicide should be ascertained and recorded. Hypochondriacal ideas are always voiced freely, but self-depreciation, ideas of guilt, subtle changes in experiencing the surroundings and other people (i.e. derealization and depersonalization) may need to be brought out. Obsessional phenomena are often concealed by the patient, as is fear of insanity, which may have to be enquired into when the patient at the end of the interview is asked to give his own ideas about his condition and its possible management. Especial care must be taken when trying to discover whether there is any evidence pointing towards a schizophrenic development. Nowadays many young psychiatrists may not have had contact with drug-free chronic schizophrenic patients, and will not have had the experience of hearing patients of this kind spontaneously describing their ideas and experiences, as if they had stepped straight from the pages of Kraepelin, Bleuler, or Fish.

The first approach should be to lead the patient gently towards the description of any 'strange or frightening experiences', towards 'any unusual feelings concerning his own actions'. Even negative suggestions may be offered, such as 'I don't suppose you ever hear any imaginary voices'. In many instances patients will in response to questions of this kind launch into fairly explicit descriptions of any hallucinations experienced, and they are quite likely to respond to attempts to elicit the precise type of their psychopathology: whether their ideas are merely over-valued, or delusional, or of a so-called true autochthonous character; whether the perceptual experiences amount to true hallucinations or only to pseudo-hallucinations, etc. Questions such as 'Do you ever feel influenced in your mind by other people in an underhand way?' 'Do you sometimes think your thoughts are not your own?' 'What do the voices say?' may have to be asked of patients right at the end of the interview, when the indirect approach had not borne fruit, but any responses obtained are more likely to be in the form of simple affirmations or denials, and may prove misleading when accepted at face value for preliminary diagnosis and for therapeutic decisions. A patient's spontaneous descriptions of his pathological thoughts and experiences are of infinitely greater value than any admissions under the most sympathetic questioning. However, some teachers (Leff & Isaacs, 1978, pp. 53–4) advocate a more direct approach, and have sought to demonstrate how the real meaning of the patient's initial response can be elicited by further questioning.

Little need be said about the assessment of the patient's level of awareness and his cognitive state, as it has been fully and excellently described recently by Lishman (1978). Attention need be drawn only to a few matters which, in my experience, are not always realized. For instance, there is little point in evaluating a patient's cognitive status without having some idea of his pre-illness level of mental ability. The school history may be falsified, but a patient's work (if of a skilled or professional kind) will exclude intelligence seriously below the average. Difficulties may arise in the case of some 'socially under-privileged' and surly people, and also with some well-spoken 'ladies and gentlemen', as the one may in fact be highly intelliigent while the others may be dullards in spite of their manner and educational veneer. Administering a brief vocabulary test of intelligence takes little time, and this should certainly be done before the results of the clinical examination of orientation, memory, language ability, etc. are interpreted as indicating cerebral deterioration. However, in comparison with either the clinician's or the psychologist's testing, incipient intellectual impairment is much more reliably suggested by an independent history describing a decline. The psychologist's tests are particularly useful because they may be repeated at relatively short intervals to refute or confirm significant deterioration or temporary confusion. It is a mistake to ask a patient only a few probing questions of the type which are sufficient to confirm the presence of advanced dementia clearly indicated by the history. Early decline is usually patchy, and questionnaires, such as that given in the Institute of Psychiatry (1973) publication, and which cover orientation, past personal and recent personal memory, as well as grasp of recent political events and dates, should be administered. If the patient's responses are recorded verbatim it becomes easier to discover some hallmarks of cerebrally caused cognitive impairment, such as perseveration, confabulation, and near-miss approximations. The differentiation of pseudo-dementia, especially when it occurs, not as part of a florid Ganser state, but in severe depression or with schizophrenic perplexity, is not as easy as is sometimes suggested: with the 'near-miss' response of brain-damaged persons the interpretation is that somewhere they know the right answer, but are not quite able to reach it, whereas with pseudo-dements it is thought that 'approximate' answers and responses are due to repression, suppression, or even near-malingering. Provided the patient is not too disturbed, a few tests for dysphasia, dyspraxia, and dysgnosia may clarify the situation. They often indicate cerebral deficits in dementing or even in temporarily confused patients, but are either well performed by pseudo-dements or produce bizarrely ridiculous answers (blue grass or a five-legged horse!) To distinguish between depressive pseudo-dementia and one of the dementias of old age may be impossible in seriously disturbed patients except on the basis of a few days' observation, but this differentiation is not necessarily of immediate therapeutic or prognostic importance (Post, 1975).

A rule should be obeyed which also holds for all other aspects of the mental state examination, but especially for the recording of a disturbed patient's cognitive state at the time of first contact: the doctor's questions and the patient's answers must be recorded verbatim; a mere note to the effect that orientation and memory were normal or slightly impaired may prove worse than useless when diagnostic problems lead to a review of previous notes which contain only opinions and judgements, but do not quote the facts on which these were based.

Finally, statements by the patient concerning his 'insight' should be recorded. For the limited value of this concept Aubrey Lewis' (1934) paper remains required reading, but changes in the degree and quality of insight during the course of a patient's illness and in relation to treatment are important indicators of progress.

Final formulation

In concluding an essay in which I have tried to offer some thoughts on clinical assessment I do not wish to leave the reader with the impression that the psychiatrist's opinions and judgement should be ignored. On the contrary, they must be formulated both in his mind and on paper as soon as the assessment has passed its preliminary stage. Once again, I would recommend giving features of the present mental state precedence over findings in the history, and suggest that a brief listing of the main psychopathological data discovered on examination should come first. Diagnostic labelling may be possible from these alone, but in most instances the way in which psychopathology had emerged from the patient's previous life and personality pattern will lead to a statement of probabilities as between a number of syndromes. A preliminary plan of treatment should follow, and here it may well be that facts from the history may be more important; the speed with which psychopathological phenomena have been increasing recently may stress the urgency and potential danger of the situation. In slowly developing conditions, the level of previous adjustment may indicate realistically limited therapeutic aims; the patient's social setting will influence numerous aspects of treatment and prognosis. The initial formulation should also comprise a list of desirable further special investigations of the patient's background, his symptomatology, his physical condition, his personality, and his cognitive structure.

It is realized that most psychiatrists have to work under pressures which do not allow for the elaborate drafting of case notes, but an explicit record of the initial mental state and of the psychiatrist's conclusions and plan of action are a required minimum and may actually prove to be timesaving in the long run.

10
The principles of treatment and therapeutic evaluation

R. H. CAWLEY

Diagnosis–treatment relationships

The clinician's main task is the treatment of his patient: his concepts of psychopathology, his understanding of the clinical phenomena of mental disorders and his assessment and diagnostic procedures all subserve this function. As elsewhere in medicine, treatment in psychiatry is not simply an application of science: intuition and artistic skills must always play their part in effective practice. But in the best treatment the use of these powers is tempered by awareness of the nature and limits of scientific evidence and of the need for making balanced judgements where uncertainty prevails.

Data available to the clinician deciding what treatment to recommend are those which have been obtained from the clinical assessment. They are of three kinds: first, the diagnosis; secondly, the information about individual characteristics of the patient, including his biographical details, personality, medical and psychiatric history, his current psychopathology, and his perceptions of his world and predicament; and thirdly, information about the patient's environment, including his social role, the nature of his interactions and expectations with significant other persons, and his material circumstances. Of these three sets of data, the first is nomothetic or categorical, denoting class membership, while the second and third are idiographic or individual, signifying the patient's uniqueness in its objectifiable and experiential aspects. In all medical practice the clinician has recourse in some degree to these three frames of reference in selecting from his therapeutic options: psychiatry differs from other specialities in their relative weightings, for the psychiatrist is continually reminded that his business is not so much to eliminate disease as to treat sick or troubled persons. While psychiatric diagnosis is of very great importance, it points the way to treatment only when considered side by side with detailed information about the patient and his life circumstances. By the same token, despite the correlations which have been firmly established, diagnosis is only a weak predictor for use in preparing detailed statements about prognosis.

In planning treatment, the clinical psychiatrist will naturally take into account the nature and extent of the resources available to him, and here the salient variables include the amount of time he has to spend with the patient, the availability of other kinds of professional help, and the resources of the patient's family, social group and community. The context of treatment is often an important determinant of its style and content.

The formal relationships between psychiatric diagnosis and treatment are convoluted because personal, environmental, and contextual variables intervene. The inconstancy is not the result of error or inaccuracy in the process of clinical assessment, diagnosis, and prescription of treatment: it is due to complexities inherent in the subject matter. Refinements in diagnostic processes, though important enough in their own right, are not aimed at eliminating irregularities in diagnosis–treatment associations. The legitimate aspiration for treatment decisions is that they should follow logically not from diagnosis alone but from balanced consideration of all the available data pertaining to the individual case.

Referral for treatment

Epidemiological studies have shown that many people who experience or exhibit significant psychopathology do not seek treatment. In a few the psychopathology leads directly to active avoidance of treatment, and such people may continue indefinitely with private suffering and deviant behaviour until their actions overstep the limits of social tolerance. More commonly the failure to seek treatment is less directly related to the psychopathology: it stems from the operation of a large number of poorly understood influences. The subgroup so affected is not restricted to those with milder illnesses or passing through the earlier stages of a disease process. A

multiplicity of social factors determines whether and when the sufferer becomes a patient, by seeking help from the medical services or having help sought on his behalf, and these factors may also determine whether the person initially consulted is the general practitioner, a psychiatric or other medical specialist, or another professional worker in the health and social services. Similarly, social and personal as well as medical and psychopathological variables can determine whether or not the patient is referred to the psychiatrist from the primary care and other services. Beyond these contingencies of treatment it must be recalled that many agencies for helping the mentally ill or emotionally disturbed exist outside the statutory medical and social services and outside the private medical sector. In most Western countries a host of voluntary organizations, 'self-help' groups, and institutions of fringe medicine hold out promise of solace or cure. Some have assured value, others seem to exist to exploit for ideological or financial gain.

Most people who seek professional help for psychopathology escape the attention of specialists in mental health care. The primary care services deal with the largest numbers of patients with neurotic illnesses, personality disorders, and low-grade morbidity in which somatic symptoms and dysfunction accompany emotional distress. Even among the most severely disturbed patients (including those with psychotic or very severe neurotic disorders) substantial numbers fail to come to the notice of psychiatrists, social workers, or clinical psychologists. On the other side of the picture, a number of people referred to psychiatrists from a variety of agencies are found to have no psychiatric abnormality. Social processes similar to those which may prevent referral of people who are by strict criteria mentally sick can also operate in the reverse direction. The referring agents are not necessarily at fault when they refer those without significant psychopathology, for a full psychiatric assessment may be needed to establish that abnormality is lacking. It may at the same time focus attention on a social problem, or even suggest that other involved persons may be psychiatrically disturbed. These considerations emphasize how important it is for the psychiatrist to adopt rigorous criteria of disorder, and to be firm in recognizing where disorder is absent.

The dimensional approach

A general comment about the objectives of medical treatment which applies with undiminished force in psychiatry is the ancient exhortation *primum non nocere*. A further aspiration is immortalized in Trousseau's *guérir quelquefois, soulager souvent, consoler toujours*. These ambitions are not modest, especially when considered alongside the interplay of phenomena of psychobiological disorder with personal idiosyncrasy which constitute the problems facing the psychiatrist.

In the strict sense the notion of 'cure' has little place in psychiatry, perhaps only a restricted place in the whole story of medical treatment, for it seems to imply complete restoration to health as a direct result of the therapeutic agent. The wise physician does well to avoid promises of cure: though he may sometimes confidently predict full recovery, he can promise no more than that he will do his best for his patient. But, given adequate time and reasonable facilities, a competent clinician working with a properly integrated team should be able to offer substantial help to a very large proportion – perhaps eighty or ninety per cent – of patients who show reasonable degrees of compliance.

In carrying out any form of treatment the psychiatrist is intervening in complex variables and their interactions. Aspects of the patient's personality or of his environment may influence critically the preferred treatment programmes. Treatment needs to be conceived as directed not only towards the mental disorder but also towards the person, the environment, and the reciprocity between these and the disorder. The subject matter of psychiatry extends beyond the conventional boundaries of medicine: psychopathology has important psychological and socio-cultural aspects, so that psychiatric studies are multidisciplinary. Psychiatric practice is correspondingly seen as a multiprofessional endeavour. The three main dimensions of treatment are first the biomedical (including pharmacotherapy and related procedures which directly influence somatic functioning); secondly the psychological (including psychotherapy in the most general sense, and specific psychological treatments focused on particular aspects of dysfunction and depending on experimental psychology or dynamic psychology); and thirdly the social and environmental (including the patient's immediate environment, and aspects of his longer-term environment and interactions). Decisions and interventions along these dimensions may take place simultaneously, but clearly need to be integrated.

The multiprofessional team includes, in addition to the psychiatrist, the psychiatric nursing staff, the social worker, the clinical psychologist, and the occupational therapist. For special purposes, other personnel may participate, such as, for example, remedial therapists, rehabilitation specialists, and workshop technicians. Three principles underlie the successful operation of the multiprofessional team: each member has his own special training, expertise, and skills, which complement those of other members; each member has clearly established functions in assembling data for clinical assessment of patients and identification of problems, for making decisions, and for administration of the treatment programme; and the whole enterprise depends on the integrated action of all members of the team. Special arrangements are necessary for liaison to achieve the requisite co-ordination of functions, and decisions and actions depend on an appropriate division of labour and recognition of roles, while careful attention to note-keeping is a feature of the most effective teamwork. Clearly there is much scope for variation in the ways in which psychiatric teams organize their work. As a general rule the team is based at a hospital, functioning in out-patient, day hospital, and ward settings, and it is becoming an increasingly common practice for members of the team to visit patients in the community.

It has been noted that most people who seek treatment for psychopathology receive it from general practitioners: others, especially social workers in the primary care team, may be involved at the same time. Among the patients referred to psychiatrists, only a small proportion is admitted to hospitals or day hospitals. In most Western countries extensive and diversified facilities exist in the community where patients living at home or in hostels serving the needs of various subgroups are managed by members of the primary care team, the psychiatric team, social services departments, professional employees of voluntary agencies, and volunteers. Thus in practice the distinction between specific treatment and help or care of a more general kind is blurred, and only a few general principles can be enunciated. Continuity of care of patients in various phases of treatment – out-patient, day patient, in-patient, community – is a desirable aim, though often difficult to implement. An effective psychiatric team maintains a satisfactory liaison with the general practitioner of each individual patient, as well as with other concerned professionals and voluntary workers in the community. The psychiatric team focuses its work not only upon the patient himself but also, when necessary and with the patient's agreement, works with family members and significant other persons in the patient's life.

Community psychiatric nurses may be based on hospital psychiatric units and work with patients in the community. It must be emphasized again that integration of the efforts of all those engaged in helping an individual patient calls for special provision for conference and communication. Demands for economy and administrative tidiness sometimes argue for particular patterns of administration and management: as a result there are risks of inflexibility and failure to accommodate the wide range of problems presented by patients with psychopathology. Detailed consideration of variables in treatment at this level overlaps with consideration of broader socio-economic and administrative themes.

General psychotherapy

Indications. All patients throughout their period of care.

Principles. In psychiatry, treatment fashions have been notoriously transient. The one form of intervention which has stood the test of time is that which depends on the most elementary and yet elusive concept: the relationship between doctor and patient and the use of this to the patient's advantage. It almost goes without saying that, throughout medicine, the establishment of confidence and trust in this relationship is a prerequisite for accurate assessment of the patient and his predicament. But in psychiatry this side of treatment has particular importance, for verbal exchanges between doctor and patient are crucial to the very essence of psychiatric assessment and treatment, and the content of the exchanges is inevitably related to the patient's most sensitive and intimate experiences which may be frightening, guilt-laden, intrusive, muddling, and otherwise unpalatable in many ways.

Signifying treatment of psychological problems by psychological means, the term psychotherapy has a general application within medicine which reaches into all circumstances in which a doctor–patient relationship proves to be established well enough to be effective in exploring or allaying a patient's anxieties. It signifies an application of the principles of good doctoring in a manner appropriate to the patient's needs and, when psychiatric disorders are at issue, this component of treatment clearly becomes a *sine qua non*. The requirement is so basic as to be definable as an aspect of professional good manners: yet it calls for the competent exercise of a complex skill, the practitioner's style depending in part on his personal characteristics and in part on his training and experience. A blend of empathy, compassion, objective appraisal, and disinterested judgement is at the core of the general psychotherapeutic approach: it embodies attentive listening, a readiness to recognize the patient's individuality and its context, and a respect for the validity of his reported experiences. It follows that this modality of treatment must be versatile, so that attempts at close definition are unlikely to succeed.

Subsumed under the heading of general psychotherapy are aspects of treatment with a host of descriptive epithets including simple, superficial, supportive, directive or non-directive, client-centred, and distributive. While widely different objectives and techniques may be employed, none of the groupings is clearly discriminatory. The common factors are the development and use with therapeutic intent of the professional relationship with form and content tailored to the needs of the individual patient as perceived by the therapist, and to the time and facilities available. The objectives are as diverse as the patients' problems: there is no unitary theoretical basis.

Every psychiatrist needs to be competent in the practice of general psychotherapy, and its uses are pervasive. There is a real sense in which treatment begins with the first encounter, for the very nature of the patient's experiences of himself and others may make it difficult or nearly impossible for him to reveal his thoughts or to describe his feelings or perceptions. An effective working relationship facilitates the eliciting of accurate information and the formulation of a realistic assessment of the patient, his disorder and the context, so that a well-reasoned programme of treatment may be devised. The patient's inclination to comply with treatment is enhanced by the knowledge that, even if he is not understood, he is at least being taken seriously. Moreover a satisfactory relationship between doctor and patient sets the scene for the patient to examine his own feelings and thoughts with a degree of application and honesty. It opens possibilities for the patient, in discussion with the doctor, to become aware of significant problems in various aspects of his life, and to recognize the extent and limits of possible change. He may be helped by a growing awareness that, although his uniqueness is respected by the therapist, others are experiencing similar types of predicament. Other definable components of general psychotherapy include the opportunity for ventilation of anxiety and distress, explanation, advice, and education, the correct use of appropriate kinds of reassurance, and mobilization of the capacity for hope.

There are no contra-indications for general psychotherapy, but adverse effects may follow incorrect or unreflective management of this side of treatment. Among these may be mentioned the raising of uncontrollable anxieties or false hopes, the inappropriate choice of topics for reassurance, the failure to allow a necessary degree of dependence and, *per contra*, the fostering of unduly passive and dependent attitudes in the patient, the failure to recognize the indications for more skilled or precisely focused intervention, the unwarranted intrusion of the therapist's own emotional reactions or value systems, and an over-ready acceptance of false and transient solutions to external or internal problems.

General psychotherapy is here described as practised by psychiatrists. Closely similar considerations apply to other members of the psychiatric team, all of whom develop relationships with the patient which are potentially therapeutic and potentially damaging. In particular psychiatric nursing, psychiatric social case work, and counselling incorporate special variants of this modality of treatment. In a psychiatric team which is functioning in an integrated fashion, the general psychotherapeutic component of treatment is a shared responsibility.

Biomedical dimensions of treatment

Drug treatments

Indications. Selected patients with certain symptoms or illnesses, often for only part of their period of care.

Principles. For centuries attempts have been made to alter mental functioning, for therapeutic, religious, and recreational purposes, by the use of drugs. The earliest therapeutic purposes were to procure sleep and to alter mood. Modern psychopharmacotherapy began in the early 1950s with the introduction of reserpine and later chlorpromazine into psychiatric practice. The wide range of drugs now available includes the antipsychotic drugs or neuroleptics (phenothiazines, butyrophenones, thioxanthenes), the minor tranquillizers, and the antidepressives, together with a miscellaneous group including the beta-adrenergic blocking agents and lithium carbonate. In addition drugs may be required to treat systemic illness or deficiency states associated with psy-

chopathology, or to treat extrapyramidal symptoms and signs induced by neuroleptic medication.

Originally adopted because of their empirical effectiveness in treating psychotic symptoms and disorders of behaviour or mood, the antipsychotic drugs and antidepressives have proved to be useful as investigative tools in animal and human pharmacology. They have an important place as quantifiable and reversible provocative agents in investigations of aspects of brain function and brain–behaviour relationships, and as such have opened immensely rewarding prospects in neuropsychopharmacological research. As a result there has been a rapid growth in knowledge about the pharmacology of the normal brain and the biological substrate of mood and behaviour; so far the most impressive advances have been concerned with the activity of neurotransmitters and the detailed pharmacology of specific transmitter systems. In parallel with these advances, various hypotheses have been successively generated concerning the pathogenesis of the major functional psychoses. At the same time the clinical effectiveness of the drugs in controlling psychotic disturbance has widened the possibilities for other modalities of treatment: most particularly it has shortened the length of stay in hospital for many patients, enabled others to avoid admission, and facilitated the operation of procedures for general psychotherapy and community care. Thus the effects on psychiatric theory and practice have been far-reaching.

The clinical prescription of these drugs is still determined by empirical considerations, but their development has received impetus from the growth of the discipline of psychopharmacology. This has in general terms provided a rationale for their use and for further development, though the relationships between clinical effectiveness, pharmacological action, and chemical structure are far from clear. The clinician's natural concern is with the factors governing individual variations in response, and it is here that pharmacokinetic studies may prove to have important practical application. Among the variables which determine the pattern and level of response are those connected with bio-availability and with plasma levels, half-life, protein binding, compartmental distribution, and concentrations at receptor sites and within cells. These variables, together with others affecting drug metabolism and receptor sensitivity, may sometimes differentiate responders from non-responders. Investigations along these lines seem likely to lead to improved techniques for monitoring drug treatment and hence greater effectiveness and precision of treatment with psychopharmacotherapeutic agents. Psycho-active drugs are prescribed with circumscribed aims: relief of certain key 'target symptoms' and constellations; relief of an underlying 'disease process'; prevention of secondary disabilities arising out of the effects of the original symptoms on the patient's life; and prevention of relapse of symptoms or disease. The neuroleptic drugs are tranquillizing and antipsychotic, though questions of specificity in antipsychotic effect remain unanswered. They may alter mood, perception, thinking, and behaviour, and vary among themselves in their sedative effects, potency, and side effects. The tricyclic antidepressive drugs are effective forms of treatment for many patients with depressive disorders; the target of treatment is generally taken to be the depressive illness though they may be useful in certain secondary depressive syndromes. Tricyclic drugs vary among themselves in sedative effects and side effects and in antidepressive efficacy. Monoamine oxidase inhibitors seem to be more effective in the treatment of certain types of anxiety than in depressive disorder.

All psycho-active drugs, including the minor tranquillizers and others, have their specific indications and absolute and relative contra-indications. The decision to prescribe depends on consideration of the disorder and of associated or intercurrent disorders and their treatment, and on the patient and the context. Prescribing a drug correctly entails offering the patient appropriate explanations, instructions, warnings, and assurances: the personal and social, as well as medical, consequences of taking the drug are anticipated. Thus compliance is more likely to be achieved if the patient knows when and how he may expect to feel the benefit and whether he is likely to experience unwanted effects; which adverse effects call for action and which have to be tolerated; for how long he should expect to continue the medication; and what activities (including driving) or foodstuffs (including alcohol) should be avoided or taken with special care. Simple dose regimes are more likely to be followed than complicated ones. Patients taking psychotropic medication should be under regular medical surveillance. As with prescribing during the acute phase, a course of maintenance treatment after symptomatic recovery (with antidepressives) or planned long-term medication (for example with lithium or neuroleptics) is to be recommended only when the likely benefits have been carefully balanced against the risks.

Electro-convulsive therapy

Indications. Carefully selected patients among those suffering from severe depressive illness, severe mania, severe catatonic states.

Principles. Early beliefs in the therapeutic value of administering electric shocks and of the administration of camphor, leading to convulsions, were followed in 1933 by Meduna's chemical convulsion therapy, by intravenous injection of camphor in oil, and later of metrazol. This was based on the current idea that schizophrenia and epilepsy were antagonistic disorders. The induction of convulsions by electricity by Cerletti and Bini in 1938 superseded the earlier method. During the following two decades electro-convulsive therapy (ECT) was widely used: since psychotropic drugs have become established the indications have become more limited, but the majority of psychiatrists retain the view that ECT is the most effective and rapid treatment for severe depressive illness. When applied in 'modified' form, with the patient under a general anaesthetic and with use of a muscle relaxant, the efficacy of the procedure seems established. It is generally used only when patients are judged to be too severely ill, and too distressed, to await the delay and greater uncertainty associated with tricyclic antidepressive medication; or else when patients have failed to respond to full courses of such medication. ECT is also reported to be an effective treatment for severe mania, and for severe catatonic excitement or stupor in the rare cases when these are resistant to treatment by drugs.

The treatment is empirically successful. The procedure is elaborate, involving premedication, anaesthetic and muscle relaxant, the passage of the current, and the cerebral excitation leading to the convulsion. The general belief, backed by evidence which is not fully conclusive, is that the convulsive activity is the essential ingredient. Animal experiments give limited and indirect support to this view, but the mechanism of action remains uncertain.

Some degree of confusion and memory loss often occurs immediately after ECT: the frequency and extent of long-term memory disorder as a sequel of repeated courses of the treatment has yet to be determined. Unilateral ECT applied to the non-dominant hemisphere is held by many to produce less short-term memory impairment than conventional (bilateral) ECT, without loss of therapeutic effectiveness, but on this point the evidence is incomplete. Procedures have been advocated for metering the strength of the impulse in accordance with the patient's convulsive threshold, which may reduce the chances of disorders of memory.

Psychosurgery

Indications. Very highly selected patients with intractable severe and distressing affective disorders and tension states, or severe behavioural disturbances associated with temporal lobe pathology.

Principles. Psychosurgery denotes selective surgical removal or destruction of neural pathways with the purpose of changing or controlling emotions or behaviour. The earlier operations involving prefrontal lobotomy, as adapted by Freeman and Watts following the suggestion of Moniz in 1935, were followed by severely disabling post-leucotomy syndromes with intellectual and personality deterioration. Operations currently in use entail more circumscribed section of nervous tissue, and are usually undertaken as stereotactic procedures using a variety of destructive agencies. It is claimed that a range of operations including frontal lobe tractotomies, limbic leucotomy, cingulotomy, and amygdalotomy are highly effective in procuring relief in the small proportion of patients who experience exceptional and lasting distress as a result of chronic affective disorders and tension states which are unrelieved by other modalities of treatment. The issue remains contentious: the exponents of the procedure stress the crucial importance of obtaining the patient's informed consent, adopting rigorous criteria for selection of patients, ensuring a high degree of surgical skill, and planning a comprehensive programme of post-operative care.

The other indication for psychosurgery is for selected patients with severe behavioural disturbances associated with temporal lobe pathology with or without fits and with EEG abnormalities. Careful medical, neurological, psychiatric, and psychosocial assessment is necessary: rigorous criteria are applied, and procedures for comprehensive post-operative treatment deemed essential.

Specific psychological treatments

Dynamic psychotherapy (individual)
Indications. Highly selected patients with neurotic difficulties which are disturbing but not severely disabling, with strong motivation to gain 'insight' and with evident assets in personality and stability in life circumstances.

Principles. The essential feature of dynamic psychotherapy is its focus on attempting to alter the balance of unconscious forces which shape current attitudes, behaviour, and inner experience. There is two-way traffic between the conscious and unconscious: in the latter, internal forces are the products of conflicting factors – inborn, developmental, and experiential – and processes such as repression, transference, and resistance have crucial importance in determining conscious behaviour and experience. Concepts of the dynamic unconscious have interested psychologists and philosophers for centuries, but it has been studied systematically as an entity having a putatively coherent organization, susceptible to change by therapeutic manoeuvres, only since Freud introduced psycho-analytic theory at the turn of the century.

Many of the concepts of psycho-analytic theory have been absorbed into the contemporary literature, language, and culture; and dynamic psychogenic constructs and reasoning have become commonplace throughout psychiatric practice. Psychoanalysis and its derivatives provide a theory of normal and abnormal mental functioning, an approach to investigating their development, a metaphysical system, and a method of treatment. The last of these has been elaborated in the formal or dynamic psychotherapies, which are based on principles concerned, for example, with the nature of anxiety and its defences, psychosexual development, ego psychology, and object relations, all of which have theoretical antecedents. The treatments are practised only by those doctors and others who have taken a specialized training in the methods, which includes not only instruction and supervised clinical work but also a personal therapeutic experience, often extending to a full psycho-analysis.

Formal psychotherapies are methods of treatment suitable only for a carefully selected subgroup of patients with neurotic illnesses or personality disorders. Criteria for selection vary, as do the specific approaches to treatment: commonly the aim is to elucidate internal conflicts and procure personality change by providing the patient with insight through his emotional experience during the course of treatment. The relationship with the therapist is the main agent for treatment: it becomes invested with special significance for the patient, and within the context of this transference relationship the therapist offers the patient interpretations of his behaviour, attitudes, and utterances. Crucial to successful treatment is the requirement that the patient should have strong motivation to gain insight, a degree of psychological awareness, and the ability and inclination to view his problems in psychological terms. Sometimes the patient's suitability is established by a trial of treatment.

Treatment varies in intensity and duration and in the extent to which it is planned, from relatively brief treatment for periods of 6–18 months to treatment of indeterminate length: the most intensive approach consists of a full psycho-analysis. Special attention may be given to preparing the patient for treatment, agreeing upon goals and establishing a therapeutic contract. The therapist generally avoids all opportunities or requests for liaison with other persons involved in the patient's life, as the focus of his treatment is confined to intra-psychic variables and personal experiences.

In contrast to the biomedical treatments, which are directed towards demonstrable mechanisms, objective explanations, and the form of psychological functioning, dynamic psychotherapy is concerned more with understanding and personal meaning and with the content of psychic experience. In so far as it aims at symptom relief (which is not its primary goal), it incorporates the assumption that psychopathological forms can be changed by manipulation of content.

Group Psychotherapy

Indications. Selected patients with neurotic disabilities manifested in symptoms, interpersonal difficulties and problems of living.

Principles. Group therapy is more economical than individual psychotherapy, but it is a treatment modality in its own right, not necessarily inferior to individual treatment, for there is a range of problems which can be dealt with more effectively in the group setting. Deriving from psycho-analytic theory and from social psychology, the study of group processes has had an impact on community relations and industrial management and on educational practice as well as psychiatry. The rationale stems from the fact that in a group a patient may recognize that he is not alone in his predicament: he may compare his own difficulties with those of other people and,

becoming gradually more involved in the interactions within the group, he gains understanding of aspects of his behaviour from observing its effects on others. The group interactions are in part reflections of the tension within each member as well as those between members, so when the group reviews and interprets its own dynamic processes, advantages may accrue to the individual participants.

The usual psychotherapeutic group consists of six to ten clients or patients with a therapist. Groups vary with respect to their constitution: some are homogeneous, consisting of people with similar problems and similar goals, but the more complex groups are heterogeneous, their membership being chosen to provide what the therapist regards as a potentially rewarding balance of attributes and problems. Thus there may be equal numbers of men and women, and the personality and attitudinal strengths of different members may be complementary in various important respects. Groups may be open, receiving new members as old ones drop out, or closed. Weekly meetings are the rule and the duration of treatment is rarely less than one year or more than three years.

The group is seen as going through various phases of development before it becomes coherent and effective. Within the framework of mutual support and group cohesiveness, frank exchanges are possible and the complex processes thought to be therapeutic begin to assert themselves. The opportunity for interpersonal learning, the re-enactment of earlier relationships, and the processes of imitation and identification all come into play in parallel with the more obvious processes of providing mutual support, reassurance concerning shared difficulties, advice and guidance, and a feeling of hope.

Groups vary in the extent to which they depend on psycho-analytic principles as well as in their goals and constitution. Consequently group processes take different courses, and are perceived and interpreted differently according to the style of the therapist, his conduct of the meetings, and the assumptive framework within which the group was established.

Patients likely to benefit from small-group psychotherapy are those who are highly motivated, not only for personal psychological change but also for experiencing this change by participating actively in a group. A degree of verbal competence is required together with an inclination to explore psychological concepts.

The principles which have been established in

small-group psychotherapy may be applied elsewhere in the hospital and community. They have implications for the management of psychiatric wards and day hospitals, and sometimes it is urged that both small and large group meetings have an important place in every psychiatric ward: it is argued that only in this way is it possible to establish the best kind of therapeutic environment. Indeed the therapeutic community may sometimes become the dominant form of treatment – this happens particularly with the management of people severely handicapped by failure of social adjustment resulting in sociopathic behaviour. Furthermore, outside the psychiatric services, a range of self-help groups is to be found, some of which have well-established networks with group meetings open to interested members of the public who express a wish for assistance of the kind proffered.

Behaviour therapy

Indications. Certain neurotic disorders; defined aspects of behaviour of a wide range of patients.

Principles. Ideas about the efficacy of reward and punishment, suggestion and practice, gradual habituation, and deliberate attempts at relaxation are as ancient as recorded history and imply that behaviour can be evoked or suppressed by appropriately planned provocative, gratifying, or quietening measures. The systematic application of these ideas in medicine emerged in the 1920s when Janet described tasks which, if practised by persons suffering from various neurotic disorders, could have a healing function. Later the study of learning processes led to the development of conditioning procedures for relief of morbid fears, and to the use of aversive conditioning in the treatment of alcohol dependence. Further application of the principles of learning theory to the treatment of neurotic patients led to the propounding of a general theory of neurosis which held that neurotic symptoms are learned maladaptive patterns of behaviour, and that strategies for unlearning or re-education will eliminate the disorder, so that there is no need to postulate any underlying process other than that which can be comprehended in terms of learning theory. Anxiety was seen as closely associated with the maladaptive behaviour and the earliest successes were associated with the reduction of anxiety responses to specific situations. The reasoning behind these propositions led to treatment procedures for a range of symptoms and maladaptive

behaviour patterns – particularly anxiety-driven avoidance responses such as phobias and obsessions, but also including examples of failure to learn adaptive responses, as in enuresis, and unwanted approach responses such as sexual deviations. The empirical success of these forms of treatment strengthened assertions that they were based on correct theory, and that the psycho-analytic theory of neurosis was thereby discredited. Much fruitless debate ensued, based on attempts at rational rather than empirical approaches to understanding neurosis.

The principles underlying behavioural therapies have lately been more firmly grounded. Their proponents adduce evidence from experimental studies in learning, cognitive, and social psychology, together with the results of clinical inquiries, and they utilize an approach to the patient's predicament which seeks to identify problems which will prove to be amenable to specific techniques. The patient's problems and circumstances are submitted to a behavioural analysis: in this the symptoms and manifest behaviour are assessed in detail, cognizance being taken of the patient's perceived problems, his thought processes, fantasies and imagery, his mood, fears, and state of autonomic arousal and the occasions of their variation, the way he responds to distress, his attitudes, motivation, and expectations. In this way a picture is obtained of how persisting abnormal behaviour is reinforced by external or internal factors. The problems are clearly delineated and placed in their context, so that realistic goals can be established. The emphasis is on concrete instances and quantifiable criteria of disorder.

Target problems most suitable for a behavioural therapeutic approach include a range of phobic conditions – simple phobias, agoraphobia, social phobias; and also obsessional rituals, anxiety manifested as somatic symptoms, psychosexual problems, and tics. Claims are also made that behaviour therapy may contribute significantly to the treatment of certain patients with marital problems, and to the control of unwanted habits, for example alcohol dependence, smoking, and overeating. The behavioural analysis leads to a formulation which sets goals, provides some idea of hierarchies of situations provoking unfavourable response, and suggests quantitative bases for assessing changes in severity of the disorder. Courses of treatment with behaviour therapy generally comprise weekly or twice weekly sessions over a period which is rarely less than six weeks or longer than six months. Treatment is closely integrated with general psychotherapeutic and social measures. Risks associated with behaviour therapy include those associated with incorrect diagnosis or incorrect formulation of treatment objectives. Particular care must be taken to ensure that the problems chosen for behavioural treatment are not features of underlying depressive, schizophrenic, or organic psychotic disorders.

Other specific psychological treatments

Applications of dynamic psychiatry, social psychology, learning theory, and cognitive psychology have led to the development of procedures for a range of approaches to *marital therapy*. The many approaches differ in terms of theoretical background and practical technique: they have in common the objective of focusing on interpersonal relations by conjoint interviews. Several conceptual frameworks or models for defining and characterizing marital pathology have been developed, based on psychoanalytic theory or on the principles of behaviour therapy or on pragmatic lines. Different aspects of the marital relationship – emotional, sexual, social, and intellectual – may be examined in the context of the marital history and current problems. The therapist may work alone or with a co-therapist of opposite sex. Sometimes two or more couples are treated as a group.

Many psychiatrists and social workers in the course of their routine work attempt to help their patients to unravel some of their marital problems: specialized approaches to marital therapy are undertaken by doctors, nurses, social workers, psychologists or others who have received a specialist training from one of the national marriage guidance councils or from centres where the appropriate techniques are being developed.

Sex therapy, directed at couples who present with sexual dysfunction, has grown since the early 1970s: increased understanding of the psychophysiology of normal and abnormal sexual functioning has combined with behavioural and psychodynamic principles to make available a number of different techniques of treatment. When appropriate, sex therapy may be included as one component of marital therapy.

Family therapy is a further example of new growth in the field of psychotherapy. The term covers a variety of approaches: the school-age adolescent or young adult may be the referred patient, several children may be included in the group, the children may be brought in only after a period of marital therapy. The practice of family therapy draws on concepts from a variety of theoretical frameworks and a number of arbitrary constructs or models may be devised to represent family interactions and their vicissitudes. Although there is no unified systematic approach, most experienced practitioners would agree on the importance of careful delineation of problems and objectives and clear formulation of the plan of treatment for each individual case.

The social dimensions of treatment

Both normal and abnormal behaviour and experience affect, and are affected by, social processes, so that the social environment is pervasively implicated in all aspects of psychopathology: aetiology, pathogenesis, identification, assessment, and diagnosis. Objective features of the social environment are important but it must be recalled that it is the individual's perception of the environment, determined by his personal characteristics and psychopathology, which most immediately determines his affective and behavioural reactions. Consequently the social environment is also of crucial importance in the management of mental disorder: whatever is done by members of the psychiatric team, they inevitably participate in the patient's social environment. It follows that these influences should as far as possible be planned deliberately to evoke some therapeutic advantage.

Principles underlying the social aspects of treatment fall under three headings: the settings where treatment may take place, the arrangements within these settings, and the procedures for longer-term rehabilitation.

The settings of treatment

When help is sought from the psychiatric team by a patient or by others acting on his behalf, the first decisions are concerned with whether he should be advised to interrupt the normal course and routines of his life. Indications for giving such advice are relative rather than absolute. Advising him to take time away from work, for example, may ease his predicament, or it may add new dimensions to his problem. Temporary alteration of aspects of his family or social life may appear to be a logical step; and established habits and circumstances may be recognised as pathogenic. Careful judgement needs to be exercised by the medical or psychiatric adviser or by other members of the team in recommending, and helping the patient to arrange, temporary changes in his life circumstances. Sometimes admission to hospital is indicated, in order to remove the patient from an environment which, in view of his psychopathology, seems noxious; or to provide a period of respite in the stable and regularized environment of the hospital; or to allow for more detailed investigation, medical, psychological, or social, than would be possible with the patient living in his normal setting. The psychopathology may be such that the patient's behaviour is severely disordered and his recognition of his predicament distorted to such an extent that there are severe dangers to his life, his health, or his personal security, or to others: in such cases, forming a small minority, compulsory admission may be advisable.

Attempts to promote relief or recovery by altering the patient's environment require clear judgement and, in their implementation, the application of the principles of general psychotherapy. The correct advice needs to be correctly conveyed to the patient and, if necessary, to his family and other associates.

The therapeutic environment

Patients may be treated at home, in other domestic settings, in psychiatric hospitals, psychiatric units in general hospitals, psychiatric day hospitals, or in hostels or 'half-way houses' in the community. A total course of treatment may include spells in several of these settings. The environment within institutions such as mental hospitals has for long been recognized as a potent influence affecting the patient's mental state and prospects of recovery for good or ill. A number of general principles have become accepted as desirable components of hospital practice: these principles derive from humanitarian considerations and from empirical knowledge influenced by the application of ideas stemming from psycho-analysis and social psychology.

General nursing care forms the backbone of inpatient management of psychiatric patients. It has investigative as well as treatment functions, for no detailed clinical assessment is complete without the opportunity for continuous observation by nursing staff. The distinct therapeutic value of admission to a ward where psychiatric nursing care is sensitive to the individual needs of the patient seems well established. A period with such management uncontaminated by drugs and other specific procedures is often

beneficial even to the most disturbed patient. It provides opportunity for detailed observation and assessment of patients and thus increases the information available when more specific treatments are planned.

Widening recognition of the use of the hospital environment as a mode of treatment has led to the development of ideas concerning the therapeutic milieu – a term of wide connotation which covers the social interactional aspects of psychiatric ward and hostel management. Verbal exchanges and behavioural responses within the patient group and between patients and staff are believed to hold therapeutic potential, and arrangements to maximize the benefits include group meetings in which their meanings are examined or interpreted. Arrangements for this kind of activity vary greatly from one institution or ward to another according to the policies and ideologies of those responsible for patient care and according to the characteristics of patients accepted in the particular setting. Although it is generally agreed that patients should be active rather than passive, that interactions between patients should be encouraged, and that nurse–patient relationships should have recourse to general psychotherapeutic principles, there is no consensus about the extent of formal organization which is desirable for social therapy. The most highly developed version of this aspect of treatment is the *therapeutic community* in which efforts are made to devolve responsibility for all matters on 'democratic' lines, to each corporate decision or consensus of the group which thereby becomes a kind of commune. Principles of permissiveness, tolerance, and egalitarianism minimize differentials between clients and paid staff: control is in the hands of the group rather than being sought by the exercise of professional skills. Some therapeutic communities exist for treatment of highly selected subgroups of patients, for example with sociopathic personality disorders who are thereby made to confront the social consequences of their behaviour. Some experts claim advantage for these principles in treating the whole range of psychiatric hospital patients. Elsewhere in the management of hospital wards, day hospitals, and hostels, recourse is had to some but not all of the principles described as governing therapeutic communities. In its fullest expression, the therapeutic community movement appears to have been an ideology fostered by a number of charismatic leaders in the context of a social climate which has proved to be transient. The history of psychiatry shows shifts of fashion between custodial and restrictive care and moral treatment in which humane principles and attention to details of the physical and social environment came to dominate the picture of inpatient care. Many psychiatrists would hold that the most important of the ideals generated by the therapeutic community movement are of ancient lineage and must inevitably continue to be represented in the institutional care of the mentally disabled.

The design of a therapeutic environment includes measures aimed at encouraging the patient's active participation in the processes directed at symptom relief and other desired change. Mention has been made of the influences of the ward milieu: in addition to psychiatric nursing procedures, *occupational therapy* has much to contribute both to assessment and to treatment of patients. In treatment its aims are to maintain a daily routine of purposeful activity of a kind which is not centred on personal psychopathology; to distract from excessive morbid self-examination; to prevent the development of secondary disabilities; to provide a framework for interactions with other patients and therapists; to inject a sense of preparation for return to normal living; and perhaps to enable the patient to learn new skills. In conjunction with ward management of the psychiatric in-patient, occupational therapy, on or off the ward, is an important aspect of milieu therapy.

The principles governing the provision of therapeutic environments hold good, with the appropriate modifications, for treatments in a wide range of settings, from the in-patient unit and the day hospital to the management of hostels. The main objectives of each type of facility are definable and within each setting procedures for ensuring patient participation, avoidance of pathological dependence, and focusing on preparation for the future are among the main guidelines for individual treatment programmes.

Procedures for longer-term rehabilitation

It is common during the early stages of treatment, whether within or outside hospital, to consider the patient's previous social functioning in relation to his psychopathology and its expected outcome, so that realistic objectives can be set for social interactions and adjustment in the longer-term future. In the simplest cases, when the illness is a circumscribed affair, the problem is one of expediting the patient's secure return to the *status quo ante*. In other cases it is not realistic to expect full resolution of the

psychopathology, because some of the major psychiatric disorders are associated with severe long-term disability. Schizophrenic illnesses, for example, have a tendency to chronicity, often with only partial recovery from acute episodes, a relapsing course, and accumulation of residual difficulties. Most of the organic psychoses of later life, and some occurring earlier, follow an intermittently or continuously downhill course with progressive disablement. Many patients with mental subnormality are disabled throughout their lives. In all such cases secondary disabilities are likely to appear, arising from the patients' increasing vulnerability and decreasing competence to meet the demands of ordinary living. Their environment – whether institutional or domestic – can itself become pathogenic, and the main focus of treatment shifts towards providing the type of human surroundings, living circumstances, daily routines, and occupational opportunity which will be therapeutic rather than harmful. The principal aims of social treatment and rehabilitation are to help the patient to reach improved levels of social functioning: to prevent or remove social disengagement on the patient's part, and to maintain or develop his capacity for adaptive behaviour. A part of the initial assessment will be concerned with the patient's social adaptation and its disorders: this assessment will guide the team to their formulation of reasonable objectives of treatment. The social worker in the team may have a special function in carrying out investigative and therapeutic procedures in this modality of patient management. The requirements are for suitably detailed information about the patient's social context to be assembled, particularly differentiating its pathogenic, protective, and therapeutic aspects. Armed with this information and supposition, the social worker and other members of the team may then proceed to attempt to alter the material or psychosocial environment in order to ameliorate the effects of maladaptive behaviour; and long-term support of patients and relatives may be arranged if they experience long-acting psychosocial difficulties.

The large number of provisions for social treatment of protracted disability include residential accommodation in hospital wards, hospital-hostels, and community hostels; half-way houses and other sheltered accommodation in the community; occupational facilities in sheltered workshops within or without the hospital setting; and recreational and social therapeutic facilities in day centres and social clubs. The principal aims for people with long-term disabling psychopathology are to provide supportive frameworks for living in circumstances as near as possible to those of a normal life. Care outside hospital is preferred to a hospital-based existence, and a range of facilities is therefore required. The whole span of community care includes the hospital services and presupposes ease of movement between hospital wards, day hospital, and extramural facilities; a crisis intervention service; and reasonable integration of care provided by statutory and voluntary agencies and volunteers. In addition a range of informal and organized procedures for self-help exist in the social networks of the community, outside the ambit of the professional service.

Treatment as a process

Treatment procedures have been differentiated as belonging to four main dimensions – the general psychotherapeutic, biomedical, specific psychological, and social. Within and between these modalities, the procedures are not mutually exclusive. General psychotherapy for example is defined as an approach required by all patients regardless of other treatments which may be exhibited, and there is some overlap between this treatment and certain components of specialized psychotherapy or behaviour therapy. Different treatments, if exhibited simultaneously, interact in various ways. Their effects may be independent, as with general psychotherapeutic methods and drug treatment; they may have additive or interactional effects, as when certain drugs are used in planned combination with a behavioural approach to a specific problem; or they may be counteractive, as is sometimes the case when psycho-active drugs are used in conjunction with specific psychotherapeutic procedures.

The planning of an individual patient's treatment is based on idiographic information deriving from the formulation of the salient characteristics of the disorder, the patient, and the context. Logical considerations suggest that a staged programme is generally the most appropriate course; for example a patient admitted to hospital with a depressive illness may begin with general psychotherapy in a therapeutic environment while his psychopathology and life circumstances are more fully assessed; a course of antidepressive medication may follow, the general psychotherapy being maintained; subsequently the patient may have achieved relief of symptoms, and an intensification of the general psychotherapeutic approach may focus on environmental or relation-

ship problems, thought to be of aetiological significance in his illness, which may call for social work intervention with longer-term aims. As a further example, a patient with a schizophrenic disorder characterized by florid paranoid delusions and associated behavioural disturbance may be treated first with general psychotherapy and phenothiazine drugs: subsequently rehabilitative measures directed towards assisting the patient to adapt to a sheltered environment may become the dominant treatment, the potential benefits and risks of long-term medication being considered at the same time.

Individualized treatment programmes have recourse to each dimension of treatment, as appropriate, in a course spread over a period of time. Often it is possible to make definite plans for only one stage ahead: a process of evaluation proceeds in parallel with the treatment, so that the prescription for later stages depends on outcome in the earlier stages, and on re-defining objectives. Continuity of treatment is thus maintained as response is reviewed at successive stages; by appraisal of progress, objectives are reformulated.

The complex activity of decision-making and intervention calls for a partnership between different members of the psychiatric team and for adequate communication and integrated action between all members of the team. Appropriate attention should be paid to record keeping: experiments are in progress in some centres with 'problem-oriented' medical records in which active and inactive problems, assets, and difficulties are entered along with brief statements about proposed action, and about further observations, by different members of the team. Progress charts of this and other kinds may supplement the narrative form of the patient's case notes.

It should be recalled that there is an educational component in effective psychiatric treatment. The patient will, in the most propitious circumstances, learn how to improve his chances of preventing recurrence of disorder: this may involve specific measures such as continued medication and medical and/or social work surveillance but a major component lies in exploiting as fully as possible the patient's potential for self-care, autonomy and self-determination. He should when appropriate learn how to perceive at an early stage the appearance or reappearance of danger signals or cues for further help-seeking. He should in any case learn to avoid the 'sick role', yet recognize the need for consultation, treatment, or help when this is indicated.

The psychiatrist as a variable

The causes of psychiatric disorders are multiple, varying from one case of a disorder to another. Possibly no causes are in themselves sufficient, very few are necessary, some are contributory, and most are uncertain. The disorders themselves are understandable only if a large measure of uncertainty can be contained, and they can be expressed in terms of diseases, patterns of social deviation, behavioural disorders, or in existential terms. Diagnostic reliability is limited and contingent variables, in personality and environment, may be all-important. Many of the common treatment measures lack specificity, though collectively they may reach a degree of success which puts them on a par with treatments in general medicine. Unified systems purporting to explain what goes wrong and how it can be corrected – whether based on disease models, behavioural theories, psychodynamic theories, or hypotheses concerning social processes – are sometimes of great theoretical interest and importance, but it is not possible to foresee a time when the whole problem of treatment of psychopathology can be incorporated into a single coherent theoretical system. A multidimensional approach to treatment is likely to remain as the only logical approach; and it follows that complexities inherent in the subject guarantee that there will be many shades of opinion among psychiatrists. A rigid conformity in the presence of so much uncertainty would surely be alarming. Systematic studies have been made of differing orientations of psychiatrists and contrasting approaches to treatment. A psychiatrist's orientation reflects aspects of his personality and cognitive style, and becomes shaped by the influence of training programmes and teachers, by variations in working circumstances and facilities, and by professional and general experience. Moreover, effective psychiatric management calls for the collaborative work of a team, and members of the team belonging to different professions may add their own perceptions of complexity to the total diversity.

Contingent variables in treatment and response

Psychiatric disorders vary in their duration and in the extent to which they pursue a self-limiting course. The notion of 'spontaneous remission' is frequently mentioned as a phenomenon which may embarrass the claims made for particular types of treatment. Patients may unaccountably recover, substantially or completely, even from a disorder of long standing, though the chances of such an outcome tend to diminish with the duration of the disorder. The concept of spontaneity of remission is not straightforward: generally speaking, biological events occur spontaneously only as a result of intrinsic processes of considerable complexity. A remission may occur because a process is inherently self-limiting, or it may take place as a result of time-related alterations in other aspects of the patient's internal or external environment; and the distinction between these is not complete, since both mechanisms may underlie any given instance of so-called spontaneous remission. In planning treatment programmes, and most particularly in evaluating treatment, it is important to have regard to the uncertain likelihood of improvement or recovery occurring as a result of circumstances which have nothing to do with the treatment.

Treatment in medicine consists of the application of an agent or process to a patient with a view to obtaining a particular result. In psychiatry special difficulties sometimes arise in defining 'agent', 'process', and 'particular result'. The treatment itself may be conceptualized with an ease and completeness which falls off as we cover the spectrum from a drug to a course of ECT or a technique of behaviour modification, a course of dynamic psychotherapy, exposure to a therapeutic milieu, and so to the more diffused and subtle agents of rehabilitation or general psychotherapy. The desired result may correspondingly elude attempts at definition, especially prescriptive definition. Nevertheless the logic of the matter assumes that there are specific links between the intervention and the sought-for amelioration.

Some effects of intervention arise from circumstances which are incidental to the treatment itself: these rather than the treatment may be the potent variables, and this phenomenon has gained recognition throughout medicine, becoming designated as the placebo response. Psychiatrists recognize that a host of contingent variables may have either positive or negative effects on outcome: the relationship of these variables to the definitive treatment may be clear or obscure, close or remote, causal or coincidental. The concepts of placebo response and placebo responder are abstractions of limited value: it is more realistic to attempt to analyse the sources and mechanisms of action of non-specific factors – i.e. factors outside the treatment itself – affecting the outcome of therapeutic interventions.

Reference has been made to the fact that many

patients with psychopathology do not enter into treatment. A variety of social factors, and sometimes in addition certain aspects of the psychopathology itself, keep them away from doctors and other formal agencies for treatment and care. Others, having become patients, may fail to accept advice or drop out of treatment before its completion. Others again accept advice irregularly and capriciously. It has been recognized in the last twenty years that co-operativeness in treatment is not a unitary factor. Having entered treatment, patients vary in the degree to which they comply with instructions or advice: hence the concept of compliance, or treatment adherence, has emerged as a quantitative variable, determined by a number of antecedent variables in the patient, his disorder, and the nature of the treatment offered. In so far as the treatment prescribed is effective, a patient who adheres to the treatment programme has a better chance of successful outcome than one who fails to participate wholeheartedly. A reasonable degree of compliance is a necessary but not sufficient condition for response to a prescribed treatment measure: but aside from this obvious fact, there are commonalities between the variables affecting compliance and those involved with non-specific effects of treatment. The underlying variables may be grouped as those which are to some extent under the therapist's control, having to do with the treatment, the therapist himself, and the setting: those which depend in some way on the patient; and those which are aspects of his illness.

Variables in the treatment, the therapist and the setting

Biomedical procedures can be studied separately from the features of the therapist himself and the setting: the three classes of variables can be distinguished and their interrelationships studied. Thus a given drug prescribed in appropriate dose may be found to be more effective in the hands of enthusiastic therapists than when prescribed by those who are sceptical; or more effective in in-patients than in comparable day hospital patients. The contrasts may be wholly or partly attributable to greater adherence when therapists are enthusiastic or when patients are under continuous supervision; further inquiry will throw more light on the extent to which therapist, setting, and treatment variables have additive or combinatorial effects. By contrast, with psychological and social treatments, the treatment may be impossible to define or comprehend without refer-

ence to the therapists and the setting. In social rehabilitation procedures, or in the therapeutic community, the therapists and the setting comprise the very essence of the treatment; in dynamic psychotherapy the relationship between patient and therapist seems to be the supreme factor. Nevertheless, whatever the treatment, the bias of the therapist, his orientation, his faith in the treatment he is applying, and the zeal with which he applies it, may all function as agents promoting (or diminishing) treatment adherence and also as non-specific variables of therapeutic significance. So may his more general attitudes and behaviour and his prestige and credibility. Equally, other staff associated with the psychiatric team have attitudes and preferences of potential significance to treatment acceptance and effectiveness. Just as enthusiasms of staff may be communicated to patients, so it may be that beliefs in effectiveness may be communicated among groups of patients treated in the same setting. In such cases it may sometimes happen that active optimistic and forceful enthusiasms, by fostering hope, encouraging confidence, and increasing the patient's willingness to rehearse solutions to his predicaments, may become the essence of treatment. A sceptical approach to some of these treatment regimes would be self-contradictory, and in such cases the issue is one not of science but of faith; the treatment has become an emblem of an ideology. But even in less extreme circumstances, the stability of the treatment setting, the quality of the doctor–patient relationship, the continuity of care from one and the same therapist or team, may all function as part-determinants of treatment adherence and treatment efficacy.

In prescribing drugs, a variety of non-specific variables have been isolated and closely studied. Psychosocial aspects of prescribing and taking medicines appear to have strong influences on adherence and effectiveness. The nature of the presentation – tablet, capsule, elixir, suppository, or injection – and, in the case of the commonest presentation, the size, shape, and colour of the tablets or capsules, apparently have some short-term effects when treatment is started. Two classes of variable are of greater importance: the precise details of the therapeutic regime, and the instructions given to the patient. Patients seem to be generally more likely to adhere to once-daily dosage schedules than to multiple daily doses, to simple rather than multiple medication, and to tablets which are conveniently packaged and clearly labelled. They are more likely to conform to instructions which are clearly stated and written and which anticipate and reassure concerning unwanted effects and delay in appearance of sought-after effects. These factors influence adherence to treatment and encourage patient participation: hence, it is sometimes argued, they are therapeutic in themselves. The correct prescribing of drugs exacts a regard for such variables as these. In particular the possibilities of non-compliance will be recognized by the wise psychiatrist, for it leads to inefficient treatment, wastage, health hazards due to storage of unused drugs, and continuing uncertainties about the effects of treatment. Adequate instructions, accompanied if necessary by such measures as counting tablets and monitoring drug intake by suitable measures for drug detection or drug marking, may be employed.

Variables in the patient

It would hardly be surprising if the patients most likely to seek professional help and comply with the proposed treatment regimes were found to be those who have a high regard for the medical and allied professions, confidence in the power of the available remedies, a belief in their own capacity to participate in such investigative and therapeutic procedures as they expect to be offered, and a view of their illness or disorder as a painful or otherwise unpleasant affliction for which relief is to be expected. These general predictions are borne out by reports of associations between treatment adherence and demographic and social variables such as age, sex, marital state, social class, occupation, and education; personality variables especially those concerning stability and suggestibility and those determining attitudes and expectations; previous experience of treatment; and the presence of relatives or friends to reinforce positive attitudes and sometimes to help or supervise with the control of medication. Sociological studies have suggested that definable attitudes and patterns of behaviour which can be construed as 'illness behaviour' and adoption of the 'sick role' influence the patient's incentives and motivations and hence contribute to the degree of rejection or acceptance of treatment programmes. Likewise there is evidence that a similar range of patient-related variables influence the extent and type of response to treatment once it is accepted. Any perceived favourable response to a form of treatment will itself be likely to reinforce both the patient's resolve to adhere to the prescribed course of action and his belief in its efficacy.

Variables in the disorder or illness

The clinical features, severity, duration, acuteness or chronicity, and previous course of the disorder have all been demonstrated to relate in some circumstances to the likelihood of treatment adherence and influence the chances of a favourable or unfavourable response to non-specific aspects of the treatment. Immediately perceived consequences of starting or discontinuing a course of treatment affect adherence for good or ill, and influence the patient's expectations and hence perhaps the outcome. The natural history of a recurrent illness may have particularly important influences of a kind which are far from simple if prophylactic measures (such as lithium carbonate or long-term neuroleptic medication) are prescribed. Nobody who feels well wishes to be medicated unnecessarily: a patient who sees himself as slightly below par may, rightly or wrongly, attribute his deficiencies to the unwanted effects of medication, as may a patient who is beginning to relapse despite the medication. These and other subtle interactions between the subjective perceptions or objective manifestations of illness and the real or supposed effects of medication may govern both degree of adherence and non-specific response. The precise details of the aspects of psychological or social treatment measures which determine treatment adherence and non-specific response tend to be buried in the complexities of the individual case: they are amenable to systematic study but present formidable methodological and practical problems.

Evaluation of treatment

In psychiatry, as elsewhere in medicine, the value which is generally assigned to a treatment method depends in part on the rationale, or theoretical considerations regarding its known or assumed mechanisms, in part on empirical evidence founded upon observed and recorded effects of the treatment, and in part upon the extent to which there is a consensus of clinical opinion. In the ideal state these three considerations would merge: each treatment would have known effectiveness, achieving its results through well understood mechanisms, and clinical opinion would reflect this certain knowledge. In the meantime some treatments are regularly employed because theoretical reasoning or belief holds that they ought to work; some are demonstrably effective; and some are acceptable on the basis of collective clinical opinion, despite the lack of empirical evidence or clear rationale.

The history of medicine and psychiatry is littered with discarded theories, and current views suggest that while theoretical and experimental biological considerations may shape the development of a treatment method, the ultimate value of the method depends not on its rationale, nor even on its mechanisms, but on the appraisal of its results. The treatment is to be judged by its effects and not by its theory: indeed its theory may be strengthened, modified, or discredited by evidence derived from careful observation of its results. One of the tasks of clinical science is the examination of empirical evidence and the advancement of methods for obtaining it. Another is the recognition and delineation of the boundaries of science, for theories or beliefs based on reasoning which does not have recourse to public evidence are generally not amenable to exploration by scientific methods. A treatment may therefore be considered scientifically established only to the extent that there is indisputable empirical evidence for its effectiveness.

The assertion that a particular treatment is effective in a given condition is essentially a comparative statement: it implies that without the treatment the outcome would in some way be less favourable. In some medical and surgical conditions the comparison is easy, when for example the course of events in the untreated case is predictable within close limits or when conditions are fatal and pursue an unremittingly downhill course. Most disease, however, is not so predictable, and psychiatric disorders are especially notable for their wayward course, their outcome being subject not only to the variations intrinsic in the disorders themselves but also to the individuality of the patient and his circumstances. The results of a particular treatment for a given condition will be obvious only if it causes immediate, pronounced, and lasting benefit or harm. Otherwise effectiveness can be assessed only by controlled inquiry in which the results of an unproven treatment are compared with those obtained from a standard treatment or placebo. Comparisons using retrospective controls are not without value in some circumstances – for example when a new treatment is expected to have striking results in a relatively rare condition in which the salient variables affecting outcome have been carefully documented. But when circumstances permit, the preferred procedure is to arrange for direct comparison by setting up a prospective trial of treatment in which a subgroup of patients receives the treatment on trial whilst a second subgroup, comparable in all significant respects, receives the standard treatment, or a placebo, or no treatment.

The conditions of the trial, including the duration of treatment, the methods of clinical assessment of severity of the disorder, the criteria of response, and the length of the follow-up period, are planned in such a way as to provide a fair test of the claims of the treatment on trial. It is necessary to ensure that the comparison is valid in that like is compared with like: and this will be so only if steps are taken to eliminate bias in the allocation of patients to one or other subgroup. The controlled trial should therefore be randomized. Furthermore, the judgement of outcome of treatment in the individual patient may be influenced by the patient's or the therapist's knowing which treatment has been exhibited: consequently the randomized controlled trial should whenever possible be double-blind, both patient and investigator remaining ignorant of the treatment group to which the patient was assigned. Even when this is not possible it can sometimes be arranged that the investigator making the clinical assessments does not know how the treatment has been allocated.

The logic of the double-blind randomized controlled clinical trial follows ineluctably from recognition that evidence for the effectiveness of a treatment can come only from a valid comparative statement. A number of variants of the standard procedure are in common use: thus it is possible to compare several treatments by allocation of a homogeneous series of patients to the appropriate number of subgroups. Economy may be achieved, and perhaps also a closer method of control, by cross-over procedures in which each sub-set of patients receives, in pre-arranged sequence, each form of treatment involved in the comparison: investigations using this design are appropriate when palliative measures, having no carry-over effects, are on trial. Sequential methods have been devised, in which the trial is terminated as soon as a statistically significant result favouring one or other treatment has been obtained or shown, by predesignated criteria, to be unobtainable: these methods are difficult to manage when several criteria of response are required. Single-case 'self-controlled' clinical trial procedures have also been described.

Application of the controlled trial procedure is often difficult, and sometimes limited, in all clinical disciplines for a variety of reasons. Ethical considerations set limits to therapeutic experimentation. Furthermore the treatment procedures may be such as to make a double-blind approach, or even blind assessments, impossible or impracticable, and there may be logistic difficulties. Nevertheless as a general rule the more closely the principles underlying the randomized clinical trial can be followed, the greater the certainty of knowledge available for therapeutic application. Important criticisms of these principles centre upon problems of statistical inference. It is argued that randomization may not be the most logical or economical form of therapeutic examination, and that conclusions drawn from application of tests of statistical significance may not legitimately be generalized because it is absurd to assume that variations attributable to multiple unknown causes are governed by the laws of probability. However, these strictures relate more to the tendency to over-generous extrapolation of the results of therapeutic trials than to the principles of carefully controlled comparison: they do not discredit the method but warn against the temptation to extend unduly the findings of necessarily circumscribed experimentation.

Special attention needs to be paid to ethical aspects of therapeutic experimentation. In this regard certain principles are easily stated though their implementation may require much thought, and some – for example the question of whether patients should be assigned to different groups before or after they are asked to choose whether or not to enter an experiment – are matters currently under debate.

(1) All patients are entitled to receive the best available treatment. Hence a serious claim that a newly-introduced (or otherwise unproven) treatment procedure is superior to others should be put to the test.

(2) In all therapies, patients are entitled to explanations about treatments they may receive: they are also entitled to choose between alternatives, and to receive guidance in making their choices. In therapeutic experimentation the patient's informed and understanding consent should be given, without duress, before the start of treatment. The patient may be informed that it is not known which of the treatments available is the best, so that it is proposed that he should have an equal chance of receiving each one.

(3) The physician will of necessity change the patient's treatment if the patient's condition deteriorates or if progress is otherwise considered unsatisfactory, or if the disadvantages of his treatment clearly outweigh the advantages.

(4) The physician is responsible for giving the best possible treatment to all of his patients; he is responsible for ensuring that all his prescriptions for treatment are supportable by the best available evidence. Yet all treatment is, in an important sense, a form of experimentation. All methods of treatment in medicine are permanently on probation: all potentially involve hazards, and a physician would not be acting responsibly if he regarded his firmly held beliefs as equivalent to established knowledge; if he failed to consider therapeutic innovation or consistently prescribed new treatments as soon as they were introduced; or if in other respects he failed to learn from his therapeutic disappointments. Just as it would be unethical to carry out unnecessary or undesirable therapeutic experiments, it would be unethical to disregard the element of experimentation inherent in all treatment, and equally unethical to refrain from carrying out the necessary experimentation in an orderly (as opposed to haphazard) fashion, so that it will yield the maximum of information in the shortest time. At the same time there are treatments which have become accepted as correct even though they have not been subjected to rigorous trial: in the absence of possibly superior alternatives, it is unethical to withhold such treatments.

(5) In all therapeutic experimentation a research protocol should be formulated, setting out details of the design and procedures, the potential benefits, hazards, and discomforts of the treatments under consideration, and the ethical considerations involved: this protocol should be submitted to a specially appointed independent committee for comment and guidance. Approval should be obtained from this committee before the work is begun.

The need for regular use of the randomized controlled trial to improve the quality of treatment is even greater in psychiatry than in other specialties of medicine, for two reasons. Most psychiatric disorders have no identifiable organic pathology, so there is no objective marker of therapeutic progress, and scrupulous and disinterested comparative clinical assessment is of the essence; and the course of psychiatric disorder is particularly likely to be influenced by the patient's personal and social circumstances and by a host of non-specific variables associated with treatment, referred to above. Indeed, much therapeutic effort in psychiatry consists of making elaborate interventions in processes which are themselves many-sided and poorly understood. Specificities, often assumed, can be established only by appeal to the kind of hard evidence which comes from controlled experimentation in which variables are manipulated or held constant as far as is possible and ethically justifiable in order to gain improved recognition of their effects and interactions.

The requirements for conducting a randomized controlled trial are summarized in table 10.1. Rigorous adherence to the procedures, tailored to the particular clinical problems and treatments under investigation, is necessary both to safeguard the ethical requirements and to avoid introducing bias for one or other treatment. Multicentre trials are often necessary to obtain sufficient patients to answer the questions under scrutiny, and in such cases special arrangements are necessary to co-ordinate work at the different centres and to ensure uniformity of procedures for treatment and assessment.

Table 10.1. *Requirements for conducting a randomized controlled trial*

1	Definition of precise objectives of the inquiry
2	Consideration of ethical needs and limitations
3	Statement of hypotheses to be supported or refuted
4	Specification of demographic, social, and clinical criteria
5	Attention to criteria of type and severity of disorder, methods of clinical assessment and measurement of change with the passage of time
6	Specification of treatment regimes being compared: nature of treatment, intensity or dosage, timing, duration, setting of treatment, and general aspects of management
7	Consideration of sources and selection of patients, sampling procedures and stratification
8	Random allocation of patients to subgroups who will receive contrasting treatment regimes
9	Clarification of practical procedures for prescribing treatment and for 'blind' clinical assessment of patients, assessment of treatment adherence, identification and surveillance of patients dropping out of treatment, and surveillance of patients needing changes of treatment before termination of trial
10	Surveillance of *all* patients admitted to series. Specification of treatment after termination or withdrawal of trial treatment
11	Analysis of results
12	Conclusions, inferences, and implications for practice and for further investigation

The procedures outlined are applicable to the simplest design, in which straightforward comparisons are made between two (or more) subgroups of patients assigned to the respective treatments being compared. Reference has already been made to the several variations on the basic theme: cross-over studies may be undertaken, where all patients receive periods on each treatment in a balanced sequence, and certain treatments with palliative rather than enduring effects can be tested; and sequential trials are of limited value in psychiatry because they are difficult to undertake when multiple criteria of response are necessary. Formal procedures for self-controlled (individual case) studies have not yet been fully developed in an acceptable style: they depend upon complex logical and statistical manipulations the credentials of which are not established. Nevertheless this approach may be valuable in the future.

When the relevance, and particular difficulties, of therapeutic experimentation by means of the randomized controlled trial are examined for each of the main dimensions of treatment, it becomes clear that ethical, methodological and practical complexities abound. *Faute de mieux*, if controlled experimentation is not feasible or ethical, it must be recalled that substantial advances could be achieved in evaluating any form of treatment, however complex, by recourse to systematic and meticulous documentation of the characteristics of patients and their psychopathology, treatment procedures, and outcome on follow-up examinations. There are strong ethical and scientific arguments for the widespread adoption of standardized methods for cataloguing these major classes of variables.

General psychotherapy

Procedures under this heading are wide-ranging and not amenable to comprehensive definition. But even if this were not so, it would be both unethical and impracticable to withhold the treatment from any patient. The procedure cannot be evaluated *in toto*, but it would be possible to apply standard methods of comparative assessment to defined aspects of treatment – for example certain kinds of counselling – for well-delineated subgroups of patients. Hence there is scope for therapeutic experimentation within the broad limits of general psychotherapy, and certain components are amenable to specific evaluation in defined circumstances. But central to the application of general psychotherapy are various assumptions, for example that it is useful to spend time with distressed people, that a capacity for empathic understanding facilitates the therapist's attempts to give relief to anxious patients, that people are reassured by the knowledge that they are not alone in their suffering, and that they are also helped by knowing that they are being treated as individuals. These propositions, though non-specific, seem indisputable, and it is doubtful whether rigorous attempts at providing scientifically acceptable evidence would be justifiable or successful.

Treatment with drugs

The randomized controlled trial has been used extensively in the evaluation of drugs of all classes used in psychopharmacotherapy once they have passed through the earlier phases of assessment by animal experiment and preliminary trials on human subjects, and after their formal release for general clinical use. It is generally agreed that to become acceptable and assimilated into everyday practice a drug has to prove itself as superior to placebo and as rivalling drugs of established worth, on the basis of a number of rigorously controlled trials. The clearest results have been those relating to the comparative effects of antidepressives and of neuroleptics in severe acute affective and schizophrenic psychoses respectively. Such results have provided a number of valuable guidelines for prescribing these drugs for very disturbed patients. For chronic and recurrent psychotic disorders therapeutic experimentation has been more difficult. The target symptoms and dysfunctions have proved elusive; the main symptoms of the illness have sometimes been overshadowed by second-order disabilities attributable to social isolation, institutionalization, unemployment, and other disturbances of the life-style consequent upon the illness; patients' motivation and compliance in treatment have been depleted; external circumstances and events may influence the course of events more decisively than drugs; and there have been difficulties in following cohorts of patients long enough to assess the therapeutic and prophylactic effects of long-term medication. Nevertheless many of the problems have been shown to be amenable in principle to the methods of the randomized controlled trial, and many practical difficulties in implementating these have been overcome. The greatest uncertainty in assessment of drug treatment in psychiatry seems to be in the use of anxiolytic drugs on a medium or long-term basis in the treatment of neurotic disorders and other low-grade morbidity. Here the problems are both methodological and practical. The drugs are over-prescribed and patients may in various ways become habituated or drop out of treatment; the target symptoms are often ill-defined and capricious; the patients are often lost to the sight of the medical services and epidemiological methods need to be combined with the trial procedures if the course of events is to be clarified to any substantial extent.

Electro-convulsive therapy

Electro-convulsive therapy (ECT) is, in the opinion of most psychiatrists, uniquely valuable in the treatment of severe depressive disorders. Its acceptance did not await controlled evaluation. The relatively small volume of evaluative research supports this view in indicating more rapid, and somewhat more certain, clinical effectiveness than the most effective drug treatments. The procedure consists of a number of components – the intravenous anaesthetic and associated nursing attention, the muscle relaxant, the passage of the electrical current, the induction of the convulsion, and the recovery phase. It is generally thought that the cerebral excitation accompanying the fit is the essential ingredient. This remains uncertain, and recent work has focused on a number of issues awaiting further therapeutic research, which could be answered by suitable adaptations of the randomized controlled trial procedure.

Ethical problems arise in ECT research, and as commonly happens, ethical objections run in both directions and the matter remains controversial. Inclusion of patients with very severe depression in a randomized trial in which a proportion of patients do not receive the treatment, or receive it only after a period on medication, is to many clinicians an unacceptable procedure. At the same time the treatment itself is regarded as unethical by a vocal minority of the population at large. The danger remains therefore that those who prejudge the issue, for or against the treatment, will prevent or delay the acquisition of more accurate knowledge.

Psychosurgery

Evaluation of psychosurgery by the randomized controlled trial presents several practical and ethical problems. On even the most generous estimate, the group of patients thought likely to benefit from the treatment is small in number and clinically heterogeneous. Several centres would be required to collaborate, using precisely similar methods of patient assessment and preparation, surgical intervention, rehabilitation, and follow-up. These are mainly logistic problems but a more severe limitation stems from the controversy surrounding the subject. Many people, including some psychiatrists, regard the treatment as, by its very nature, unethical: they would remain uninfluenced by empirical demonstrations of benefit, patient satisfaction, and the lack of untoward effects. On the other hand firm exponents of the practice of psychosurgery may be over-enthusiastic in their advocacy of one or other technique, even to the extent of showing unwillingness to submit the procedure to a properly randomized trial. Thus the matter tends to be prejudged in one or other direction, and ethical experimentation is thereby prohibited.

Dynamic psychotherapy

Among the many ingredients of dynamic psychotherapies, the therapist–patient relationship is by general consent the principal component of treatment: it makes it possible for the patient to explore his conflicts and interpersonal difficulties and in doing so to undergo emotional experiences as a result of which it is hoped he will expand his comprehension, acceptance, control, and self-fulfilment. These are the principal aims of treatment and it is these rather than more objectively measurable variables which must be established if treatment is to be assessed. Thus there are major unsolved problems in choice of criteria of therapeutic success. However there are further problems of a different order. For example, as the main agent of the treatment, the therapist is himself deeply involved to such an extent that he must be strongly committed to a belief in its efficacy. This commitment is underlined by the fact that he has survived the selection procedures and undertaken the prescribed training, which includes a personal 'therapeutic experience'. Because of the selection and training requirements necessary for practising this type of treatment, the psychotherapist's capacity for scepticism is blunted. He may doubt certain aspects of theory and he may assert his inability to help all comers, but he inevitably accepts the value of dynamic psychotherapy as a form of treatment for selected patients. He is therefore unable, for ethical reasons, to participate in a randomized controlled trial of treatment: to do so would entail either denial of his commitment to a belief in the practice of psychotherapy, or unethical behaviour. It may be argued that it is possible to submit certain components of dynamic psychotherapy to critical

research, or to compare different procedures among the many that are available. Nevertheless the treatment is essentially private and personal to the therapist, and it may be that in pooling data the essential components of treatment would be lost to sight. Meanwhile other kinds of investigative work seem possible – and likely to yield more useful information if undertaken by psychotherapists collaborating with those outside the specialty – but it is difficult to see how decisive results can be obtained about specific therapeutic effectiveness while the principle of random allocation is unacceptable. Consequently dynamic psychotherapy remains as one of the treatments for which the legitimate claims are matters for assertion linked to belief in specific therapeutic techniques rather than evidence based on comparative data.

Group psychotherapy

A large array of approaches is employed in small-group psychotherapy. The approaches are in principle amenable to assessment by the randomized controlled trial, although certain practical problems pose difficulties. A matched control group of patients may receive other treatment and have the same methods of assessment, over the same period of time, as those which are applied to the patients participating in the group treatment. But any significant dropout from either treatment will invalidate the comparison; double-blind assessment is virtually impossible; the criteria of successful outcome may be elusive; and long-term follow-up of patients requires strenuous measures.

Behaviour therapy

Behavioural methods of treatment embody detailed specification of methods of intervention and close definition of objectives of treatment. In these respects they are peculiarly amenable to therapeutic evaluation; indeed many of those who have been concerned with developments of these forms of treatment have based much of their reasoning on the need for replicable results and the importance of identifying the critical components of contrasting treatment regimes. Intricate designs have been worked out, as variants of the randomized controlled trial, to gain the maximum of information from small samples of patients.

Other specialized psychological treatments

Marital, sexual, and family psychotherapies vary in the extent to which objectives are defined at the start of treatment; and their methods also vary in the degree to which they draw on models and assumptions from dynamic psychotherapies and behaviour therapies respectively. Insofar as they utilize methods derived from behaviour therapy, they are amenable to therapeutic evaluation in regard to their defined objectives.

Social treatments

Scientific evaluation of social treatments is bedevilled by the very complexity of treatment objectives, the difficulty of stating objectives in advance of treatment, and the elaborate and often hidden properties of the treatment procedures themselves. Comparative studies of defined components of treatment are possible: the whole procedure of social treatment is open to investigation within the limits of what is practicable and what is ethical, but problems of replicability may limit the value of some assessment procedures.

Psychiatric services: organization and evaluation

A multidimensional approach to treatment is needed both for patients with acute disorders and for those with lasting disabilities. The latter group is large and diverse in its requirements, and it often happens that the nature of the disability is such that special living arrangements, occupational facilities, and social support are needed: if these are not provided the tendency for patients suffering from long-term psychiatric disorder to develop secondary disabilities and further impairment of functioning becomes increasingly pronounced, distressing, and inconvenient. It follows that medical services, within the traditional framework comprising general practitioner, hospital out-patients department, and hospital wards, are insufficient. Complex patterns of care are required, over and above the routine primary care and hospital service, to provide the whole extent of the necessary medico-social measures. Reference has to be made to the range of provisions necessary for the social dimensions of treatment, such as (in addition to the general practitioner and hospital service), psychiatric day hospitals, hospital-hostels providing shelter and supervision for certain classes of hospital patients; a range of hostels and group homes in the community where the mentally disabled may live reasonably normal lives with varying degrees of practical help and social support; day centres for regular attendance by those living at home or in hostels who would

otherwise become isolated or helpless; 'walk-in' clinics and arrangements for crisis intervention, and special remedial centres for more specific subgroups of people requiring particular forms of management. In practical terms the need is for accommodation, physical facilities, transport, and, most important of all, a suitable variety of trained and highly motivated personnel. Local demographic and social circumstances may shape local needs to some extent: often the best arrangements for inner city areas will not be the best for sparsely populated rural areas. But the general requirement still holds: a suitable framework for integrated social care and social and medical treatments.

Such facilities clearly need to be planned in relation to a geographically or otherwise designated population or community. And they can be planned only by recourse to a series of demographic, social, and clinical assumptions which in the best circumstances are derived from hard data. Thus it is important to know the present and projected size and age-structure of the population being served, and to be able to make forecasts of future prevalence of disability of various kinds and degrees. Economic considerations also enter the equation, since the provisions for social and medical care are generally seen as correctly and inevitably chargeable in some way to the community, generally to the public services supplemented to some extent by services and facilities provided by voluntary bodies and volunteers.

The planning of services thus relates to a defined community, and hence there is an epidemiological base to which reference may be made when estimating the present and likely future prevalence of disabilities of various kinds. The services will be effective and efficient only if they are planned in accordance with the known facts about the community and the types and degrees of disability it contains. And among the necessary facts which serve as a basis for planning, information is needed about the past achievements and deficiencies of the services for the mentally disabled. It follows that, if the services are to provide the best resources within the limits of what is available, they need to be monitored; they can be monitored effectively only if attention is specifically devoted to methods of evaluation of services.

The evaluation of the psychiatric service of a community is a conceptually and technically difficult venture which calls for exercise of a range of methods of epidemiological research and social inquiry. The principles of the randomized controlled trial have relatively little to offer: they are applicable only in relation to restricted components of the service. We are concerned more with assessing the efficiency of the arrangements for mental health care than with establishing the effectiveness of circumscribed treatment procedures. For the greater part of this enterprise, careful and comprehensive data collection is required. The excellence of the method of evaluation, and hence of the planning of the services, is a function of the way in which the data-gathering is designed and executed. The required data are those which refer to the patients in the community (including those resident in hospitals and other institutions), characterizing their disorders in terms of diagnoses and levels of functional disability, and to their domicile – home, hostel, hospital, reception centre, homeless – and also to the facilities at present deployed in their care. It is necessary, moreover, to take special steps to update this information, in order to provide an accurate running account of the problems and the methods in use for controlling them and also in order to assess management policies. Consequently, for completeness it is necessary to establish and maintain a register of the psychiatrically disturbed and disabled. In doing this, due regard must be paid to sampling and survey methods for primary collection of data; procedures for checking the accuracy of information and ensuring its completeness; the methods of categorizing diagnoses, leading clinical features, and functional disability; and the process for storage of data and obtaining access in order to answer questions central to the planning process.

Interpretation of trends revealed by successive sets of data is a necessary part of evaluation, and may be an elaborate process. At first sight an effective and efficient service would reduce the prevalence of the morbidity at which it was aimed. With chronic disability the picture is complicated because of the nature of the social processes involved with the personal pathology. A good service may attract potential clients who had hitherto resisted suggestions that they should enter the treatment and caring network and it may also slow down the progression of a process of deterioration so that certain demands increase, for example for day care and episodes of acute medical care of patients living satisfactorily in domestic surroundings. Furthermore it may preserve life and hence survival into old age of larger numbers of people with physical as well as mental infirmities. Such considerations are among those which underline the need for the planning process to take a comprehensive view of the whole of the population at risk and the distributions within the population of levels of disability, the resources available, and the comparative use of different types of resource.

The requirements are for comprehensive services for a defined population, in which a wide range of facilities is planned, monitored, and revised in a co-ordinated fashion in accordance with good epidemiological and social survey methods. These requirements are elaborate and expensive, and cannot always be met. It is necessary, therefore, for information obtained from those areas or districts where services are closely monitored to be applied, with appropriate modifications, to other communities. For this reason, and also because there is scope for experimenting with simple alternative systems, the methodology for evaluation of psychiatric services has far-reaching implications for ensuring that effective components of mental health care are adequately supplied and efficiently utilized.

References

Introduction

Alinstein, P. (1965) Theoretical models. *Brit. J. Philosophy Sci.* **16**, 102–20

Beech, H. R. & Vaughan, M. (1978) *Behavioural Treatment of Obsessional States.* Chichester: Wiley

Bolton, N. (1979) (Ed.) *Philosophical Problems in Psychology.* London: Methuen

Brazier, M. A. B. (1979) (Ed.) *Brain Mechanisms in Memory and Learning: From the Single Neuron to Man.* International Brain Research Organisation Monograph Series. Vol. 4. New York: Raven Press

Broadhurst, P. A. (1978) *Drugs and the Inheritance of Behaviour.* New York: Plenum Press

Carlsson, A. (1977) Does dopamine play a role in schizophrenia? *Psychol. Med.,* **7**, 583–97

Cawley, R. H. (1970) Evaluation of psychotherapy. *Psychol. Med.,* **1**, 101–3

Commission on Terminology (1969) Clinical and electroencephalographic classification of epileptic seizures. *Epilepsie* **10**, Supp. S.2

Fisher, S. & Greenberg, R. P. (1977) *The Scientific Credibility of Freud's Theories and Therapies.* Hassocks: Harvester Press

Freyhan, F. A. (1978) Treatment-resistant or intractable? *Compr. Psychiatry,* **19**, No. 2, 97–101

Gantt, W. H. (1944) *Experimental Basis for Neurotic Behaviour'.* New York: Harper

Ginsburg, B. E. (1971) The role of genic activity in the determination of sensitive periods in the development of aggressive behaviour. In *Dynamics of Violence,* ed. Fawcett, J., pp. 165–75. Chicago: American Medical Association

Ginsburg, B. E., Becker, R. E., Trattner, A., Dutson, J. & Bareggi, S. R. (1976) Genetic variation in drug responses in hybrid dogs: a possible model for the hyperkinetic syndrome. *Behav. Genet.* **6**, 107

Ginsburg, B. E., Cowen, J. S., Maxson, S. C. & Sze, P. Y. (1969) Neurochemical effects of gene mutations associated with audiogenic seizures. In *Progress in Neurogenetics*, ed. Barbeau, A. & Brunette, J. R., pp. 695–701.

Ginsburg, B. E., Yanai, J. & Sze, P. Y. (1975) A developmental genetic study of the effects of alcohol consumed by parent mice on the behaviour and development of their offspring. In *Research, Treatment & Prevention*, pp. 183–204. Washington D.C.: NIAAA

Gjessing, R. V. (1976) *Contribution to the Somatology of Periodic Catatonia*. Oxford: Pergamon Press

Hartmann, H. (1964) Understanding & explanation. In *Essays on Ego-Psychology. Selected Problems in Psychoanalytic Theory*, pp. 369–403 London: Hogarth Press

Hinde, R. A. & Davies, L. (1972) Removing infant rhesus from mother for 13 days compared with removing mother from infant'. *J. child Psychol.*, **13**, 227–37

Jaspers, K. (1963) *General Psychopathology*, 7th ed., transl. Hoenig, J. & Hamilton, M. W. Manchester: Manchester University Press

Johnstone, E. C. (1975) Relationship between acetylator status and response to phenelzine. In *Genetics and Psychopharmacology. Modern Problems of Pharmacopsychiatry*, vol. 10, ed. Mendlewicz, J., pp. 30–7. Basle: Karger

Kuhn, T. (1970) *The Structure of Scientific Revolutions*, 2nd ed. International Encyclopaedia of Unified Science, vol. 2, no. 2. Chicago: University of Chicago Press

Legg, N. J. (1978) (Ed.) *Neurotransmitter Systems and their Clinical Disorders*. London: Academic Press

Lynch, J. C., Mountcastle, V. B., Talbot, W. H. & Yin, Y. C. T. (1977) Parietal lobe mechanisms for directed visual attention. *J. Neurophysiol.* **40**, 362.

Lynn, R. (1963) Russian theory and research on schizophrenia. *Psychol. Bull.*, **60**, 486–98

Maas, J. W. (1975) Catecholamines & depression: a further specification of the catecholamine hypothesis of the affective disorders. In *Catecholamines & Behaviour*, ed. Friedhoff, A. J., vol. 2, pp. 119–33. New York: Plenum Press

Maher, B. (1970) *Introduction to Research in Psychopathology*. New York: McGraw-Hill

Mainz, F. (1955) Foundations of Biology. In *International Encyclopaedia of Unified Science*, vol. 1, no. 9. Chicago: University of Chicago Press

Margolis, J. (1978) *Persons and Minds*. Boston Studies in the Philosophy of Science, vol. LVII. Dordrecht: Reidel

Marks, I. M. (1969) *Fears and Phobias*. London: Academic Press

Matthysse, S. (1977) Animal models of human cognitive processes. In *Animal Models in Psychiatry and Neurology*, ed. Hanin, I. & Usdin E. pp. 75–82. Oxford: Pergamon Press

— (1978) A theory of the relation between dopamine and attention. *J. psychiat. Res.*, **14**, 241–8

Matthysse, S. & Haber, S. (1975) Animal models of schizophrenia. In *Model Systems in Biological Psychiatry*, ed. Ingle, D. J. & Schein, H. M., p. 4. Cambridge, Mass.: MIT Press

Matthysse, S., Spring, B. J. & Sugarman, J. (1979) (Eds.) *Attention and Information Processing in Schizophrenia*. Oxford: Pergamon Press

Menninger, K. (1963) *The Vital Balance*. New York: Viking

Miller, W. R., Rossellini, R. A. & Seligman, M. E. P. (1977) (Eds.) Learned helplessness and depression. In *Psychopathology: Experimental Models*, ed. Maser, J. D. & Seligman, M. E. P., p. 104–30. San Francisco: Freeman

Monod, J. (1971) The meaning of science. In *The Social Impact of Modern Biology*, ed. Fuller, W. p. 12. London/Henley on Thames: Routledge & Kegan Paul

Oakeshott, M. (1978) *Experience and its Modes*. London: Cambridge University Press

Racagni, G., Cattabeni, F. & Paoletti, R. (1977) A biochemical analysis of strain differences in narcotic action. In *Animal Models in Psychiatry and Neurology*, ed. Hanin, I. & Usdin, E., pp. 315–19. Oxford: Pergamon Press

Rosenthal, D. & Kety, S. S. (1968) (Eds.) *The Transmission of Schizophrenia*. Oxford: Pergamon Press

Shepherd, M. (1978) Epidemiology and clinical psychiatry. *Brit. J. Psychiat.* **133**, 289–98

Shepherd, M., Lader, M. H. & Rodnight, R. (1968) *Clinical Psychopharmacology*. London: English Universities Press

Spitz, R. A. (1946) Anaclitic depression. *Psychoanal. Study Child*, **2**, 313–47

Squire, L. S. (1976) Amnesia and the biology of memory. In *Current Developments in Psychopharmacology*, ed. Essman, W. B. & Valzelli, L., vol. 3, pp. 1–23. New York: Spectrum Publications

Suomi, S. J. & Harlow, H. F. (1977) Production and alleviation of depressive behaviours in monkeys. In *Psychopathology: Experimental Models*, ed. Maser, J. D. & Seligman, M. E. P. pp. 131–73 San Francisco: Freeman

Thorpe, W. H. (1974) *Animal Nature and Human Nature*. London: Methuen

Zubin, J. (1972) Scientific models for psychopathology in the 1970s. In *Seminars in Psychiatry*, **4**, No. 3, 283–96

Chapter 1

Ackerknecht, E. H. (1950) History of legal medicine. *Ciba Symposia*, **11**, 1286–1304

— (1967) *Medicine at the Paris Hospital 1794–1848*. Baltimore: Johns Hopkins University Press

— (1968) *A Short History of Psychiatry*, 2nd ed, trans. Wolff, Sula. New York: Hafner

Alexander, F. & Selsnick, S. (1966) *The History of Psychiatry*. New York: Harper & Row

Allderidge, P. H. (1974) Criminal insanity: Bethlem to Broadmoor. *Proc. Roy. Soc. Med.*, **67**, 897–904

Allen, G. (1976) Genetics, eugenics and society: internalists and externalists in contemporary history of science. *Soc. Stud. Sci.* **6**, 105–22

Altschule, M. D. (1977) *Origins of Concepts in Human Behavior: social and cultural factors*. Washington and London: Hemisphere

Aurelianus, Caelius (1950) *On Acute Diseases and on Chronic Diseases*, trans. Drabkin, I. E. Chicago: University of Chicago Press

Ayd, F. J., Jr. & Blackwell, B. (1970) Eds. *Discoveries in Biological Psychiatry*. Philadelphia: Lippincott

Babb, L. (1951) *The Elizabethan Malady: A Study of Melancholia in English Literature from 1580 to 1640*. East Lansing: Michigan State University Press

— (1959) *Sanity in Bedlam: A Study of Robert Burton's Anatomy of Melancholy*. East Lansing: Michigan State University Press

Ballester, L. Garcia (1974) Diseases of the soul in Galen: the impossibility of a Galenic psychotherapy. *Clio Med.*, **9**, 35–43

Bamborough, J. B. (1952) *The Little World of Man*. London: Longman, Green

Bannister, R. C. (1979) *Social Darwinism: Science and Myth in Anglo-American Thought*. Philadelphia: Temple University Press

Baruk, H. (1967) *La Psychiatrie français de Pinel à nos Jours*. Paris: Presses Universitaires de France

Batisse, F. (1962) *Montaigne et la médecine*. Paris: Les Belles Lettres

Battie, W. (1962) *A Treatise on Madness;* and Monro, John, *Remarks on Dr. Battie's Treatise on Madness.* Intro. by Hunter, R. & Macalpine, I. London: Dawson (Reprint of 1758 eds.)

Bleuler, E. (1950) *Dementia Praecox, or the Group of Schizophrenias.* trans. Zinkin, J. New York: International Universities Press

Bleuler, M. (1979) Ed. *Beiträge zur Schizophrenielehre der Zürcher psychiatrischen Universitätsklinik Burghölzli (1902–1971).* Darmstadt: Wissenschaftliche Buchgesellschaft

Bloch, S. & Reddaway, P. (1977) *Russia's Political Hospitals: the Abuse of Psychiatry in the Soviet Union.* London: Gollancz

Bloomfield, M. W. (1967) *The Seven Deadly Sins.* Michigan: State University Press

Boring, E. G. (1950) *A History of Experimental Psychology.* 2nd ed. New York: Appleton-Century-Crofts

Boss, J. M. N. (1979) The seventeenth-century transformation of the hysteric affection, and Sydenham's Baconian medicine. *Psychol. Med.,* **9,** 221–34

Boyer, P. & Nissenbaum, S. (1974) *Salem Possessed: The Social Orgins of Witchcraft.* Cambridge, Mass.: Harvard University Press

Bradley, A. C. (1955) *Shakespearean Tragedy.* New York: Meridian Books

Brody, B. A. & Engelhardt, H. T., Jr. (1980) Eds. *Mental Illness: Law and Public Policy.* Dordrecht and Boston: Reidel

Bromberg, W. (1954) *Man Above Humanity. A History of Psychotherapy.* Philadelphia: Lippincott

Burdett, H. C. (1893) *Hospitals and Asylums of the World: Their Origin, History, Construction, Administration, Management and Legislation.* 4 vols. London: Churchill

Burke, P. (1978) *Popular Culture in Early Modern Europe.* London: Temple Smith

Burnham, J. G. (1967) *Psychoanalysis and American Medicine, 1894–1918: Medicine, Science, and Culture.* New York: International Universities Press

Burton, R. (1955) *The Anatomy of Melancholy,* ed. Dell F. & Jordan-Smith, P. New York: Tudor

Bynum, W. F. (1968) Chronic alcoholism in the first half of the nineteenth century. *Bull. Hist. Med.,* **42,** 160–185

— (1972) Varieties of Cartesian experience in early nineteenth century physiology. In *Philosophical Dimensions of the Neuromedical Sciences,* ed. Spicker, S. F. & Engelhardt, H. T., Jr. Dordrecht and Boston: Reidel

— (1973) The anatomical method, natural theology, and the functions of the brain. *Isis,* **54,** 445–68.

— (1974) Rationales for therapy in British psychiatry: 1780–1835. *Med. Hist.,* **18,** 317–34

— (1980) Health, disease and medical care. In *The Ferment of Knowledge,* ed. Rousseau, G. & Porter, R. S. Cambridge: Cambridge University Press

Byrd, M. (1974) *Visits to Bedlam.* Columbia: University of South Carolina Press

Cantor, G. N. (1975) Phrenology in early nineteenth century Edinburgh: an historiographical discussion. *Ann. Sci.,* **32,** 195–218

Carlson, E. T. (1956–7) Amariah Brigham: 1. Life and works, and 2. Psychiatric thought and practice. *Amer. J. Psychiat.,* **112,** 831–6 and **113,** 911–16

Chamberlain, A. S. (1966) Early mental hospitals in Spain. *Amer. J. Psychiat.,* **123,** 143–9

Checkland, S. G. & Checkland, E. O. A. (1974) Eds. *The Poor Law Report of 1834.* Harmondsworth: Penguin

Chesney, E. (1977) The theme of folly in Rabelais and Ariosto. *J. Med. Renaiss. Stud.,* **7,** 67–93

Cheyne, G. (1733) *The English Malady: or, a Treatise of Nervous Diseases of All Kinds.* London: Strahan & Leake

Clare, A. (1976) *Psychiatry in Dissent.* London: Tavistock

Clarke, B. (1975) *Mental Disorder in Earlier Britain.* Cardiff: University of Wales Press

Clarke, E. S. & Dewhurst, Kenneth (1972) *An Illustrated History of Brain Function.* Oxford: Sandford Publications

Clarke, E. S. & O'Malley, C. D. (1968) Eds. *The Human Brain and Spinal Cord.* Berkeley: University of California Press

Clements, R. D. (1967) Physiological–psychological thought in Juan Luis Vives. *J. Hist. behav. Sci.,* **3,** 219–35

Cobben, J. J. (1976) *Jan Wier, Devils, Witches and Magic.* Trans. Prins, S. A. Philadelphia: Dorrance

Cohn, N. (1970) *The Pursuit of the Millennium.* London: Paladin

— (1976) *Europe's Inner Demons.* London: Paladin

Conolly, J. (1964) *An Inquiry Concerning the Indications of Insanity.* Intro. by Hunter R. & Macalpine, I. London: Dawsons. (Reprint of 1830 ed.)

— (1968) *The Construction and Government of Lunatic Asylums and Hospitals for the Insane.* Intro. by Hunter, R. & Macalpine I. London: Dawsons (Reprint of 1847 ed.)

— (1973) *Treatment of the Insane without Mechanical Restraints.* Intro. by Hunter, R. MacAlpine, I. London: Dawsons (Reprint of 1856 ed.)

Cooter, R. J. (1976) Phrenology and British alienists circa 1825–1845. *Med. Hist.,* **20,** 1–21, 135–51

Coulter, H. L. (1973–77) *Divided Legacy: a History of Schism in Medical Thought.* 3 vols. Washington: Wehawken Book Company

Cranefield, P. F. & Federn, W. (1970) Paulus Zacchias on mental deficiency and on deafness. *Bull. N.Y. Acad. Med.,* **46,** 3–21

Dain, N. (1964) *Concepts of Insanity in the United States, 1789–1865.* New Brunswick: Rutgers University Press

Debus, A. G. (1974) Ed. *Medicine in Seventeenth Century England.* Berkeley: University of California Press

— (1978) *Man and Nature in the Renaissance.* Cambridge: Cambridge University Press

Decker, H. S. (1977) *Freud in Germany: Revolution and Reaction in Science, 1893–1907.* New York: International Universities Press

De Porte, M. V. (1974) *Nightmares and Hobbyhorses. Swift, Sterne, and Augustan Ideas of Madness.* San Marino, California: Huntington Library

Descartes, R. (1967) *The Philosophical Works of Descartes.* Trans. Haldane, E. S. & Ross, G. R. T. 2 vols. Cambridge: Cambridge University Press

— (1972) *Treatise of Man.* Trans. and ed. Hall, T. S. Cambridge, Mass.: Harvard University Press

Deutsch, A. (1949) *The Mentally Ill in America.* 2nd ed. New York: Columbia University Press

Dewhurst, K. (1966) *Dr. Thomas Sydenham (1624–1689): His Life and Original Writings.* London: Wellcome Institute for the History of Medicine

Diderot, D. (1966) *Rameau's Nephew; D'Alembert's Dream.* Trans. Tancock, L. W. Harmondsworth: Penguin

Diethelm, O. (1971) *Medical Dissertations of Psychiatric Interest Printed before 1750.* Basle: Karger

Diethelm, O. & Heffernan, T. F. (1965) Felix Platter and psychiatry. *J. Hist. behav. Sci.,* **1,** 10–23

Dodds, E. R. (1951) *The Greeks and the Irrational.* Berkeley and London: University of California Press

Doerner, K. (1981) *Madmen and the Bourgeoisie.* Trans. Neugroschel, J. & Steinberg, J. Oxford: Blackwell

Dominguez, E. J. (1967) The Hospital of Innocents. Humane treatment of the mentally ill in Spain, 1409–1512. *Bull. Menninger Clin.*, **31**, 285–97

Doob, P. B. R. (1974) *Nebuchadnezzar's Children. Conventions of Madness in Middle English Literature*. New Haven and London: Yale University Press

Dover, K. J. (1978) *Greek Homosexuality*. London: Duckworth

Drabkin, I. E. (1955) Remarks on ancient psychopathology. *Isis*, **46**, 223–34

Eggert, G. H. (1977) *Wernicke's Works on Aphasia, a Sourcebook and Review*. The Hague: Mouton

Eliade, M. (1964) *Shamanism: Archaic Technique of Ecstasy*. New York: Pantheon

Ellenberger, H. (1970) *The Discovery of the Unconscious*. New York: Basic Books

— (1974) Psychiatry from Ancient to Modern Times. In *American Handbook of Psychiatry*, ed. Arieti, S., 2nd ed. New York: Basic Books

Engelhardt, H. T. Jr. (1975) John Hughlings Jackson and the mind–body relationship. *Bull. Hist. Med.* **49**, 137–651

Engelhardt, H. T. Jr. & Spicker, S. (1976) Eds. *Mental Health: Philosophical Perspectives*. Dordrecht: Reidel

Entralgo, P. Lain (1955) *Mind and Body. Psychosomatic Pathology*. Trans. Espinosa, A. M. London: Harvill

— (1970) *The Therapy of the Word in Classical Antiquity*. Trans. Rather, L. J. & Sharp, J. M. New Haven: Yale University Press

Evans, B. (1972) *The Psychiatry of Robert Burton*. New York: Octagon Books

Favazza, A. R. & Oman, M. (1977). *Anthropological and Cross-Cultural Themes in Mental Health: an Annotated Bibliography, 1925–1974*. Columbia and London: University of Missouri Press

Fischer-Homberger, E. (1970) *Hypochondrie, Melancholie bis Neurose, Krankheiten und Zustandsbilder*. Berne: Huber

— (1972) Hypochondriasis of the eighteenth century – neurosis of the present century. *Bull. Hist. Med.*, **46**, 391–401

— (1975) *Die traumatische Neurose. Vom somatischen zum sozialen Leiden*. Berne: Huber

Fisher, S. & Greenberg, R. P. (1978) Eds. *The Scientific Evaluation of Freud's Theories and Therapy*. Hassocks: Harvester Press

Flashar, H. (1966) *Melancholie und Melancholiker in den medizinischen Theorien der Antike*. Berlin: de Gruyter

Foucault, Michel (1971) *Madness and Civilization. A History of Insanity in the Age of Reason*. Trans. Howard, R. London: Tavistock

Fox, Richard W. (1978) *So far Disordered in Mind. Insanity in California, 1870–1930*. Berkeley: University of California Press

Freud, S. (1954) *The Origins of Psycho-analysis*. Ed. Bonaparte, Marie, *et al.*; trans. Mosbacher, E. & Strachey, J. London: Imago

Friedlander, R. (1973) *Benedict–Augustin Morel and the Development of the Theory of Degenerescence: The Introduction of Anthropology into Psychiatry*. University of California, San Francisco, Ph. D. thesis

Friedreich, J. B. (1830) *Versuch einer Literärgeschichte der Pathologie und Therapie der psychischen Krankheiten*. Würzburg: Strecker

— (1836) *Historisch-kritische Darstellung der Theorien über das Wesen und den Sitz der psychischen Krankheiten*. Leipzig: Wigand

Fullinwider, S. P. (1975) Insanity as the loss of self: the moral insanity controversy revisited. *Bull. Hist. Med.*, **49**, 87–101

Galen (1928) *On the Natural Faculties*. Trans. Brock, A. J. London: Heinemann (Loeb Classical Library)

— (1956) *In Hippocratis Epidemiorum*. Trans. Wenkebach, E. & Pfaff, F. Berlin: Corpus Medicorum Graecorum

— (1963) *On the Passions and Errors of the Soul*. Trans. Harkins, P. Intro. Riese, W. Columbus: Ohio State University Press

— (1968) *On the Usefulness of the Parts of the Body*. Trans. May, M. T. 2 vols. Ithaca: Cornell University Press

Gay, P. (1967–9) *The Enlightenment: An Interpretation*. 2 vols. New York: Knopf

George, M. D. (1966) *London Life in the Eighteenth Century*. Harmondsworth: Penguin

Geschwind, N. (1974) Carl Wernicke, the Breslau School and the history of aphasia. *Boston Stud. Philos. Sci.*, **16**, 42–61

Gifford, G. J., Jr. (1978) Ed. *Psychoanalysis, Psychotherapy and the New England Medical Scene, 1894–1944*. New York: Science History Publications

Gilbert, A. N. (1975) Doctor, patient, and onanist diseases in the nineteenth century. *J. Hist. Med. allied Sci.*, **30**, 217–34

Glaser, G. H. (1978) Epilepsy, hysteria, and 'possession'. *J. nerv. ment. Dis.*, **166**, 268–74

Goodman, N. G. (1934) *Benjamin Rush, Physician and Citizen, 1746–1813*. Philadelphia: University of Pennsylvania Press

Gould, S. J. (1977) *Ontogeny and Phylogeny*. Cambridge, Mass: Harvard University Press

Grange, K. (1961) Pinel and eighteenth century psychiatry. *Bull. Hist. Med.*, **35**, 442–53

— (1963) Pinel or Chiarugi? *Med. Hist.*, **7**, 371–80

Gregory, F. (1977) *Scientific Materialism in Nineteenth Century Germany*. Dordrecht and Boston: Reidel

Grob, G. (1962) Samuel B. Woodward and the practice of psychiatry in early nineteenth century America. *Bull. Hist. Med.*, **36**, 420–43

— (1966) *The State and the Mentally Ill: A History of Worcester State Hospital in Massachusetts, 1830–1920*. Chapel Hill: University of North Carolina Press

— (1973) *Mental Institutions in America*. New York: Free Press

Hale, N. G., Jr. (1971a) *James Jackson Putnam and Psychoanalysis*. Cambridge, Mass: Harvard University Press

— (1971b) *Freud and the Americans: The Beginnings of Psychoanalysis in the United States, 1876–1917*. New York: Oxford University Press

Haller, A. v. (1936) *A Dissertation on the Sensible and Irritable Parts of Animals*. Intro. by Temkin, Owsei. Baltimore: Johns Hopkins University Press

Haller, M. H. (1963) *Eugenics: Hereditarian Attitudes in American Thought*. New Brunswick, New Jersey: Rutgers University Press

Hansen, J. (1900) *Zauberwahn, Inquisition und Hexenprozess im Mittelalter*. Munich: Historische Bibliothek

Hare, E. H. (1962) Masturbatory insanity: the history of an idea. *J. ment. Sci.*, **108**, 1–25

Harms, E. (1959) An attempt to formulate a system of psychotherapy in 1818. *Amer. J. Psychother.*, **13**, 269–82

Harris, C. R. S. (1973) *The Heart and the Vascular System in Ancient Greek Medicine*. Oxford: Clarendon Press

Havens, L. L. (1973) *Approaches to the Mind: Movement of the Psychiatric Schools from Sects toward Science*. Boston: Little, Brown

Hearnshaw, L. S. (1964) *A Short History of British Psychology, 1840–1940*. London: Methuen

Hearst, E. (1979) Ed. *The First Century of Experimental Psychology*. Hillsdale, New Jersey: Erlbaum

Henderson, D. (1963) *The Evolution of Psychiatry in Scotland*. Edinburgh: Livingstone

Hierons, R. (1967) Willis's contributions to clinical medicine and neurology. *J. neurol. Sci.*, **4**, 1–13

Hill, D. (1969) *Psychiatry in Medicine; Retrospect and Prospect*. London: Nuffield Provincial Hospitals Trust

Hippocrates (1923–31) *Works*. Trans. Jones, W. H. S. & Withington, E. T. London: Heinemann (Loeb Classical Library)

Hirsch, S. R. & Shepherd, M. (1974) Eds. *Themes and Variations in European Psychiatry*. Bristol: Wright

Hirschmüller, A. (1978) *Physiologie und Psychoanalyse in Leben und Werk Josef Breuers*. Berne: Huber

Hoeldtke, R. (1967) The history of associationism and British medical psychology. *Med. Hist.*, **11**, 46–65

Hofstadter, R. (1955) *Social Darwinism in American Thought*. Boston: Beacon Press

Howells, J. G. (1975) Ed. *World History of Psychiatry*. New York: Brunner Mazel

Hunter, R. A. & Macalpine, I. (1963) *Three Hundred Years of Psychiatry, 1535–1860*. London: Oxford University Press

— (1974) *Psychiatry for the Poor. 1851 Colney Hatch Asylum, Friern Hospital 1973: A Medical and Social History*. London: Dawsons

Hurd, H. M. (1916–17) Ed. *The Institutional Care of the Insane in the United States and Canada*. 4 vols. Baltimore: Johns Hopkins University Press

Ignatieff, M. (1978) *A Just Measure of Pain. The Penitentiary in the Industrial Revolution, 1750–1850*. London: Macmillan

Isler, H. (1968) *Thomas Willis, 1621–1675, Doctor and Scientist*. New York: Hafner

Jackson, S. W. (1969) Galen – on Mental Disorders. *J. Hist. behav. Sci.*, **5**, 365–84

— (1972) Unusual mental states in medieval Europe. 1. Medical syndromes of mental disorder: 400–1100A.D. *J. Hist. Med. allied Sci.*, **27**, 262–97

— (1978) Melancholia and the waning of the humoral theory. *J. Hist. Med. allied Sci.*, **33**, 367–76.

Jaeger, W. (1939–45) *Paideia: the Ideas of Greek Culture*. 3 vols. Oxford: Blackwell

Jaspers, K. (1963) *General Psychopathology*. Trans. J. Hoenig and M. W. Hamilton from the seventh German ed. Manchester: Manchester University Press; Chicago: Chicago University Press

Jetter, D. (1971) *Geschichte des Hospitals, vol. 2: Zur Typologie des Irrenhauses in Frankreich und Deutschland (1780–1840)*. Wiesbaden: Steiner

Jobe, T. H. (1976) Medical theories of melancholia in the seventeenth and early eighteenth centuries. *Clio Med.*, **11**, 217–31

Jones, E. (1949) *Hamlet and Oedipus*. New York: Norton

— (1956–7) *Sigmund Freud: Life and Work*. 3 vols. London: Hogarth Press

— (1959) *Free Associations*. London: Hogarth Press

Jones, K. (1972) *A History of the Mental Health Services*. London: Routledge & Kegan Paul

Kahlbaum, K. L. (1973) *Catatonia*. Intro. by Mora, George. Baltimore: Johns Hopkins University Press

Kieckhefer, R. (1976) *European Witch-Trials: their Foundations in Popular and Learned Culture, 1300–1500*. London and Berkeley: University of California Press

Kiell, N. (1965) *Psychiatry and Psychology in the Visual Arts and Aesthetics. A Bibliography*. Madison: University of Wisconsin Press

Kiev, A., ed. (1964) *Magic, Faith, and Healing*. New York: Free Press

King, L. S. (1978) *The Philosophy of Medicine. The Early Eighteenth Century*. Cambridge, Mass: Harvard University Press

Kleist, K. (1959) Carl Wernicke. In *Grosse Nervenärzte*, ed. Kolle, K., vol. 2. Stuttgart: Thieme

Klibansky, R., Panofsky, E. & Saxl, F. (1964) *Saturn and Melancholy*. London: Nelson

Kraepelin, E. (1962) *One Hundred Years of Psychiatry*. trans. Baskin, W. London: Owen

Kroll, J. (1973) A reappraisal of psychiatry in the Middle Ages. *Arch. gen. Psychiat.*, **29**, 276–83

Kudlien, F. (1967) *Der Beginn des medizinischen Denkens*. Zürich: Artemis

Laehr, H. (1900) Ed. *Die Literatur der Psychiatrie, Neurologie und Psychologie von 1459–1799*. 3 vols. Berlin: Reimer

Lain Entralgo, see Entralgo

Lange-Eichbaum, W. (1931) *The Problem of Genius*. Trans. Paul, E. & C. London: Kegan Paul

Lassek, A. M. (1970) *The Unique Legacy of Doctor Hughlings Jackson*. Springfield: Thomas

Laurentius, M. A. (1938) *A Discourse of the Preservation of the Sight: of Melancholike Diseases; of Rheumes, and of Old Age*. Intro. Larkey, S. V. (1599 ed.). Oxford: The Shakespeare Association

Lawrence, C. J. (1979) The nervous system and society in the Scottish Enlightenment. In *Natural Order: Historical Studies of Scientific Culture*, ed. Barnes, B. & Shapin, J. London: Sage Publications

Leibbrand, W. & Wettley, A. (1961) *Der Wahnsinn: Geschichte der abendländischen Psychopathologie*. Munich: Alber

Leidesdorf, M. (1865) *Lehrbuch der psychischen Krankheiten*. 2nd ed. Erlangen: Enke

Leigh, D. (1961) *The Historical Development of British Psychiatry*. Oxford: Pergamon Press

Lesky, E. (1976) *The Vienna Medical School of the 19th Century*. Baltimore: Johns Hopkins University Press

Levi, A. (1964) *French Moralists: the Theory of the Passions, 1585 to 1649*. Oxford: Clarendon Press

Levin, K. (1978) *Freud's Early Theory of the Neuroses. A Historical Perspective*. Hassocks: Harvester Press

Levine, H. G. (1978) The discovery of addiction. Changing conceptions of habitual drunkenness in America. *J. Stud. Alcohol*, **39**, 143–74

Lewis, A. (1959) J. C. Reil's Concepts of Brain Function. See Poynter, F. N. L. (1959) Ed.

— (1967) *The State of Psychiatry*. London: Routledge & Kegan Paul

— (1979) *The Later Papers of Sir Aubrey Lewis*. Oxford: Oxford University Press

Lidz, T. (1976) *Hamlet's Enemy: Madness and Myth in Hamlet*. London: Vision Press

Littman, R. A. (1979) Social and intellectual origins of experimental psychology. In *The First Century of Experimental Psychology*, ed. Hearst, E. Hillsdale, N.J.: Erlbaum

Locke, J. (1890) *An Essay Concerning Human Understanding*, ed. Fraser, A. C. 2 vols. Oxford: Clarendon Press

Lopez Piñero, J. M. (1963) *Orígenes históricos del concepto de neurosis*. Valencia: Instituto de Historia de la Medicina

Lopez Piñero, J. M. & Morales Meseguer, J. M. (1970) *Neurosis y psicoterapia; un estudio histórico*. Madrid: Espasa-Calpe

Lyons, B. G. (1971) *Voices of Melancholy. Studies in Literary Treat-*

ments of Melancholy in Renaissance England. London: Routledge & Kegan Paul

Macalpine, I. & Hunter, R. (1969) *George III and the Mad-Business*. London: Allen Lane

MacDonald, M. (1977) The inner side of wisdom: suicide in early modern England. *Psychol. Med.*, **7**, 565–82

— (1981) *Mystical Bedlam: Madness, Anxiety, and Healing in Seventeenth-Century England*. Cambridge: Cambridge University Press

Macfarlane, A. D. J. (1970) *Witchcraft in Tudor and Stuart England*. London: Routledge & Kegan Paul

McGuire, W. (1974) Ed. *The Freud/Jung Letters*. trans. Mannheim, R. & Hull, R. F. C. Princeton: Princeton University Press

Macmillan, M. B. (1976) Beard's concept of neurasthenia and Freud's concept of the actual neuroses. *J. Hist. behav. Sci.*, **12**, 376–90

Marx, O. M. (1965) A re-evaluation of the mentalists in early 19th century German psychiatry. *Amer. J. Psychiat.*, **121**, 752–60

— (1970) Nineteenth-century medical psychology, theoretical problems in the work of Griesinger, Meynert, and Wernicke. *Isis*, **61**, 355–70

— (1971) Psychiatry on a neuropathological basis: Theodore Meynert's application for the extension of his venia legendi. *Clio Med.*, **6**, 139–58

— (1972) Wilhelm Griesinger and the history of psychiatry: a reassessment. *Bull. Hist. Med.*, **46**, 519–44

Mellett, D. J. (1981) Bureaucracy and mental illness: The Commissioners in Lunacy 1845–90. *Med. Hist.*, **25**, 221–50

Merton, R. K. (1970) *Science, Technology and Society in Seventeenth-Century England*. New York: Harper

Mette, A. (1976) *Wilhelm Griesinger: der Begründer der wissenschaftlichen Psychiatrie in Deutschland*. Leipzig: Teubrier

Meyer, A. (1973) Frederick Mott, founder of the Maudsley Laboratories. *Brit. J. Psychiat.*, **122**, 497–516

Meyer, A. & Hierons, R. (1965) On Thomas Willis's concepts of neurophysiology. *Med. Hist.*, **9**, 1–15, 142–55

Midelfort, H. C. E. (1972) *Witch-hunting in Southwestern Germany, 1562–1684*. Stanford: Stanford University Press

— (1980) Madness and Civilisation in early modern Europe. In *After the Reformation. Essays in Honor of J. H. Hexter*, ed. Malamont, B. Philadelphia: University of Pennsylvania Press

Monter, E. W. (1976) *Witchcraft in France and Switzerland: The Borderlands During the Reformation*. Ithaca and London: Cornell University Press

— (1972) The historiography of European witchcraft: progress and prospects. *J. interdiscip. Hist.*, **2**, 435–51

Mora, G. (1966) The history of psychiatry: a cultural and bibliographical survey. *Psychoanal. Rev.*, **52**, 335–56

— (1970) The psychiatrist's approach to the history of psychiatry. In *Psychiatry and its History. Methodological Problems in Research*, ed. Mora, G. & Brand, J. L. Springfield: Thomas

— (1972) On the bicentenary of the birth of Esquirol (1772–1840): the first complete psychiatrist. *Amer. J. Psychiat.*, **129**, 562–67

— (1975) Historical and theoretical trends in psychiatry. In *Comprehensive Textbook of Psychiatry*, ed. Kaplan, H. I. & Sadock, B. J. 2nd ed. Baltimore: Williams & Wilkins

— (1977) Juan Huarte. The Examination of Men's Wits (1575). *J. Hist. behav. Sci.*, **13**, 67–78

— (1978) Mind-body concepts in the Middle Ages: Part. 1. *J. Hist. behav. Sci.*, **14**, 344–61

— (1979) French ideology at the dawn of the American nation: Cabanis and Jefferson on psychology and mental health care. See Riese, H. ed.

Mora, G. and Brand, J. L. (1970) (Eds.) *Psychiatry and its History. Methodological Problems in Research*. Springfield: Thomas

Morris, A. D. (1958) The Hoxton Madhouses. March, Cambridgeshire: For the Author

Mullahy, P. (1970) *The Beginnings of Modern American Psychiatry: the Ideas of Harry Stack Sullivan*. Boston: Houghton Mifflin

Neu, J. (1977) *Emotion, Thought and Therapy*. London: Routledge & Kegan Paul

Neuburger, M (1943) *The Doctrine of the Healing Power of Nature*. Trans. Boyd, L. J. New York: n.p.

Neugebauer, R. (1979) Medieval and early modern theories of mental illness. *Arch. gen. Psychiat.*, **36**, 477–83

Neuman, R. P. (1975) Masturbation, madness, and the modern concepts of childhood and adolescence. *J. soc. Hist.*, **8**, 1–27

Noel, P. S. & Carlson, E. T. (1973) The faculty psychology of Benjamin Rush. *J. Hist. behav. Sci.*, **9**, 369–77

North, H. (1966) *Sophrosyne: Self-Knowledge and Self-restraint in Greek Literature*. Ithaca: Cornell University Press

Ober, W. B. (1979) Madness and poetry: A note on Collins, Cowper, and Smart. In *Boswell's Clap and other Essays*. Carbondale, Ill: Southern Illinois University Press

O'Donoghue, E. G. (1914) *The Story of Bethlehem Hospital, from its Foundation in 1247*. London: Fisher Unwin

Owen, A. R. G. (1971) *Hysteria, Hypnosis and Healing: the Work of J. M. Charcot*. London: Dobson

Pagel, W. (1958) *Paracelsus. An Introduction to Philosophical Medicine in the Era of the Renaissance*. Basle: Karger

— (1967) *William Harvey's Biological Ideas*. Basle and New York: Karger

Paracelsus (1941) *Four Treatises*, ed. Sigerist, H. E. Trans. Temkin, C. L. *et al*. Baltimore: Johns Hopkins University Press

Parry-Jones, W. L. (1972) *The Trade in Lunacy*. London: Routledge & Kegan Paul

Passmore, J. (1951) *Ralph Cudworth*. Cambridge: Cambridge University Press

— (1970) *The Perfectibility of Man*. London: Duckworth

Peters, R. S. (1962) *Brett's History of Psychology*. Cambridge, Mass: M.I.T. Press

Phillips, H. Temple (1973) *The History of the Old Private Lunatic Asylum at Fishponds Bristol, 1740–1859*. Bristol: University of Bristol M.Sc. Thesis

Pickett, R. C. (1952) *Mental Affliction and Church Law*. Ottawa: University of Ottawa Press

Pinel, Ph. (1962) *A Treatise on Insanity*, trans. Davis, D. D. New York: Hafner (Reprint of 1806 ed.)

Porter, R. S. (1980) Was there a moral therapy in the eighteenth century? Paper delivered at a Symposium on *History and Mental Disorder*, Wellcome Institute for the History of Medicine, 26 September 1980

Poynter, F. N. L. (1959) Ed. *The History and Philosophy of Knowledge of the Brain and its Functions*. Oxford: Blackwell

Prévost, C. M. (1973) *Janet, Freud et la psychologie clinique*. Paris: Petite Bibliothèque Payot

Pribram, K. H. & Gill, M. M. (1976) *Freud's 'Project' Reassessed*. London: Hutchinson

Prichard, J. C. (1835) *A Treatise on Insanity and Other Disorders affecting the Mind*. London: Sherwood *et al*

Quen, J. M. (1974) Isaac Ray: have we learned his lessons? *Bull. Amer. Acad. Psychiat. Law*, **2**, 137–47

Rabb, T. K. (1975) *The Struggle for Stability in Early Modern Europe*. New York: Oxford University Press

Randall, J. H., Jr. (1961) *The School of Padua and the Emergence of Modern Science*. Padua: Antenore

Reed, R. R., Jr. (1952) *Bedlam on the Jacobean Stage*. Cambridge, Mass: Harvard University Press

Reynolds, D. K. (1976) *Morita Psychotherapy*. Berkeley and London: University of California Press

Reynolds, L. D. & Wilson, N. G. (1974) *Scribes and Scholars. A Guide to the Transmission of Greek and Latin Literature*. 2nd ed. Oxford: Clarendon Press

Rieber, R. W. & Salzinger, K. (1977) Eds. The roots of American psychology: historical influences and implications for the future. *Ann. N.Y. Acad. Sci.*, **291**, 1–394

Rieff, P. (1979) *Freud: the Mind of the Moralist*. 3rd ed. Chicago: Chicago University Press

Riese, H. (1979) Ed. *Historical Explorations in Medicine and Psychiatry*. New York: Springer

Riese, W. (1965) *La Théorie des passions à la lumière de la pensée médicale du xviie siècle*. Basle: Karger

Risse, G. B. (1970) The Brownian system of medicine: its theoretical and practical implications. *Clio Med.*, **5**, 45–51

Rohde, E. (1925) *Psyche: the Cult of Souls and Belief in Immortality among the Greeks*. London: Kegan Paul

Roosens, E. (1979) *Des fous dans la ville? Gheel et sa thérapie séculaire*. Paris: Presses Universitaires de France

Rosen, G. (1968) *Madness in Society. Chapters in the Historical Sociology of Mental Illness*. London: Routledge & Kegan Paul

— (1971) History in the study of suicide. *Psychol. Med.*, **1**, 267–85

— (1975) Nostalgia: a 'forgotten' psychological disorder. *Psychol. Med.*, **5**, 340–54

Rosenberg, C. E. (1968) *The Trial of the Assassin Guiteau*. Chicago: University of Chicago Press

— (1974) The bitter fruit: heredity, disease, and social thought in nineteenth-century America. *Perspect. Amer. Hist.*, **8**, 189–235.

Rosenkrantz, B. G. & Vinovskis, M. A. (1978) The invisible lunatics: old age and insanity in mid-nineteenth century Massachusetts. In *Aging and the Family*, ed. Spicker, S. et al. Atlantic Highlands, N.J.: Humanities Press

Rothman, D. (1971) *The Discovery of the Asylum*. Boston: Little, Brown

Rousseau, G. S. (1976) Nerves, spirits and fibres: towards defining the origins of sensibility; with a postscript, 1976. *The Blue Guitar*, **2**, 125–53

— (1980) Psychology. In *The Ferment of Knowledge*, ed. Rousseau, G. S. & Porter, R. S. Cambridge: Cambridge University Press

Russell, J. B. (1972) *Witchcraft in the Middle Ages*. Ithaca and London: Cornell University Press

Scheff, T. J. (1966) *Being Mentally Ill*. Chicago: Aldine

Schneck, J. N. (1960) *A History of Psychiatry*. Springfield: Thomas

— (1975) United States of America. In Howells (1975)

Schoeneman, T. J. (1977) The role of mental illness in the European Witch Hunts of the 16th and 17th centuries: an assessment. *J. Hist. behav. Sci.*, **13**, 337–51

Schofield, R. E. (1970) *Mechanism and Materialism: British Natural Philosophy in an Age of Reason*. Princeton: Princeton University Press

Schur, M. (1972) *Freud: Living and Dying*. New York: International Universities Press

Screech, M. A. (1979) *Rabelais*. London: Duckworth

Scull, A. (1975) From madness to mental illness. Medical men as moral entrepreneurs. *Arch. Europ. Sociol.*, **16**, 218–51

— (1977) *Decarceration*. Englewood Cliffs: Prentice-Hall

— (1970) *Museums of Madness*. London: Allen Lane

— (1981) Ed. *Madhouses, Mad-doctors, and Madmen: the Social History of Psychiatry in the Victorian Era*. Philadelphia: University of Pennsylvania Press

Searle, G. R. (1976) *Eugenics and Politics in Britain, 1900–1914*. Leyden: Noordhoff

Sémelaigne, R. (1930) *Les Pionniers de la psychiatrie française*. Paris: Baillière

Sérieux, P. (1921) *V. Magnan, (1835–1916). Sa vie et son oeuvre*. Paris: Masson

Shapin, S. (1975) Phrenological knowledge and the social structure of early nineteenth century Edinburgh. *Ann. Sci.*, **32**, 219–43

Shepherd, M. (1977) *The Career and Contributions of Sir Aubrey Lewis*. London: Bethlem Royal and Maudsley Hospitals

Sherrington, C. S. (1946) *The Endeavour of Jean Fernel*. Cambridge: Cambridge University Press

Sicherman, B. (1977) The uses of a diagnosis: doctors, patients, and neurasthenia. *J. Hist. Med.*, **32**, 33–54

Simon, B. (1978) *Mind and Madness in Ancient Greece*. Ithaca: Cornell University Press

Skultans, V. (1979) *English Madness: Ideas on Insanity, 1580–1890*. London: Routledge & Kegan Paul

Smith, R. (1979) Mental disorder, criminal responsibility and the social history of theories of volition. *Psychol. Med.*, **2**, 13–19

— (1981) *Trial by Medicine. Insanity and Responsibility in Victorian Trials*. Edinburgh: Edinburgh University Press

Starobinski, J. (1960) Geschichte der Melancholiebehandlung von den Anfängen bis 1900. *Documenta Giegy, Acta psychosom.*, **4**

Stengel, E. (1963) Hughlings Jackson's influence in psychiatry. *Brit. J. Psychiat.*, **109**, 348–55

Stone, L. (1977) *The Family, Sex and Marriage in England, 1500–1800*. London: Weidenfeld & Nicolson

Szasz, T. S. (1973) *The Manufacture of Madness*. London: Paladin

Taylor, F. Kräupl (1979) *The Concepts of Illness, Disease and Morbus*. Cambridge: Cambridge University Press

Temkin, O. (1947) Gall and the phrenological movement. *Bull. Hist. Med.*, **21**, 275–321

— (1973) *Galenism: Rise and Decline of a Medical Philosophy*. Ithaca & London: Cornell University Press

— (1977) On Galen's Pneumatology. In *The Double Face of Janus*. Baltimore and London: Johns Hopkins University Press

Thomas, K. (1973) *Religion and the Decline of Magic*. Harmondsworth: Penguin

Thompson, J. D. & Goldin, G. (1975) *The Hospital: A Social and Architectural History*. New Haven and London: Yale University Press

Thorndike, L. (1923–58) *A History of Magic and Experimental Science*. 8 vols. New York: Columbia University Press

Townsend, J. M. (1978) *Cultural Conceptions and Mental Illness. A Comparison of Germany and America*. Chicago and London: University of Chicago Press

Trevor-Roper, H. R. (1967) The European witch-craze of the sixteenth and seventeenth centuries. In *Religion, the Reformation and Social Change*. London: Macmillan

Tuke, D. H. (1882) *Chapters in the History of the Insane in the British Isles*. London: Kegan Paul

Tuke, S. (1964) *A Description of the Retreat*. Intro. by Hunter, R. and Macalpine, I. London: Dawsons. (Reprint of 1813 ed.)

Tuveson, E. (1960) *The Imagination as Means of Grace*. Los Angeles: University of California Press

Tyor, P. L. & Zainaldin, J. S. (1979) Asylum and society: an approach to institutional change. *J. soc. Hist.*, **13**, 23–48

Vartanian, A. (1953) *Diderot and Descartes: a Study of Scientific Naturalism in the Enlightenment*. Princeton: Princeton University Press

Veith, I. (1965) *Hysteria: the History of a Disease*. Chicago: University of Chicago Press

Villeneuve, R. (1956) Lycanthropie et vampirisme. *Aesculape*, **39**, 2–63

Waldinger, R. J. (1979) Sleep of reason: John P. Gray and the challenge of moral insanity. *J. Hist. Med.*, **34**, 163–79

Walk, A. (1954) Some aspects of the 'moral treatment' of the insane up to 1854. *J. ment. Sci.*, **100**, 807–37

— (1959) On the state of lunacy, 1859–1959. *J. ment. Sci.*, **105**, 879–92

— (1961) Gloucester and the beginnings of the R.M.P.A. *J. ment. Sci.*, **107**, 604–32

— (1970) Lincoln and non-restraint. *Brit. J. Psychiat.*, **117**, 481–96

— (1978) 'Forty years of wanderings' – the Medico-Psychological Association, 1855–1894. *Brit. J. Psychiat.*, **132**, 530–47

Walker, D. P. (1958) *Spiritual and Demonic Magic from Ficino to Campanella*. London: Warburg Institute

Walker, N. (1968) *Crime and Insanity in England. Vol. 1. The Historical Perspective*. Edinburgh: Edinburgh University Press

Walser, H. H. (1968) (Ed.) *August Forel. Briefe. Correspondance, 1864–1927*. Berne: Huber

Walton, J. K. (1979) Lunacy in the Industrial Revolution: a study of asylum admissions in Lancashire, 1848–50. *J. soc. Hist.*, **13**, 1–22.

Warren, H. C. (1921) *A History of Association Psychology*. London: Constable

Weber, M. (1930) *The Protestant Ethic and the Spirit of Capitalism*. Trans. Parsons, T. London: Unwin University Books

Webster, C. (1975) *The Great Instauration. Science, Medicine and Reform, 1626–1660*. London: Duckworth

Wenzel, S. (1961) Petrarch's accidia. *Stud. Renaissance*, **8**, 37–48

— (1967) *The Sin of Sloth: Acedia in Medieval Thought and Literature*. Chapel Hill: University of North Carolina Press

Werlinder, H. (1978) *Psychopathy: A History of the Concepts*. Stockholm: Almqvist & Wiksell

West, D. J. & Walk, A. (1977) *Daniel McNaughton: his Trial and the Aftermath*. Ashford: Gaskell Books

Wettley, A. (1953) *August Forel*. Salzburg: Müller

Wilson, J. D. (1935) *What Happens in Hamlet*. Cambridge: Cambridge University Press

Wing, J. K. (1978) *Reasoning about Madness*. London: Oxford University Press

Wolf, H. B. (1976) *Zur Entdeckung des Patellarsehnen-reflexes durch Erb und Westphal*. Münster: Institut für Theorie und Geschichte der Medizin

Wolfe, D. E. (1961) Sydenham and Locke on the limits of anatomy. *Bull. Hist. Med.*, **35**, 193–220

Young, R. M. (1970) *Mind, Brain and Adaptation in the Nineteenth Century*. Oxford: Clarendon Press

— (1973) Association of Ideas. In *Dictionary of the History of Ideas*, ed. Wiener, P. P. 4 vols. New York: Scribner

Zilboorg, G. (1935) *The Medical Man and the Witch in the Renaissance*. Baltimore: Johns Hopkins Press

— (1941) *A History of Medical Psychology*. New York: Norton

Chapter 2.1

Birnbaum, K. (1923) *Der Aufbau der Psychose. Grundzüge der psychiatrischen Strukturanalyse*. Berlin: Springer

Bleuler, E. (1911) *Dementia praecox oder Gruppe der Schizophrenien*. Leipzig, Vienna: Deuticke

Bonhoeffer, K. (1910) *Die symptomatische Psychose im Gefolge von akuten Infektionen und inneren Erkrankungen*. Leipzig, Vienna: Deuticke

Faergeman, P. M. (1963) *Psychogenic psychoses. A Description and Follow-up of Psychoses following Psychological Stress*. London: Butterworth

Feuchtersleben, E. V. (1845) *Lehrbuch der ärztlichen Seelenkunde*. Vienna: Gerold

Freud, S. (1968) *Das Ich und das Es*. Orig. ed. 1924. *Gesammelte Werke*, vol. XIII. Frankfurt: Fischer

Griesinger, W. (1861) *Die Pathologie und Therapie der psychischen Krankheiten*. 2nd ed. Stuttgart: Krabbe

Heinroth, J. C. (1818–25) *Lehrbuch der Störungen des Seelenlebens oder der Seelenstörungen und ihre Behandlung, vom rationalen Standpunkt aus entworfen*. Liepzig: Vogel

Jaspers, K. (1910) Eifersuchtswahn. Ein Beitrag zur Frage: 'Entwicklung einer Persönlichkeit' oder 'Prozess'? *Z. ges. Neurol. Psychiat.*, Orig. **1**, 402–452

— (1913) Kausale und 'verständliche' Zusammenhänge zwischen Schicksal und Psychose bei der Dementia praecox (Schizophrenie). *Z. ges. Neurol. Psychiat.*, Orig. **14**, 158–263

— (1959) *Allgemeine Psychopathologie*. 7th ed. Berlin, Göttingen, Heidelberg: Springer

Kleist, K. (1908) *Untersuchungen zur Kenntnis der psychomotorischen Bewegungsstörungen bei Geisteskranken*. Leipzig: Vogel

Kraepelin, E. (1887) *Psychiatrie*. 1st ed. Leipzig: Barth

Meynert, Th. (1884) *Psychiatrie. Lehrbuch der Erkrankungen des Vorderhirnes, begründet auf dessen Bau, Leistungen und Ernährung*. Vienna: Braumüller

Möbius, P. J. (1886) *Allgemeine Diagnostik der Nervenkrankheiten*. Leipzig: Vogel

Neumann, K. G. (1822) *Die Krankheiten des Vorstellungsvermögens*. Leipzig: Cnobloch

Scharfetter, Ch. (1970) *Symbiontische Psychosen. Studie über schizophrenieartige 'induzierte Psychosen'*. Berne, Stuttgart, Vienna: Huber

Schneider, K. (1967) *Klinische Psychopathologie*. 8 ed. Stuttgart: Thieme

Wernicke, C. (1881–3) *Lehrbuch der Gehirnkrankheiten*. Kassel, Berlin: Fischer

Zeller, A. (1840) Zweiter Bericht über die Wirksamkeit der Heilanstalt Winnenthal. *Med. Korrespondenzbl. Württemberg. aerztl. Verein.* **10**, 129, 137, 145

Chapter 2.2

Secondary references (primary references are given in text)

Ellenberger, H. F. (1970) The discovery of the Unconscious. New York: Basic Books

Fischer-Homberger, E. (1972) Hypochondriasis of the eighteenth century – neurosis of the present century. *Bull. Hist. Med.* **46** 391–401

— (1975) Die traumatische Neurose. Vom somatischen zum sozialen Leiden. Berne, Stuttgart, Vienna: Huber

Knoff, W. F. (1970) A history of the concept of neurosis, with a memoir of William Cullen. *Amer. J. Psychiat.* **127** 80–84

Levin, K. (1978) Freud's Early Psychology of the Neuroses. A Historical Perspective. Pittsburgh: Pittsburgh University Press

López Piñero, J. M. (1963) Orígenes históricos del concepto de neurosis. *Cuadernos Valencianos de historia de la medicina,* 1. Valencia: Catedra e Instituto de Historia de la Medicina

López Piñero, J. M. & Morales Meseguer, J. M. (1970) Neurosis y psicoterapia, un estudio histórico. *Monografías de psicología normal y patológica,* 11. Madrid: España-Calpe

Macmillan, M. B. (1976) Beard's concept of neurasthenia and Freud's concept of the actual neuroses. *J. Hist. behav. Sci.* **12** 376–90

Maier, J. S. (1948) Beitrag zur Geschichte des Neurosebegriffes von 1778–1887. *Med. Diss. Erlangen*

Schafer, M. L. (1972) *Der Neurosebegriff. Ein Beitrag zu seiner historischen Entwicklung.* (Das wissenschaftliche Taschenbuch, Abt. Medizin 29). Munich: Goldmann

Sims A. (1975) The English concept of neurosis: a short historical account. *Midl. med. Rev.* **11** (1975) 51–7

Chapter 2.3

1 Plato, Phaedrus, 244 B.C.
2 See Dodds, E. R. (1975) *The Greeks and the Irrational.* Berkeley, Los Angeles, London: University of California Press
3 *The Extant Works of Aretaeus, the Cappadocian* (1856) Ed. and transl. Adams, Francis. London: The Sydenham Society
4 Caelius Aurelianus (1950) *On Acute Diseases and On Chronic Diseases,* ed. and transl. Drabkin, I. E., pp. 534–63. Chicago: University of Chicago Press
5 Pinel, Ph. (1800) *Traité philosophique sur l'aliénation mentale.* Paris, *an IX.* (Engl. transl. Davis, D. D., *A Treatise on Insanity,* 1806. London)
6 Bleuler, E. (1911) *Dementia praecox, oder Gruppe der Schizophrenien.* Leipzig, Vienna: Deuticke (Engl. transl. Zinkin, Joseph & Lewis, Nolan D. C., 1950. New York: International Universities Press)
7 Haslam, J. H. (1798) *Observations on Insanity.* London
8 Beddoes, T. (1802) *Hygéia: or Essays, Moral and Medical* (. . .). 3 vol. Bristol
9 Guislain, J. G. (1833) *Traité sur les phrénopathies ou doctrine nouvelle des maladies mentales.* Brussels
10 Griesinger, W. G. (1945) *Pathologie und Therapie der psychischen Krankheiten.* Stuttgart. (Engl. transl. Robertson, C. & Rutherford, J. 1867 London)
11 Falret, J.-P. F. (1851) *De la folie circulaire ou forme de maladie mentale caractérisée par l'alternative régulière de la manie et de la mélancholie.* Paris. (Later published in *Des Maladies mentales et des asiles d'aliénés,* 1864. Paris, London)
12 Kahlbaum, K. L. (1882) Ueber zyklisches Irresein, *Irrenfreund,* No. 10.

13 (Ps) Aristotle *Problemata,* xxx, 1.
14 Ficino, M. (1489) *De vita triplici,* in *Opera Omnia* (1576), vol. i, p. 493. Basle. (See Klibansky, R., Panofsky E. & Saxl, F., 1964, *Saturn and Melancholy.* Nelson)
15 Galen (1904) *De Temperamentis,* libri III. Ed. Helmreich, Georg. Leipzig
16 Burton, R. (1621) *The Anatomy of Melancholy.* London (Modern ed. Holbrook Jackson, London: Dent)
17 See Temkin, O. (1973) *Galenism. Rise and Decline of a Medical Philosophy.* Cornell University Press
18 Sauvages de la Croix, F Boissier de (1768) *Nosologia methodica, sistens morborum classes, genera et species.* 5 vol. Amsterdam
19 Linné (Linnaeus), Carl von (1763) *Genera morborum in auditorum usum.* Uppsala
20 Cullen, W. (1769) *Synopsis nosologiae methodicae.* Edinburgh. (Several English translations)
21 Darwin, Erasmus (1794–6) *Zoonomia; or the Laws of Organic Life.* 2 vol. London
22 Pinel, Ph. (1813) *Nosographie philosophique.* 5th ed. 3 vol. Paris
23 Esquirol, J. E. D. (1838) *Des maladies mentales.* 2 vol. Paris (Engl. transl. Hunt, E. K., 1845. Philadelphia)
24 Kraepelin, E. (1913) *Psychiatrie.* 8th ed., pp. 1284–1303. 4 vols. Leipzig
25 See reference (5)
26 Heinroth, J. C. A. (1818) *Lehrbuch der Störungen des Seelenlebens.* Leipzig
27 Meynert, T. H. (1884) *Psychiatrie. Klinik der Erkrankungen des Vorderhirns.* Vienna
28 Freud, S. (1917) Trauer und Melancholie. In *Gesammelte Werke,* vol. x, 1946, pp. 428–46. (English transl.: Standard edition of the *Complete Works of Sigmund Freud,* vol. 14, pp. 243–58, 1957. London: Hogarth Press)
29 Binswanger, L. (1960) *Melancholie und Manie.* Pfullingen

Chapter 2.4

Bleuler, E. (1911) *Dementia praecox oder Gruppe der Schizophrenien.* Leipzig, Vienna: Deuticke

Diem, O. (1903) Die einfach demente Form der Dementia praecox. *Arch. Psychiat.,* **37,**, 111–87

Fink, E. (1881) Beitrag zur Kenntnis des Jugendirreseins. *Allg. Z. Psychiat.,* **37,** 490–520

Hecker, E. (1871) Die Hebephrenie. *Virchows Arch. pathol. Anat.,* **52,** 394–429

Kahlbaum, K. L. (1874) *Die Katatonie oder das Spannungsirresein.* Berlin: Hirschwald

Kraepelin, E. (1909) *Psychiatrie.* 8th ed. Leipzig: Barth (1st ed. 1887; 6th ed. 1899)

Morel, B. A. (1852) *Etudes cliniques: traité théorique et pratique des maladies mentales.* Paris: Masson

— (1860) *Traité des maladies mentales.* Paris: Masson

Pick, A. (1891) *Über primäre Demenz.* Wandervorträge

Pinel, Ph. (1801) *Traité médico-philosophique sur l'aliénation mentale.* Paris: R. Caille, Ravier

Scharfetter, Ch. (1976) *Allgemeine Psychopathologie.* Stuttgart: Thieme

Schneider, K. (1950) *Klinische Psychopathologie.* 3rd ed. Stuttgart: Thieme

Snell, L. (1865) Uber Monomanie als primäre Form der Seelenstörung. *Allg. Z. Psychiat.,* **22,** 368–81

World Health Organization (1973) *The International Pilot Study on Schizophrenia.* Geneva: WHO
— (1977) *Manual of the International Statistical Classification of Diseases, Injuries and Causes of Death.* Geneva: WHO

Chapter 2.5

Berner, P. (1965) *Das paranoische Syndrom.* Berlin: Springer
Freud, S. (1968) Psychoanalytische Bemerkungen über einen autobiographisch beschriebenen Fall von Paranoia (dementia paranoides). (Orig. 1911) *Ges. Werke,* vol. 8. Frankfurt/M.: Fischer
Gaupp, R. (1920) Der Fall Wagner. Eine Katamnese, zugleich ein Beitrag zur Lehre von der Paranoia. *Z. Neurol.,* **60,** 312–27
Griesinger, W. (1861) *Die Pathologie und Therapie der psychischen Krankheiten.* 2nd ed. (1st ed. 1860). Stuttgart: Krabbe
Heinroth, D. F. E. U. (1818) *Störungen des Seelenlebens.* Leipzig: Vogel
Kehrer, F. (1928) Paranoische Zustände. In *Handbuch der Geisteskrankheiten.* Ed. Bumke, O., vol. VI, Spez. T.2., pp. 232–364 *Berlin: Springer*
Kolle, K. (1931) *Die primäre Verrücktheit.* Leipzig: Thieme
Kraepelin, E. (1896) *Psychiatrie.* 5th ed. (8th ed. 1909–13). Leipzig: Barth
Kretschmer, E. (1950) *Der sensitive Beziehungswahn.* 3rd ed. (1st ed. 1918). Berlin, Göttingen, Heidelberg: Springer
Lewis, A. (1970) Paranoia and paranoid: a historical perspective. *Psychol. Med.,* **1,** 2–12
Snell, L. (1865) Über Monomanie als primäre Form der Seelenstörung. *Allg. Z. Psychiat.,* **22,** 368–81

Chapter 2.6
Secondary references (primary references are given in text)

Fischer-Homberger, E. (1970) Hypochondrie. *Melancholie bis Neurose: Krankheiten und Zustandsbilder.* Berne, Stuttgart, Vienna: Huber
Keyserlingk, H. V. & Opitz, B. (1968) Von der Hypochondrie zum hypochondrischen Symptomenkomplex. Ein medizinhistorischer Versuch. *Psychiat. Neurol. med. Psychol. (Lpz.),* **20,** 121–9.
Ladee, G. A. (1966)*Hypochondriacal syndromes,* pp. 7–39. Amsterdam, London, New York: Elsevier (Historical survey of the concept of hypochondriasis)
Wollenberg, R. (1904) Die Hypochondrie. In *Specielle Pathologie und Therapie,* ed. Nothnagel, H., vol. 12, part 1,3, pp. 1–17. (Einleitung: Geschichtliches etc.) Vienna: Hölder

Chapter 2.7

Benjamin, H. (1966) *The Transsexual Phenomenon.* New York: Julian Press
Bieber, I. (1962) *Homosexuality: A Psychological Study.* New York: Basic Books
Binswanger, L. (1949/50) *Sinn und Gehalt der Sexuellen Perversionen. Psyche* **3,** 881–909
Boss, M. (1966) *Sinn und Gehalt der sexuellen Perversionen* 3rd ed. Berne, Stuttgart: Huber
Comfort, A. (1972) *Joy of Sex.* New York: Simon & Fisher
Ehrhard, A. A., Epstein, R., & Money, J. (1968) Fetal androgens and female gender/identity in the early-treated androgenital syndrome *Johns Hopkins Med. J.,* **122,** 160–67

Freud, S. (1943) *Drei Abhandlungen zur Sexualtheorie.* 7th ed. Vienna: Deuticke
Gebsattel, E. V. von (1932) Über süchtiges Verhalten im Gebiet Sexueller Verirrungen. *Monatschr. Psychiat. Neurol.,* **82,** 113–77
Hare, E. H. (1962) Masturbatory insanity: the history of an idea *J. ment. Sci.,* **108,** 2–25
Häussler, J. (1826) *Über die Beziehungen des Sexualsystems zur Psyche überhaupt und zum Kretinismus im Besonderen.* Würzburg
Hoenig, J. (1976) Sigmund Freud's views on the sexual disorders in historical perspective *Brit. J. Psychiat.,* **129,** 193–200
— (1977a) The development of sexology during the second half of the 19th century. In *Handbook of Sexology,* ed. Money, J. & Musaph, H., pp. 5–20. Amsterdam: Excerpta medica, North Holland, Elsevier
— (1977b) Dramatis personae: selected biographical sketches of 19th century pioneers in sexology In *Handbook of Sexology,* ed. Money, J. & Musaph, H. pp. 21–43. Amsterdam: Excerpta medica, North Holland, Elsevier
Jirásek, J. E. (1967) The relationship between the structure of the testis and differentiation of the external genitalia and phenotype in man. *Ciba Found. Colloq. Endocrinol. (Proc.),* **16,** 3–30
Kaan, Heinrich (1844) *Was ist die Psychopathia Sexualis?* Leipzig.
Kiernan, J. G. (1888) Sexual perversion and the Whitechapel murders. *Med. Standard,* Chicago, **4,** 170–72
Krafft-Ebing, R. v. (1886) *Psychopathia Sexualis.* Stuttgart: Enke
Kunz, H. (1942) Zur Theorie der Perversionen *Monatschr. Psychiat. Neurol.,* **105,** 1–101
Lorenz, K. (1953) Die Entwicklung der vergleichenden Verhaltensforschung in den letzten 12 Jahren. *Verh. Deutsch. Zool. Ges. Freiburg.* Leipzig: Akad. Verlag
Lydston, G. F. (1889) Sexual perversion, satyriasis and nymphomania. *Med. Surg. Reporter,* Philadelphia, **61,** 253–81
Masters, W. H. & Johnson, V. E. (1966) *Human Sexual Response.* Boston: Little Brown
Money, J., Hampson, J. C. & Hampson, J. L. (1955) Hermaphroditism *Bull. Johns Hopkins Hosp.,* **97,** 284–300
Schwartz, O. (1935) *Sexualpathologie* Vienna
Strauss, E. (1930) *Geschehnis und Erlebnis* Berlin: Springer
Tarnowsky, B. (1886) *Die krankhaften Erscheinungen des Geschlechtssinnes.* Berlin: Hirschwald
Tinbergen, N. (1951) *The Study of Instinct.* Oxford: Clarendon Press
Tissot, S. (1766) *L'Onanisme ou dissertation physique sur les maladies produites par la masturbation.* Paris. (Transl. Hume, A. London)
Ulrichs, C. H. (1898) *Gladius furens.* Leipzig: Spohr
Wettley, A. (1959a) Die Trieblehre Auguste Comtes. *Confinia Psychiat.* **2,** 37–55.
— (1959b) Zur Problemgeschichte des Entartungsbegriffes im 19. Jahrhundert. *Sudhoff's Archiv.* 43, 3, 193–212
Wettley, A. & Leibbrand, W. (1959) Von der 'Psychopathia sexualis' zur Sexualwissenschaft. *Beitr. Sexualforsch.,* **17.** Stuttgart: Enke

Chapter 2.8

Berger, H. (1929) Ueber das Elektrenkephalogram des Menschen. *Arch. Psychiat. Nervenkrankh.,* **87,** 527–70
Jackson, J. H. (1873) On the anatomical, physiological, and pathological investigation of epilepsies. *The West Riding Lunatic Asylum Medical Reports,* **3,** 315–39

Temkin, O. (1971) *The Falling Sickness: A History of Epilepsy from the Greeks to the Beginnings of Modern Neurology.* 2nd ed. Baltimore and London: Johns Hopkins University Press

Chapter 2.9

Ackerknecht, E. H. (1968) *A Short History of Psychiatry,* 2nd ed., trans. Wolff, S. New York: Hafner.

Brain, Lord (1964) Psychosomatic medicine and the brain-mind relationship. *Lancet,* **ii,** 325–8

Burtt, E. A. (1932) *The Metaphysical Foundations of Modern Physical Science.* London: Kegan Paul

Cannon, W. B. (1915) *Bodily Changes in Pain, Hunger, Fear and Rage.* New York: Appleton Century

Cobb, S., Miles, H. H. W., & Shands, H. C. (1952) *Case Histories in Psychosomatic Medicine.* New York: Norton

Dijksterhuis, E. J. (1961) *The Mechanization of the World Picture.* Trans. Dikshoorn, C. Oxford: Clarendon Press

Entralgo, P. Lain (1955) *Mind and Body: Psychosomatic Pathology.* Trans. Espinosa, A. M. London: Harvill

Havens, L. L. (1973) *Approaches to the Mind: Movement of the Psychiatric Schools from Sects towards Science.* Boston: Little Brown

Heinroth, J. C. (1818) *Lehrbuch der Störungen des Seelenlebens, oder der Seelenstörungen und ihrer Behandlung.* Leipzig: Vogel

Jacobi, K. W. M. (1822) *Sammlungen für die Heilkunde der Gemütskrankheiten.* Elberfeld: Schonian

James, W. (1884) What is an emotion? *Mind,* **9,** 188–205

Kaplan, H. I. (1980) History of psychosomatic medicine. In *Comprehensive Textbook of Psychiatry,* ed. Kaplan, H. I., Freedman, A. M. & Sadock, B. J. 3rd ed. Baltimore: Williams & Wilkins

Kollar, E. J. & Alcalay, M. (1967) The physiological basis for psychosomatic medicine. A historical view. *Arch. int. Med.,* **67,** 883–95

Lange, C. G. (1887) *Uber Gemüthsbewegungen.* Trans. Kurella, H. Leipzig: Thomas

Lewis, A. (1967) Aspects of psychosomatic medicine. In *Inquiries in Psychiatry.* New York: Science House

Lipowski, Z. J. Lipsitt, D. R., & Whybrow, P. C. (1977) *Psychosomatic Medicine: Current Trends and Clinical Applications.* New York: Oxford University Press

Mayne, R. G. (1860) *An Expository Lexicon of the Terms, Ancient and Modern, in Medical and General Science.* London: Churchill

Rather, L. J. (1965) *Mind and Body in Eighteenth Century Medicine. A Study Based on Jerome Gaub's De regimine mentis.* London: Wellcome Historical Medical Library

Seyle, H. (1950) *The Physiology and Pathology of Exposure to Stress.* Montreal: Acta

Titchener, E. B. (1914) An historical note on the James–Lange theory of emotion. *Amer. J. Psychol.,* **3,** 285–98

Walker, N. (1956) The definition of psychosomatic disorder. *Brit. J. Philos. Sci.,* **6,** 265–99

Wolff, H. G. (1953) *Stress and Disease.* Springfield: Thomas

Chapter 3

Ackner, B. (1954) Depersonalization. *J. ment. Sci.,* **100,** 838–72

Aggernaes, A. (1972a) The experienced reality of hallucinations and other psychological phenomena. *Acta psychiat. scand.,* **48,** 220–38

— (1972b). The difference between the experienced reality of hallucinations in young drug abusers and schizophrenic patients. *Acta psychiat. scand.,* **48,** 287–99

Allison, R. S. (1962) *The Senile Brain. A Clinical Study.* London: Arnold

Allport, G. W. (1925) Eidetic imagery. *Brit. J. Psychol.,* **15,** 99–120

Anand, B. K., Chhina, G. S. & Singh, B. (1961) Studies on Shri Rananand Yogi during his stay in an airtight box. *Indian. J. med. Res.,* **49,** 82–9

Anderson, E. W., Trethowan, W. H. & Kenna, J. C. (1959) An experimental investigation of simulation and pseudodementia. *Acta psychiat. neurol. scand.,* supp. **132,** 1–42

Arkin, A. M., Toth, M. F., Baker, J. & Hastey, J. M. (1970) The frequency of sleep talking in the laboratory among chronic sleep talkers and good dream recallers. *J. nerv. ment. Dis.,* **151,** 369–74

Babinski, J. (1914) Contribution à l'étude des troubles mentaux dans l'hémiplégie organique cérébrale (anosognosie). *Rev. Neurol.,* **27,** 845–8

Backman, E. L. (1952) *Religious Dances in the Christian Church and in Popular Medicine.* London: Allen & Unwin

Bartlett, F. C. (1932) *Remembering.* Cambridge: Cambridge University Press,

Belbin, E. (1950) The influence of interpolated recall upon recognition. *Q. J. exper. Psychol.,* **2,** 163–9

Bender, L. & Vogel, B. F. (1941) Imaginary companions of children. *Amer. J. Orthopsychiat.,* **11,** 58–65

Benjamin, H. (1966) *The Transsexual Phenomenon.* New York: Julian Press

Bennet, G. (1973) Medical and psychological problems in the 1972 singlehanded transatlantic yacht race. *Lancet,* **ii,** 749–54

Benton, A. L. (1977) The Amusias. In *Music and the Brain. Studies in the Neurology of Music,* ed. Critchley, MacDonald & Henson, R. A., chap. 22. London: William Heinemann

Berlyne, N. (1972) Confabulation. *Brit. J. Psychiat.,* **120,** 31–9

Berrington, W. P., Liddell, D. W. & Foulds, G. A. (1956) A re-evaluation of the fugue. *J. ment. Sci.,* **102,** 280–86

Bexton, W. H., Heron, W. & Scott, T. H. (1954) Effects of decreased variation in the sensory environment. *Can. J. Psychol.,* **8,** 70–76

Bing, R. (1923) Uber einige bemerkenswerte Begleiterscheinungen der extra-pyramidalen Rigidität. (Akathisia-Mikrographie-Kinesia paradoxa). *Schweiz. med. Wochenschr.,* 4, 167–171

Biot, R. (1962) *The Riddle of the Stigmata.* London: Burns Oates

Bishop, P. M. F. (1966) Intersexual states and allied conditions. *Brit. med. J.,* **1,** 1255–62

Bivin, G. D. & Klinger, M. P. (1937) *Pseudocyesis.* Bloomington, Ind.: Principia Press

Black, P., Jeffries, J. J., Blumer, D., Wellner, A. & Walker, A. E. (1969) The Post-traumatic Syndrome in Children. In *The Late Effects of Head Injury,* ed. Walker, A. E., Caveness, W. F. & Critchley, M., chap. 14. Springfield, Ill.: Thomas

Bodamer, J. (1947) Die Prosop-Agnosie. (Die Agnosie des Physiognomienerkennen.) *Arch. Psychiat. Nervenkr.* 179, 6–53

Bonhoeffer, K. (1904) Der Korsakowsche Symptomenkomplex in seinen Beziehungen zu den verschiedenen Krankheitsformen. *Allg. Z. Psychiat.,* **61,** 744–52

Boulougouris, J. C., Marks, I. M. & Marset, P. (1971) The superiority of flooding (implosion) to desensitisation for reducing pathological fear. *Behav. Res. Ther.,* **9,** 7–16

Bower, T. G. R. (1966) The visual world of infants. *Sci. Amer.,* **215,** 80–92

— (1971) Early learning and behaviour. *Times Lit. Suppl.*, May, 523–4

Brain, Sir Russell (1956) The thirtieth Maudsley lecture: perception and imperception. *J. ment. Sci.*, **102**, 221–32

— (1961) *Speech Disorders. Aphasia, Apraxia and Agnosia.* London: Butterworths

Brentano, F. (1874) *Psychologie vom empirischen Standpunkt.* Leipzig: Duncker & Humblot. (Subsequent enlarged editions: Hamburg: Meiner, 1955, 1959)

Brindley, G. S. & Lewin, W. S. (1968) The sensations produced by electrical stimulation of the visual cortex. *J. Physiol.*, **196**, 479–93

Brown, J. (1964) Short-term memory. *Brit. med. Bull.*, **20**, 8–11

Burton, R. (1641, orig. 1621) *The Anatomy of Melancholy.* 6th ed. Oxford and London. Reprinted 1932, London: Dent

Burwell, C. S., Robin, E. D., Whaley, R. D. & Bickelmann, A. G. (1956) Extreme obesity associated with alveolar hypoventilation – a Pickwickian syndrome. *Amer. J. Med.*, **21**, 811–18

Cantwell, D. (1976) Hyperkinetic Syndrome. In *Child Psychiatry. Modern Approaches*, ed. Rutter M. & Hersov, L., chap. 22. Oxford: Blackwell

Carothers, J. C. (1947) A study of mental derangement in Africans, and an attempt to explain its peculiarities, more especially in relation to the African attitude to life. *J. ment. Sci.*, **93**, 548–97

Chapman, J. (1966) The early symptoms of schizophrenia. *Brit. J. Psychiat.*, **112**, 225–51

Chapman, J. & McGhie, A. (1964) Echopraxia in schizophrenia. *Brit. J. Psychiat.*, **110**, 365–74

Clérambault, G. G. de (1942) Le Psychoses passionelles. Paris: Presses Universitaires

Cotard, J. (1882) Du délire des négations. *Arch. Neurol., Paris*, **4**, 152–70, 282–96. (Transl. as 'Nihilistic delusions' and repub. in *Themes and Variations in European Psychiatry*, ed. Hirsch, S. R. & Shepherd, M. Bristol: Wright, 1974)

Crane, G. E. (1973) Persistent dyskinesia. *Brit. J. Psychiat.*, **122**, 395–405

Crisp, A. H. & Kalucy, R. S. (1974) Aspects of the perceptual disorder in anorexia nervosa. *Brit. J. med. Psychol.*, **47**, 349–61

Critchley, M. (1950) The body image in neurology. Lancet, i, 335–40

— (1951) Types of visual perseveration: 'paliopsia' and 'illusory visual spread'. *Brain*, **74**, 267–99

— (1953) *The Parietal Lobes.* London: Arnold,

— (1965) Acquired anomalies of colour perception of central origin. *Brain*, **88**, 711–24

— (1970) *The Dislexic Child.* 2nd ed. London: Heinemann

Dewhurst, C. J. & Gordon, R. R. (1963) Change of sex. Lancet, **88**, 1213–16

Dewhurst, K. & Pearson, J. (1955) Visual hallucinations of the self in organic diseases. *J. Neurol. Neurosurg. Psychiat.*, **18**, 53–7

Donath, J. (1897) Zur Kenntnis des Anancasmus. (Psychische Zwangszustände). *Arch. Psychiat. Nervenkr.*, **29**, 211–24

Edwards, G. & Gross, M. M. (1976) Alcohol dependence: provisional description of a clinical syndrome. *Brit. med. J.*, **1**, 1058–61

Eelkema, R. C., Brosseau, J., Koshnik, R. & McGee, C. (1970) A statistical study on the relationship between mental illness and traffic accidents – a pilot study. *Amer. J. pub. Hlth*, **60**, 459–69

Ekbom, K. A. (1945) *Restless Legs.* Stockholm: Ivar Hoeggströms

— (1950) Restless legs. A report of 70 new cases. *Acta. med. scand.*, Supp. 246, 64–8

Ellenberger, H. F. (1970) *The Discovery of the Unconscious. The History and Evolution of Dynamic Psychiatry.* London: Allen Lane, Penguin Press

Fenton, G. W. (1975) Clinical disorders of sleep. *Brit. J. hosp. Med.*, **14**, 120–45

Fisher, C. M. & Adams, R. D. (1964) Transient global amnesia. *Acta neurol. scand.*, Supp. 9, 7–83

Franz, S. I. (1933) *Persons One and Three. A Study in Multiple personalities.* New York: McGraw-Hill

Freedman, A. M. & Kaplan, H. I. (1967) *Comprehensive Textbook of Psychiatry.* Baltimore: Williams & Wilkins

French, N. R. & Steinberg, J. C. (1947) Factors governing the intelligibility of speech sounds. *J. acoust. Soc. Amer.*, **19**, 90–119 (Quoted from Miller, G. A.: *Language and Communication*, p. 64. New York: McGraw-Hill, 1951

Freud, S. (1891) *Zur Auffassung der Aphasien. Eine kritische Studie.* Leipzig: Deuticke (Transl. Stengel, E. in *On Aphasia*, p. 78. London: Imago, 1953)

Ganser, S. J. M. (1898) Uber einen eigenartigen hysterischen Dämmerzustand. *Arch. Psychiat. Nervenkr.*, **30**, 633–40. (Transl. Schorer, C. E. (1965): A peculiar hysterical state. *Brit. J. Crim.*, **5**, 120–26. Republished in *Themes and Variations in European Psychiatry*, ed. Hirsch, S. R. & Shepherd, M., chap 4. Bristol: Wright, 1974)

Gelder, M. G., Bancroft, J. H. J., Gath, D. H., Johnston, D. W., Mathews, A. M. & Shaw, P. M. (1973) Specific and non-specific factors in behaviour therapy. *Brit. J. Psychiat.*, **123**, 445–62

Gelder, M. G. & Marks, I. M. (1966) Severe agoraphobia. A controlled prospective trial of behaviour therapy. *Brit. J. Psychiat.*, **112**, 309–19

Gibbens, T. C. N., Palmer, C. & Prince, J. (1971) Mental health aspects of shoplifting. *Brit. med. J.*, **2**, 612–15

Gibbens, T. C. N. & Prince, J. (1962) *Shoplifting.* London: Institute for the Study and Treatment of Delinquency

Gibbens, T. C. N. & Silberman, M. (1960) The clients of prostitutes. *Brit. J. vener. Dis.*, **36**, 113–17

Glatt, M. M. (1974) *A Guide to Addiction and its Treatment.* Lancaster, Engl.: Medical and Technical Publishing

Goldstein, K. (1942) *Aftereffects of Brain Injuries in War. Their Evaluation and Treatment. The Application of Psychologic Methods in the Clinic.* London: Heinemann

Goodwin, D. W., Crane, J. B. & Guze, S. B. (1969a) Alcoholic blackouts: a review and clinical study of 100 alcoholics. *Amer. J. Psychiat.*, **126**, 191–8

— (1969b) Phenomenological aspects of the alcoholic 'blackout'. *Brit. J. Psychiat.*, **115**, 1033–8

Goodwin, D. W., Powell, B., Bremer, D., Heine, H. & Stern, J. (1969c) Alcohol and recall: state-dependent effects in man. *Science*, **163**, 1358–60

Gordon, E. E., Januszko, D. M. & Kaufman, L. (1967) A critical survey of stiff man syndrome. *Amer. J. Med.*, **42**, 582–99

Gralnick, A. (1942) Folie à deux: the psychosis of association. *Psychiat. Q.*, **16**, 230–63

Gregory, R. L. (1974) *Concepts and Mechanisms of Perception.* London: Duckworth

Grünthal, E. & Störring, G. E. (1930a) Uber das Verhalten umschriebener, völliger Merkunfähigkeit. *Monatsschr. Psychiat. Neurol.*, **74**, 254–69

— (1930b) Ergänzende Beobachtungen und Bemerkungen zu

dem im Band 74 (1930) dieser Zeitschrift beschriebenen Fall mit reiner Merkunfähigkeit. *Monatsschr. Psychiat. Neurol.*, **77**, 374–82

Gunn, J. (1976) Sexual offenders. *Brit. J. hosp. Med.*, **15**, 57–65

Haber, R. N. (1969) Eidetic images. *Sci. Amer.*, **220**, 36–44

Haggard, E. A., Brekstad, A. & Skard, Å G. (1960) On the reliability of the anamnestic interview. *J. abn. soc. Psychol.*, **61**, 311–18

Halmi, K. A., Goldberg, S. C. & Cunningham, S. (1977) Perceptual distortion of body image in adolescence. *Psychol. Med.*, **7**, 253–7

Hamilton, M. (1959) The assessment of anxiety states by rating. *Brit. J. med. Psychol.*, **32**, 50–55

— (1974) (Ed.) *Fish's Clinical Psychopathology. Signs and Symptoms in Psychiatry*. Bristol: Wright

Hare, E. H. (1973) A short note on pseudo-hallucinations. *Brit. J. Psychiat.*, **122**, 469–76

Harris, A. (1959) Sensory deprivation and schizophrenia. *J. ment. Sci.*, **105**, 235–7

Haškovec, L. (1901) L'akathisie. *Rev. Neurol.*, **9**, 1107–9

— (1904) Weitere Bemerkungen über die Akathisie. *Wien. med. Wochenschr.*, **54**, 525–9, 582–6

Hay, G. G. (1970a) Psychiatric aspects of cosmetic nasal operations. *Brit. J. Psychiat.*, **116**, 85–97

— (1970b) Dysmorphophobia. *Brit. J. Psychiat.*, **116**, 399–406

Hay, G. G. & Heather, B. B. (1973) Changes of psychometric test results following cosmetic nasal operations. *Brit. J. Psychiat.*, **122**, 89–90

Head, H. (1920) *Studies in Neurology*. London: Frowde

Hebb, D. D. (1949) *The Organization of Behavior. A Neuropsychological Theory*. New York: Wiley

Heller, T. (1930) Uber dementia infantilis. *Z. Kinderforschung*, **37**, 661. (Transl. and reprinted in *Modern Perspectives in International Child Psychiatry*, ed. Howells, J. G. Edinburgh: Oliver & Boyd, 1969)

Hill, A. L. (1975) An investigation of calendar calculating by an idiot savant. *Amer. J. Psychol.*, **132**, 557–60

Hoenig, J. (1968) Medical research on Yoga. *Confinia psychiat.*, **11**, 69–89

Hoffer, W. (1946) Diaries of adolescent schizophrenics (hebephrenics). *Psychoanal. Stud. Child*, **2**, 293–312

Hunter, J. M. L. (1957) Memory, Facts and Fallacies. Harmondsworth: Penguin

Jackson, J. Hughlings (1876) Case of large cerebral tumour without optic neuritis and with left hemiplegia and imperception. *Roy. Lond. Ophthalm. Hosp. Rep.*, **8**, 434. (Reprinted in *Selected Writings*, ed. Taylor, J. **2**, 146–52 London: Hodder & Stoughton 1932)

Jaensch, E. R. (1930) *Eidetic Imagery*. London: Kegan Paul

James, W. (1890) *The Principles of Psychology*. New York: Holt; London: Macmillan

Jaspers, K. (1948) *Allegemeine Psychopathologie*. 5 ed. Berlin and Heidelberg: Springer (Orig. 1913) (Transl. as *General Psychopathology* by Hoenig, J. & Hamilton, M. W. Manchester University Press, 1962

Jones, H. S. & Oswald I (1968) Two cases of healthy insomnia. *Electroenceph. clin. Neurophysiol.*, **24**, 378–80

Jung, C. G. (1902) On the psychology and pathology of so-called *occult phenomena*. In *Collected Works*, **1**, 3–92. London: Routledge & Kegan Paul, 1957

— (1905) Cryptomnesia. In *Collected Works*, **1**, 95–106. London: Routledge & Kegan Paul,

Kandinsky, V. (1885) *Kritische und klinische Betrachtungen im Gebiete der Sinnestäuschungen*. Berlin: Friedlaender

Kelly, D., Guirguis, W., Frommer, E., Mitchell-Heggs, N. & Sargant, W. (1970) Treatment of phobic states with antidepressants. A retrospective study of 246 patients. *Brit. J. Psychiat.*, **116**, 387–98

Kendell, R. E. (1975) The concept of disease and its implications for psychiatry. *Brit. J. Psychiat.*, **127**, 305–15

Kenyon, F. E.: Hypochondriacal states. *Brit. J. Psychiat.*, 1976, **129**, 1–14

Kleine, W. (1925) Periodische Schlafsucht. *Monatsschr. Psychiat. Neurol.*, **57**, 285–320

Klüver, H. (1931) Eidetic Imagery. In *A Handbook of Child Psychology*, ed. Murchison, C. Worcester, Mass.: Clark University Press

— (1966) *Mescal and Mechanisms of Hallucinations*. Chicago: University of Chicago Press,

Kral, V. A. (1952) Psychiatric observations under severe chronic stress. *Amer. J. Psychiat.*, **108**, 185–92

— (1962) Senescent forgetfulness: benign and malignant. *Can. Med. Assoc. J.*, **86**, 257–60

Leff, J. P. (1968) Perceptual phenomena and personality in sensory deprivation. *Brit. J. Psychiat.*, **114**, 1499–1508

Levin, M. (1936) Periodic somnolence and morbid hunger: a new syndrome. *Brain*, **59**, 494–504

Lewis, A. (1934) Melancholia: a clinical survey of depressive states. *J. ment. Sci.*, **80**, 277–378. (Reprinted in Sir Aubrey Lewis: *Inquiries in Psychiatry. Clinical and Social Investigations*, pp. 30–117. London: Routledge & Kegan Paul, 1967)

— (1957) Obsessional illness. *Acta. neuropsiquiat. argent.*, **3**, 323–35. (Reprinted as above, pp. 157–72)

Lewis, H. E., Harries, J. M., Lewis, D. H. & de Monchaux, C. (1964) Voluntary solitude. Studies of men in a single-handed transatlantic sailing race. *Lancet*, **1**, 1431–5

Lhermitte, J. (1951) Visual hallucinations of the self. *Brit. med. J.*, **1**, 431–4

Lishman, W. A. (1978) *Organic Psychiatry. The Psychological Consequences of Cerebral Disorder*. Oxford: Blackwell

Lorenz, K. Z. (1935) Der Kumpan in der Umwelt des Vogels. *J. Ornith.*, **83**, 137–213, 289–413

— (1958) The evolution of behavior. *Sci. Amer.*, **199**, 67–78

Lukianowicz, N. (1958) Autoscopic phenomena. *Arch. Neurol. Psychiat.*, **80**, 199–220

— (1967) 'Body image' disturbances in psychiatric disorders. *Brit. J. Psychiat.*, **113**, 31–47

Luria, A. R. (1960) Memory and the structure of mental processes. (A psychological study of the case of an exceptional memory). *Problems of Psychology* (Pergamon), **1**, 81–93. (Transl. Elliott, G. K. from the Russian original in *Vopr. Psikhol.*, 1960, **1**, 145–55)

— (1969) *The Mind of a Mnemonist*. London: Jonathan Cape

McFarland, R. A. & Moore, R. D. (1957) Human factors in highway safety: a review and evaluation. *New Engl. J. Med.*, 1957, **256**, 792–799

McGaugh, J. L. (1966) Time-dependent processes in memory storage. *Science*, **153**, 1351–8

McGhie, A. & Russell, S. M. (1962) The subjective assessment of normal sleep patterns. *J. ment. Sci.*, **108**, 642–54

Maher, B. (1972) The language of schizophrenia: a review and interpretation. *Brit. J. Psychiat.*, **120**, 3–17

Marks, I. M. (1969) *Fears and Phobias*. London: Heinemann, (1970) The classification of phobic disorders. *Brit. J. Psychiat.*, **116**, 377–86

Marks, I. M. & Gelder, M. G. (1966) Different onset ages in varieties of phobia. *Amer. J. Psychiat.*, **123**, 218–21

Mayer-Gross, W. (1935) Depersonalization. *Brit. J. med. Psychol.*, **15**, 103–22

Mental Health Act, 1959. London: HMSO

Milner, B. (1966) Amnesia Following Operation on the Temporal Lobes. In *Amnesia*, ed. Whitty, C. W. M. & Zangwill, O. L. chap. 5. London: Butterworths

Moersch, F. P. & Woltman, H. W. (1956) Progressive fluctuating muscular rigidity and spasm (stiff-man syndrome). *Proc. Staff Meet. Mayo Clin.*, **31**, 421–7

Money, J., Hampson, J. G. & Hampson, J. L. (1955) Hermaphroditism: recommendations concerning assignment of sex, change of sex, and psychological management. *Johns Hopkins Hosp. Bull.*, **97**, 284–300

— (1955) An examination of some basic sexual concepts: the evidence of human hermaphroditism. *Johns Hopkins Hosp. Bull.*, **97**, 301–19

— (1956) Sexual incongruities and psychopathology: the evidence of human hermaphroditism. *Johns Hopkins Hosp. Bull.*, **98**, 43–57

Moody, R. L. (1946) Bodily changes during abreaction. Lancet, **ii**, 934–935

Moran, E. (1970a) Varieties of pathological gambling. *Brit. J. Psychiat.*, **116**, 593–8

— (1970b) Pathological gambling. *Brit. J. hosp. Med.*, **4**, 59–70. (Revised repub. in *Contemporary Psychiatry*, ed. Silverstone, T. & Barraclough, B., pp. 416–28. Asford, Kent: Headley, 1975)

O'Connor, N. & Tizard, J. (1956) *The Social Problem of Mental Deficiency*. London: Oxford University Press

Opie, I. & Opie, P. (1959) *Lore and Language of School Children*. Oxford University Press

Oster, G. (1970) Phosphenes. *Sci. Amer.*, **222**, 83–7

Oxbury, J. M., Oxbury, S. M. & Humphrey, N. K. (1969) Varieties of colour anomia. *Brain*, **92**, 847–60

Pavlov, I. P. (1927) *Conditioned Reflexes. An Investigation of the Physiological Activity of the Cerebral Cortex*. Oxford: Oxford University Press, (Repub. New York: Dover, 1960)

Penrose, L. S. (1963) *The Biology of Mental Defect*. 3rd ed. London: Sidgwick & Jackson

— (1970) Measurement in mental deficiency. *Brit. J. Psychiat.*, **116**, 369–75

Peterson, L. R. (1966) Short-term memory. *Sci. Amer.*, **215**, 90–95

Pick, A. (1903) On reduplicative paramnesia. *Brain*, **26**, 260–67

Pierloot, R. A. & Houben, M. E. (1978) Estimation of body dimensions in anorexia nervosa. *Psychol. Med.*, **8**, 317–24

Post, F. (1962) The Significance of Affective Symptoms in Old Age. Maudsley Monograph No. 10. London: Oxford University Press

— (1965) *The Clinical Psychiatry of Late Life*. London: Pergamon

Rancurello, A. C. (1968) *A Study of Franz Brentano. His Psychological Standpoint and His Significance in the History of Psychology*. New York and London: Academic Press

Randell, J. B. (1959) Transvestitism and trans-sexualism. *Brit. med. J.*, **2**, 1448–52

Rechtschaffen, A., Goodenough, D. R. & Shapiro, A. (1962) Patterns of sleep talking. *Arch. gen. Psychiat.*, **7**, 418–26

Rechtschaffen, A., Wolpert, E. A., Dement, W. C., Mitchell, S. A. & Fisher, C. (1963) Nocturnal sleep of narcoleptics. *Electroenceph. clin. Neurophysiol.*, **15**, 599–609

Reding, G. R., Zepelin, H., Robinson, J. E., Zimmerman, S. O. & Smith, V. H. (1968) Nocturnal teeth-grinding: all-night psychophysiologic studies. *J. dent. Res.*, **47**, 786–97

Rees, J. R. (1947) (Ed.) *The Case of Rudolf Hess*. London: Heinemann

Révész, G. (1953) *Introduction to the Psychology of Music*. (Transl. de Courcy, G. I. C) London: Longmans, Green

Richards, W. (1971) The fortification illusions of migraines. *Sci. Amer.*, **224**, 89–95

Ritter, C. (1900) *A Woman in the Polar Night*. New York: Century

Roth, B., Nevsimalova, S. & Rechtschaffen, A. (1972) Hypersomnia with sleep drunkenness. *Arch. gen. Psychiat.*, **26**, 456–62

Rothstein, H. J. (1941) *A Study of Aments with Special Abilities*. M.A. Thesis, Columbia University

Rutter, M. (1966) *Children of Sick Parents: An Environmental and Psychiatric Study*. Maudsley Monograph No. 16. London: Oxford University Press

— (1976) Infantile Autism and Other Child Psychoses. In *Child Psychiatry. Modern Approaches*, ed. Rutter, M. & Hersov, L., chap. 30 Oxford: Blackwell

Rutter, M. & Yule, W. (1976) Reading Difficulties. In *Child Psychiatry. Modern Approaches*, ed. Rutter, M. & Hersov, L., chap. 23. Oxford: Blackwell

Sainsbury, P. (1968) Suicide and Depression. In *Recent Developments in Affective Disorders*, ed. Coppen, A. & Walk, A. chap. 1. *Brit. J. Psychiat. Spec. Publ.*, No. 2

Sargant, W. (1957) *Battle for the Mind. A Physiology of Conversion and Brainwashing*. London: Heinemann

— (1969) Physical Treatments of Anxiety. In *Studies of Anxiety*, ed. Lader, M. H., chap. 1. *Brit. J. Psychiat. Spec. Publ.*, No. 3,

Satoh, T. & Harada, Y. (1971) Tooth-grinding during sleep as an arousal reaction. *Experientia*, **27**, 785–6

Scadding, J. G. (1967) Diagnosis: The clinician and the computer. *Lancet*, **ii**, 877–82

Schapira, K., Kerr, T. A. & Roth, M. (1970) Phobias and affective illness. *Brit. J. Psychiat.*, **117**, 25–32

Scheerer, M., Rothmann, E. & Goldstein, K. (1945) A case of 'idiot savant': an experimental study of personality organization. *Psychol. Monog.*, **58**, No. 4

Schilder, P. (1935) *The Image and Appearance of the Human Body*. Psyche Monog. No. 4. London: Kegan Paul, Trench, Trubner

Scott, P. D. (1960) The treatment of psychopaths. *Brit. med. J.*, **1**, 1641–6

— (1965) The Ganser syndrome. *Brit. J. Crim.*, **5**, 127–34

Sedman, G. (1966) A comparative study of pseudohallucinations, imagery and true hallucinations. *Brit. J. Psychiat.*, **112**, 9–17

Shaffer, D. (1974) Suicide in childhood and early adolescence. *J. child Psychol. Psychiat.*, **15**, 275–92

Shepherd, M., Lader, M. & Rodnight, R. (1968) *Clinical Psychopharmacology*. London: English Universities Press

Siegel, R. K. (1977) Hallucinations. *Sci. Amer.*, **237**, 132–40

Silverman, G. (1972) Psycholinguistics of schizophrenic language. *Psychol. Med.*, **2**, 254–9

— (1973) Redundancy, repetition and pausing in schizophrenic speech. *Brit. J. Psychiat.*, **122**, 407–13

Simpson, L. & McKellar, P. (1955) Types of synaesthesia. *J. ment. Sci.*, **101**, 141–7

Skinner, B. F. (1938) *The Behavior of Organisms*. New York: Appleton-Century-Crofts

— (1953) *Science and Human Behavior*. New York: Macmillan

Slade, P. D. & Russell, G. F. M. (1973) Awareness of body dimensions in anorexia nervosa: cross-sectional and longitudinal studies. *Psychol. Med.*, **3**, 188–9

Snaith, R. P. (1968) A clinical investigation of phobias. *Brit. J. Psychiat.*, **114**, 673–97

Sours, J. A., Frumkin, P. & Indermill, R. R. (1963) Somnambulism: its clinical significance and dynamic meaning in late adolescence and adulthood. *Arch. gen. Psychiat.*, **9**, 400–413

Steiner, F. (1956) *Taboo*. London: Cohen & West

Stengel, E. (1941) On the aetiology of the fugue states. *J. ment. Sci.*, **87**, 572–99

— (1943) Further studies on pathological wandering. (Fugues with the impulse to wander.) *J. ment. Sci.*, **89**, 224–41

— (1947) A clinical and psychological study of echo-reactions. *J. ment. Sci.*, **93**, 598–612

— (1948) The syndrome of visual alexia with colour agnosia. *J. ment. Sci.*, **94**, 46–58

Stern, W. (1939) The psychology of testimony. *J. abn. soc. Psychol.*, **34**, 3–20

Svendsen, M. (1934) Children's imaginary companions. *Arch. Neurol. Psychiat.*, **32**, 985–99

Talland, G. A. (1965) *Deranged Memory. A Psychonomic Study of the Amnesic Syndrome*. New York and London: Academic Press

Taylor, F. Kräupl (1956) Collective emotions and mental epidemics. *New Scient.*, No. 4, 40–42

— (1965) Cryptomnesia and plagiarism. *Brit. J. Psychiat.*, **111**, 1111–18

— (1971) A logical analysis of the medico-psychological concept of disease. *Psychol. Med.*, **1**, 356–64

— (1976) The medical model of the disease concept. *Brit. J. Psychiat.*, **128**, 588–94

— (1978) Phobic partner-specific impotence in women. *Acta psychiat. scand.*, **58**, 80–87

— (1979a) *The Concepts of Illness, Disease and Morbus*. Cambridge: Cambridge University Press

— (1979b) *Psychopathology. Its Causes and Symptoms*. (Revised Edition). London: Quartermaine House; Baltimore: Johns Hopkins University Press

Thipgen, C. H. & Cleckley, H. (1957) *The Three Faces of Eve*. New York: McGraw-Hill

Tramer, M. (1934) Elektiver Mutismus bei Kindern. *Z. Kinderpsychiat.*, **1**, 30–35

Tune, G. S. (1968) Sleep and wakefulness in normal human adults. *Brit. med. J.*, **2**, 269–71

Walker, L. (1959) The prognosis for affective illness with overt anxiety. *J. Neurol. Neurosurg. Psychiat.*, **22**, 338–41

Wallace, R. K. & Benson, H. (1972) The physiology of meditation. *Sci. Amer.*, **226**, 85–90

Weinstein, E. A., Kahn, R. L., Malitz, S. & Rozanski, J. (1954) Delusional reduplication of parts of the body. *Brain*, **77**, 45–60

Weiskrantz, L. (1966) Experimental Studies of Amnesia. In *Amnesia*, ed. Whitty, C. W. M. & Zangwill, O. L. London: Butterworths

West, D. J. (1977) *Homosexuality Re-examined*. London: Duckworth

Whitlock, F. A. (1967) The Ganser syndrome. *Brit. J. Psychiat.*, **113**, 19–29

Whitlock, F. A. & Hynes, J. V. (1978) Religious stigmatization: an historical and psychophysiological enquiry. *Psychol. Med.*, **8**, 185–202

Wing, J. K., Cooper, J. E. & Sartorius, N. (1974) *The Measurement and Classification of Psychiatric Symptoms*. Cambridge: Cambridge University Press

Yap, P.-M. (1951) Mental diseases peculiar to certain cultures: a survey of comparative psychiatry. *J. ment. Sci.*, **97**, 313–27

— (1952) The latah reaction: its pathodynamics and nosological position. *J. ment. Sci.*, **98**, 515–64

Zangwill, O. L. (1941) On a peculiarity of recognition in three cases of Korsakow's psychosis. *Brit. J. Psychol.*, **31**, 230–48

— (1967) The Grünthal-Störring case of amnesic syndrome. *Brit. J. Psychiat.*, **113**, 113–28

Chapter 4.1 and 4.2

Abeles, M. & Schilder, P. (1935) Psychogenic loss of personal identity. *Arch. Neurol. Psychiat., Chicago*, **34**, 587–604

Abercrombie, J. (1867) *Inquiries concerning the Intellectual Powers and Investigation of Truth*. 7th ed. Edinburgh: Waugh & Innes

Albert, M. S., Butters, N. & Levin, J. (1979) Temporal gradients in the retrograde amnesia of patients with alcoholic Korsakoff's disease. *Arch. Neurol.*, **36**, 211–16

Allison, R. S. (1962) *The Senile Brain: A Clinical Study*. London: Arnold

Banister, H. & Zangwill, O. L. (1941a) Experimentally induced visual paramnesias. *Brit. J. Psychol.*, **32**, 30–51

— (1941b) Experimentally induced olfactory paramnesias. *Brit. J. Psychol.*, **32**, 155–75

Benson, D. F., Gardner, H. & Meadows, J. C. (1976) Reduplicative paramnesia. *Neurol., Minneapolis*, **26**, 147–51

Benson, D. F. & Geschwind, N. (1967) Shrinking retrograde amnesia. *J. Neurol. Neurosurg. Psychiat.*, **30**, 539–44

Berlyne, N. (1972) Confabulation. *Brit. J. Psychiat.*, **120**, 31–9

Bleuler, E. (1924) *Textbook of Psychiatry*. Transl. Brill, A. A. New York: Macmillan

Bonhöffer, K. (1901) *Die akuten Geisteskrankheiten der Gewohnheitstrinker*, Jena: Fisher

Brierley, J. B. (1961) Clinico-psychological correlations in amnesia. *Geront. Clin.*, **3**, 97

— (1965) The influence of brain swelling, age and hypotension upon the pattern of cerebral damage in hypoxia. *Proc. 5th Int. Congr. Neuropathol.*, Zürich

— (1977) Neuropathology of amnesic states. In *Amnesia: Clinical, Psychological and Medico-legal Aspects*, ed. Whitty, C. W. M. & Zangwill, O. L., 2nd ed., pp. 199–243. London: Butterworths

Brodie, Sir Benjamin (1856) *Psychological Inquiries*, 3rd ed. London: Longman, Brown, Green, Longman

Brodmann, K. (1902; 1904) Experimenteller und klinischer Beitrag zur Psychopathologie der polyneuritischen Psychose. *J. Psychol. Neurol.*, **1**, 225–47 (1902); **3**, 1–48 (1904)

Brody, M. B. (1944) Prolonged memory defects following E.C.T. *J. ment. Sci.*, **90**, 777–9

Busse, E. W. (1962) Findings from the Duke Geriatric Research Project: the effects of aging on the nervous system. In *Medical and Clinical Aspects of Ageing*, ed. Blumenthal, H. T., pp. 115–23. New York: Columbia University Press

Butters, L. & Albert, M. S. (1982) Processes underlying failures to recall remote events. In *Human Memory and Amnesia*, ed. Cermak, L. S. Hillside, New Jersey: Erlbaum (in press)

Chapman, L. F., Thetford, W. N., Berlin, L., Guthrie, T. C. & Wolff, H. G. (1958) Highest integrative functions in man during stress. *Ass. Res. nerv. ment. Dis.*, **36**, 491–534

Charcot, J. M. (1892) Sur un cas d'amnésie rétro-antérograde problablement d'origine hystérique. (Cited by P. Janet, 1911,

L'Etat Mental des Hystériques, 2nd ed., pp. 78–90. Paris: Alcan)

Claparède, E. (1911) Récognition et moiïté. *Arch. Psychol.,* (Genève), **11,** 79–90

Cole, M. & Zangwill, O. L. (1963) *Déjà Vu* in temporal lobe epilepsy. *J. Neurol. Neurosurg. Psychiat.,* **26,** 37–8

Conrad, K. (1953) Uber einen Fall von 'Minuten-Gedächtnis'. Beitrag zum Problem des amnestischen Symptomenkomplexes. *Arch. Psychiat. u. Z. Neurol.,* **190,** 471–502

Coriab, I. H. (1904) Reduplicative paramnesia. *J. nerv. ment. Dis.* **31,** 577–87; 639–58

Corsellis, J. A. N. (1970) The limbic areas in Alzheimer's disease and in other conditions associated with dementia. In *Alzheimer's Disease and Related Conditions,* Ciba Foundation Symposium, ed. Wolstenholme, G. E. W. & O'Connor, M. London: Churchill

Cronholm, B. & Blomquist, C. (1959) Memory disturbances after E.C.T. *Acta psychiat. neurol. scand.,* **34,** 18–25

Cronholm, B. & Molander, L. (1957) Memory disturbances after E.C.T. *Acta. psychiat. neurol. scand.,* **32,** 280–306

Davidson, G. M. (1948) Psychosomatic aspects of the Korsakoff syndrome. *Psychiat. Q.,* **22,** 1–17

Delay, J. & Brion, S. (1954) Syndrome de Korsakoff et corps mamillaires. *L'Encéphale,* **43,** 193

D'Elia, G. (1970) Unilateral electro-convulsive therapy. *Acta psychiat. scand.,* **46,** Supp. 215

— (1976) Memory changes after electroconvulsive therapy with different electrode positions. *Cortex,* **12,** 280–89

Dornbush, R. L., Abrams, E. & Fink, M. (1971) Memory changes after unilateral and bilateral E.C.T. *Brit. J. Psychiat.,* **119,** 75–8

Drachman, D. A. & Arbit, J. (1966) Memory and the hippocampal complex. *Arch. Neurol.,* **15,** 52–61

Ebbinghaus, H. (1885) *Uber das Gedächtnis.* Leipzig: Duncker

Ewald, G. (1940) Zur Frage der Lokalisation des amnestischen Symptomenkomplexes. *Allg. Z. Psychiat.,* **115,** 220–37

Flament, S. (1957) La fabulation dans le syndrome de Korsakov d'étiologie traumatique. *Arch. neurol. psychiat. belgica,* **57,** 119–61

Gaffan, D. (1972) Loss of recognition memory with lesions of the fornix. *Neuropsychologia,* **10,** 327–41

— (1974) Recognition impaired and association intact in the memory of monkeys after transection of the fornix. *J. comp. physiol. Psychol.,* **86,** 1100–9

Gellerstedt, N. (1933) Zur Kenntnis der Hirnveränderungen bei der normalen Altersinvolution. *Läk. För. Forh,* **38,** 193 (Cited by Brierley, 1977)

Geschwind, N. (1965) Disconnexion syndromes in animals and man. *Brain,* **88,** 237–94; 585–652

Gregor, A. (1909) Beiträge zur Psychopathologie des Gedächtnisses. *Monatschr. Psychiat. Neurol.,* **25,** 218–55; 330–86

Gregor, A. & Römer, H. (1906) Zur Kenntnis der Auffassung einfacher optischer Sinneseindrücke bei alkoholischen Geistesstörungen, insbesondre bei der Korsakoffschen Psychose. *Neurol. Centralbl.,* **25,** 339–51

Grünthal, E. (1923) Zur Kenntnis der Psychopathologie der Korsakowschen Symptomenkomplexes. *Monatschr. Psychiat. Neurol.,* **53,** 85–132

Grünthal, E. & Störring, G. E. (1930a) Uber das Verhalten bei umschriebener völliger Merkunfähigkeit. *Monatschr. Psychiat. Neurol.,* **74,** 354–69

(1930b) Ergänzende Beobachtungen zu den beschriebenen

Fall mit reiner Merkunfähigkeit. *Monatschr. Psychiat. Neurol.,* **72,** 374–82

— (1950) Volliger isolierter Verlust der Merkfähigkeit: Organische Schädigung oder hysterischer Verdrängung? *Nervenarzt,* **21,** 522–4

— (1956) Abschliessende Stellungsnahme zu den vorstehenden Arbeit von H. Völkel und R. Stolze über den Fall B. *Monatschr. Neurol. Psychiat.,* **132,** 309–11

Halliday, A. M., Davison, K., Browne, M. N. & Kreeger, L. C. (1968) A comparison of the effects on depression and memory of bilateral ECT and unilateral ECT to the dominant and non-dominant hemispheres. *Brit. J. Psychiat.,* **114,** 997–1012

Head, H. (1926) *Aphasia and Kindred Disorders of Speech,* vol. 2, p. 494. London: Cambridge University Press

Hering, E. (1870) *Uber das Gedächtnis als eine allgemeine Funktion der organisierte Materie.* Vienna: Gerold

Hetherington, R. (1956) The effects of ECT on efficiency and retentivity. *Brit. J. med. Psychol.,* **29,** 258–69

Horel, J. A. (1978) The neuroanatomy of amnesia: a critique of the hippocampal memory hypothesis. *Brain,* **101,** 403–45

Huppert, F. A. (1980) Personal Communication.

Huppert, F. A. & Piercy, M. (1976) Recognition memory in amnesic patients: effects of temporal context and familiarity of material. *Cortex,* **12,** 3–20

— (1978) The role of trace strength in recency judgments by amnesic and control subjects. *Q. J. exp. Psychol.,* **30,** 347–54

— (1979) Normal and abnormal forgetting in organic amnesia. Effect of locus of lesion. *Cortex,* **15,** 383–90

Inglis, J. A. (1970) Shock, surgery and cerebral asymmetry. *Brit. J. Psychiat.,* **117,** 143–8

Jackson, J. Hughlings (with Purves Stewart, J.) (1931) On a particular variety of epilepsy ('intellectual aura'). One case with symptoms of organic brain disease (1879). In *Selected Writings of John Hughlings Jackson,* ed. Taylor, J., vol. 1, 385–405. London: Hodder & Stoughton

Jackson, J. Hughlings (1931) Remarks on evolution and dissolution of the nervous system (1887). In *Selected Writings of John Hughlings Jackson,* ed. Taylor, J., vol. 2, pp. 92–118. London: Hodder & Stoughton

Janet, P. (1911) *L'Etat mental des hystériques,* 2nd ed., pp. 78–90. Paris: Alcan

— (1928) *L'Evolution de la mémoire et de la notion du temps,* pp. 372–8. Paris: Chahine

Kanzer, M. (1939) Amnesia. *Amer. J. Psychiat.,* **96,** 711–18

Katzaroff, D. (1911) Contribution a l'étude de la récognition. *Arch. Psychol. (Génève),* **11,** 1–78

Konorski, J. (1959) A new method of physiological investigation of recent memory in animals. *Bull. Acad. Pol. Sci. (Biol.),* **7,** 115–17

Korsakoff, S. S. (1889) Etude médico-psychologique sur une forme des maladies de la mémoire. *Rev. Phil.,* **28,** 501–30

— (1890) Uber eine besondere Form psychischer Störung combinirt mit multipler Neuritis. *Arch. Psychiat.,* **21,** 669–704

Kraepelin, E. (1886;1887) Uber Erinnerungsfälschungen. *Arch. Psychiat.,* **17,** 830–43 (1886); **18,** 199–239; 395–436 (1887)

— (1890) Uber die Merkfähigkeit. *Monatschr. Psychiat. Neurol.,* **8,** 245–50

Krauss, R. (1904) Uber Auffassungs-und Merk-Versuche bei einem Falle von polyneuritische Psychose. *Psychol. Arbeiten,* **4,** 513–37

Lashley, K. S. (1929) *Brain Mechanisms and Intelligence.* Chicago: University of Chicago Press

— (1950) In search of the engram. In *Physiological Mechanisms in Animal Behaviour*, ed. Danielli, J. F. & Brown, R., pp. 454–82. Cambridge: Cambridge University Press

Lewis, A. (1953) Hysterical dissociation in dementia paralytica. *Monatschr. Psychiat. Neurol.*, **125**, 589

— (1961) Discussion on amnesic syndromes: the psychopathological aspect. *Proc. R. Soc. Med.*, **54**, 955

Lhermitte, F. & Signoret, J. L. (1972) Analyse neuropsychologique et différenciation des syndromes amnésiques. *Rev. Neurol.*, **126**, 161–78

Liepmann, H. (1910) Beitrag zur Kenntnis des amnestischen Symptomenkomplexes. *Neurol. Zbl.*, **29**, 1147–61

Lishman, W. A. (1978) *Organic Psychiatry: The Psychological Consequences of Cerebral Disease*. Oxford: Blackwell

Lishman, W. A., Ron, M. & Acker, W. (1980) Computed tomography of the brain and psychometric assessment of alcoholic patients – a British study. In *Addiction and Brain Damage*, ed Richter, D., pp. 215–27. London: Croom Helm

Mabille, H. & Pitres, A. (1913) Sur un cas d'amnésie de fixation post-apoplectique ayant persisté pendant 23 ans. mort-autopsie-réflexions. *Rev. méd.*, **33**, 257

MacCurdy, J. T. (1928) *Common Principles in Psychology and Physiology*, pp. 112–30. Cambridge: Cambridge University Press

Mair, W. G. P., Warrington, E. K. & Weiskrantz, L. (1979) Memory disorder in Korsakoff's psychosis: a neuropathological and neuropsychological investigation of two cases. *Brain*, **102**, 749–83

Marslen-Wilson, W. D. & Teuber, H. L. (1975) Memory for remote events in anterograde amnesia: recognition of public figures from news photographs. *Neuropsychologia*, **13**, 353–64

Mayer-Gross, W. (1943) Retrograde amnesia: some experiments. *Lancet*, **ii**, 603–5

Meggendorfer, F. (1928) Intoxikationspsychosen. In *Handbuch der Geisteskrankheiten*, ed. Bumke, O., vol. 7, pp. 272–85. Berlin: Springer

Meyer, V. & Yates, A. J. (1955) Intellectual changes following temporal lobectomy for psychomotor epilepsy: preliminary communication. *J. Neurol. Neurosurg. Psychiat.*, **18**, 44–52

Miller, E. (1971) On the nature of the memory disorder in presenile dementia. *Neuropsychologia*, **9**, 75–81

— (1972) Efficiency of coding and the short-term memory defect in presenile dementia. *Neuropsychologia*, **10**, 133–6

— (1973) Short- and long-term memory in patients with presenile dementia. *Psychol. Med.*, **3**, 221–4

Milner, B. (1968a) Disorders of memory after brain lesions in man: material specific and generalized memory loss. *Neuropsychologia*, **6**, 175–9

— (1968b) Visual recognition and recall after right temporal-lobe excisions in man. *Neuropsychologia*, **6**, 191–209

— (1972) Disorders of learning and memory after temporal lobe lesions in man. *Clin. Neurosurg.*, **19**, 421–46

Milner, B., Corkin, S. & Teuber, H-L. (1968) Further analysis of the hippocampal syndrome: 14-year follow-up study of H.M. *Neuropsychologia*, **6**, 215–34

Mullan, S. & Penfield, W. (1959) Illusions of comparative interpretation and emotion. *A.M.A. Arch. Neurol. Psychiat.*, **81**, 269–84

Newcombe, F., Oldfield, R. C. & Wingfield, A. (1965) Object naming by dysphasic patients. *Nature, Lond.*, **207**, 1217–18

Oldfield, R. C. (1966) Things, words and the brain. *Q.J. exp. Psychol.*, **18**, 340–53

Ottoson, J. O. (1970) Age and memory impairment after ECT. *Acta psychiat. scand.*, Supp. 219

Parfitt, D. N. & Gall, C. M. (1944) Psychogenic amnesia: the refusal to remember. *J. ment. Sci.*, **90**, 511–15

Paterson, A. & Zangwill, O. L. (1944) Recovery of spatial orientation in the post-traumatic and confusional state. *Brain*, **67**, 54–68

Pick, A. (1903) On reduplicative paramnesia. *Brain*, **26**, 260–67 (1903)

— (1915) Beiträge zur Pathologie des Denkverlaufes beim Korsakow. *Z. Neurol. Psychiat.* **28**, 344–83

Piercy, M. (1977) Experimental studies of the organic amnesic syndrome. In *Amnesia: Clinical, Psychological and Medico-Legal Aspects*, ed. Whitty, C. W. M. & O. L. Zangwill, pp. 1–51. London: Butterworths

Piercy, M. & Huppert, F. A. (1964) Efficient recognition of pictures in organic amnesia. *Nature, Lond.*, **240**, 564

Pratt, R. T. C. (1977) Psychogenic loss of memory. In *Amnesia: Clinical, Psychological and Medico-Legal Aspects*, ed. Whitty, C. W.M. & Zangwill, O. L., 2nd ed., pp. 224–32. London: Butterworths

Prisco, L. Cited by Milner, B. (1972) *Clin. Neurosurg.*, 19, 421–46 (see above)

Ribot, E. (1882) *Diseases of Memory: An Essay in the Positive Psychology*. London: Kegan Paul, Trench

Rieger, C. (1888–9) Beschreibung der Intelligenzstörungen in Folge eine Hirnverletzung nebst einem Entwurf zu einer allgemein anwendbaren Methode der Intelligenz-Prüfung. *Verhandl. physik. med. Gesellschaft zu Würzburg NF.* **22**, 65

Rochford, D. G. & Williams, M. (1962, 1963, 1964) Studies in the development and breakdown of the use of names. *J. Neurol. Neurosurg. Psychiat.*, **25** (1962), 222–7 and 228–33 (1962); **26**, 377–81 (1963); **27**, 407–13 (1964)

Rose, F. C. & Symonds, C. P. (1960) Persistent memory defect following encephalitis. *Brain*, **83**, 195–212

Russell, W. R. (1971) *The Traumatic Amnesias*. Oxford: Oxford University Press

Russell, W. R. & Nathan, P. U. (1946) Traumatic amnesia. *Brain*, **69**, 280–301

Russell, W. R. & Smith, A. (1961) Post-traumatic amnesia in closed head injury. *Arch. Neurol.*, **5**, 4–17

Ryan, C. & Butters, N. (1980) Learning and memory impairments in young and old alcoholics: evidence for the premature ageing hypothesis. *Clin. exp. Res.*, **4**, 288–93

Sanders, H. I. & Warrington, E. K. (1971) Memory for remote events in amnesic patients. *Brain*, **94**, 661–8

Sargant, W. & Slater, E. (1941) Amnesic syndromes in war. *Proc. R. Soc. Med.*, **34**, 757–64

Scheller, H. (1950) Volliger isolierter Verlust der Merkfähigkeit: organische CO-Schädigung oder hysterische Verdrängung. Nachuntersuchung des Falles Br. von Grünthal und Störring. *Nervenarzt*, **21**, 49–56

— (1956) Ein sekunden Gedächtnis? Kritische Beobachtungen und neue Ermittlung zum Fall Br. von Grünthal und Störring. *Nervenarzt*, **27**, 216–18

Scoville, W. B. & Milner, B. (1957) Loss of recent memory after bilateral hippocampal lesions. *J. Neurol. Neurosurg. Psychiat.*, **20**, 11–21

Seltzer, B. & Benson, D. F. (1974) The temporal pattern of retrograde amnesia in Korsakoff's disease. *Neurology, Minneapolis*, **24**, 527–30

Small, I. F. (1974) Inhalant convulsive therapy. In *Psychobiology of ECT*, ed. Fink, E. New York: Wiley

Sperry, R. W., Gazzaniga, M. S. & Bogen, J. E. (1969) Interhemispheric relationships: the neocortical syndromes: hemisphere disconnection. In *Handbook of Clinical Neurology*, ed. Vinken, P. H. & Bruyn, G. W. Amsterdam: N. Holland

Starr, A. & Phillips, L. (1970) Verbal and motor memory in the amnesic syndrome. *Neuropsychologia*, 8, 75–88

Stengel, E. (1941) The aetiology of fugue states. *J. ment. Sci.*, 87, 572–99

— (1951) Intensive electro-convulsive therapy. *J. ment. Sci.*, 97, 139–42

— (1966) Psychogenic loss of memory. In *Amnesia*, ed. Whitty, C. W. M. and Zangwill, O. L., 1st ed., pp. 181–91. London: Butterworths

Strain, J. J., Brunschwig, L., Duffy, J. P. Agle, D. P., Rosenbaum, A. L. & Bidder, T. G. (1968) Comparison of therapeutic effects and memory changes with bilateral and unilateral ECT. *Amer. J. Psychiat.*, 125, 294–304

Syz, H. (1936) Posttraumatic loss of reproductive memory and its restoration through hypnosis and analysis. *Med. Rec.*, October p. 12

— (1937) Recovery from loss of mnemic retention after head trauma. *J. gen. Psychol.*, 17, 355–87 (1937)

Talland, G. A. (1961) Confabulation in the Wernicke-Korsakoff syndrome. *J. nerv. ment. Dis.*, 132, 361–81

— (1965) *Deranged Memory*. New York and London: Academic Press

Tomlinson, B. E. (1979) The ageing brain. In *Recent Advances in Neuropathology*, ed. Smith, W. T. & Cavanagh, J. B., no. 1, pp. 129–59. London, Churchill Livingstone

van der Horst, L. (1932) Uber die Psychologie des Korsakow Syndroms. *Monatschr. Psychiat. Neurol.*, 83, 65–84

— (1956) Le sens de la temporalisation pour la mémoire et pour l'orientation. *L'Évolution psychiatrique*, 1, 189–205

Victor, M. & Yakovlev, P. I. (1955) S. S. Korsakoff's Psychic Disorder in Conjunction with Peripheral Neuritis. A translation of Korsakoff's original article with brief comments on the author and his contribution to clinical medicine. *Neurology, Minneapolis*, 5, 394–406

Victor, M., Adams, R. D. & Collins, G. H. (1971) *The Wernicke-Korsakoff Syndrome: A Clinical and Psychological Study of 245 Patients, 82 with Post-Mortem Examinations*. Oxford: Blackwell

Walton, J. N. (1953) The Korsakoff syndrome in spontaneous subarachnoid haemorrhage. *J. ment. Sci.*, 99, 521–30

Warrington, E. K. (1971) Neurological disorders of memory. *Brit. med. Bull.*, 27 (3), 243–7. London: British Council

Warrington, E. K. & Sanders, H. I. (1971) The fate of old memories. *Q. J. exp. Psychol.*, 23, 432–442

Warrington, E. K. & Silberstein, M. (1970) A questionnaire technique for investigating very long-term memory. *Q.J. exp. Psychol.*, 22, 508–12

Warrington, E. K. & Weiskrantz, L. (1968) New method of testing long-term retention with special reference to amnesic patients. *Nature*, 217, 972–4

— (1970) A study of forgetting in amnesic patients. *Neuropsychologia*, 8, 281–8

— (1973) An analysis of short-term and long-term memory defects in man. In *The Physiological Basis of Memory*, ed. Deutsch, J. A., pp. 363–92. New York and London: Academic Press

— (1979) Conditioning in amnesic patients. *Neuropsychologia*, 17, 187–94

Wechsler, D. (1917) A study of retention in Korsakoff's psychosis. *Psychiat. Bull.*, 2 (4), 403–51

Weinstein, E. A. & Kahn, R. L. (1951) Patterns of disorientation in organic brain disease. *J. Neuropathol. clin. Neurol.*, 1, 214–221

— (1955) *Denial of Illness*. Springfield: Thomas

Weiskrantz, L. & Warrington, E. K. (1970) Amnesic Syndrome: consolidation or retrieval? *Nature*, 228, 622–63

Whitty, C. W. M., Stores, G. & Lishman, W. A. (1977) Amnesia in Cerebral Disease. In *Amnesia: Clinical, Psychological and Medico-Legal Aspects*, ed. Whitty, C. W. M. & Zangwill, O. L. London: Butterworths

Whitty, C. W. M. & Zangwill, O. L. (1977) Traumatic Amnesia. In *Amnesia: Clinical Psychological and Medico-Legal Aspects*, ed. Whitty, C. W. M. & Zangwill, O. L., 2nd ed., pp. 93–103. London: Butterworths

Wigan, A. L. (1844) *The Duality of the Mind*, London

Williams, M. (1953) Investigation of amnesic defects by progressive prompting. *J. Neurol. Neurosurg. Psychiat.*, 16, 14–18

— (1977) Memory disorders associated with electro-convulsive therapy. In *Amnesia: Clinical, Psychological and Medico-Legal Aspects*, ed. Whitty, C. W. M. & Zangwill, O. L., 2nd ed. pp. 193–8. London and Boston: Butterworths

— (1979) *Brain Damage, Behaviour and the Mind*, pp. 45, 53. Chichester and New York: Wiley

Williams, H. W. & Rupp. C. (1938) Observations on Confabulation. *Amer. J. Psychiat.* 95, 395–405

Williams, M. & Zangwill, O. L. (1952) Memory defects after head injury. *J. Neurol. Neurosurg. Psychiat.*, 15, 54–8

Wilson, S. A. K. (1928) *Modern Problems in Neurology*, chap. 4. London: Arnold

Winslow, Forbes (1860). *On Obscure Diseases of the Brain and Disorders of Mind*, pp. 364–98. London: Churchill

Zangwill, O. L. (1941) On a peculiarity of recognition in three cases of Korsakoff's psychosis. *Brit. J. Psychol.*, 31, 230–48

— (1943) Clinical tests of memory impairment. *Proc. R. Soc. Med.*, 36, 566–80

— (1945) A case of paramnesia in Nathaniel Hawthorne. *Character and Personality*, 13, 246–60

— (1950) Amnesia and the generic image. *Q. J. exp. Psychol.*, 2, 7–12

— (1953) Disorientation for age. *J. ment. Sci.*, 99, 698–702

— (1960) Lashley's principle of cerebral mass action. In *Current Problems in Animal Behaviour*, ed. Thorpe, W. H. & Zangwill, O. L., pp. 59–86. Cambridge: Cambridge University Press

— (1961) Psychological studies of amnesic states. *Proc. 3rd World Congr. Psychiat.*, 3, 219–22

— (1967) The Grünthal-Störring case of amnesic syndrome. *Brit. J. Psychiat.*, 113, 113–28

— (1977) The Amnesic Syndrome. In *Amnesia: Clinical, Psychological and Medico-Legal Aspects*, ed. Whitty, C. W. M. & Zangwill, O. L., 2nd ed., pp. 104–17. London: Butterworths

Chapter 4.3

Basso, A., De Renzi, E., Faglioni, P., Scotti, G. & Spinnler, H. (1973) Neuropsychological evidence for the existence of cerebral areas critical to the performance of intelligence tasks. *Brain*, 96, 715–28

Blakemore, C. B. & Falconer, M. A. (1967) Long-term effects of anterior temporal lobectomy on certain cognitive functions. *J. Neurol., Neurosurg. Psychiat.*, 30, 364–7

Blessed, G., Tomlinson, B. E. & Roth, M. (1968) The association between qualitative measures of dementia and of senile change in the cerebral grey matter of elderly subjects. *Brit. J. Psychiat.*, **114**, 797–811

Botwinick, J. (1977) Intellectual abilities. In *Handbook of the Psychology of Aging*, ed., Birren, J. E. & Schaie, K. W., pp. 580–605. New York: Van Norstrand Reinhold

Butcher, H. J. (1968) *Human Intelligence*. London: Methuen

Cooper, J. E., Kendell, R. E., Gurland, B. J., Sharpe, L., Copeland, J. R. M. & Simon, R. (1972) *Psychiatric Diagnosis in New York and London*. Maudsley Monograph No. 20. London: Oxford University Press

Crow, T. J., Johnstone, E. C. & Owen, F. (1979) Research on schizophrenia. In *Recent Advances in Clinical Psychiatry*, No. 3, ed. Granville-Grossman, K., pp. 26–32. Edinburgh: Churchill Livingstone

Crow, T. J. & Mitchell, W. S. (1975) Subjective age in chronic schizophrenia: evidence for a sub-group of patients with defective learning capacity. *Brit. J. Psychiat.*, **126**, 360–3

Crow, T. J. & Stevens, M. (1978) Age disorientation in chronic schizophrenia: the nature of the cognitive deficit. *Brit. J. Psychiat.*, **133**, 137–42

De Renzi, E., Pieczulo, A. & Vignolo, L. A. (1968) Ideational apraxia: a quantitative study. *Neuropsychologia*, **6**, 41–52

Dixon, J. C. (1965) Cognitive structure in senile conditions with some suggestions for developing a brief screening test of mental status. *J. Gerontol.*, **20**, 41–9

Dorken, H. & Greenbloom, G. C. (1953) Psychological investigations of senile dementia. II. The Wechsler-Bellevue Adult Intelligence Scale. *Geriatrics*, **8**, 324–33

Golden, C. J., Moses, J. A., Zelazowski, R., Graber, B., Zatz, L. M., Horvath, T. B. & Berger, P. A. (1980) Cerebral ventricular size and neuropsychological impairment in young chronic schizophrenics. *Arch. gen. Psychiat.*, **37**, 619–23

Goodglass, H. & Kaplan, E. (1963) Disturbance of gesture and pantomime in aphasia. *Brain*, **86**, 703–20

Griffiths, R. M., Estes, B. W. & Zerof, S. A. (1962) Intellectual impairment in schizophrenia. *J. consult. Psychol.*, **26**, 336–9

Gustafson, L. & Hagberg, B. (1975) Dementia with onset in the presenile period: a cross sectional study. *Acta psychiat. Scand. Suppl.* No. 257

Hearnshaw, L. S. (1979) *Cyril Burt, Psychologist*. London: Hodder & Stoughton

Hécaen, H. & Albert, M. (1978) *Human Neuropsychology*. New York: Wiley

Husen, T. (1951) The influence of schooling upon IQ. *Theoria*, **17**, 61–88

Jensen, A. (1980) *Bias in Mental Testing*. New York: Free Press

Johnstone, E. C., Crow, T. J., Frith, C. D., Stevens, M., Kreel, L. & Husband, J. (1978) The dementia of dementia praecox. *Acta psychiat. scand.*, **57**, 305–24.

Lilliston, L. (1973) Schizophrenic symptomatology as a function of probability of cerebral damage. *J. abnorm. Psychol.*, **82**, 377–81

McFie, J. & Piercy, M. F. (1952) Intellectual impairment with localized cerebral lesions. *Brain*, **75**, 292–311

Mason, C. F. (1956) Pre-illness intelligence of mental hospital patients. *J. consult. Psychol.*, **20**, 297–300

Meyer, V. (1959) Cognitive changes following temporal lobectomy for temporal lobe epilepsy. *Arch. Neurol. Psychiat.*, **81**, 299–309

Miller, E. (1972) *Clinical Neuropsychology*. Harmondsworth: Penguin

— (1974) Dementia as an accelerated ageing of the nervous system: some psychological and methodological considerations. *Age and Ageing*, **3**, 197–202

— (1977) *Abnormal Ageing*. Chichester: Wiley

— (1979) The long-term consequences of head injury: a discussion of the evidence with special reference to the preparation of legal reports. *Brit. J. soc. clin. Psychol.*, **18**, 87–98

Miller, W. R. (1975) Psychological deficit in depression. *Psychol. Bull.*, **82**, 238–60

Milner, B. (1958) Psychological defects produced by temporal lobe excision. *Res. Pub. Assoc. Res. Nerv. Ment. Dis.*, **6**, 191–210

— (1964) Some effects of frontal lobectomy in man. In *The Frontal Granular Cortex and Behavior*, ed. Warren, J. M. & Akert, K., pp. 136–74. New York: McGraw-Hill

Munsinger, H. (1975) The adopted child's IQ: a critical review. *Psychol. Bull.*, **82**, 623–59

Owens, W. A. (1966) Age and mental abilities: a second adult follow-up. *J. educ. Psychol.*, **57**, 311–25

Palmore, E. & Cleveland, W. (1976) Aging, terminal decline and terminal drop. *J. Gerontol*, **31**, 76–81

Payne, R. W. (1973) Cognitive abnormalities. In *Handbook of Abnormal Psychology*, ed. Eysenck, H. J., 2nd ed., pp. 420–83. London: Pitman

Piercy, M. F. (1969) Neurological aspects of intelligence. In *Handbook of Clinical Neurology*, vol. 3, ed. Vinken, P. J. & Bruyn, H. W., pp. 296–315. Amsterdam: North Holland

Riegel, K. F. & Riegel, R. M. (1972) Development, drop, and death. *Dev. Psychol.*, **6**, 306–19

Schaie, K. W. & Strother, C. R. (1968a) The effect of time and cohort differences upon age changes in cognitive behavior. *Multivariate behav. Res.*, **3**, 259–94

— (1968b) A cross-sequential study of age changes in cognitive behavior. *Psychol. Bull.*, **70**, 671–80

Smith, A. (1966) Intellectual functions in patients with lateralized frontal tumours. *J. Neurol. Neurosurg. Psychiat.*, **29**, 52–9

Stevens, M., Crow, T. J., Bowman, M. J. & Coles, E. C. (1978) Age disorientation in schizophrenia: a constant prevalence of 25 per cent in a chronic mental hospital population? *Brit. J. Psychiat.*, **133**, 130–6

Talland, G. A. (1965) *Deranged Memory: A Psychonomic Study of the Amnesia Syndrome*. New York: Academic Press

Vernon, P. E. (1979) *Intelligence, Heredity and Environment*. San Francisco: Freeman

Walsh, K. W. (1978) *Neuropsychology: A Clinical Approach*. Edinburgh: Churchill Livingstone

Wechsler, D. (1955) *Manual for the Wechsler Adult Intelligence Scale*. New York: The Psychological Corporation

Wells, C. (1977) *Dementia*, 2nd ed. Philadelphia: Davis

Whitehead, A. (1973) The pattern of WAIS performance in elderly psychiatric patients. *Brit. J. soc. clin. Psychol.*, **12**, 435–6

Wilkie, F. & Eisdorfer, C. (1971) Intelligence and blood pressure in the aged. *Science*, **172**, 959–62

Zangwill, O. L. (1964) Intelligence in aphasia. In *Disorders of Language*, ed. de Reuck, A. V. S. & O'Connor, M., pp. 261–74. London: Churchill

— (1969) Intellectual status in aphasia. In *Handbook of Clinical Neurology*, ed. Vinken, P. J. & Bruyn, G. W., vol. 4, pp. 105–11. Amsterdam: North Holland

— (1977) The amnesic syndrome. In *Amnesia; Clinical, Psychological and Medico-Legal Aspects*, ed. Whitty, C. W. M. & Zangwill, O. L., 2nd ed., pp. 104–17. London: Butterworths

Chapter 4.4

Akert, D., Gruesen, R. A., Woolsey, C. N. & Meyer, D. R. (1961) Kluver-Bucy syndrome in monkeys with neocortical ablations of temporal lobe. *Brain, 84*, 480–98.

Amassian, V. E. (1951) Fiber groups and spinal pathways of cortically represented visceral afferents. *J. Neurophysiol., 14*, 445–60

Anisman, H. (1975) Time-dependent variations in aversively motivated behaviors: non-associative effects of cholinergic and catecholaminergic activity. *Psychol. Rev., 82*, 359–85

Antelman, S. M. & Caggiula, A. R. (1977) Norepinephrine–dopamine interactions and behavior. *Science, 195*, 646–53

Antelman, S. M., Szechtman, H., Chin, P. & Fisher, A. E. (1975) Tail-pinch-induced eating, gnawing and licking behavior in rats: dependence on the nigrostriatal dopamine system. *Brain Res., 99*, 319–37

Averill, J. R. (1969) Autonomic response patterns during sadness and mirth. *Psychophysiol., 5*, 399–414

Ax, A. F. (1953) The physiological differentiation of fear and anger in humans. *Psychosom. Med., 15*, 433–42

Azmitia, E. C. (1978) The serotonin-producing neurons of the midbrain median and dorsal raphe nuclei. In *Handbook of Psychopharmacology*, ed. Iversen, L. L., Iversen, S. D. & Snyder, S. H., vol. 9, pp. 233–314. New York: Plenum Press

Bacelli, G., Guazzi, M., Libretti, A. & Zanchetti, A. (1965) Pressoceptive and chemoceptive aortic reflexes in decorticate and in decerebrate cats. *Amer. J. Physiol., 208*, 708–14

Bagshaw, M. H. & Benzies, S. (1968) Multiple measures of the orienting reaction and their dissociation after amygdalectomy in monkeys. *Exp. Neurol., 20*, 175–87

Bagshaw, M. H., Kimble, D. P. & Pribram, K. H. (1965) The GSR of monkeys during orienting and habituation and after ablation of the amygdala, hippocampus and inferotemporal cortex. *Neuropsychologia, 3*, 111–19

Bagshaw, M. H. & Pribram, J. D. (1968) Effect of amygdalectomy on stimulus threshold of the monkey. *Exp. Neurol., 20*, 197–202

Bailey, P. & Bremer, F. (1938) A sensory cortical representation of the vagus nerve. *J. Neurophysiol., 1*, 405–12

Ball, G. G. (1972) Self-stimulation in the ventromedial hypothalamus. *Science, 178*, 72–3

Bard, P. (1928) A diencephalic mechanism for the expression of rage with specific reference to the sympathetic nervous system. *Amer. J. Physiol., 84*, 490–515

— (1929) The central representation of the sympathetic nervous system as indicated by certain physiologic observations. *Arch. Neurol. Psychiat. 22*, 230–46.

— (1939). Central nervous mechanisms for emotional behavior patterns in animals. *Res. Pub. Res. nerv. ment. Dis., 19*, 190–218.

Barrett, J. E. & Spealman, R. D. (1978) Behavior simultaneously maintained by both presentation and termination of noxious stimuli. *J. exp. Anal. Behav., 29*, 375–83

Bear, D. M. (1979) The temporal lobes: an approach to the study of organic behavioural changes. In *Handbook of Behavioral Neurobiology*, vol. 2, ed. Gazzaniga, M. S. pp. 75–95. New York: Plenum Press

Berger, B. & Thompson, R. F. (1977) Limbic system interrelations: functional differences among hippocampal–septal connections. *Science*, 197, 587–9

Berlyne, D. E. (1967) Arousal and Reinforcement. In *Nebraska Symposium on motivation*, ed. Levine, D., pp. 1–110. Lincoln: University of Nebraska Press

Bingley, T., Leksell, L., Meyerson, B. A. & Rylander, G. (1973) Stereotactic anterior capsulotomy in anxiety and obsessive-compulsive states. In *Surgical Approaches to Psychiatry*, ed. Laitinen, L. V. & Livingston, K. E., pp. 159–64. Lancaster: Medical & Technical Publishing

Brady, J. V. (1967). Emotion and sensitivity of psychoendocrine systems. In *Neurophysiology and Emotion*, ed. Glass, D. C., pp. 70–95. New York: Rockefeller University Press and Russell Sage Foundation

Brener, J. (1977) Visceral perception. In *Biofeedback and Behavior*, ed. Beatty J. & Legewie, H., pp. 235–59. New York: Plenum Press

Brown, S. & Schäfer, E. A. (1888) An investigation into the functions of the occipital and temporal lobes of the monkey's brain. *Philos. Trans. R. Soc. London (B), 179*, 303–27

Buss, A. H. (1962) Critique and notes: two anxiety factors in psychiatric patients. *J. abnorm. soc. Psychol., 65*, 426–7

Cannon, J. T., Liebeskind, J. C. & Frenk, H. (1978) Neural and neurochemical mechanisms of pain inhibition. In *The Psychology of Pain*, ed. Sternbach, R. A., pp. 27–47. New York: Raven Press

Cannon, W. B. (1927) The James–Lange theory of emotions. *Amer. J. Psychol., 39*, 115–24

— (1929) *Bodily Changes in Pain, Hunger, Fear and Rage*. 2nd ed. Boston: Brandford

— (1931) Again the James–Lange and the thalamic theories of emotion. *Psychol. Rev., 38*, 281–95

Chi, C. C. & Flynn, J. D. (1971) Neural pathways associated with hypothalamically elicited attack behavior in cats. *Science, 171*, 703–5

Ciba Foundation Symposium (1972) 8. *Physiology, Emotion and Psychosomatic Illness*, ed. Porter, R. & Knight, J. Amsterdam: Elsevier, Excerpta Medica, North Holland

— (1978) *Functions of the Septo-hippocampal System*, ed. Porter, R. & Knight, J. Amsterdam: Elsevier, Excerpta Medica, North Holland

Clark, F. C. & Smith, J. B. (1977) Schedules of food postponement. II. Maintenance of behavior by food postponement and effects of the schedule parameter. *J. exp. Analysis Behav., 28*, 253–69

Darwin, C. (1872) *The Expression of the Emotions in Man and Animals*. London: Murray

Dell, P. C. (1957) Humoral effects on the brain stem reticular formation. In *Reticular Formation of the Brain*, ed. Jasper, H. K., Procter, L. D., Knighton, R. S., Noshay, W. C. & Costello, R. T., pp. 365–408. London: Churchill

Denny-Brown, D. (1951) The frontal lobes and their functions. In *Modern Trends in Neurology*, ed. Feiling, A., pp. 13–58. London: Butterworths

Douglas, R. J. & Pribram, K. H. (1966) Learning and limbic lesions. *Neuropsychologia, 4*, 197–220

Duffy, E. A. (1934) 'Emotion': an example of the need for reorientation in psychology. *Psychol. Rev., 41*, 184–98

— (1962) *Activation and Behavior*. New York: Wiley

Egger, M. D. & Flynn, J. P. (1963) Effects of electrical stimulation of the amygdala on hypothalamically elicited attack behavior in cats. *J. Neurophysiol., 26*, 705–20

Ervin, F. R. & Mark, V. H. (1969) Behavioral and affective responses to brain stimulation in man. In *Neurobiological*

Aspects of Psychopathology, ed. Zubin, J. & Shagass, C., pp. 54–65. New York: Grune & Stratton

Fehr, F. S. & Stern, J. A. (1970) Peripheral physiological variables and emotion. The James–Lange Theory revisited. *Psychol. Bull.*, **74**, 411–24

Feldman, S. M. & Waller, H. J. (1962) Dissociation of behavioural electrocortical activation and behavioural arousal, *Nature*, **196**, 1320–22

Fenz, W. D. & Epstein, S. (1965) Manifest anxiety: unifactorial or multifactorial composition? *Percep. mot. Skills*, **20**, 773–80
— (1967) Gradients of physiological arousal in parachutists as a function of the approaching jump. *Psychosom. Med.*, **29**, 33–51

Flanigin, H. F., Nashold, B. S. Jr., Wilson, W. P. & Nebes, R. (1976) Stimulation of the temporal lobe and thalamus in man and its relation to memory and behavior. In *Brain Stimulation Reward*, ed. Wauquier, A. & Rolls, E. T. pp. 521–6. New York: North Holland American Elsevier

Flynn, J. P., Vanegas, H., Foote, W. & Edwards, S. (1970) Neural mechanisms involved in a cat's attack on a rat. In *Neural Control of Behavior*, ed. Whalen, R. E., Thompson, R. F., Verzeano, M. & Weinberger, N. M., pp. 135–73. New York: Academic Press

Freeman, W. J. (1949) Transorbital leucotomy: the deep frontal cut. *Proc. R. Soc. Med.*, **42**, Supp. 8–12

Fulton, J. F. (1949) Functional localisation in the frontal lobes and cerebellum. London: Oxford University Press

Funkenstein, D. H. (1956) Nor-epinephrine-like and epinephrine-like substances in relation to human behavior. *J. nerv. ment. Dis.*, **124**, 58–68

Gaffan, D. (1972) Loss of recognition memory in rats with lesion of the fornix. *Neuropsychologia*, **10**, 327–41
— (1974) Recognition impaired and association intact in the memory of monkeys after transection of the fornix. *J. comp. physiol. Psychol.*, **86**, 1100–1109

Gainotti, G. (1972) Emotional behavior and the hemispheric side of the lesion. *Cortex*, **8**, 41–55

Gardner, H., Ling, P. K., Flamm, L. & Silverman, J. (1975) Comprehension and appreciation of humorous material following brain damage. *Brain*, **98**, 399–412

Gellhorn, E. (1964) Motion and emotion: the role of proprioception in the physiology and pathology of the emotions. *Psychol. Rev.*, **71**, 457–72

Geschwind, N. (1965) Disconnection syndromes in animals and man. *Brain*, **88**, 237–94

Glanzer, M. & Clark, E. O. (1979) Cerebral mechanisms of information storage: the problem of memory. In *Handbook of Behavioral Neurobiology*, vol. 2, ed. Gazzaniga, M. S., p. 465–93. New York: Plenum Press

Gloor, P. (1960) Amygdala. In *Handbook of Physiology, Section I, Neurophysiology*, ed. Field, J. Vol. II ed Magoun, H. W. & Hall, V. E. pp. 1395–1420. Washington: American Physiological Society

Gray, J. A. (1972) The structure of the emotions and the limbic system. In *Physiology, Emotion and Psychosomatic Illness*. Ciba Foundation Symposium, pp. 87–120. Amsterdam: Elsevier, Excerpta Medica, North Holland

Gray, J. A., Feldon, J., Rawlins, J. N. P. Owen, S. & McNaughton, N. (1978) The role of the septo-hippocampal system and its noradrenergic afferents in behavioural responses to non-reward. In *Functions of the Septo-Hippocampal System*. Ciba Foundation Symposium, pp. 275–300. Amsterdam: Elsevier, Excerpta Medica, North Holland

Gray, J. A., Rawlins, J. N. P. & Feldon, J. (1979) Brain mechanisms in the inhibition of behavior. In *Mechanisms of Learning and Motivation*, ed. Dickinson, A. & Boakes, R. A., pp. 295–316. Hillsdale: Wiley

Gregory, R. L. (1966) *Eye and Brain*. London: Weidenfeld & Nicholson

Grossmman, S. P. (1966) The VMH: a center for affective reactions, satiety or both? *Physiol. Behav.*, **1**, 1–10
— (1978) An experimental 'dissection' of the septal syndrome. In *Functions of the septo-hippocampal system*. Ciba *Foundation symposium*, pp. 227–73. Amsterdam: Elsevier, Excerpta Medica, North Holland

Gruzelier, J. H. (1978) Bimodal states of arousal and lateralised dysfunction in schizophrenia; effects of chlorpromazine. In *The Nature of Schizophrenia*, ed. Wynne, L. C., Cromwell, R. L. & Matthysse, S., pp. 167–87. New York: Wiley

Hassler, R. E. & Dieckman, G. (1973). Relief of obsessive-compulsive disorders, phobias and tics by stereotactic coagulation of the rostral intralaminar and medial thalamic nuclei. In *Surgical Approaches to Psychiatry*, ed. Laitinen, L. V. & Livingston, K. E., pp. 206–12. Lancaster: Medical & Technical Publishing

Hebb, D. O. (1955) Drives and the C.N.S. (Conceptual Nervous System). *Psychol. Rev.*, **62**, 243–54

Hess, W. (1954) *Diencephalon*. London: Heineman

Hilgard, E. R. (1978) Hypnosis and pain. In *The Psychology of Pain*, ed. Sternbach, R. A., pp. 241–64. New York: Raven Press

Hodgson, R. & Rachman, S. (1974) II. Desynchrony in measures of fear. *Behav. Res. Ther.*, **12**, 319–26

Hohmann, G. W. (1966) Some effects of spinal cord lesions on experienced emotional feelings. *Psychophysiol.*, **3**, 143–56

Holloway, F. A. & Parsons, O. A. (1972) Physiological concomitants of reaction time performance in normal and brain-damaged subjects. *Psychophysiol.*, 9, 189–98

Hull, C. L. (1943) *Principles of Behavior*. New York: Appleton-Century-Crofts

Hunsperger, R. W. (1968) Commentary. In *Biological Foundations of Emotion*, ed Gellhorn, E., pp. 14–24. Illinois: Scott, Foresman

Ingram, W. R. (1960) Central autonomic mechanisms. In *Handbook of Physiology, Section 1 Neurophysiology*, ed Field, J. Vol. II, ed. Magoun, H. W. & Hall, V. E. , pp. 951–78. Washington: American Physiological Society

Isaacson, R. L. (1974) *The Limbic System*. New York: Plenum Press

James, W. (1884) What is an emotion? *Mind*, **9**, 188–205
— (1890) The emotions. In *Principles of Psychology*, vol. 2, Chap. 25. New York: Holt

Jones, B. & Mishkin, M. (1972) Limbic lesions and the problem of stimulus-reinforcement associations. *Exp. Neurol.*, **36**, 362–77

Jouvet, M. (1978) Neuropharmacology of the sleep-waking cycle. In *Handbook of Psychopharmacology*, ed. Iversen, L. L., Iversen, S. D. & Snyder, S. H., vol. 8, pp. 233–93. New York: Plenum Press

Kaada, B. R. (1960). Cingulate, posterior orbital, anterior insular and temporal pole cortex. In *Handbook of Physiology, Section 1, Neurophysiology*, ed. Field J. Vol. II, ed. Magoun, H. W. & Hall, V. E., pp. 1345–72. Washington: American Physiological Society

Kling, A., Lancaster, J. & Benitone, J. (1970) Amygdalectomy in the free-ranging vervet (Cercopithecus athliops). *J. psychiat. Res.*, **7**, 191–9

Kluver, H. & Bucy, P. C. (1937) 'Psychic blindness' and other symptoms following bilateral temporal lobectomy in rhesus monkeys. *Amer. J. Physiol.*, **119**, 352–3

Koob, G. F., Fray, P. J. & Iversen, S. D. (1978) Self-stimulation at the lateral hypothalamus and locus coeruleus after specific unilateral lesions of the dopaminergic system. *Brain Res.*, **146**, 123–40

Lang, P. J. (1978) Anxiety: towards a psychophysiological definition. In *Psychiatric Diagnosis*, ed. Akiskal, H. S. & Webb, W. L., pp. 365–89. New York: Spectrum

Lange, C. G. and James, W. (1922) *The Emotions*, pp. 33–90. Baltimore: Williams & Wilkins

Ledoux, J. E., Wilson, D. K. & Gazzaniga, M. S. (1979) Beyond commissurotomy; clues to consciousness. In *Handbook of Behavioral Neurobiology*, vol. 2, ed. Gazzaniga, M. S., pp. 543–54: New York: Plenum Press

Le Gros Clark, W. E. & Meyer, M. (1950) Anatomical relationships between the cerebral cortex and the hypothalamus. *Brit. med. Bull.*, **6**, 341–4

Levine, S., Weinberg, J. & Ursin, H. (1978) Definition of the coping process and statement of the problem. In *Psychobiology of Stress*, ed. Ursin, H., Baade, E. & Levine, S., pp. 3–21. London; Academic Press

Lewin, W. (1973). Selective leucotomy: a review. In *Surgical Approaches to Psychiatry*, ed. Laitinen, L. V. & Livingston, K. E., pp. 69–74. Lancaster; Medical & Technical Publishing

Lewis, P. R. & Shute, C. C. D. (1978) Cholinergic pathways in CNS. In *Handbook of Psychopharmacology*, ed. Iversen, L. L., Iversen, S. D. & Snyder, S. H., vol. 9, pp. 315–55. New York: Plenum Press

Lindsley, D. B. (1951) Emotion. In *Handbook of Experimental Psychology*, ed. Stevens, S. S. pp. 473–516. New York: Wiley

Lindvall, O. & Björklund, A. (1978) Organisation of catecholamine neurons in the rat central nervous system. In *Handbook of Psychopharmacology*, ed. Iversen, L. L., Iversen, S. D. & Snyder, S. H., vol. 9, pp. 139–231. New York: Plenum Press

Lord, B. J., King, M. & Pfister, M. D. (1976) Chemical sympathectomy and two-way escape and avoidance learning in the rat. *J. comp. physiol. Psychol.*, **90**, 303–16

Lyon, M. & Robbins, T. (1975) The action of central nervous system stimulant drugs: a general theory concerning amphetamine effects In: *Current Developments in Psychopharmacology*, vol. 2, ed. Essmann, W. B. & Valzelli, L., pp. 79–163. New York: Spectrum

McEntee, W. J. & Mair, R. W. (1978) Memory impairment in Korsakoff's psychosis: a correlation with brain noradrenergic activity. *Science*, **202**, 905–7

McEwen, B. S., Gerlach, J. L. & Micco, D. J. (1977) Putative glucocorticoid receptors in hippocampus and other regions of rat brain. In *The Hippocampus*, ed. Isaacson, R. L. & Pribram, K. H., vol. 1, pp. 285–322. New York: Plenum Press

McKilligott, J. W. V. (1959) Autonomic functions and affective states in spinal cord injury. Unpublished Ph.D. Thesis, University of California, cited in van Toller, C. (1979) *The Nervous Body*. Chichester: Wiley

MacLean, P. D. (1958) The limbic system with respect to self-preservation and the preservation of the species. *J. nerv. ment. Dis.*, **127**, 1–11

— (1975) An ongoing analysis of hippocampal inputs and outputs: microelectrode and neuroanatomical fundings in squirrel monkeys. In *The Hippocampus*, vol. 1, ed. Isaacson, R. L. & Pribram, K. H., pp. 177–211. New York: Plenum Press

Mahl, G. F., Rothenberg, A., Delgado, J. M. R. & Hamlin, H.

(1964) Psychological responses in the human to intracerebral electric stimulation, *Psychosom. Med.*, **26**, 337–68

Malmo, R. B. (1959) Activation: a neuropsychological dimension, *Psychol. Rev.*, **66**, 367–86

Mandler, G. (1975) *Mind and Emotion*. New York: Wiley

Mandler, G. & Kremen, I. (1958) Automatic feedback: a correlational study. *J. Pers.*, **26**, 388–99

Mandler, G., Mandler, J. M. & Uviller, E. T. (1958) Autonomic feedback: the perception of autonomic activity. *J. abnor. soc. Psychol.*, **56**, 367–73

Marañon, G. (1924) Contribution à l'étude de l'action émotive de l'adrénaline. *Rev. Fr. Endocrinol.* **2**, 301–25

Marlowe, W. B., Mancall, E. L. & Thomas, J. J. (1975) Complete Kluver–Bucy syndrome in man. *Cortex*, **11**, 53–9

Marshall, J. F. (1975) Increased orientation to sensory stimuli following medial hypothalamic damage in rats. *Brain Res.*, **86**, 373–87

Marshall, J. F. & Teitelbaum, P. (1977) New considerations in the neuropsychology of motivated behavior. In *Handbook of Psychopharmacology*, ed. Iversen, L. L., Iversen, S. D. & Snyder, S. H., vol. 7, pp. 201–29. New York: Plenum Press

Mason, S. T. & Iversen, S. D. (1975) Learning in the absence of forebrain noradrenaline. *Nature*, **258**, 422–4

Melzack, R. & Casey, K. L. (1970) The affective dimension of pain. In *Feelings and Emotions* ed. Arnold, M. B., pp. 55–68. New York: Academic Press

Melzack, R. & Dennis, S. G. (1978) Neurophysiological foundations of pain. In *The Psychology of Pain*, ed. Sternbach, R. A., pp. 1–26. New York: Raven Press

Meyer, G., Mcelhaney, M., Martin, W. & McGraw, C. P. (1973) Stereotactic cingulotomy with results of acute stimulation and serial psychological testing. In *Surgical Approaches to Psychiatry*, ed. Laitinen, L. V. & Livingston, K. E., pp. 39–58. Lancaster: Medical & Technical Publishing

Millenson, J. (1967) *Principles of Behavioral Analysis*. New York: Macmillan

Miller, G. A., Galanter, E. & Pribram, K. H. (1960) *Plans and the Structure of Behaviour*. London: Holt, Rinehart & Winston

Mishkin, M. & Pribram, K. H. (1954) Visual discrimination performance following partial ablations of the temporal lobe. 1. Ventral vs. lateral, *J. comp. physiol. Psychol.*, **47**, 14–20

Molina de, F. & Hunsperger, R. W. (1962) Organisation of the subcortical system governing defence and flight reactions in the cat. *J. Physiol.*, **160**, 200–13

Morse, W. H. & Kelleher, R. T. (1977) Determinants of reinforcement and punishment. In *Handbook of Operant Behavior*, ed. Honig, W. K. & Staddon, J. E. R., pp. 174–200. New Jersey: Prentice-Hall

Morse, W. H., Mead, R. N. & Kelleher, R. T. (1967) Modulation of elicited behavior by a fixed-interval schedule of electric shock presentation. *Science*, **157**, 215–17

Mowrer, O. H. (1960) *Learning Theory and Behavior*. New York: Wiley

Nádvornik, P., Pogády, J. & Sramka, M. (1973). The results of stereotaxic treatment of the aggressive syndrome. In *Surgical Approaches to Psychiatry*, ed. Laitinen, L. V. & Livingston, K. E., pp. 125–8. Lancaster: Medical & Technical Publishing

Narabayashi, H. & Shima, F. (1973) Which is the better amygdala target, the medial or lateral nuclei? In *Surgical Approaches to Psychiatry*, ed. Laitinen, L. V. & Livingston, K. E., pp. 129–37. Lancaster: Medical & Technical Publishing

Narabayashi, H., Nagao, T., Saito, Y., Yoshida, M. & Nagahuata,

M. (1963) Stereotoxic amygdalectomy for behaviour disorders. *Arch. Neurol.* **9**, 1–16

Nauta, W. J. H. (1971) The problem of the frontal lobe: a reinter-
pretation. *J. psychiat. Res.*, **8**, 167–87

— (1973) Connections of the frontal lobe with the limbic sys-
tem. In *Surgical Approaches to Psychiatry*, ed. Laitinen,
L. V. & Livingston, K. E., pp. 303–14. Lancaster: Medical &
Technical Publishing

Nauta, W. J. H. & Kuypers, H. G. J. M. (1957) Some ascending
pathways in the brain stem reticular formation. In *Reticular
Formation of the Brain*, ed. Jasper, H. H. Procter, L. D.,
Knighton, R. S., Noshay, W. C. & Costello, R. T., pp. 1–30.
London: Churchill

O'Keefe, J. & Nadel, L. (1978) *The Hippocampus as a Cognitive Map*.
Oxford: Clarendon Press

Olds, J. (1970) The behaviour of hippocampal neurons during conditioning experiments. In *Neural Control of Behavior*, ed.
Whalen, R. E., Thompson, R. F., Verzeano, M. & Weinberger, N. M., pp. 257–93. New York: Academic Press

— (1976) Reward and drive neurons: 1975. In *Brain Stimulation
Reward*, ed. Wauquier, A. & Rolls, E. T., pp. 1–27. New
York: NorthHolland American Elsevier

Olds, J. & Milner, P. (1954) Positive reinforcement produced by
electrical stimulation of septal area and other regions of rat
brain. *J. comp. physiol. Psychol.*, **47**, 419–27

Olds, J. & Olds, M. (1965). Drives rewards and the brain. In *New
Directions in Psychology*, ii, pp. 329–410, New York: Holt,
Rinehart & Winston.

Ortiz, A. (1973) The role of the limbic lobe in central pain mechanisms, an hypothesis relating to the gate control theory of
pain. In *Surgical Approaches to Psychiatry*, ed. Laitinen,
L. V. & Livingston, K. E., pp. 59–64. Lancaster: Medical &
Technical Publishing

Palkovitz, M. (1979) Central control of blood pressure. In *Catechol-
amines: Basic and Clinical Frontiers*, ed. Usdin, E., Kopin,
I. J. & Barchas, J., vol. 2, pp. 1411–15. New York: Pergamon
Press

Panksepp, J. (1971) Aggression elicited by electrical stimulation of
the hypothalamus in albino rats. *Physiol. Behav.*, **6**, 321–9

Papez, J. W. (1937) A proposed mechanism of emotion. *Arch. Neurol. Psychiat.*, **38**, 725–43

Pátkai, P. (1971) Catecholamine excretion in pleasant and unpleasant situations. *Acta psychol.*, **35**, 352–63

Penfield, W. & Jasper, H. (1954) *Epilepsy and the Functional Anatomy of the Human Brain*. London: Churchill

Penfield, W. & Rasmussen, T. (1950) *The Cerebral Cortex of Man*.
New York: Macmillan

Phillips, A. G., Carter, D. A. & Fibiger, H. C. (1976) Dopaminergic
substrates of intracranial self-stimulation in the caudate-
putamen. *Brain Res.*, **104**, 221–32

Pick, J. (1970) The *Autonomic Nervous System: Morphological, Comparative and Surgical Aspects*. New York: Lippincott

Plutchik, R. & Ax, A. F. (1962) A critique of Determinants of emotional state by Schachter and Singer (1962). *Psychophysiol.*
4, 79–82

Poeck, K. (1969) Pathophysiology of emotional disorders associated
with brain damage. In *Handbook of Clinical Neurology*, ed.
P. J. Vinken & G. W. Bruyn, vol. 3, pp. 343–67. Amsterdam: NorthHolland

Praag, H. M. van (1978) Amine hypothesis of affective disorders.
In *Handbook of Psychopharmacology*, ed. Iversen, L. L., Iver-
sen, S. D. & Snyder, S. H., vol. 13, pp. 187–297. New York:
Plenum Press

Pribram, K. H. (1971). *Languages of the brain*. New Jersey, Prentice-
Hall

Pribram, K. H. & Bagshaw, M. H. (1953) Further analysis of the
temporal lobe syndrome utilizing frontotemporal ablations
in monkeys *J. comp. physiol. Psychol.*, **99**, 347–75

Pribram, K. H. & Fulton, J. F. (1954) An experimental critique of
the effects of anterior cingulate ablations in monkeys.
Brain, **77**, 34–44

Pribram, K. H. & McGuinness, D. (1975) Arousal, activation and
effort in the control of attention. *Psychol. Rev.*, **82**, 116–49

Randrup, A., Munkvad, I., Fog, R., Gerlach, J., Molander, L.,
Kjellberg, B. & Scheel-Kruger, J. (1975) Mania, depression
and brain dopamine, In *Current Developments in Psychopharmacology*, ed. Essman, W. B. & Valzelli, L., vol. 2,
207–48, New York: Spectrum

Rapoport, J. L., Buchsbaum, M. S., Weingartner, H., Zahn, T. P.,
Ludlow, C. & Mikkelsen, E. J. (1980) Dextro-amphetamine-
Its cognitive and behavioural effects in normal and hyperactive boys and normal men. *Arch. gen. Psychiat.*, **37**, 933–
43

Reeves, A. G. & Plum, F. (1969) Hyperphagia, rage and dementia
accompanying a ventromedial hypothalamic neoplasm.
Arch. Neurol., **20**, 616–24

Roberts, W. W. (1970) Hypothalamic mechanisms for motivational
and species typical behavior. In *Neural Control of Behaviour*,
ed. Whalen, R. E., Thompson, R. F., Verzeano, M. & Weinberger, N. M., pp. 175–206. New York: Academic Press

Robbins, T. W. & Sahakian, B. J. (1980). Animal models of mania.
In *Mania, an Evolving Concept*, ed. Belmaker, R. H. &
Praag, H. van. New York: Spectrum

Rubins, J. L. & Friedman, E. D. (1948) Asymbolia for pain. *Arch.
Neurol. Psychiat.*, **60**, 554–73

Ryle, G. (1949) *The concept of mind*. New York: Hutchinson

Sacks, O. (1973) *Awakenings*. London: Duckworth

Schachter, S. (1966) The interaction of cognitive and physiological
determinants of emotional state. In *Anxiety & Behavior*, ed.
Spielberger, C. D., pp. 193–224. London: Academic Press

Schachter, S. & Singer, J. (1962) Cognitive, social and physiological
determinants of emotional states. *Psychol. Rev.*, **69**,378–99

Schildkraut, J. & Kety, S. (1967) Biogenic amines and emotion. *Science*, **156**, 21–30

Schwartz, G. E., Davidson, R. J. & Maer, F. (1975) Right hemisphere lateralisation for emotion in the human brain: interaction with cognition. *Science*, **190**, 286–8

Schwartzbaum, J. S. (1960) Changes in reinforcing properties of
stimuli following ablation of the amygdaloid complex in
monkeys. *J. comp. physiol. Psychol.*, **53**, 388–95

Seligman, M. E. P. (1975) *Helplessness*. San Francisco: Freeman

Sem-Jacobsen, C. W. (1976) Electrical stimulation and self-stimulation in man with chronic implanted electrodes. Interpretation and pitfalls of results. In *Brain Stimulation Reward*, ed.
Wauquier, A. & Rolls, E. T., pp. 505–20. New York: North-
Holland American Elsevier

Sideroff, S. & Bindra, D. (1976) Neural correlates of discriminative
conditioning: separation of associational and motivational
properties *Brain Res.*, **101**, 378–82

Sokolov, Ye. N. (1960) Neuronal models and the orienting reflex. In
The Central Nervous System and Behavior, ed. Brazier,
M. A. B., pp. 187–276. New York: Josiah Macy Jr. Founda-
tion

Sparber, S. B. & Tilson, H. A. (1972) Schedule controlled and drug
induced release of norepinephrine-7-^{3}H into the lateral ventricle of rats. *Neuropharmacol.*, **11**, 453–64

Spealman, R. D. (1979) Behavior maintained by termination of a schedule of self-administered cocaine. *Science*, **204**, 1231–3

Sperry, R. W. & Gazzaniga, M. S. (1967) Language following surgical disconnection of the hemispheres. In *Brain Mechanisms underlying Speech and Language*, ed. Darley, F. L. New York: Grune & Stratton

Sprague, J. M., Chambers, W. W. & Stellar, E. (1961) Attentive, affective and adaptive behavior in the cat. *Science*, **133**, 165–73

Squires, R. F. & Braestrup, C. (1977) Benzodiazepine receptors in rat brain. *Nature*, **266**, 732–4

Stein, L. & Wise, C. D. (1969) Release of norepinephrine from hypothalamus and amygdala by rewarding forebrain stimulation and amphetamine. *J. comp. physiol. Psychol.*, **67**, 189–98

Steiner, S. S., Beer, B. & Shaffer, M. M. (1969) Escape from self-produced rates of brain stimulation. *Science*, **163**, 90–91

Sternbach, R. A. (1978) Clinical aspects of pain. In *The Psychology of Pain*, ed. Sternbach, R. A., pp. 241–64. New York: Raven Press

Stolk, J. M., Conner, R. L., Levine, S. & Barchas, J. D. (1974) Brain norepinephrine metabolism and shock-induced fighting, behavior in rats; differential effects of shock and fighting on the neurochemical response to a common footshock stimulus. *J. Pharmacol. exper. Ther.*, **190**, 51–9

Strongman, K. T. (1978) *The Psychology of Emotion*. Chichester: Wiley

Swanson, L. W. (1978) The anatomical organisation of septo-hippocampal projections. In *Functions of the Septo-Hippocampal System*. Ciba Foundation Symposium, pp. 25–48. Amsterdam: Elsevier, Exerpta Medica, North Holland

Sweet, W. H. (1959) Pain. In *Handbook of Physiology*, Section 1 *Neurophysiology*, ed. Field, J. vol. ı, ed. Magoun, H. W. & Hall, V. E.

Taylor, J. (1958) Ed. *Selected writings of John Hughlings Jackson*, vols. *1 & 2*. London: Staples Press

Tye, N. C., Everitt, B. J. & Iversen, S. D. (1977) 5-hydroxytryptamine and punishment. *Nature*, **268**, 741–3

Tyrer, P. J. (1976) *The role of bodily feelings in anxiety*. Maudsley Monograph, No. 23. London: Oxford University Press

Ungerstedt, U. (1971) Stereotaxic mapping of the monoamine pathways in the rat brain. *Acta physiol. scand., Supp.*, 267, 1–48

Ursin, H. & Kaada, B. R. (1960) Functional localisation within the amygdaloid complex in the cat. *Electroenceph. clin. Neurophysiol.*, **23**, 41–9

Valenstein, E. (1973) *Brain Control*. New York: Wiley

Valenstein, E. S. & Valenstein, T. (1964) Interaction of positive and negative reinforcing systems. *Science*, **145**, 1456–8

Valenstein, E. S., Cox, V. C. & Kakolewski, T. W. (1970) Re-examination of the role of the hypothalamus in motivation. *Psychol. Rev.*, **77**, 16–31

Valins, S. (1970) The perception and labeling of bodily changes as determinants of emotional behavior. In *Physiological Correlates of Emotion*, ed. Black, P., pp. 229–43. New York: Academic Press

van Praag, see Praag

Vinogradova, O. S. & Brazhnik, E. S. (1978) Neuronal aspects of septo-hippocampal relations. In *Functions of the Septo-Hippocampal System*. Ciba Foundation Symposium, pp. 145–71. Amsterdam: Elsevier, Excerpta Medica, North-Holland

Wall, P. D. & Davis, G. D. (1951) Three cerebral cortical systems affecting autonomic functions, *J. Neurophysiol.*, **14**, 507–17

Wasman, M. & Flynn, J. P. (1962) Directed attack elicited from hypothalamus. *Arch. Neurol.*, **6**, 220–27

Weiskrantz, L. (1956) Behavioral changes associated with ablation of the amygdaloid complex in monkeys. *J. comp. physiol. Psychol.*, **49**, 381–91

— (1960) Effects of medial temporal lesions on taste preference in the monkey. *Nature*, **187**, 879–80

— (1977) Trying to bridge some neuropsychological gaps between monkey and man. *Brit. J. Psychol.*, **68**, 431–45

— (1978) A comparison of hippocampal pathology in man and other animals. In *Functions of the Septo-hippocampal System*. Ciba Foundation Symposium, pp. 383–7. Amsterdam: Elsevier, Excerpta Medica, North Holland

Weiss, J. M. (1972) Influence of psychological variables on stress-induced pathology. In *Ciba Foundation Symposium 8. Physiology, Emotion and Psychosomatic Illness*, ed. Porter, R. & Knight, J., pp. 253–79. Amsterdam: Elsevier, Excerpta Medica, North Holland

Weiss, J. M., Glazer, H. I., Pohorecky, L. A., Brick, J. & Miller, N. E. (1975) Effect of chronic exposure to stressors on avoidance escape behaviour and brain norepinephrine. *Psychosom. Med.*, **37**, 522–34

Williams, D. (1956) The structure of emotions reflected in epileptic experiences. *Brain*, **79**, 29–67

Winkler, H. & Smith, A. D. (1972) Phaeochromocytoma and other catecholamine producing tumours. In *Catecholamines*, ed. Blashko, H. & Maschcoll, E., pp. 900–33. Berlin: Springer

Wynne, L. C. & Solomon, R. L. (1955) Traumatic avoidance learning: acquisition and extinction in dogs deprived of normal peripheral autonomic function. *Genet. Psychol. Monogr.*, **52**, 241–84

Yakovlev, P. I. (1948) Motility, behavior and the brain: stereodynamic organization and neural co-ordination of behavior. *J. nerv. ment. Dis.*, **107**, 313–35

Zanchetti, A. (1967) Subcortical and cortical mechanisms in arousal and emotional behavior. In *The Neurosciences, a Study Program*, ed. Quarton, G. C., Melnechuk, T. & Schmitt, F. O., pp. 602–14. New York: Rockefeller University Press

Zangwill, O. L. (1977) The amnesic syndrome. In *Amnesia: Clinical, Psychological and Medico-Legal Aspects*, ed. Whitty, C. M. W. & Zangwill, O. L., 2nd ed., pp. 104–17. London: Butterworths

Zeman, W. & King, F. A. (1959) Tumors of the septum pellucidium and adjacent structures with abnormal affective behavior: an anterior midline structure syndrome. *J. nerv. ment. Dis.*, **127**, 490–502

Chapter 4.5

Alajouanine, T., Castaigne, P., Sabouraud, O. & Contamin, F. (1959) Palilalie paroxystique et vocalisations interatives au cours de crises épileptiques par lésion intéressant l'aire motrice supplémentaire. *Rev. Neurol.*, **101**, 685–97

Alajouanine, T. H. & Lhermitte, F. (1965) Acquired aphasia in children. *Brain*, **88**, 653–62

Annett, M. (1972) The distribution of manual asymmetry. *Brit. J. Psychol.*, **63**, 343–58

— (1973) Laterality of childhood hemiplegia and the growth of speech and intelligence. *Cortex*, **9**, 4–33

— (1979) Family handedness in three generations predicted by the right shift theory. *Ann. hum. Genet.*, **42**, 479–91

Basser, L. S. (1962) Hemiplegia of early onset and the faculty of speech, with special reference to the effects of hemispherectomy. *Brain*, **85**, 427–60

Benson, D. F. (1975) Disorders of verbal expression. In *Psychiatric Aspects of Neurological Disease*, ed. Benson, D. F. & Blumer, D., pp. 121–36. New York, San Francisco, London: Grune & Stratton

— (1979) *Aphasia, Alexia and Agraphia*. New York, Edinburgh, London: Churchill Livingstone

Benson, D. F. & Geschwind, N. (1971) The aphasias and related disturbances. In *Clinical Neurology*, vol. 1, ed. Barer, A. B., pp. 1–25. New York: Harper

Benson, D. F., Sheremata, W. A., Bouchard, R., Segarra, J. M., Price, D. & Geschwind, N. (1973) Conduction aphasia. *Neurol.*, **28**, 339–46

Benton, A. L. (1964) Psychological evaluation; a differential diagnosis. In *Mental Retardation*, ed. Stevens, H. A. & Heber, R., pp. 16–56. Chicago and London: University of Chicago Press

— (1978) The cognitive functioning of children with developmental dysphasia. In *Developmental Dysphasia*, ed. Wyke, M. A., pp. 43–62. London: Academic Press

Brain, R. (1961) *Speech Disorders–Aphasia, Apraxia and Agnosia*. London: Butterworths

Brown, J. W. (1972) *Aphasia, Apraxia and Agnosia: Clinical and Theoretical Aspects*. Springfield, Ill.: Thomas

— (1979) Thalamic mechanisms in language. In *Handbook of Behavioral Neurobiology*, vol. 2, Neuropsychology, ed. Gassaniga, M. S., pp. 215–36. New York & London: Plenum Press

Butler, R. B. & Benson, F. (1974) Aphasia: a clinical anatomical correlation. *Brit. J. hosp. Med.*, **12**, 211–17

Butler, S. R. & Norrsell, U. (1968) Vocalization possibly initiated by the minor hemisphere. *Nature*, **220**, 793–4

Cantwell, D. P., Baker, L. & Rutter, M. D. (1979) Families of autistic and dysphasic children. *Arch. gen. Psychiat.*, **36**, 682–6

Cappa, S. F., & Vignolo, L. A. (1979) 'Transcortical' features of aphasia following left thalamic hemorrhage. *Cortex*, **15**, 121–30

Ciemins, V. (1970) Localized thalamic hemorrhage. A cause of aphasia. *Neurol., Minneapolis*, **20**, 776–82

Collignon, R., Hécaen, H. & Angelergues, G. A. (1968) À propos de 12 cas d'aphasie acquise chez l'enfant. *Acta neurol. psychiat belg.*, **68**, 245–77

Collins, R. L. (1977) Origins of the sense of asymmetry: Mendelian and non-Mendelian models of inheritance. In *Evolution and Lateralization of the Brain*, ed. Diamond, S. J. & Blizard, D. A., pp. 283–305. New York Academy of Sciences

Coltheart, M. & Wyke, M. A. Reading defects in conduction aphasia (to be published).

Cooper, I. S., Amin, I., Chandra, R. & Waltz, J. M. (1973) A surgical investigation of clinical physiology of the pulvinar complex in man. *J. neurol. Sci.*, **18**, 89–110

Critchley, M. (1970) *True Acquired Aphasia as occurring in Childhood. Aphasiology, and other Aspects of Language*. London: Arnold

Cromer, R. (1978) The basis of childhood dysphasia; a linguistic approach. In *Developmental Dysphasia*, ed. Wyke, M. A., pp. 85–134. London: Academic Press

Darley, F. L., Brown, J. R., & Swenson, W. M. (1975) Language changes after neurosurgery for Parkinsonism. *Brain Lang.*, **2**, 65–9

Denes, G. & Semenza, C. (1975) Auditory modality-specific anomia; evidence from a case of pure word deafness. *Cortex*, **11**, 305–38

Dennis, M. & Whitaker, H. A. (1976) Language acquisition following hemidecortication: linguistic superiority of the left over the right hemisphere. *Brain Lang.*, **3**, 404–33

Diamond, S. J. & Blizard, D. A. (eds.) (1977) *Evolution and Lateralization of the Brain*. New York: New York Academy of Sciences

DiSimoni, F. G., Darley, F. L. & Aronson, A. E. (1977) Patterns of dysfunction in schizophrenic patients on an aphasic test battery. *J. speech hear. Disord.*, **42**, 498–513

Doehring, D. B. (1960) Visual spatial memory in aphasic children. *J. speech hear. Res.*, **3**, 138–49

Dubois, J., Hécaen, H., Angelergues, R., Maufras du Chatelier, A., & Marcie, P. (1964) Etude neurolinguistique de l'aphasie de conduction. *Neuropsychologia*, **2**, 9–44

Eisenson, J. (1968) Developmental aphasia: A speculative view with therapeutic implications. *J. speech hear Disord*, **33**, 3–13

Fazio, C., Sacco, G. & Bugiani, O. (1973) The thalamic hemorrhage. An anatomical study. *Europ. Neurol.*, **9**, 30–43

Fedio, P. & van Buren, J. M. (1974) Memory deficits during electrical stimulation of the speech cortex in conscious man. *Brain Lang.*, **1**, 29–42

— (1975) Memory and perceptual deficits during electrical stimulation in the left and right thalamus and parietal subcortex. *Brain Lang.*, **2**, 78–100

Furth, H. G. (1964) *Thinking without Language*. New York: Free Press

Galaburda, A. M., Le May, M., Kemper, T. L. & Geschwind, N. (1978) Right-left asymmetries in the brain. *Science*, **199**, 852–6

Gardiner, M. F. & Walter, D. O. (1977) Evidence of hemispheric specialization from infant EEG. In *Lateralization in the Nervous System*, ed. Harnard, S., Doty, R. W., Goldstein, L., Jaynes, J. & Krauthamer, G., pp. 481–500. London: Academic Press

Gascon, G., Victor, D., Lombroso, C. T., & Goodglass, H. (1973) Language disorder, convulsive disorder and electroencephalographic abnormalities. *Arch. Neurol.*, **28**, 156–62

Gazzaniga, M. S. & Hillyard, S. A. (1971) Language and speech capacity of the right hemisphere. *Neuropsychologia*, **9**, 273–80

Gazzaniga, M. S. & Sperry, R. W. (1967) Language after section of the cerebral commissures. *Brain*, **90**, 131–48

Gazzaniga, M. S., Velleri Glass, A., Sarno, M. T. & Posner, J. B. (1973) Pure word deafness and hemispheric dynamics: a case history. *Cortex*, **9**, 136–43

Gerson, S. N., Benson, D. F. & Frazier, S. H. (1977) Diagnosis: schizophrenia versus posterior aphasia. *Amer. J. Psychiat.*, **134**, 966–9

Geschwind, N. (1964) Non-aphasic disorders of speech. *Int. J. Neurol.*, **4**, 207–14

— (1965) Disconnexion syndromes in animals and man. *Brain*, **88**, 237–94

— (1972) Language and the brain. *Sci. Amer.*, **266**, 76–83

Goodglass, H., Barton, M. I. & Kaplan, E. F. (1968) Sensory modality and object-naming in aphasia. *J. speech hear. Res.*, **11**, 488–96

Goodglass, H. & Kaplan, E. (1972) *The Assessment of Aphasia and related Disorders*. Philadelphia: Lea & Febinger

Green, E. & Howes, D. (1977) Conduction aphasia. In *Studies in*

Neurolinguistics, ed. Whitaker, H. A. & Whitaker, H. vol. 3, pp. 123–56. London: Academic Press

Griffiths, P. (1972) *Developmental Aphasia: An Introduction*. London: Invalid Children's Aid Association

Guiot, G., Hertzog, E., Randot, P. & Molina, P. (1961) Arrest of acceleration of speech evoked by thalamic stimulations in the course of stereotaxis procedures for Parkinsonism *Brain*, **84**, 363–79

Guttmann, E. (1942) Aphasia in children. *Brain*, **65**, 205–19

Harnard, S., Doty, R. W., Goldstein, L., Jaynes, J. & Krauthamer, G. (1977) (Eds.) *Lateralization in the Nervous System*. London: Academic Press

Hécaen, H. (1976) Acquired aphasia in children and the ontogenesis of hemispheric functional specialization. *Brain Lang.*, **3**, 114–34

— (1979) Aphasias. In *Handbook of Behavioral Neurobiology*, vol. 2, Neuropsychology, ed. Gazzaniga, M. S., pp. 239–86. New York and London: Plenum Press

Hillier, W. F. jun. (1954) Total left cerebral hemispherectomy for malignant glioma. *Neurol, Minneapolis*, **4**, 718–21

Hiskey, M. S. (1955) *The Hiskey-Nebraska Test for Learning Aptitude* (rev.). Lincoln, Neb.: University of Nebraska

Hochberg, F. H. & Le May, M. (1975) Arteriographic correlates of handedness. *Neurol.*, **25**, 218–22

Kertesz, A. (1979) *Aphasia and Associated Disorders*. New York: Grune & Stratton

Kinsbourne, M. (1971) The minor cerebral hemisphere. *Arch. Neurol.*, **25**, 302–6

— (1972) Behavioural analysis of the repetition deficit in conduction aphasia. *Neurol.*, **22**, 1126–32

— (1975) The ontogeny of cerebral dominance. In Developmental Psycholinguistic and Communication Disorders, ed. Aaranson, D. & Rieber, R. E. *Ann. N.Y. Acad. Sci.*, **263**, 244–50

Koepp, P. & Lagenstein, I. (1978) Acquired epileptic aphasia. *J. Pediat.*, **92**, 1964–5.

Kornhuber, H. T., Brunner, R. J. & Wallesch, C. W. (1979) Basal ganglia participation in aphasia. In *Hearing Mechanism and Speech*, ed. Creutzfeld, O., Scheich, H. & Schreiner, Chr. Experimental Brain Research Supplement II, pp. 183–8. Berlin, Heidelberg: Springer

Krashen, S. (1973) Lateralization, language learning and the critical period. Some new evidence. *Language Learning*, **23**, 63–74

Landau, W. M. & Kleffner, F. R. (1957) Syndrome of acquired aphasia with convulsive disorder in children. *Neurol.*, **10**, 915–21

Lashley, K. S. (1951) The problem of serial order in behaviour. In *Cerebral Mechanisms in Behaviour*, ed. Jeffress, L. A., pp. 111–36. New York: Wiley

Le May, M. & Culebras, A. (1972) Human brain – morphologic differences in the hemispheres demonstrable by carotid arteriography. *New Eng. J. Med.*, **287**, 168–70

Lenneberg, E. H. (1967) *Biological Foundations of Language*. New York: Wiley

Levy, C. B. & Menyuk, P. (1975) Cognitive and linguistic skills of children with normal and deviant language development. Paper presented at meeting of American Speech and Hearing Assoc., Washington, D.C.

Levy, J. & Nagylaki, T. (1972) A model for the genetics of handedness. *Genetics*, **72**, 117–28

Levy, J., Nebes, R. D. & Sperry, R. W. (1971) Expressive language in the surgically separated minor hemisphere. *Cortex*, **7**, 49–58

McFie, J. (1961) Intellectual impairment in children with localized postinfantile cerebral lesions. *J. Neurol. Neurosurg. Psychiat.* **24**, 361–5

McRae, D. L., Branch, C. L. & Milner, B. (1968) The occipital horns and cerebral dominance. *Nuerol.*, **18**, 95–8

McReynolds, L. V. (1966) Operant conditioning for investigating speech sound discrimination in aphasic children. *J. speech hear. Res.*, **9**, 519–28

Milner, B., Branch, C. & Rasmussen, T. (1964) In *Ciba Foundation Symposium on Disorders of Language*, ed. de Reuck, A. V. S. & O'Connor, M. London: Churchill

Mohr, J. P., Pessin, M. S., Finkelstein, S., Funkestein, H. H., Duncan, G. W. & Davis, K. R. (1978) Broca's aphasia: pathologic and clinical. *Neurol.*, **28**, 311–24

Mohr, J. P., Watters, W. C. & Duncan, G. W. (1975) Thalamic hemorrhage and aphasia. *Brain Lang.*, **2**, 3–17

Molfese, D. L. (1977) Infant cerebral asymmetry. In *Language Development and Neurological Theory*, ed. Segalowitz S. J. & Gruber, F. A., pp. 21–35. New York, San Francisco, London: Academic Press

Monsees, E. K. (1961) Aphasia in children. *J. speech hear. Disord*, **26**, 83–6

Morgan, M. (1977) Embryology and inheritance of asymmetry. In *Lateralization in the Nervous System*, ed. Harnard, S., Doty, R. W. Goldstein, L., Jaynes, J. & Krauthamer, G., pp. 173–94. London: Academic Press

Naeser, M. A. & Hayward, R. W.. (1978) Lesion localization in aphasia with cranial computed tomography and the Boston Diagnostic Aphasia Examination. *Neurol.*, **28**, 545–51

Newcombe, F. B., Oldfield, R. C. & Wingfield, A. (1965) Object-naming by dysphasic patients. *Nature*, **207**, 1217–18

O'Connor, N. & Hermelin, B. (1971) Cognitive deficits in children. In *Cognitive Psychology*, ed. Summerfield, A., pp. 227–31. London: British Medical Bulletin

Ojemann, G. A. (ed.) (1975a) The thalamus and language. *Brain Lang.*, **2**, 1–120

— (1975b) Language and the thalamus. Object naming and recall during and after thalamic stimulation. *Brain Lang.*, **2**, 101–20

— (1975c) Subcortical language mechanisms. In *Studies in Neurolinguistics*, ed. Whitaker, H. & Whitaker, H. A. vol. 1 New York: Academic Press

Ojemann, G. A., Fedio, P. & Van Buren, J. M. (1968) Anomia from pulvinar and subcortical parietal stimulation. *Brain*, **91**, 99–116

Ojemann, G. A. & Ward, A. A. (1971) Speech representation in ventrolateral thalamus. *Brain*, **94**, 669–80

Oxbury, J. M., Oxbury, S. M. & Humphrey, N. K. (1969) Variety of colour anomia. *Brain*, **92**, 847–60

Penfield, W. & Roberts, L. (1959) *Speech and Brain Mechanisms*. Princeton, N.J.: Princeton University Press

Poppen, R., Stark, J., Eisenson, J., Forrest, T. & Wertheim, G. (1969) Visual sequencing performance of aphasic children. *J. speech hear. Res.*, **12**, 288–300

Rapin, I., Mattis, S., Rowan, A. J. & Golden, G. G. (1977) Verbal auditory agnosia in children. *Dev. Med. child Neurol.*, **19**, 192–220

Rapin, I. & Wilson, B. (1978) Children with developmental language disability: neurological aspects and assessment. In

Developmental Dysphasia, ed. Wyke, M. A., pp. 13–41. London: Academic Press

Raven, J. C. (1962) *Coloured Progressive Matrices*. London: Lewis

Reynolds, A. F., Harris, A. B., Ojemann, G. A. & Turner, P. T. (1978) Aphasia and left thalamic hemorrhage. *J. Neurosurg.*, **48**, 570–74

Riklan, M. & Cooper, I. S. (1975) Psychometric studies of verbal functions following thalamic lesions in humans. *Brain Lang.*, **2**, 45–64

Riklan, M., Levita, E., Zimmerman, J. & Cooper, I. (1969) Thalamic correlates of language and speech. *J. Neurol. Sci.*, **8**, 307–28

Rochester, S. & Martin, J. R. (1979) *Crazy Talk*. New York and London; Plenum Press

Rosenthal, W. S. & Eisenson, J. (1970) Auditory temporal order in aphasic children as a function of selected stimulus features. *Paper delivered at the 46th Annual Convention of the American Speech and Hearing Association, New York (November)*

Rubens, A. B. (1977) Anatomical asymmetries of human cerebral cortex. In *Lateralization in the Nervous System*, ed. Harnard, S., Doty, R. W., Goldstein, L., Haynes, J. & Krauthamer, G., pp. 503–16. New York, San Francisco, London: Academic Press

Rubens, A. B., Mahowald, M. & Hutton, T. (1976) Asymmetry of the lateral (Sylvian) fissure in man. *Neurol.*, **26**, 620–24

Rutter, M., (1971) (Ed.) *Infantile Autism: Concepts, Characteristics and Treatment*. Edinburgh and London: Churchill Livingstone

Shallice, T. & Warrington, E. K. (1970) Independent functioning of verbal memory stores: a neuropsychological study. *Q. J. exp. Psychol.*, **22**, 261–73

Slater, E. & Roth, M. (1972) *Clinical Psychiatry*. London: Bailliere, Tindall & Cassell

Smith, A. (1966) Speech and other functions after left (dominant) hemispherectomy. *J. Neurol., Neurosurg. Psychiat.*, **29**, 467–71

— (1972) Dominant and non-dominant hemispherectomy. In *Drugs Development and Cerebral Fucnction*, ed. Smith, W. L., pp. 37–68. Springfield: Thomas

Sperry, R. W. (1974) Lateral specialization in the surgically separated hemispheres. In *The Neurosciences Third Study Program*, ed. Schmitt, F. O. & Worden, F. G., chap. I, pp. 5–19. Cambridge, Mass: MIT Press

Sperry, R. W. & Gazzaniga, M. S. (1967) Language following surgical disconnection of the hemispheres. In *Brain Mechanisms underlying Speech and Language*, ed. Darley, F. L., p. 13. New York: Grune & Stratton

Stark, J. (1967) A comparison of the performance of aphasic children on three sequencing tests. *J. commun. Disord*, **1**, 31–4

Strub, R. L. & Gardner, H. (1974) The repetition in conduction aphasia: mnestic or linguistic? *Brain Lang.*, **1**, 241–55

Szentagothai, J. (1974) Plasticity in the central nervous system. *Neurosci. Res. Prog. Bull.*, **12**, 534–6

Tallal, P. & Piercy, M. (1978) Defects of auditory perception in children with developmental dysphasia. In *Developmental Dysphasia*, ed. Wyke, M. A., pp. 63–84. London; Academic Press

Teszner, D., Tzavaras, A., Gruner, J. & Hécaen, H. (1972) L'asymétrie droit-gauche du *planum temporale* à propos de l'étude anatomique de 100 cerveaux. *Rev. Neurol.*, **126**, 444–9

Tzortzis, C. & Albert, M. L. (1974) Impairment of memory for sequences in conduction aphasia. *Neuropsychologia*, **12**, 355–66

van Buren, J. M. (1975) Question of thalamic participation in speech mechanisms. *Brain Lang.*, **2**, 31–44

Vilkki, J. & Laitinen, L. V. (1974) Differential effect of left and right ventrolateral thalamotomy on receptive and expressive verbal performances and face matching. *Neuropsychologia*, **12**, 11–19

Wada, J. A., Clarke, R. & Hamon, A. (1975) Cerebral hemispheric asymmetry in humano-cortical speech zones in 100 adult and 100 infant brains. *Arch. Neurol.*, **32**(4), 239–46

Warrington, E. K., Logue, V. & Pratt, R. T. C. (1971) The anatomical localization of selective impairment of auditory verbal short-term memory. *Neuropsychologia*, **9**, 377–87

Warrington, E. K. & Shallice, T. (1969) The selective impairment of auditory verbal short-term memory. *Brain*, **92**, 885–96

Whitaker, H. A. & Ojemann, G. A. (1977) Graded localization of naming from electrical stimulation mapping of left cerebral cortex. *Nature*, **270**, 50–51

Wilson, P. J. E. (1970) Cerebral hemispherectomy for infantile hemiplegia: a report of 50 cases. *Brain*, **93**, 147–80

Withrow, F. R. (1964) Immediate recall by aphasic, deaf and normal children for visual forms presented simultaneously and sequentially. *American speech hearing Assoc.*, **6**, 386

Wittelson, S. F. & Pallis, W. (1973) Left hemisphere specialization for language in the new-born. *Brain*, **96**, 641–6

Woods, B. & Teuber, H. L. (1973) Early onset of complementary specialization of cerebral hemispheres in man. *Trans. Amer. Neurol. Assoc.*, **98**, 113–17

Wyke, M. (1962) An experimental study of verbal association in dysphasic subjects. *Brain*, **85**, 679–86

— (1971) Dysphasia: a review of recent progress. *Brit. med. Bull.*, **27**, 211–17

— (1978) (Ed.) *Developmental Dysphasia*. London: Academic Press

Wyke, M. A. & Asso, D. (1979) Perception and memory for spatial relations in children with developmental dysphasia. *Neuropsychol.*, **17**, 231–9

Zaidel, E. (1975) A technique for presenting lateralized visual input with prolonged exposure. *Vision Res.*, **15**, 283–9

— (1976) Auditory vocabulary of the right hemisphere following brain bisection or hemidecortication. *Cortex*, **12**, 191–211

— (1977) Unilateral auditory language comprehension on the token test following cerebral commisurotomy and hemispherectomy. *Neuropsychologia*, **15**, 1–17

Zangwill, O. L. (1975) Excision of the Broca's area without persistent aphasia. In *Cerebral Localization*, ed. Zulch, K. J., Creutzfeldt, O. & Galbraith, G. C., pp. 258–63. Berlin, Heidelberg, New York: Springer Verlag

Chapter 5

Bleuler, E. (1950) *Dementia Praecox, or the group of Schizophrenias*. English translation. New York: International Universities Press

Bourguignon, E. (1973) *Religion, Altered States of Consciousness and Social Change*. Columbus: Ohio State University Press

Carstairs, M. (1954) Daru and Bhang; cultural factors in the choice of an intoxicant. *Q. J. Stud. Alcohol* **15**, 220–25

Cawte, J. E. (1972) *Cruel, Poor and Brutal Nations*. Honolulu: University Press of Hawaii

Cooper, J. E., Kendell, R. E., Gurland, B. J., Sharpe, L., Copeland, J. R. M. & Simon, R. (1972) *Psychiatric Diagnosis in New*

York and London. Maudsley Monograph No. 20 London: Oxford University Press

Dewhurst, K. (1969) The neurosyphilitic psychoses today. *Brit. J. Psychiat.,* **115,** 31–8

Eaton, J. W. & Weil, R. J. (1955) *Culture and Mental Disorders.* Glencoe, Ill.: Free Press

Ey, H. (1950) Bouffées délirantes et psychoses hallucinatoires aiguës. In *Etudes psychiatriques,* vol. III, 201–324. Paris: Desclée de Brower

Fraser, R. (1947) *The Incidence of Neurosis among Factory Workers.* MRC Industrial Health Research Board Report No. 90. London: HMSO

Goldstein, K. (1959) Functional disturbances in brain damage. In *American Handbook of Psychiatry,* ed. Arieti, S., 1st ed. pp. 770–96. New York: Basic Books

Hirsch, S. J. & Hollender, M. H. (1969) Hysterical psychosis; clarification of the concept. *Amer. J. Psychiat.,* **125,** 909–15

Hollingshead, A. B. & Redlich, F. C. (1958) *Social Class and Mental Illness.* New York: Wiley

Jellinek, E. M. (1960) *The Disease Concept of Alcoholism.* New Haven, Conn.: Hillhouse Press

Kino, F. F. (1951) Alien's paranoid reaction. *J. ment. Sci.,* **97,** 589–93

Kluckhohn, C. (1952) Culture; a critical review of concepts and definitions. *Papers of the Peabody Museum* **41,** 181–95

Kretschmer, E. (1927) *Der sensitive Beziehungswahn.* 2nd ed. Berlin: Springer

Lambo, T. A. (1962) Malignant anxiety in Africans. *J. ment. Sci.,* **108,** 256–64

Lebra, T. S. & Lebra, W. P. (1974). *Japanese Culture and Behavior: Selected Readings.* Honolulu: University Press of Hawaii

Marmot, M. G. & Syme, S. L. (1976) Acculturation and coronary heart disease in Japanese Americans. *Amer. J. Epidemiol.,* **104,** 225–47

McClelland, D. C. Davis, W. N., Kalin R. & Wanner, L. (1972) (Eds) *The Drinking Man.* New York: Free Press

Murphy, H. B. M. (1973) History and the evolution of syndromes: The striking case of *latah* and *amok.* In *Psychopathology,* ed. Hammer, M., Salzinger, K. & Sutton, S. New York: Wiley

— (1976) Notes for a theory on *latah.* In *Culture-bound Syndromes, Ethnopsychiatry, and Alternate Therapies,* ed. Lebra, W. P. Honolulu: University Press of Hawaii

— (1978) The advent of guilt feelings as a common depressive symptom: a historical comparison on two continents. *Psychiatry* **41**(3) 229–42

Murphy, H. B. M., Wittkower, E. D., Fried, J. & Ellenberger, H. (1963) A cross-cultural survey of schizophrenic symptomarology. *Int. J. soc. Psychiat.,* **9,** 237–49

Parker, S. & Kleiner, S. J. (1966) *Mental Illness in the Urban Negro Community.* Glencoe, Ill.: Free Press

Robins, L. N. (1974) *The Vietnam Drug User Returns.* Special Action Office Monograph, Series A, No. 2. Washington, D.C.: US Government Printing Office

Rutter, M., Mule, B., Quinton, D., Rowlands, O., Yule, W. & Berger, M. (1975) Attainment and adjustment in two geographic areas: III. Some factors accounting for area differences. *Brit. J. Psychiat.,* **126,** 520–33

Rutter, M. & Madge, N. (1976) *Cycles of Disadvantage.* London: Heinemann

Scotch, N. A. & Geiger, H. J. (1962) The epidemiology of essential hypertension. *J. chron. Dis.,* **16,** 1183–1213

Segal, S. P. & Aviram, U. (1978) *The Mentally-Ill in Community-based, Sheltered Care.* New York: Wiley

Slater, P. E. & Slater D. A. (1965) Maternal ambivalence and narcissism; a cross-cultural study. *Merrill-Palmer Q. Behav. Dev.,* **11,** 241–59

Spiegel, J. P. (1957) The resolution of role conflict within the family. In *The Patient and the Mental Hospital,* ed. Greenblatt, M., Levison, D. J. & Williams, R. H., pp. 545–64. Glencoe, Ill.: Free Press

Tonnies, F. (1957) *Community and Society (Gemeinschaft und Gesellschaft).* English translation. East Lansing, Mich.: University of Michigan Press

Wastrell, C. (1972) *Chronic Duodenal Ulcer.* London: Butterworths

WHO (1973) *The International Pilot Study of Schizophrenia* Geneva: World Health Organization

— (1979) *Schizophrenia; an International Follow-Up Study.* New York: Wiley

Chapter 6

Böker, W. & Häfner, H. (1973) *Gewaltaten Geistesgestörten.* Berlin: Springer
See also Gibbens, T. C. N. *Psychol. Med.* 1977, **7,** 731–6, Review article
also Häfner, H. & Böker, W., (1973) Mentally disordered violent offenders. *Soc. Psychiat.,* **8,** 220–29

Bratty (1961) 3 WLR 965. 3 All E.R. 523

Butler Committee (1975) *Report of the Committee on Mentally Abnormal Offenders.* Cmd 6244. London: HMSO

Charlson (1955) 1 WLR 317. 1 All E.R. 859

Cloninger, C. R. & Guze, S. (1970) Psychiatric illness and female criminality: the role of sociopathy and hysteria in the antisocial woman. *Amer. J. Psychiat.,* **127,** 303–11

Criminal Law Revision Committee (1980) *Offences against the Person.* Home Office. II London: HMSO

Dalgard, O. S. & Kringlen, I. (1976) A Norwegian twin study of criminality. *Brit. J. Crim.,* **16,** No. 3, 213–32

General Register Office (1968) *Studies in Medical and Population Subjects.* No. 22. Glossary of Mental Disorders. London: HMSO

Gibbens, T. C. N. (1972) Violence to children. *Howard J. Penol.,* **13,** No. 3, 212–19

Gibbens, T. C. N., Briscoe, O., & Dell, S. (1968) Psychopathic and neurotic offenders in mental hospitals. In *The Mentally Abnormal Offender,* ed. de Reuck, A. V. S. & Porter, R., pp. 143–51. Ciba Foundation. London: Churchill

Gibbens, T. C. N., Pond, D. A. & Stafford-Clark, D. (1959) Follow-up study of criminal psychopaths. *J. ment. Sci.,* **105,** 108

Gibbens, T. C. N., Soothill, K. L. & Way, C. (1980) Child molestation. In *Sexual Offenders in the Criminal Justice System.* 12th Cropwood Conference. Cambridge: Institute of Criminology

Goldberg, D., (1972) *The Detection of Psychiatric Illness by Questionnaire.* Maudsley Monograph No. 21. Oxford: Oxford University Press

Gunn, J. C. (1976) Psychopathic personality: a conceptual problem. *Psychol. Med.,* **6,** 631–4

— (1978a) *Psychiatric Aspects of Imprisonment.* London: Academic Press

— (1978b) Epileptic homicide: a case report. *Brit. J. Psychiat.,* **132,** 510–13

Guze, S. (1976) *Criminality and Psychiatric Disorder.* Oxford: Oxford University Press

Halsey, A. H. (1978) *Change in British Society.* Oxford: Oxford University Press

Hill, D., Sargant, W. & Heppenstall, M. E. (1943) A case of matricide. *Lancet,* **i,** 526–7

Kemp (1956) 3 WLR 724. 3 All E.R. 249

Kutchinsky, O. (1974) *Pornography, Law and Crime. The Danish Experience.* London: Robertson

Lipman (1969) 3 WLR 819

O'Connell, P. (1960) Amnesia and homicide. *Brit. J. Delinq.*, **10**, 263–76

Palmer, T. (1974) The community treatment project in perspective 1961–1973. *Youth Authority Q.* **26**, 3. Sacramento, California

Pincus, J. (1978) The hyperventilation syndrome. *Brit. J. hosp. Med.* April, 312–13

Policy Advisory Committee on Sexual Offences (1979) *Working paper on the Age of Consent in relation to Sexual Offences.* London: HMSO

Quick (1973) 3 WLR 26

Review of the Mental Health Act (1978) London: HMSO

Robins, L. N. (1966) *Deviant Children Grown Up.* Baltimore: Williams

Royal Commission on Capital Punishment (1953) Report of the Royal Commission on Capital Punishment, 1949–53. London: HMSO

Rutter, M., Lebovici, S., Eisenberg, L., Sneznevskij, A. V., Sadoun, R., Brooke, E., & Tsung-Yi Lin (1969) A tri-axial classification of mental disorders in childhood. An international study. *J. child Psychol. Psychiat.*, **10**, 41–61

Schofield, M (1965) *The Sexual Behaviour of Young People.* London: Longmans Green

Scott, P. D. (1965) Juvenile delinquency. In *Modern Perspectives in Child Psychiatry*, ed. Howells, J. London: Oliver & Boyd

Shepherd, M. (1961) Morbid jealousy: some clinical and social aspects of a psychological symptom. *J. ment. Sci.*, **107**, 687–753

Shepherd, M. & Sartorius, N. (1974) Personality disorder and the International Classification of Diseases. *Psychol. Med.*, **4**, No. 2, 141–6

Virkkunen, M. (1974) Incest offences and alcoholism. *Med. Sci. Law*, **14**, 124–8

Walker, N., & McCabe, S. (1973) *Crime and Insanity in England*, p. 234. Edinburgh: Edinburgh University Press

Warren, M. Q. (1969) The case for differential treatment of delinquents. *Ann. Amer. Acad. Pol. Sci., Philadelphia*, **381**, 47–59

Watmore v. Jenkins (1962) 3 WLR 463

Weeks, H. A. (1958) *Youthful Offenders at Highfields.* Ann Arbor: University of Michigan Press

West, D. J. & Farrington, D. P. (1977) *The Delinquent Way of Life.* London: Heinemann

Whitty, C. W. M. (1978) Loss of memory as a clinical problem. *Brit. J. hosp. Med.*, Sept., 276–8

Williams Committee (1980) *Report of the Committee on Obscenity and Film Censorship.* Cmd.7772. London: HMSO

Wolfenden Committee (1957) *Report of the Committee on Homosexual Offences and Prostitution.* London: HMSO

World Health Organization (1971) *Draft Glossary of Psychiatric Disorders.* Geneva: World Health Organization

Chapter 7

American Psychiatric Association (1980) *Diagnostic and Statistical Manual of Mental Disorders.* 3rd ed. Washington, D.C.: APA

Essen-Möller, E. (1971) Suggestions for further improvement of the international classification of mental disorders. *Psychol. Med.*, **1**, 308–11

Menninger, K. (1963) *The Vital Balance: The Life Process in Mental Health and Illness.* New York: Viking Press

Ottosson, J. O. & Perris, C. (1973) Multidimensional classification of mental disorders. *Psychol. Med.*, **3**, 238–43

Rutter, M., Lebovici, S., Eisenberg, L., Sneznevskij, A. V., Sadoun, R., Brooke, E. & Lin, T. (1969) A triaxial classification of mental disorders in childhood. *J. child Psychol. Psychiat.*, **10**, 41–61

Scadding, J. G. (1967) Diagnosis: the clinician and the computer. *Lancet*, **ii**, 877–82

World Health Organization (1978) *Mental Disorders: Glossary and Guide to their Classification in accordance with the Ninth Revision of the International Classification of Diseases.* Geneva: WHO

Chapter 8

APA (1968) *Diagnostic and Statistical Manual of Mental Disorders (DSM-II).* Washington, DC: American Psychiatric Association

— (1980) *Diagnostic and Statistical Manual of Mental Disorders.* 3rd ed. Washington, DC: American Psychiatric Association

Bartlett, F. C. (1932) *Remembering.* (Paperback edition, 1967) London: Cambridge University Press

Beck, A. T. (1962) Reliability of psychiatric diagnoses; a critique of systematic studies. *Amer. J. Psychiat.*, **119**, 210–16

Beck, A. T., Ward, C., Mendelson, M., Mock, J. & Erbaugh, J. (1961) An inventory for measuring depression. *Arch. gen. Psychiat.*, **4**, 561–71

Cooper, J. E., Kendell, R. E., Gurland, B. J., Sharpe, L., Copeland, J. R. M. & Simon, R. (1972) *Psychiatric Diagnosis in New York and London* Maudsley Monograph No. 20. London: Oxford University Press

Edwards, W., Lindman, H., & Savage, L. J. (1963) Bayesan statistical inference for psychological research. *Psychol. Rev.*, **70**, 193–242

Elstein, A. S., Kagan, N., Shulman, L. S., Hilliard, J. & Loupe, M. J. (1972) Methods and theory in the study of medical inquiry. *J. med. Educ.*, **47**, 85–92

Endicott, J., & Spitzer, R. L., (1978). A diagnostic interview: the schedule for affective disorders and schizophrenia. *Arch. gen. Psychiat.*, **35**, 837–44

Feighner, J. P., Robins, E., Guze, S. B., Woodruff, R. A., Winokur, G. & Munoz, R. (1972) Diagnostic criteria for use in psychiatric research. *Arch. gen. Psychiat.*, **26**, 57–63

Fiedler, F. E. (1950) A comparison of therapeutic relationships in psychoanalytic, nondirective and Adlerian therapy. *J. consult. Psychol.*, **14**, 436–45

Fleiss, J. L., Spitzer, R. L., Cohen, J. & Endicott, J. (1972) Three computer diagnosis methods compared. *Arch. gen. Psychiat.*, **27**, 643–9

Gauron, E. F. & Dickinson, J. K. (1966) Diagnostic decision making in psychiatry. *Arch. gen. Psychiat.*, **14**, 225–37

— (1969) The influence of seeing the patient first on diagnostic decision making in psychiatry. *Amer. J. Psychiat.*, **126**, 199–205

Goldberg, D., Cooper, B., Eastwood, M. R., Kedward, H. B. & Shepherd, M. (1970) A standardised psychiatric interview for use in community surveys. *Brit. J. prev. soc. Med.*, **24**, 18–24

Grinker, R. R., Miller, J., Sabshin, M., Nunn, R. & Munally, J. C. (1961) *The Phenomena of Depressions.* New York: Hoeber

Grosz, H. J. & Grossman, K. G. (1968) Clinician's response style. *J. abnorm. soc. Psychol.*, **73**, 207–14

Guilford, J. P. (1954) *Psychometric Methods.* New York: McGraw-Hill

Hamilton, M. (1960) A rating scale for depression. *J. Neurol. Neurosurg. Psychiat.*, **23**, 56–62

HMSO (1968) *A Glossary of Mental Disorders; Studies on Medical and Population Subjects, No. 22.* London

Institute of Psychiatry (1973) *Notes on Eliciting and Recording Clinical Information.* Prepared by the Department of Psychiatry Teaching Committee, Institute of Psychiatry, University of London. Oxford: Oxford University Press

Katz, M., Cole, J. O. & Lowery, H. A. (1969) Studies of the diagnostic process: the influence of symptom perception, past experience and ethnic background on diagnostic decisions. *Amer. J. Psychiat.*, **125**, 937–47

Kendell, R. E., Everitt, B., Cooper, J. E., Sartorius, N. & David, M. E. (1968) The reliability of the 'Present State Examination'. *Soc. Psychiat.*, **3**, 123–29
Brit. J. Psychiat., **122**, 437–45
— (1975) *The Role of Diagnosis in Psychiatry.* London: Blackwell

Kendell, R. E., Everitt, B., Cooper, J. E., Sartorius, N. & David, M. E. (1968) The reliability of the 'Present State Examination'. *Soc. Psychiat.*, **3**, 123–29

Kramer, M. (1961) Some problems for international research suggested by observations on differences in first admission rates to the mental hospitals of England and Wales and of the United States. In *Proceedings of the Third World Congress of Psychiatry*, vol. 3, pp. 153–60. Montreal: Toronto University Press

Kreitman, N. (1961) The reliability of psychiatric diagnosis. *J ment. Sci.*, **107**, 876–86

Leaper, D. J., Gill, P. W., Staniland, J. R., Horrocks, J. C. & De Dombal, F. T. (1973) Clinical diagnostic process: an analysis. *Brit. med. J.*, **3**, 569–74

Leff, J. P. & Isaacs, A. D. (1968) *Psychiatric Examination in Clinical Practice.* London: Blackwell

Lehmann, H. E., Ban, T. A. & Donald, M. (1965) Rating the rater. *Arch. gen. Psychiat.*, **13**, 67–75

Lewis, A. J. (1946) Ageing and senility: a major problem of psychiatry. *J. ment. Sci.*, **92**, 150–70

Lorr, M. & Klett, C. J. (1967) *Inpatient Multidimensional Psychiatric Scale.* Palo Alto, California: Consulting Psychologist Press

Marquis, K. H., Cannell, C. F. & Laurent, A. (1972) Reporting health events in a household interview: effects of reinforcement, question length and re-interviews. In *Vital Health and Statistics series 2, No. 45.* U.S. Dept. of Health, Education and Welfare

Matarazzo, J. & Weins, A. N. (1972) *The Interview: Research on its Anatomy and Structure.* Chicago: Aldine Press

Mechanic, D. (1961) The concept of illness behaviour. *J. chron. Dis.*, **15**, 189–194
— (1978) *Medical Sociology: a Selective View.* 2nd ed. New York: Free Press

Menninger, K. (1963) *The Vital Balance: the Life Process in Mental Health and Illness.* New York: Viking Press

Newcomb, T. M. (1931) An experiment designed to test the validity of a rating technique. *J. educ. Psychol.* **22**, 279–89
— (1950) *Social Psychology.* London: Routledge & Kegan Paul

Overall, J. E. & Gorham, D. R. (1962) The brief psychiatric rating scale. *Psychol. Rep.*, **10**, 799–812

Parsons, T. (1951) *The Social System.* Chicago: Free Press

Raines, G. N. & Rohrer, J. H. (1954) The operational matrix of psychiatric practice. *Amer. J. Psychiat.*, **111**, 721–33

Sandifer, M. G., Hordern, A. & Green, L. M. (1970) The psychiatric interview: the impact of the first three minutes. *Amer. J. Psychiat.*, **126**, 968–73

Sandifer, M. G., Hordern, A., Timbury, G. C. & Green, L. M. (1968) Psychiatric diagnosis: a comparative study in North Carolina, London and Glasgow. *Brit. J. Psychiat.*, **114**, 1–9

Slater, E. T. O. (1935) The incidence of mental disorder. *Ann. Eugen.*, **6**, 172–84

Spitzer, R. L. & Endicott, J. (1969) DIAGNO II: further developments in a computer program for psychiatric diagnosis. *Amer. J. Psychiat.*, **125** (January supplement) 12–20

Spitzer, R. L., Endicott, J., & Fleiss, J. (1967) Instruments and recording forms for evaluating psychiatric status and history: rationale, method of development and description. *Compr. Psychiat.*, **8**, 321–43

Spitzer, R. L., Endicott, J., Robins, E. (1978) Research diagnostic criteria: rationale and reliability. *Arch. gen. Psychiat.*, **35**, 773–82

Thorndike, E. L. (1920) A constant error in psychological ratings. *J. educ. Psychol.*, **4**, 25–9

Truax, C. B. (1966) Reinforcement and non-reinforcement in Rogerian psychotherapy. *J. abnorm. Psychol.*, **71**, 1–9

WHO (1973) *The International Pilot Study of Schizophrenia*, vol. 1. Geneva: World Health Organization
— (1974) *Glossary of Mental Disorders and Guide to their Classification.* Geneva: World Health Organization
— (1978) *Mental Disorders: Glossary and Guide to their Classification in Accordance with the Ninth Revision of the International Classification of Diseases.* Geneva: World Health Organization

Wing, J. K., Birley, J. L. T., Cooper, J. E., Graham, P. & Isaacs, A. D. (1967). Reliability of a procedure for measuring and classifying 'Present Psychiatric State'. *Brit. J. Psychiat.*, **113**, 499–515

Wing, J. K., Cooper, J. E., Sartorius, N. (1974) *The Measurement and Classification of Psychiatric Symptoms.* Cambridge: Cambridge University Press

World Health Organization see WHO

Zubin, J. (1967) Classification of the behaviour disorders. *Ann. Rev. Psychol.*, **18**, 373–406

Chapter 9

Bailey, J. & Coppen, A. (1976) A comparison between the Hamilton Rating Scale and the Beck Inventory in the measurement of depression. *Brit. J. Psychiat.*, **128**, 486–9

Bannister, D. (1970) *Perspectives in Personal Construct Theory.* London, New York: Academic Press

Bannister, D. & Fransella, F. (1966) A grid test of schizophrenic thought disorder. *Brit. J. soc. clin. Psychol.*, **5**, 95–102

Beck, A. T., Ward, C. N., Mendelson, M., Mock, J. & Erbaugh, J. (1961) An inventory for measuring depression. *Arch. gen. Psychiat.*, **4**, 561–71

Biggs, J. T., Wylie, L. T. & Ziegler, V. E. (1978) Validity of the Zung self-rating depression scale. *Brit. J. Psychiat.*, **132**, 381–5

Blessed, G., Tomlinson, B. E. & Roth, M. (1968) The association between quantitative measures of dementia and of senile change in the cerebral grey matter of elderly subjects. *Brit. J. Psychiat.*, **114**, 797–812

Copeland, J. R. M. (1978) Evaluation of diagnostic methods: An international comparison. In *Studies in Geriatric Psychiatry*, ed. Isaacs, A. D. & Post, F. Chichester, New York, Brisbane, Toronto: Wiley

Copeland, J. R. M., Kelleher, M. J., Kellet, J. M., Gourlay, A. J., Gurland, B. J., Fleiss, J. L. & Sharpe, L. (1976) A semi-structured clinical interview for the assessment of diagnosis and mental state in the elderly: the Geriatric Mental State Schedule. *Psychol. Med.*, **6**, 439–49

Gilleard, C. J. & Pattie, A. H. (1977) The Stockton geriatric rating scale: A shortened version with British normative data. *Brit. J. Psychiat.*, **131**, 90–4

Hamilton, M. (1960) A rating scale for depression. *J. Neurol., Neurosurg. Psychiat.*, **23**, 56–62

— (1976) Clinical evaluation of depression: clinical criteria and rating scales: In *Depression*, ed. Gallant, D. M. & Simpson, G. M. New York: Spectrum Publications

Hill, D. (1974) Non-verbal behaviour in mental illness. *Brit. J. Psychiat.*, **124**, 221–30

Institute of Psychiatry, London (1973) *Notes on Eliciting and Recording Clinical Information.* London, New York, Toronto: Oxford University Press

Jaspers, K. (1959) *General Psychopathology.* (Transl. Hoenig, J. & Hamilton, M. W. 1963). Manchester: Manchester University Press

Kelly, G. A. (1963) *A Theory of Personality: The Psychology of Personal Constructs.* New York: Norton

Kind, H. (1973) *Leitfaden für die psychiatrische Untersuchung.* Berlin, Heidelberg, New York: Springer

Knesevich, J. W., Biggs, J. T., Clayton, P. J. & Ziegler, V. E. (1977) Validity of the Hamilton rating scale for depression. *Brit. J. Psychiat.*, **131**, 49–52

Leff, J. (1977) International variations in the diagnosis of psychiatric illness. *Brit. J. Psychiat.*, **131**, 329–38

— (1978) Diagnosis of psychiatric illness. (Letter to) *Brit. J. Psychiat.*, **132**, 319–20

Leff, J. P. & Isaacs, A. D. (1978) *Psychiatric Examination in Clinical Practice.* London, Edinburgh, Melbourne: Blackwell

Lewis, A. J. (1934) The psychopathology of insight. *Brit. J. med. Psychol.*, **14**, 332–48

Lishman, W. A. (1978) *Organic Psychiatry.* Oxford, London, Edinburgh, Melbourne: Blackwell

Lorr, M., Klett, C. H., McNair, P. M. & Lasky, J. (1963) *In-patient Multidimensional Psychiatric Scale (Manual).* Palo Alto: Consulting Psychologists Press

Marks, I. M. (1978a) Behaviour therapy in adult neurosis. In *Handbook of Psychotherapy and Behaviour Change*, ed. Garfield, S. L. & Bergin, A. E. New York: Wiley

— (1978b) Exposure treatment. In *Behaviour Modifications: Principles and Clinical Applications*, ed. Agras, W. J. 2nd ed. Boston: Little, Brown

Meer, B. & Baker, L. A. (1966) The Stockton geriatric rating scale. *J. Gerontol.*, **21**, 393–403

Overall, J. E. & Gorham, D. R. (1962) The brief psychiatric rating scale. *Psychol. Reports*, **10**, 799–812

Pattie, A. H. & Gilleard, C. J. (1975) A brief psychogeriatric assessment schedule: validation against psychiatric diagnosis and discharge from hospital. *Brit. J. Psychiat.*, **127**, 489–93

— (1978) The two-year predictive validity of the Clifton assessment schedule and the shortened Stockton geriatric rating scale. *Brit. J. Psychiat.*, **133**, 457–60

Perris, C. (1974) A study of cycloid psychoses. *Acta psychiat. scand.* Supp. 253

Post, F. (1971) Schizo-affective symptomatology in late life. *Brit. J. Psychiat.*, **118**, 437–45

— (1972) The management and nature of depressive illness in late life. *Brit. J. Psychiat.*, **121**, 393–404

— (1975) Dementia, depression and pseudo-dementia. In *Psychiatric Aspects of Neurological Disease*, ed. Benson, D. F. & Blumer, D. New York: Grune & Stratton

— (1980) Paranoid, schizophrenia-like and schizophrenic states in the aged. In *Handbook of Mental Health and Aging*, ed. Birren, J. E. & Sloane, R. B., pp. 591–615. Englewood Cliffs, N.J.: Prentice-Hall

Procci, W. R. (1976) Schizo-affective psychosis: fact or fiction? *Arch. gen. Psychiat.*, **33**, 1167–78

Shapiro, M. B. (1969) A clinically orientated strategy in individual-centred research. *Brit. J. soc. clin. Psychol.*, **8**, 290–91

Shapiro, M. B., Litman, G. K., Nias, D. K. B. & Hendry, E. R. (1973) A clinician's approach to experimental research. *J. clin. Psychol.*, **29**, 165–9

Shapiro, M. B. & Post, F. (1974) Comparison of self-ratings of psychiatric patients with ratings made by a psychiatrist. *Brit. J. Psychiat.*, **125**, 36–41

Sheldrick, C., Jablensky, A., Sartorius, N. & Shepherd, M. (1977) Schizophrenia succeeded by affective illness. Catamnestic study and statistical enquiry. *Psychol. Med.*, **7**, 619–24

Taylor, J. A. A. (1953) A personality scale of manifest anxiety. *J. abnorm. soc. Psychol.*, **48**, 285–90

WHO see World Health Organization

Wing, J. K., Cooper, J. E. & Sartorius, N. (1974) *Measurement and Classification of Psychiatric Symptoms.* London, New York: Cambridge University Press

Wittenborn, J. R. (1955) *Wittenborn Psychiatric Rating Scales.* New York: Psychological Corporation

World Health Organization (1973) *Report of the International Pilot Study of Schizophrenia.* Vol. 1. Geneva: WHO

Zung, W. W. K. (1965) A self-rating depression scale. *Arch. gen. Psychiat.*, **12**, 63–70

Chapter 10

Methods of treatment referred to in Chapter 10 are described in detail in the appropriate chapters of volumes 2–4 of the Handbook of Psychiatry. The following references have a bearing on the principles underlying treatment and its evaluation, as reviewed in Chapter 10.

Beech, H. R. & Vaughan, M. (1978) *Behavioural Treatment of Obsessional States.* Chichester: Wiley

Bernard, Claude (1865) *An Introduction to the Study of Experimental Medicine*, trans. Green, H. C. New York: Dover

Blackwell, B. (1976) Treatment Adherence. *Brit. J. Psychiat.*, **129**, 513–31

Candy, J., Balfour S. H. G., Cawley, R. H., Hildebrand, H. P., Malan, D. H., Marks, I. M. & Wilson J. (1972) A feasibility study for a controlled trial of formal psychotherapy. *Psychol. Med.*, **2**, 345–62

Chassan, J. B. (1979) *Experimental Design in Clinical Psychology and Psychiatry* 2nd ed. New York: Irvington

Cochrane, A. L. (1972) *Effectiveness and Efficiency: Random Reflections on Health Services.* London: The Nuffield Provincial Hospitals Trust

Cranberg, L. (1979) Do retrospective controls make clinical trials 'inherently fallacious'? *Brit. med. J.*, **2**, 1265–6

Crow, T. J. (1979) The scientific status of electro-convulsive therapy. *Psychol. Med.*, **9**, 401–8

Ellenberger, H. F. (1970) *The Discovery of the Unconscious.* London: Allen Lane, Penguin Press

Feinstein, A. R. (1967) *Clinical Judgment.* Baltimore: Williams & Wilkins

Frank, J. D. (1973) *Persuasion and Healing: a Comparative Study of Psychotherapy.* 2nd ed. Baltimore: John Hopkins University Press

Garfield, S. L. & Bergin, A. E. (1978) (Eds.) *Handbook of Psychotherapy and Behaviour Change: An Empirical Analysis.* 2nd ed. New York: Wiley

Hill, A. Bradford (1960) (Ed.) *Controlled Clinical Trials.* Oxford: Oxford University Press

— (1962) *Statistical Methods in Clinical and Preventive Medicine.* Edinburgh: Livingstone

— (1977) *A Short Textbook of Medical Statistics.* London: Hodder & Stoughton

Hoch, P. H. & Zubin, J. (1964) *The Evaluation of Psychiatric Treatment.* New York: Grune & Stratton

Hogben, Lancelot (1963) The Assessment of Remedies. In *Science in Authority* by Hogben, Lancelot, chap. 5, reprinted from *Medical Press,* 1954, **232.** London: Unwin

Honigfeld, G. (1964) Non-specific factors in treatment. I. Review of placebo reactions and placebo reactors. II. Review of social-psychological factors. *Dis. nerv. Syst.,* **25,** 145–56, 225–39

Janet, P. (1925) *Psychological Healing.* London: Allen & Unwin

Jaspers, K. (1963) *General Psychopathology,* 7th ed, trans. Hoenig, J. & Hamilton, M. W. Manchester: Manchester University Press

Lewis, Aubrey (1967) Empirical or rational? The nature and basis of psychiatry. *Lancet,* **ii,** 1–9

Marks, I. M. (1979) Cure and care of neurosis. *Psychol. Med.,* **9,** 629–60

Medical Research Council (1965) Report of Clinical Psychiatry Committee: Clinical trial of the treatment of depressive illness. *British med. J.,* **1,** 881–6

Mindham, R. H. S., Howland, C. & Shepherd, M. (1973) An evaluation of continuation therapy with tricyclic antidepressants in depressive illness. *Psychol. Med.,* **3,** 5–17

Taylor, F. K. (1961) *The Analysis of Therapeutic Groups.* Maudsley Monograph No. 8. London: Oxford University Press

Wrighton, R. F. (1973). *Elementary Principles of Probability and Information.* London: Academic Press

Zelen, M. (1979) A new design for randomised clinical trials. *New Eng. J. Med.,* **300,** 1242–5

Cross-references to other volumes in the series

CROSS-REFERENCES

In addition to specific references given below, the reader is referred to volume 2 for the relationship between mental disorder and somatic illness, to volume 3 for a study of psychoses of uncertain aetiology, with particular reference to schizophrenias, affective psychoses, paranoid states, and psychoses with origin specific to childhood, to volume 4 for a review of the neuroses and personality disorders, and to volume 5 for a discussion of the scientific foundations of psychiatry.

(See also the key to volumes and chapters.)

Author index

Subject index